SPORTS-SPECIFIC
Rehabilitation

Robert Donatelli, PhD, PT, OCS
National Director
Physiotherapy Associates
Sports Specific Rehabilitation
Developer
Strengthen Your Game Rehabilitation and Performance
Enhancement Programs for Athletes
Las Vegas, Nevada

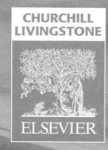

CHURCHILL
LIVINGSTONE

ELSEVIER

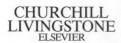

CHURCHILL LIVINGSTONE
ELSEVIER

11830 Westline Industrial Drive
St. Louis, Missouri 63146

ISBN-13: 978-0-443-06642-9
ISBN-10: 0-443-06642-6

Publishing Director: Linda Duncan
Acquisitions Editor: Kathy Falk
Developmental Editor: Melissa Kuster Deutsch
Publishing Services Manager: Julie Eddy
Project Manager: Gail Michaels
Text Designers: Bill Drone, Jyotika Shroff

Printed in the United States of America

Last digit is the print number: 9   8   7   6   5   4   3   2   1

I would like to dedicate this book to my beautiful wife and soul mate, Georgi, for her support and understanding, and to my new special gifts from God, Robby and Briana.

Contributors

Ronnie G. Bernard, MS, ATC, CSCS
Director of Athletic Training and Sports Relations
Southern Orthpaedic Specialists, LLC
Atlanta, Georgia
Appendix A: Approach to Differential Diagnosis in Orthopedics

Kenji Carp, PT, OCS, ATC, Certified Vestibular Therapist
Certified VestiClinic Director
Physiotherapy Associates
Eugene, Oregon
Chapter 12: Evaluation of the Trunk and Hip CORE

Donald A. Chu, PhD, PT, ATC, CSCS
Graduate Program Director
Rocky Mountain University
Provo, Utah
Chapter 14: Plyometrics in Rehabilitation

Ozgur Dede, MD
Research Fellow
Department of Bioengineering
Musculoskeletal Research Center
University of Pittsburgh
Pittsburgh, Pennsylvania
Chapter 1: Basic Science of Ligaments and Tendons Related to Rehabilitation

Robert Deppen, ATC, MS, PT
Physical Therapist
Hamot Medical Center; Sports Medicine
Erie, Pennsylvania
Chapter 10: From the CORE to the Floor—Interrelationships

Donn Dimond, PT, OCS
Physical Therapist
PT Associates
Beaverton, Oregon
Chapter 13: Strength Training Concepts in the Athlete
Appendix B: Rehabilitation through Performance Training: Cases in Sport

Todd S. Ellenbecker, DPT, MS, SCS, OCS, CSCS
Clinic Director
National Director of Clinical Research
Physiotherapy Associates Scottsdale Sports Clinic
Scottsdale, Arizona
Chapter 11: Evaluation of Glenohumeral, Acromioclavicular, and Scapulothoracic Joints in the Overhead-Throwing Athlete

Wendy J. Hurd, PT, MS, SCS
Doctoral Candidate
Graduate Program in Biomechanics and Movement Science
Department of Physical Therapy
University of Delaware
Newark, Delaware
Chapter 15: Neuromuscular Training

Jacob Irwin, DPT, MTC
Clinic Director
Physiotherapy Associates
Suwanee, Georgia
Appendix B: Surgical Considerations in the Athlete

Christopher Kuchta, PT, SCS, CSCS
Director of Aquatic Physical Therapy
PRO Physical Therapy
Wilmington, Delaware
Chapter 4: Aerobic Metabolism during Exercise

Eyal Lederman, DO, PhD
Visiting Professor
Unitec
Auckland, New Zealand
Director
Centre for Professional Development in Osteopathy and Manual Therapy
London, UK
Chapter 16: Manual Therapy in Sports Rehabilitation

Jaclyn Maurer, PhD, RD
Senior Research Specialist
Nutritional Sciences
University of Arizona
Tucson, Arizona
Chapter 17: Nutrition for the Athlete

Daniel K. Moon, MS
Research Fellow
Department of Bioengineering
Musculoskeletal Research Center
University of Pittsburgh
Pittsburgh, Pennsylvania
Chapter 1: Basic Science of Ligaments and Tendons Related
    to Rehabilitation

Stephanie Petterson, PhD, MPT
Post-Doctoral Researcher
Department of Physical Therapy
University of Delaware
Newark, Delaware
Chapter 4: Aerobic Metabolism during Exercise

Sharon Ann Plowman, PhD
Professor Emeritus
Dept. of Kinesiology and Physical Education
Northern Illinois University
Dekalb, Illinois
Chapter 2: Understanding Muscle Contraction
Chapter 3: Anaerobic Metabolism during Exercise
Chapter 7: Physiological Effects of Overtraining and
    Detraining

Jay Shiner, CSCS
Strength and Conditioning Coordinator
Minor Leagues/Player Development
Baltimore Orioles
Baltimore, Maryland
Chapter 14: Plyometrics in Rehabilitation

Denise Smith, PhD
Professor and Chair
Department of Exercise Science
Skidmore College
Saratoga Springs, New York
Chapter 2: Understanding Muscle Contraction
Chapter 3: Anaerobic Metabolism during Exercise
Chapter 7: Physiological Effects of Overtraining and
    Detraining

Lynn Snyder-Mackler, PT, ScD, ATC, SCS
Professor
Alumni Distinguished
Department of Physical Therapy
Academic Director
Graduate Program in Biomechanics and Movement Science
University of Delaware
Newark, Delaware
Chapter 4: Aerobic Metabolism during Exercise
Chapter 15: Neuromuscular Training

Vijay B. Vad, MD
Assistant Professor of Rehabilitation Medicine
Hospital for Special Surgery
Cornell University Medical Center
New York, New York
Chapter 8: Pathophysiology of Injury to the Overhead-
    Throwing Athlete

**Harvey W. Wallmann, PT, DPTSc, SCS, LAT,
ATC, CSCS**
Associate Professor
Department of Physical Therapy
University of Nevada, Las Vegas
Las Vegas, Nevada
Chapter 5: Muscle Fatigue

Joseph S. Wilkes, MD
Associate Clinical Professor of Orthopaedic Surgery
Department of Orthopaedics
Emory University School of Medicine
Orthopedic Surgeon
Atlanta, Georgia
Appendix A: Approach to Differential Diagnosis in Orthopedics

Savio L-Y Woo, PhD, DSc
Center Director, Whiteford Professor
Department of Bioengineering
Musculoskeletal Research Center
University of Pittsburgh
Pittsburgh, Pennsylvania
Chapter 1: Basic Science of Ligaments and Tendons Related
    to Rehabilitation

Michael S. Zazzali, DSc, PT, OCS
Co-Director and Partner
Physical Therapy Associates of New York
New York, New York
Chapter 8: Pathophysiology of Injury to the Overhead-
    Throwing Athlete

Foreword

As the proud father of tennis champion Andy Roddick, I met Dr. Robert Donatelli in 2000 during Andy's first ATP victory in Atlanta, Georgia. At the time, Andy was experiencing some severe shoulder and elbow pain that had been ongoing for some time. Dr. Donatelli started working with Andy and insisted the elbow pain was a direct result of the shoulder problems. Dr. Donatelli was the only person that told us the elbow problem was coming from his shoulder problems.

After evaluating Andy, Dr. Donatelli put together an upper body exercise and conditioning program that within 1 year eliminated the elbow and shoulder pain. The Donatelli program is unique in many ways. Dr. Donatelli evaluates Andy twice a year, checking for strengths and weaknesses throughout the entire body. With these results, Dr. Donatelli creates a specific program for the next 6 months. Each of Andy's evaluations have shown improvement. The last evaluation shows Andy scoring 5 and 5+ in all categories, based on a scale of 1-5. I realized early on this was exactly what Andy needed to do to stay healthy. Dr. Donatelli worked on not only preventing injury but increasing Andy's overall strength and agility. We saw his serve, as Dr. Donatelli predicted, go from 139 mph to an astonishing world record 155 mph, smashing the old record by a full 8 mph!

It has been a true pleasure to work with a fellow as knowledgeable and helpful as Dr. Donatelli. Under his guidance, Andy has been virtually injury free. So go ahead kick it up a notch—work with the best, Las Vegas style!

Jerry Roddick

Preface

The physical demands of the modern daily athlete are destructive to the skeletal, muscular, and neural systems. The athletes grow up learning how to play with pain, by making adaptations. Those adaptations may lead to serious injury and cause the athlete to miss long periods of performing or cause them to retire at a young age.

The mission of *Sports-Specific Rehabilitation* is to introduce a scientifically-based clinical approach to treating the athlete. Sporting activities require a state of readiness, which means the athlete, is strong, powerful, and requires a basic level of fitness. For an athlete to perform at the highest level, the musculoskeletal and neuromuscular systems must be functioning without limitations.

Sports-specific rehabilitation is not only the treatment of the injured athlete but also identification of musculoskeletal and neuromuscular deficits of which the athlete is unaware. A specific evaluation needs to be performed to determine these deficits. Evaluation skills, manual therapy skills, and the knowledge to design a specific exercise program are critical for implementing a sports-specific rehabilitation program to improve the athlete's performance.

The goal of this text is to offer scientific evidence on how to evaluate and treat the musculoskeletal and neuromuscular systems. Understanding how the skeletal, muscular, and neural systems function separately and together to bring about movement of any type is critical. In addition, for muscles to contract, they must continually produce energy (ATP), which means the metabolic system and the cardiovascular system are responsible for muscle contraction and, ultimately, athletic performance. Specificity of an evaluation of the muscles, joints, neuromuscular, cardiovascular, and metabolic systems will lead to specificity of exercise prescription.

This textbook combines the knowledge of several difference disciplines, exercise physiology, strength and conditioning, rehabilitation, and sports specific training. The text is divided into eight parts.

Part I covers the basic science of ligaments and tendons related to rehabilitation.

Part II contains topics related to muscle physiology as it pertains to exercise prescription, including a cellular understanding of muscle contraction and anaerobic and aerobic metabolism during exercise.

Part III discusses the damaging effect of overtraining, muscle fatigue, and eccentric exercises.

Part IV, the Pathophysiology of Overuse Injury in the Athlete, details the pathophysiology of injury to the overhead-throwing athlete, the anatomy of the hip and trunk core, and the connection of the core (hip and trunk) to the foot.

Part V describes and demonstrated detailed evaluations of the upper and lower core.

Part VI is the Physiological Basis of Exercise Specific to Sport. The chapters cover strength training concepts, including the muscular and metabolic adaptations to exercise, including neuromuscular changes, muscle hypertrophy, and converting type II muscle fibers. In addition, plyometrics and neuromuscular training concepts are discussed in detail.

Part VII is Special Considerations for the Athlete. The first chapter in this part is a refreshing look at manual therapy as an evidence-based treatment approach, and the second chapter discusses the newest information on nutritional guidance for gaining strength and peaking performance.

Finally, the appendixes present patient case studies. The first group of patient cases is focused on determining a medical diagnosis. The second group of patient cases demonstrates soft tissue diagnosis and includes a detailed discussion and display of treatment approaches in the athlete, including examples of periodization and neuromuscular training concepts. The neuromuscular training programs presented provide examples of perturbation and plyometric exercises.

Contents

PART 1: **BASIC SCIENCE OF SOFT TISSUES,** *1*

Chapter 1: **Basic Science of Ligaments and Tendons Related to Rehabilitation,** *1*
Savio L-Y Woo, Daniel K. Moon, and Ozgur Dede

PART 2: **MUSCLE PHYSIOLOGY: THE FOUNDATION FOR EXERCISE PRESCRIPTION,** *15*

Chapter 2: **Understanding Muscle Contraction,** *15*
Denise Louise Smith and Sharon Ann Plowman

Chapter 3: **Anaerobic Metabolism during Exercise,** *39*
Sharon Ann Plowman and Denise Louise Smith

Chapter 4: **Aerobic Metabolism during Exercise,** *65*
Stephanie Petterson, Christopher Kuchta, and Lynn Snyder-Mackler

PART 3: **MUSCLE FATIGUE, MUSCLE DAMAGE, AND OVERTRAINING CONCEPTS,** *87*

Chapter 5: **Muscle Fatigue,** *87*
Harvey W. Wallmann

Chapter 6: **Overuse Injury and Muscle Damage,** *97*
Robert A. Donatelli

Chapter 7: **Physiological Effects of Overtraining and Detraining,** *105*
Sharon Ann Plowman and Denise Louise Smith

PART 4: **PATHOPHYSIOLOGY OF OVERUSE INJURY IN THE ATHLETE,** *123*

Chapter 8: **Pathophysiology of Injury to the Overhead-Throwing Athlete,** *123*
Michael S. Zazzali, Robert A. Donatelli, and Vijay B. Vad

Chapter 9: **The Anatomy and Pathophysiology of the CORE,** *135*
Robert A. Donatelli

Chapter 10: **From the CORE to the Floor—Interrelationships,** *145*
Robert Deppen

PART 5:   CORE EVALUATION: SPORTS-SPECIFIC TESTING, *175*

**Chapter 11:   Evaluation of Glenohumeral, Acromioclavicular, and Scapulothoracic Joints in the
Overhead-Throwing Athlete,** *175*
Todd S. Ellenbecker

Chapter 12:   Evaluation of the Trunk and Hip CORE, *193*
Robert A. Donatelli and Kenji Carp

PART 6:   PHYSIOLOGICAL BASIS OF EXERCISE SPECIFIC TO SPORT, *223*

Chapter 13:   Strength Training Concepts in the Athlete, *223*
Robert A. Donatelli and Donn Dimond

Chapter 14:   Plyometrics in Rehabilitation, *233*
Donald A. Chu and Jay Shiner

Chapter 15:   Neuromuscular Training, *247*
Wendy J. Hurd and Lynn Snyder-Mackler

Chapter 16:   Manual Therapy in Sports Rehabilitation, *259*
Eyal Lederman

PART 7:   SPECIAL CONSIDERATIONS FOR THE ATHLETE, *279*

Chapter 17:   Nutrition for the Athlete, *279*
Jaclyn Maurer

APPENDIXES, *293*

Appendix A: Approach to Differential Diagnosis in Orthopedics, *295*
Joseph S. Wilkes and Ronnie Bernard

Appendix B: Rehabilitation through Performance Training: Cases in Sport, *303*
Donn Dimond and Jacob Irwin

Glossary, *329*

SPORTS-SPECIFIC
Rehabilitation

CHAPTER

1

Savio L-Y. Woo, Daniel K. Moon, and Ozgur Dede

Basic Science of Ligaments and Tendons Related to Rehabilitation

LEARNING OBJECTIVES

After studying this chapter, the reader will be able to do the following:

1. Recognize the complexity of the biology and biomechanics of ligaments and tendons
2. Use an understanding of the biology and biomechanics of ligaments and tendons in treatment after injury and rehabilitation on healing
3. Appreciate new trends in the management of ligament and tendon injuries

Ligaments and tendons traverse diarthrodial joints to provide stability and to mediate normal joint motion. The structure and composition of ligaments and tendons give them the flexibility and tensile strength required to perform their functions. Tendons connect muscles to bones and transmit muscle forces to generate joint movement. Tendons also absorb shock to prevent damage to the muscle. Ligaments help to position the bones in appropriate alignment for muscle action and also guide joint motion. In the case of excessive external loading, the stiffness of the ligament would increase and thereby limit excessive displacements between bones so that joint loads would not damage soft tissues, such as the articular cartilage and meniscus. Because of their respective functions, ligaments and tendons display slight differences in their histomorphologies, biochemical compositions, biomechanical properties, and intrinsic healing response. Furthermore, biological factors, such as age, homeostatic responses secondary to immobilization or mobilization of the joint, tension, and exercise, can affect their properties.[1-5]

Injuries to ligaments and tendons resulting from excessive forces or overuse can disrupt the balance between mobility and joint stability, resulting in damage to soft tissues in and around the joint that leads to pain, morbidity, and even osteoarthritis. The incidence of ligament and tendon injuries in the United States has reached epidemic proportions and affects daily function in both occupational and athletic settings. Ligaments, particularly the knee ligaments, are especially susceptible to injury during sports activities. As many as 150,000 new anterior cruciate ligament (ACL) injuries occur annually in the United States.[6] In addition, approximately 100,000 medial collateral ligament (MCL) and 25,000 posterior cruciate ligament injuries occur annually.[7] The incidence of tendon injuries has also increased over the past few decades. For example, tendinopathy accounts for an estimated 30% to 50% of all sports injuries.[8]

Treatment of these injuries ranges from rest or passive immobilization for MCL and some tendon injuries to surgical reconstruction for ACL injuries using tendon autografts and allografts. These treatment options vary on the basis of the ligament or tendon's intrinsic ability to heal or lack of it. However, current treatment modalities have been shown to result in healing tissues that have inferior properties and cannot entirely restore normal joint function.[9,10] Hence the basic science behind ligament and tendon function, injury mechanism, and healing process needs to be better understood so that treatment strategies can be developed.

This chapter provides an overview of the basic science of ligaments and tendons with emphasis toward rehabilitation science. The healing of ligaments and tendons is described, with the MCL and the flexor tendons used as examples. The biological and biomechanical changes that occur in the ACL replacement grafts after a reconstruction are then discussed. Finally, new developments in the field of functional tissue engineering to enhance the quality, rate, and completeness of healing are presented. Future directions, such as potential new treatment strategies to enhance the healing of ligament and tendon injuries, are suggested.

BASIC SCIENCE

Biology and Biochemical Composition

Ligaments and tendons have a highly organized extracellular matrix (ECM) of densely packed collagen fiber bundles. The alignment of these collagen fiber bundles generally follows the lines of tension applied to the ligament or tendon. These bundles are composed of tropocollagen as the basic molecular component. Tropocollagen molecules are systematically arranged into a hierarchic structure of microfibrils, subfibrils, fibrils, and fibers (Figure 1-1, *A*).[11] Inspection of ligaments and tendons under polarized light microscopy reveals that the

arrangement of collagen fibrils within the bundles has a sinusoidal wave or crimp pattern that can elongate easily when a force is applied (Figure 1-1, *B*). When the force is removed, the fibers recoil and return to the original crimp pattern configuration.

Insertions of ligaments and tendons into the bone consist of transitional zones from soft to hard tissues in order to minimize stress concentrations. Morphologically, these insertions can be direct or indirect. In a direct insertion, there are four distinct zones of transition: ligament or tendon, uncalcified fibrocartilage, calcified fibrocartilage, and finally bone (Figure 1-2, *A*).[12,13] In indirect insertions the superficial layers of the ligament or tendon connect with the periosteum, whereas the deeper layers connect directly to bone via Sharpey's fibers

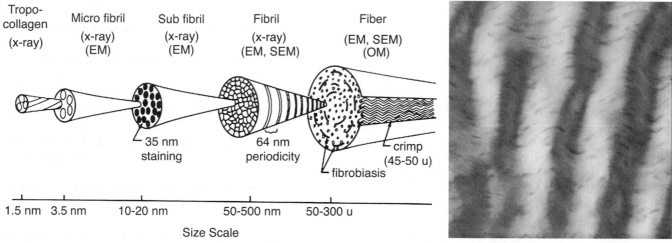

Figure 1-1 A, Ligament architectural hierarchy. **B,** Photomicrograph in polarized light of the relaxed medial collateral ligament fiber bundles exhibiting crimp. (From Woo SL-Y, Buckwalter JA, editors: *Injury and repair of musculoskeletal soft tissues,* Park Ridge, IL, 1988, American Academy of Orthopaedic Surgeons.)

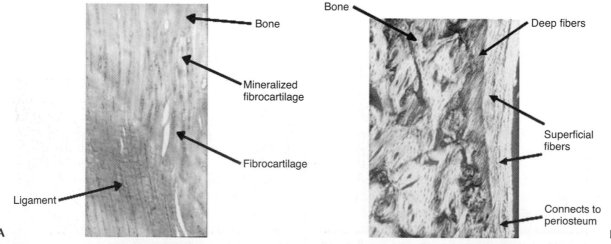

Figure 1-2 A, Photomicrograph demonstrating direct insertion (i.e., the femoral insertion of rabbit medial collateral ligament [MCL]). The ligament passes acutely into bone through a well-defined zone of fibrocartilage (hematoxylin and eosin, ×50). **B,** Photomicrograph demonstrating indirect insertion (i.e., the tibial insertion of rabbit MCL). The superficial fibrils of the ligament course parallel with the bone and insert in the periosteum. The deeper fibrils course obliquely and insert in the underlying bone (hematoxylin and eosin, ×50). (**B,** From Woo SL, Gomez MA, Sites TJ, et al: *J Bone Joint Surg Am* 69(8):1200-1211, 1987.)

(Figure 1-2, *B*).[12,13] The MCL of the knee is an example of a ligament that exhibits both types of insertions (i.e., its femoral insertion is direct while its tibial insertion is indirect).

Ligaments and tendons are relatively hypocellular, with fibroblasts interspersed throughout the tissue matrix. Fibroblasts are responsible for the maintenance and remodeling of the ECM through the secretion of macromolecules, such as collagen, elastin, and proteoglycans.[14] Collagen type I (70% to 90% of the dry weight) is the main component of ligaments and tendons and is the main contributor to their tensile stiffness and strength. Many other collagen types, such as III, V, IX, X, XI, and XII, also exist, but only in lesser amounts. Although the significance of some of these minor collagen types is not completely clear, some recent findings have helped to elucidate their roles within the tissue. For example, type V collagen is believed to exist in association with type I collagen and serves as a regulator of collagen fibril diameter,[15,16] whereas type III collagen is thought to be elevated during healing.[17] Type XIV collagen provides lubrication between collagen fibers.[18] Collagen has the ability to form covalent intramolecular (aldol) and intermolecular (Schiff base) cross-links, which are key contributors to its tensile strength and resistance to chemical or enzymatic breakdown.[19]

Elastin, another fibrous protein present in ligaments and tendons (usually <1% of the dry weight), allows the tissue to return to its prestretched length following physiological loading. Other constituents include proteoglycans and glycosaminoglycans. They form only a small portion of the macromolecular framework of the ligament (<1%), but they have a significant role in the formation and organization of the ECM. The chemical structure, intermolecular cross-linking of the collagen, and its interaction with other ECM macromolecules bring a hydrophilic nature to maintain the high water content (65% to 70% of the total weight) that is crucial to the unique function of these tissues.[14]

Biomechanics

Because ligaments and tendons function to resist tensile loads, uniaxial tensile tests are performed on these tissues to characterize their biomechanical behavior, as well as their relative contribution to joint kinematics. Generally, a bone-ligament-bone complex or bone-tendon-muscle complex is tested, and the resulting load-elongation curve exhibits nonlinearity that has an initial nonlinear region called the "toe region" of lower stiffness. With further loading, the curve gradually stiffens into a "linear region" (where the slope of the curve becomes constant). Finally, continuous increase in loading will eventually cause the specimen to fail (Figure 1-3, *A*). The load-elongation curves represent the tensile behavior of the whole structure including bony or muscle insertions, or both (i.e., to mimic ligament or tendon function in vivo). Parameters representing the structural properties (load-elongation curve) including stiffness, ultimate load, ultimate elongation, and energy absorbed at failure, are obtained. The definitions of these parameters (see Figure 1-3, *A*) are listed as follows:

- Stiffness (N/mm): the slope of the linear portion of the load-elongation curve
- Ultimate load (N): the highest load observed on the load-elongation curve immediately before tissue failure during a tensile test
- Ultimate elongation (mm): the maximum length a tissue can be elongated from its initial reference length before failure
- Energy absorbed at failure (N-mm): the entire area under the load-elongation curve that represents energy stored in the complex before failure

To assess the quality of a ligament or tendon, a stress-strain curve representing the mechanical properties must be obtained so that the properties of different tissues can be compared. Mechanical properties yield a better description of the effects of biological factors and mechanical factors on the quality of the

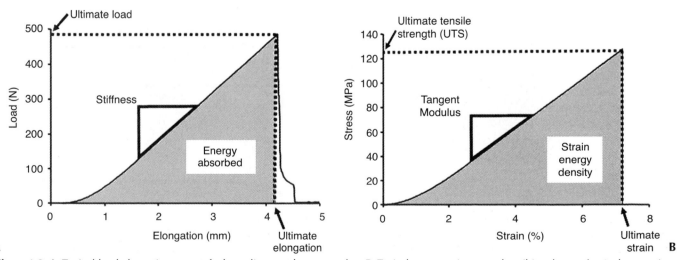

Figure 1-3 A, Typical load-elongation curve of a bone-ligament-bone complex. **B,** Typical stress-strain curve describing the mechanical properties of the ligament substance.

tissues. The stresses and strains of a defined region of the ligament or tendon substance can be calculated from a uniaxial tensile test, as described previously. Stresses can be obtained by normalizing the load with respect to the cross-sectional area whereas strain is measured on the basis of the change in length of the specimen with respect to the original (gauge) length of the specimen. To perform these measurements, it is best to determine the cross-sectional area of the specimen by using a laser micrometer system.[20,21] For strain, video cameras and a video dimensional analysis system are used to track the position of reflective surface markers placed on the ligament.[22] Thus measuring stress and strain is possible without making physical contact with these soft tissues. From the stress-strain curves, the parameters representing mechanical properties including tangent modulus, tensile strength, ultimate strain, and strain energy density of the ligament or tendon substance, are obtained. The definitions of these parameters (Figure 1-3, B) are listed as follows:

- Tangent modulus (MPa): the slope of the linear portion of the stress-strain curve
- Ultimate tensile strength (MPa): the highest stress observed on the stress-strain curve immediately before tissue failure during a tensile test
- Ultimate strain (% or mm/mm): the maximum strain at failure of the ligament substance
- Strain energy density (MPa): the entire area under the stress-strain curve

Ligaments and tendons also display time- and history-dependent viscoelastic properties that reflect the complex interactions among collagen, elastin, proteoglycans, and water.[23,24] For example, the loading and unloading curves of these tissues do not follow the same path but instead form a hysteresis loop representing internal energy dissipation following a cycle of loading and unloading (Figure 1-4). However, over the course of several cycles, the area of hysteresis is reduced, and the curves become more repeatable. Because the mechanical behavior of a tissue tested after the first cycle

will differ from that of a tissue tested at the tenth cycle, the specimen must be preconditioned by a number of cycles to obtain more consistent data. Other important viscoelastic characteristics of ligaments and tendons include creep, an increase in deformation over time under a constant load or stress, and stress relaxation, a decline in stress over time under a constant deformation or stress (Figure 1-5).

The viscoelastic behavior of ligaments and tendons has important clinical significance. For example, during walking or jogging, cyclic stress relaxation decreases a tissue's resistance to strain, resulting in a continuous decrease in peak stress for each cycle.[14,25] This phenomenon may help prevent fatigue failure of ligaments and tendons. Similarly, cyclic creep can be used to demonstrate how warm-up exercises and stretching can increase flexibility of a joint as a constant applied stress during stretching increases the length of the ligaments and tendons.

Tissue Homeostasis

Ligaments and tendons respond to physical stimuli in vivo and undergo changes accordingly. A generalized statement similar to Wolff's law[26] for bone can be made for ligaments and tendons because they do respond to these physiological stress and motion through remodeling of their morphological appearance and biochemical constituents, as well as biomechanical properties. In the past, ligament injuries were treated with prolonged immobilization of joints followed by a delayed therapeutic exercise after surgery. In time, as the detrimental effects of immobilization were elucidated by laboratory and clinical studies, the clinical paradigm shifted toward the introduction

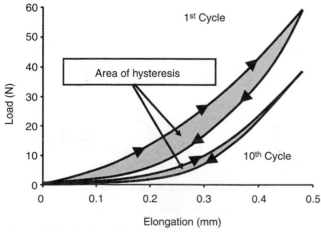

Figure 1-4 The loading and unloading curves for a ligament or tendon do not follow the same path, forming a hysteresis loop. Note the decrease in the area of hysteresis by the tenth cycle of loading and unloading.

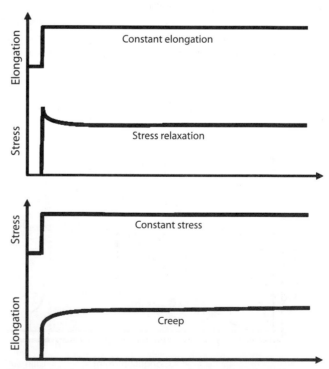

Figure 1-5 Schematic representation of stress-relaxation (decreasing stress over time under a constant deformation) and creep (increasing deformation over time under a constant load).

of stress as rapidly as possible to limit the damage to the joint, as well as to improve its healing. On the other hand, overzealous therapeutic approaches that introduce excessive stress or motion can cause further injury and retard recovery. Hence observing the time course for immobilization and mobilization are important for an athlete or worker to effectively return to sport or work after suffering an injury. Any rehabilitation procedure begs the question of how soon and how much. The answers must be tailored to the age and physical state of the patient, as well as the location and severity of injury.

Immobilization

Immobilization of a joint induces concomitant stress deprivation of surrounding healthy structures, which can adversely affect them.[14] For example, immobilization can cause intra-articular changes including pannus formation, which leads to necrosis and erosion and ulceration of the articular cartilage.[27,28] Increased joint stiffness is also commonly observed clinically and has been demonstrated quantitatively in experimental animals.[29,30] After 9 weeks of immobilization, the amount of torque required to initially extend a rabbit knee is significantly increased.[29] Immobilization also causes the other tissues, such as joint capsule, to be cross-linked, which contributes to joint stiffness.[29]

In ligaments and tendons, alterations in collagen cross-linking, synthesis, and degradation occur following immobilization.[31] These changes lead to decreased stiffness and ultimate load of a ligament or tendon complex (Figure 1-6). The ultimate loads and energy absorbed at failure of the femur-MCL-tibia complexes (FMTC) are only 31% and 18%, respectively, of the contralateral nonimmobilized controls.[13] The tangent modulus of the MCL substance is significantly decreased, revealing a softening of the ligament substance after immobilization. Failures occur at the tibial insertion rather than at the midsubstance because of increasing osteoclastic activities at the insertion sites.[32] Different ligaments such as the ACL experience fewer changes in tensile properties than the MCL of the same knee after 9 weeks of immobilization.[33] Therefore it appears that different soft tissue structures are affected differently by immobilization, and care must be exercised when generalizing specific results to all ligaments or tendons.

Remobilization of the knee joint following immobilization reveals that the mechanical properties of the MCL substance in the functional range return to normal values relatively rapidly.[13] The mode of failure for the remobilized limb continues to occur by disruption at the bony insertion sites, suggesting recovery at these sites remains incomplete. These findings imply an asynchronous rate of recovery between the ligament and bony insertion, which has strong implications for how to develop appropriate rehabilitation strategies.[34]

Exercise

The effects of exercise can have specific influence on different ligaments and tendons. In a study of the effect of short-term (3 months) and long-term (12 months) exercise on the biomechanical properties of swine digital tendons, short-term exercise demonstrated little or no effect on the digital extensor tendon properties, whereas long-term exercise resulted in positive changes including an increase in cross-sectional area, as well as a 22% increase in tensile strength.[35,36] On the other hand, for the digital flexor tendons, the mechanical properties of the tendon substance exhibited no statistical changes for both short-term and long-term exercise, whereas the ultimate load of the exercised flexor-tendon complexes increased by 6% in the short-term exercised group and 19% in the long-term exercised group secondary to changes at the bony insertion sites.[5]

On the basis of these findings, a spectrum may exist for tissue response to different activity levels to maintain homeostasis. Figure 1-7 shows a hypothetical curve that describes

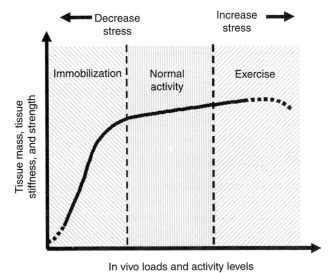

Figure 1-6 Schematic diagram illustrating ligament homeostatis secondary to stress and motion. (From Woo SL, Chan SS, Yamaji T: *J Biomechics* 30(5):431-439, 1997.)

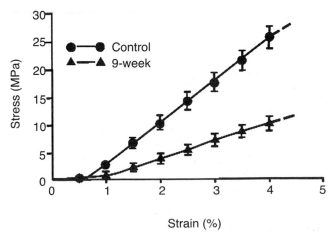

Figure 1-7 Mechanical properties of rabbit MCL from control and 9-week immobilization groups. (From Woo SL, Gomez MA, Sites TJ, et al: *J Bone Joint Surg Am* 69(8):1200-1211, 1987.)

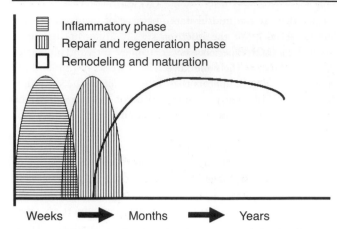

Figure 1-8 Schematic showing the time course of the overlapping phases of healing for ligaments and tendons. (From Hunter LY, Funk FJ, editors: *Rehabilitation of the injured knee*, St Louis, 1984, Mosby, Proc AAOS.)

the homeostatic responses for soft tissues, such as ligaments and tendons. The relationship between the level and duration of stress and motion and the in vivo biological responses in tissue properties and tissue mass is represented by a highly nonlinear curve. With stress and motion deprivation (immobilization), a rapid reduction in tissue properties and mass occurs. In contrast, the gains following exercise training are much less pronounced. Experts also know that the functional integrity of an immobilized ligament can return to its normal mechanical characteristics quite rapidly following remobilization.[13] However, the recovery of the ligament-bone junction is much slower than that of the ligament substance.

Effects of Aging

Biomechanical changes associated with skeletal maturation and senescence have been documented in the MCL, ACL, and patellar tendon using animal models, as well as human cadavers.[1,2,37,38] These studies show that different soft tissue structures are affected differently by aging. Significant increases in the linear stiffness, ultimate load, and energy absorbed at failure of the FMTC were noted in both the male and female rabbits during skeletal maturation. Afterward, only slight decreases in these properties were found with increasing age. The modes of failure correlated well with closure of the epiphyses in both sexes (i.e., tibial avulsion failure for the skeletally immature groups and ligament midsubstance for the skeletally mature groups). The tangent modulus of the rabbit MCL substance increased during maturation for both sexes until 12 months of age and then gradually declined until 48 months. The ultimate tensile strength also remained relatively constant after 12 months of age and reduced slightly at 48 months. Thus the rate of skeletal maturation is a significant contributor to the differences in the tensile properties of both the male and female rabbits.[39]

In the case of ACL, data on age-related changes have been obtained from human cadavers. In a study using pairs of human cadaveric knees obtained from young donors (22 to

41 years, mean age 35 years) and older donors (60 to 97 years, mean age 76 years), there was a rapid decline in the stiffness and ultimate load in the femur-ACL-tibia complex as a function of age.[2] These differences in the biomechanical properties for older individuals may be due to a decrease in the level of activity with advancing age, the changes in hormone levels, and other physiological or geometric changes of the joints.

For the rabbit patellar tendon, a decrease in maximum stress was found between 1- and 4-year-old rabbits whereas minimal differences were found for other biomechanical parameters.[37] The age-related changes in tensile and viscoelastic properties were investigated using fresh-frozen human patellar tendons. Specimens for the younger group were from individuals 29 to 50 years of age, whereas those from the older group were from individuals 64 to 93 years of age. Except for ultimate tensile strength, which was 17% less for the older group than the younger group, minimal differences in tensile and viscoelastic properties existed between younger and older groups.[38] Another study evaluated the biomechanical properties of patellar tendon allografts from donors aged 18 to 55 years. There was no significant correlation between age and any of the mechanical properties.[40] The data from these studies imply that patellar tendon allografts harvested from individuals up to 55 years of age can be used for ACL reconstruction without a significant loss in the mechanical properties.

LIGAMENT AND TENDON HEALING

Ligaments and tendons have different capability of healing. The MCL of the knee is an excellent model for studying ligament healing because of its ability to heal spontaneously without surgical intervention. In addition, its uniform cross-sectional area with a relatively large aspect ratio is suitable for uniaxial tensile testing.[41,42] As a result, extensive studies have been done to elucidate the complex process of ligament healing. Generally, the process involves overlapping but distinct phases of acute inflammation, repair, and remodeling that last for 1 or more years after injury (Figure 1-8). The following section reviews the changes in the histological appearance, biochemical composition, and biomechanical properties of the healing MCL, as well as the factors (e.g., repair versus conservative treatment, mobilization versus immobilization, increased stresses, multiple ligament injuries) affecting MCL healing.

Medial Collateral Ligament Healing

After a midsubstance rupture of the MCL (characterized by the mop-end appearance of its torn ends), hemorrhage begins and a hematoma forms between the retracting ligament ends. Inflammatory and monocytic cells migrate to the injury site to convert the clot into granulation tissue and phagocytose necrotic tissue. These events cause swelling, erythema, increased temperature, pain, and impaired function, the five cardinal signs of inflammation. Inflammation begins immediately after injury with the release of inflammatory mediators from damaged cells. These mediators promote vascular dilation and increase vascular permeability. Blood escaping from the damaged vessels forms a hematoma that temporarily fills the injured site. Fibrin accumulates within the hematoma, and platelets bind to fibrillar collagen, thereby achieving hemostasis and forming a clot consisting of fibrin, platelets, red blood cells, and debris. The participation of platelets in clot formation is marked by their release of vasoactive mediators, cytokines, and growth factors including transforming growth factor beta (TGF-β), platelet-derived growth factor (PDGF), and many others.[14,43]

Within about 2 weeks, the granulation tissue is replaced with a continuous network of immature collagen fibers with randomly oriented fibroblasts that connect the ligament. At this point the torn ends of the ligament are no longer distinguishable, and angiogenesis begins, while fibroblasts continue to actively produce extracellular matrix.[14,43] During the next several weeks, the biochemical composition of the repair tissue changes as repair progresses. Water, glycosaminoglycans, and type III collagen concentrations decline, inflammatory cells disappear, and the concentration of type I collagen increases as newly synthesized collagen fibrils increase in size and begin to form tightly packed bundles. The tensile strength of the repair tissue increases as the collagen content, especially type I collagen, increases.[14,43]

In most ligaments, evidence of remodeling appears within several weeks of injury as the numbers of fibroblasts and macrophages decrease, fibroblast synthetic activity decreases, and the fibroblasts and collagen fibrils assume a more organized appearance. In the months following injury, the volume of the repair tissue decreases and the remodeling process is marked by increased alignment of collagen fibers along the long axis of the ligament and continued collagen maturation. The longitudinal alignment of these fibers has been shown to correlate directly with an improvement in the structural properties of the bone-ligament complex.[14,43]

The extracellular matrix of the healing ligament exhibits a number of important changes including elevated water content and glycosaminoglycan levels and differences in elastin and other glycoproteins. The ligament also contains more type III and V collagen than do normal ligaments.[10,44] Recent work performed in our research center demonstrated in rabbits that the ratios of collagen types V/I and III/I in the healing MCL increased by 84% and 138%, respectively.[44] By 52 weeks, the ratio of collagen type III/I returned to normal levels, but collagen type V/I remained elevated. This persistent elevation of the type V/I ratio serves to explain the uniform distribution of small collagen fibrils,[45] as both collagen types III and V have been postulated to hinder cross-sectional growth of collagen fibrils.[15,16,46-48] Furthermore, the number of mature collagen cross-links is only 45% of normal values after 1 year.[47] A relationship has also been demonstrated between inferior mechanical properties of the MCL and the smaller number of collagen cross-links, as well as the decrease in mass and diameter of the collagen fibers.[47,49]

Although the healing ligament remodels over time, long-term animal studies show that the histological and morpho-

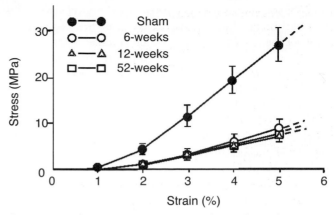

Figure 1-9 Stress-strain curves representing the mechanical properties of the MCL substance for sham-operated and healing MCLs at time periods of 6 ($n = 6$), 12 ($n = 6$), and 52 ($n = 4$) weeks. (From Ohland KJ, Weiss JA, Anderson DR, et al: *Transactions of the 37th Annual Meeting of the Orthopaedic Research Society*, 16(1):158, 1991.)

logical appearance of healed ligaments fails to return to its preinjury state. As demonstrated with transmission electron microscopy, the number of collagen fibrils increases in comparison with the uninjured ligament, but the diameters are uniformly small. This condition remains even after 2 years of healing.[45,50] Additionally, the "crimp" patterns and collagen fiber alignment of the healing ligament remain abnormal for up to 1 year.[43,50]

Biomechanically, the structural properties of the FMTC differ from normal at 6 weeks after injury, but the stiffness approaches normal levels by 12 weeks after injury. The valgus knee rotation improves from more than doubled as compared with sham operated controls, to approximately 20% greater than controls.[41] Interestingly, the mechanical properties of the healed tissue have been found to be much inferior to normal at 6 weeks and remain so for up to 2 years (Figure 1-9).[34,51,52] Therefore the return of the structural function to near normal level is largely due to an increase in the cross-sectional area of the inferior healing tissue to as much as 2.5 times the size of normal MCL at 1 year.[52] Overall, the healed MCL can be described as a larger quantity of lesser-quality ligamentous tissue.

In addition, healing ligaments and tendons have been shown to display abnormal viscoelastic properties. Under static and cyclic loading, the healing MCLs from rabbits and goats stress relax significantly more compared with sham controls.[53,54] Such altered viscoelastic behavior may be due to increased water content in the healing tissue, as well as alterations of other biochemical composition, such as changes in glycosaminoglycans, elastin, other glycoproteins, and collagen.

Conservative Treatment versus Repair

For an MCL injury, studies have demonstrated that nonoperative treatment yields better results than surgical repair followed by immobilization. In a canine model, a transected MCL healed spontaneously without surgical treatment or immobilization.[34] When compared with surgical repair plus 6 weeks' immobilization, the healed tissue had better alignment of the fibroblasts and more longitudinal fibers than the repaired ligaments at 12 weeks. However, by 48 weeks both the repaired and nonrepaired tissues became similar, although neither resembled the normal MCL. Biomechanical data indicated that valgus knee rotation, the stiffness, and ultimate load of the FMTC for the nonrepair group were closer to controls throughout the study (6, 12, and 48 weeks). Nevertheless, the quality of the healed tissue (mechanical properties) of both the nonrepaired and surgically repaired MCLs did not improve with time and remained significantly different from the normal MCL.

Similar results were obtained using a "mop-end" tear of the rabbit MCL substance.[41] No statistically significant differences in biomechanical properties could be demonstrated between the repaired and nonrepaired groups at 6 or 12 weeks after injury. These structural properties of the FMTC, the mechanical properties of the MCL midsubstance, and varus-valgus knee rotation were similar. These findings help to solidify the clinical management of grade III MCL tear by nonoperative treatment followed by early motion and functional rehabilitation. Positive outcomes have been shown as the paradigm shifts to nonoperative management for isolated grade III injuries of the MCL as the preferred method of treatment.[55]

Immobilization versus Passive Controlled Mobilization

Unlike the MCL, a lacerated digital flexor tendon needs surgical repair. Canine forepaws were used to study the effects of postoperative immobilization versus controlled passive mobilization on its healing. With controlled passive mobilization, tendons had a higher survival rate, and the strength at the repair site was improved as the ultimate loads were significantly higher than those of the immobilized controls. Controlled passive mobilization can also significantly minimize adhesion formation between the repaired tendon and the surrounding sheath, thus providing better gliding function of the digits.[35]

Stress and Exercise

Increasing the stress levels experienced by a healing ligament can elicit positive changes in its biomechanical properties.[4] In an experimental study, increased tension on the healing rabbit MCL was accomplished by inserting a stainless steel pin beneath the MCL perpendicular to the long axis of the ligament representing a 2- to 3.5-fold increase of the in situ load and stress over those of controls. At 6 weeks, joints with the stainless steel pin (increased stress) had lower varus-valgus laxity compared with those for the nonstressed group, although the difference diminished at 12 weeks. Nevertheless, the tangent moduli of the stressed group were higher at 12 weeks, and its collagen content was closer to normal MCL. The histological appearance of healed ligament was also improved.[4]

Exercise has also been shown to have a positive effect on the healing properties of MCL. In a rat model, collagen synthesis and tensile strength of the healed MCL were found to be increased following exercise, compared with immobilized controls.[56]

Multiple Ligament Injuries

Clinical management of multiple ligamentous injuries to the knee remains controversial. In the case of a combined ACL/MCL injury, some have reported satisfactory results with nonoperative treatment,[57] whereas others advocate surgical reconstruction of the ACL with repair of the MCL to adequately restore knee stability.[58] Still others choose to surgically reconstruct the ACL without addressing the MCL.[59] Regardless, the prognosis for such injuries is generally worse than for the isolated MCL injury.

In our research center the effects of ACL deficiency on the healing of the injured MCL have been studied by using canine, rabbit, and goat models.[60-62] It has been demonstrated that repairing the rabbit MCL in combination with ACL reconstruction can help to restore the valgus laxity of the knee initially. However, at longer term (52 weeks), the advantages of the surgical repair disappear. The biomechanical properties of the FMTC are also better following repair, but in the long term there are no differences between the repair and nonrepair groups.[61]

ACL reconstructions can be done more precisely by using a larger animal model (i.e., the goat) than a rabbit model.[63,64] A series of studies performed in our research center investigated the healing of a combined injury treated with ACL reconstruction using this model.[62] It was demonstrated that from time 0 to 6 weeks the initially high in situ force in the ACL graft was transferred to the healing MCL. The results suggest that the strong ACL graft could stabilize the knee initially. But with graft remodeling, loads are transferred to the healing MCL. As a result, the healing MCL suffers from excess loads and hypertrophies with tissue of lesser quality. This is supported by a large cross-sectional area of the healing ligament, with a concomitant decrease in the structural properties of the healing FMTC and even poorer mechanical properties of the healing MCL.[42,62] These findings prove that in combined ACL/MCL injuries, healing of the MCL depends on the quality of ACL reconstruction, illustrating the important role the ACL plays in maintaining valgus knee stability. It is apparent that only reconstruction of the ACL is necessary for the MCL to heal.

Anterior Cruciate Ligament Reconstruction

An injury to intra-articular ligaments, such as midsubstance tears of the ACL and PCL, generally fails to heal successfully. Reasons including the hostile synovial environment, limited vascular ingrowth, and fibroblast migration from surrounding tissues, as well as the high mechanical demand, have been postulated.[14] As a result, surgeons use tissue autografts or allografts to reconstruct the failed ACL. Currently the most commonly used autografts are bone-patellar tendon-bone grafts and the hamstring tendon grafts (semitendinosus and/or gracilis tendons). As for allografts, the Achilles tendon has also been used as an allograft for failed ACL reconstructions.

From a historical standpoint, graft selection has been based on the structural properties, such as stiffness and ultimate load of the available graft complexes.[2,9,65,66] However, despite their comparable high stiffness and ultimate load at the time of implantation, the biomechanical properties of these grafts have been shown to decline after the grafts are placed in the intra-articular environment and do not recover to their original levels or near to those of the normal ACL. In animal studies the stiffness and ultimate load of a patellar tendon autograft were only 24% and 15% of the control, respectively, at 30 weeks. At 52 weeks post ACL reconstruction, these values further reduced to 13% and 11% of the control, respectively. Similar trends have been observed in the canine and goat models.[63,67]

Early integration of the ACL replacement graft with the bone at the tunnels is also important to the success of the reconstruction. The bone-patellar tendon-bone graft has bony ends allowing for bone-to-bone healing and more rapid integration of the graft into the joint. This could allow for earlier rehabilitation. On the other hand, the hamstring tendon grafts lack bony ends, resulting in a soft tissue–to–hard tissue interface that is weaker and takes a longer time to integrate. Animal studies have revealed that the tendon-bone interface requires more than 12 weeks of healing before sufficient mechanical strength of interface can be achieved.[68,69] As a result, several investigators are exploring the possibility of using growth factors to improve the stiffness and strength of the tendon-bone interface.[70,71]

FUNCTIONAL TISSUE ENGINEERING FOR TENDON AND LIGAMENT HEALING

Because of the inability of ligaments and tendons to heal with properties close to those for their native tissues, clinicians and researchers are looking into alternative treatment modalities to enhance these properties. With the recent advances in the fields of molecular biology, biochemistry, and functional tissue engineering, potential use of growth factors, gene therapy, cell therapy, and biological tissue scaffolds are being explored.

Growth Factors

Because growth factors have been known to regulate cell migration, proliferation, differentiation, and increase in matrix synthesis, they have been explored in aiding the repair of ligaments and tendons.[72-75] In our research center in vitro studies were conducted in which TGF-β_1 was found to promote collagen synthesis by both MCL and ACL fibroblasts[73] while PDGF-BB and epidermal growth factor could significantly increase fibroblast cell proliferation.[72,75] Follow-up in vivo studies with the application of these growth factors were done. Unfortunately, different outcomes including minimal changes in the biomechanical properties of healing ligaments were found.[76] With careful examination, it became clear that the responses of healing MCL fibroblasts to various growth factors are different than for normal fibroblasts.[77] The phenotype of fibroblasts from the healing MCL also changed during the

healing process with concomitant changes in the healing milieu, plus too much growth factor (e.g. TGF-β_1) could have a negative impact on MCL healing.[76] It is no wonder that no enhancement in the healing MCL occurred. In other words, it is extremely difficult to know what, when, and how much growth factor to apply, a common but serious problem. Much more work remains in order to find the role of growth factors in improving the healing of ligaments.

Growth factors have been used in attempts to accelerate tendon-to-bone healing and following ACL reconstruction in animal models with some success.[70,71] Treating the autograft with bone-growth factors can result in an 80% increase in ultimate load of the ACL graft construct at 8 weeks after surgery compared with untreated controls.[70] Bone morphogenetic protein-2 delivered to the bone-tendon interface with an adenovirus-mediated viral gene transfer technique resulted in an improved integration of semitendinosus tendon grafts in rabbits.[71] The stiffness and the ultimate load of the femur-ACL-tibia complexes were significantly increased in the specimens with bone morphogenetic protein-2 compared with untreated controls.

Gene Therapy

Gene therapy has been used to deliver growth factors and proteins to the cells in order to alter their function.[78,79] In our research center, the LacZ marker gene has been successfully introduced and expressed in the MCL and ACL of rabbits, using both retroviral and adenoviral vectors on allogenic fibroblasts.[80] Expression of the LacZ gene product, β-galactosidase, could be detected using X-gal staining between 10 days and 6 weeks in the normal MCL, as well as injured MCL. Expression time did not differ in the ruptured and uninjured medial collateral ligaments with use of adenoviral in vivo gene transfer. Although these results are encouraging, much work still needs to be done, such as choosing the appropriate genes to regulate and the time of application. In addition, because of possible clinical risks from potential immune responses to adenoviruses, low in vivo transduction efficiency, and the ability of retroviruses to transfer genes only to dividing cells, safer and more efficient methods such as lipidic gene transfer systems need to be developed.

Antisense mediated gene inhibition of those proteins (e.g., collagen types III and V and decorin) that are excessively expressed during healing has been investigated as a potential approach to enhancing properties of the healing ligament. Antisense (AS) oligonucleotides (ODNs) are synthetic oligonucleotides complementary to specific mRNA sequences and have been found to limit expression of these specific genes by binding to their target mRNA. Introduction of AS-decorin-ODNs to the healing MCL via hemagglutinating virus of Japan-liposome vector complexes led to the formation of larger-diameter collagen fibrils and an increase in tensile strength at 6 weeks.[81] In our research center, AS-collagen types III and V-ODNs were transfected into human patellar tendon fibroblasts (HPTFs) in vitro by using lipofectamine, a nonviral lipidic vector.[78,82] The results showed that AS-ODNs were

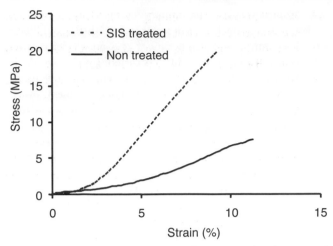

Figure 1-10 Typical stress-strain curves for SIS-treated and nontreated groups at 12 weeks. (From Musahl V, Abramowitch SD, Gilbert TW, et al: *J Orthop Res* 22(1):214-220, 2004.)

effective in inhibiting collagens type III and type V synthesis and mRNA levels with respect to sense and missense controls.[78,82,83] These studies show that antisense gene therapy may be a promising approach to successfully down-regulating the expression of decorin, type III and V collagen that could improve the quality of the healing ligaments.

Cell Therapy

In recent years there has been an increasing interest in stem cell research because mesenchymal stem cells (MSC) have been shown to contribute to the healing of tissues, such as bone, cartilage, muscle, ligament, tendon, adipose, and marrow stroma. One strategy to enhance ligament and tendon healing is autologous transplantation of MSCs because they can be introduced into the healing area without eliciting an immune response. MSCs can be isolated from bone marrow, expanded in culture, and transduced with genes. The hypothesis is that these multipotent progenitor cells can differentiate into fibroblast-like cells once transplanted into the healing ligament or tendon and therefore may aid in the ligament healing process. Using a rat model, one study found that MSCs transplanted into the healing MCL could be detected for up to 28 days, with their shapes similar to the surrounding fibroblasts,[84] indicating that MSCs can potentially serve as vehicles for the delivery of therapeutic agents to enhance the healing process.

Bone marrow–derived MSCs suspended in a collagen-gel matrix have also been implanted into the Achilles tendon gap defect model and central patellar tendon defect models in rabbits.[85-88] MSC stem cell–implanted repairs of Achilles tendon gap defects showed better mechanical properties than control repairs that were closer to the properties of the normal contralateral tendon.[85] Bone marrow–derived stem cells have also been shown to have positive effects on central third patellar tendon defects. In a rabbit study, central patellar tendon defects were repaired using MSC-seeded and acellular collagen gel constructs. MSC-seeded repairs showed better

mechanical and structural properties than the acellular repairs, and these values were closer to the properties of the central third of the normal patellar tendon.[88] These studies demonstrate the potential of stem cell–based therapies for improving ligament and tendon healing.

Bioscaffolds

Scaffolding materials can serve as the necessary matrix to guide cells to make new tissues, as well as to provide mechanical support. In recent years, one of the biological scaffolds, namely the porcine small intestinal submucosa (SIS), has received much attention. SIS is composed mainly of collagen (90% of dry weight), with its fiber alignment largely in the longitudinal direction.[89] It has been found to contain a small amount of growth factors, such as fibroblast growth factor, TGF-β, and vascular endothelial growth factor.[90] SIS was previously used to repair a segmental defect in the dog Achilles tendon. The SIS remodeled healing tendons were stronger than the musculotendinous origin or the bony insertion at 12 weeks after surgery, and the healed tendon had organized collagen-rich connective tissue similar to the contralateral normal tendons.[90,91]

In our research center, SIS has been shown to enhance MCL healing by improving the mechanical properties of the healing rabbit MCL at 12 and 26 weeks (Figure 1-10).[92-94] SIS-treated MCLs had a tangent modulus and tensile strength nearly two times greater than the nontreated MCLs.[92] Furthermore, a concomitant decrease in collagen type V levels and an increase in collagen fibril diameter were found in SIS-treated healing MCLs compared with nontreated MCLs.[93] Although previous studies have shown that healing involved only an increased amount of inferior tissue mass to restore its function, a successfully improved quality of the healed MCL midsubstance has generated much excitement and offers many possibilities to further enhance healing in ligaments.

SUMMARY AND FUTURE DIRECTIONS

Extensive laboratory and clinical research has resulted in a better understanding of the process of ligament and tendon healing. More importantly, such knowledge has led to new and improved paradigms for clinical managements (i.e., better treatment methods and rehabilitation protocols). Healing of ligaments and tendons is now recognized as an extremely complicated process that involves multiple factors including extent of injury and the effects of biomechanical and biochemical environments. Because management of ligament and tendon injuries has not had universally favorable outcomes, significant efforts must continue.

Advances in molecular and cell biology have opened the door to the possibility of manipulating the healing environment and the cells within it, thus enhancing the properties of the healing tissue. In vitro data have shown that some growth factors have stimulatory effects on cell proliferation, as well as on the mechanical properties of ligaments.[73] Gene and cell therapy could be a valuable biological intervention in ligament and tendon healing.[81,86] Functional tissue engineering including the use of bioscaffolds has also been shown to have potential to enhance healing of ligaments and tendons.[90,92-94] Ultimately, solutions will likely come from combining several of these approaches.

Scientific research has clearly led to a greater appreciation and respect for ligaments and tendons as living and dynamic tissue. Team research involving multidisciplinary collaboration among molecular biologists, biochemists, bioengineers, therapists, and clinicians is necessary so that the complicated issues can be understood and appropriate methodologies for treatment regimen developed to improve clinical outcome for patients with ligament and tendon injuries.

REFERENCES

1. Woo SL, Orlando CA, Gomez MA, et al: Tensile properties of the medial collateral ligament as a function of age, *J Orthop Res* 4(2):133-141, 1986.

2. Woo SL-Y, Hollis JM, Adams DJ, et al: Tensile properties of the human femur-anterior cruciate ligament-tibia complex. The effects of specimen age and orientation, *Am J Sports Med* 19(3):217-225, 1991.

3. Woo SL, Gomez MA, Woo YK, et al: Mechanical properties of tendons and ligaments. II. The relationships of immobilization and exercise on tissue remodeling, *Biorheology* 19(3):397-408, 1982.

4. Gomez MA, Woo SL, Amiel D, et al: The effects of increased tension on healing medical collateral ligaments, *Am J Sports Med* 19(4):347-354, 1991.

5. Woo SL, Gomez MA, Amiel D, et al: The effects of exercise on the biomechanical and biochemical properties of swine digital flexor tendons, *J Biomech Eng* 103(1):51-56, 1981.

6. Beaty J, editor: *Knee and leg: soft tissue trauma.* Volume 6. Rosemont, IL, 1999, American Academy of Orthopaedic Surgeons.

7. Miyasaka KC, Daniel DM, Stone ML, et al: The incidence of knee ligament injuries in the general population, *Am J Knee Surg* 4:3-8, 1991.

8. Kannus P, Natri A: Etiology and pathophysiology of tendon ruptures in sports, *Scand J Med Sci Sports* 7(2):107-112, 1997.

9. Woo SL-Y, Kanamori A, Zeminski J, et al: The effectiveness of anterior cruciate ligament reconstruction by hamstrings and patellar tendon: a cadaveric study comparing anterior tibial load versus rotational loads, *J Bone Joint Surg* 84A(6):907-914, 2002.

10. Frank C, Woo SL-Y, Amiel D, et al: Medial collateral ligament healing. A multidisciplinary assessment in rabbits, *Am J Sports Med* 11(6):379-389, 1983.

11. Kastelic J, Galeski A, Baer E: The multicomposite structure of tendon, *Connect Tissue Res* 6(1):11-23, 1978.

12. Cooper RR, Misol S: Tendon and ligament insertion. A light and electron microscopic study, *J Bone Joint Surg Am* 52(1):1-20, 1970.

13. Woo SL, Gomez MA, Sites TJ, et al: The biomechanical and morphological changes in the medial collateral ligament of the rabbit after immobilization and remobilization, *J Bone Joint Surg Am* 69(8):1200-1211, 1987.

14. Woo S, An K-N, Frank C, et al: Anatomy, biology and biomechanics of tendon and ligaments. In Buckwalter J, Einhorn T, Simon SR, editors: *Orthopaedic basic science,* ed 2, pp. 581-616, Rosemont, IL, 2000, American Academy of Orthopaedic Surgeons.

15. Birk DE, Mayne R: Localization of collagen types I, III and V during tendon development. Changes in collagen types I and III are correlated with changes in fibril diameter. Eur J Cell Biol 72(4):352-361, 1997.

16. Linsenmayer TF, Gibney E, Igoe F, et al: Type V collagen: molecular structure and fibrillar organization of the chicken a1(V) NH2-terminal domain, a putative regulator of corneal fibrillogenesis. *J Cell Biol* 121(5):1181-1189, 1993.

17. Liu SH, Yang RS, al-Shaikh R, et al: Collagen in tendon, ligament, and bone healing. A current review. *Clin Orthop Rel Res* 318:265-278, 1995.

18. Niyibizi C, Visconti CS, Kavalkovich K, et al: Collagens in an adult bovine medial collateral ligament: Immunofluorescence localization by confocal microscopy reveals that type XIV collagen predominates at the ligament-bone junction. *Matrix Biol* 14(9):743-751, 1995.

19. Tanzer ML. Cross-linking of collagen. *Science*; 180(86):561-566, 1973.

20. Lee TQ, Woo SL-Y: A new method for determining cross-sectional shape and area of soft tissues. *J Biomech Eng* 110(2):110-114, 1988.

21. Woo SL-Y, Danto MI, Ohland KJ, et al: The use of a laser micrometer system to determine the cross-sectional shape and area of ligaments: a comparative study with two existing methods. *J Biomech Eng* 112(4):426-431, 1990.

22. Smutz WP, Drexler M, Berglund LJ, et al: Accuracy of a video strain measurement system. *J Biomechics* 29(6):813-817, 1996.

23. Woo SL-Y. Mechanical properties of tendons and ligaments: I. Quasi-static and nonlinear viscoelastic properties. *Biorheology* 19(3):385-396, 1982.

24. Johnson GA, Livesay GA, Woo SL-Y, et al: A single integral finite strain viscoelastic model of ligaments and tendons. *J Biomech Eng* 118(2):221-226, 1996.

25. Woo SL-Y, Gomez MA, Akeson WH: The time and history-dependent viscoelastic properties of the canine medical collateral ligament. *J Biomech Eng* 103(4):293-298, 1981.

26. Wolff J: *Das gesetz der transformation der kochen.* Hirschwald, Berlin, 1882.

27. Evans EB, Eggers GWN, Butler JK, et al: Experimental immobilization and remobilization of rat knee joints. *J Bone Joint Surg* 42A:737-758, 1960.

28. Salter RB, Field P: The effects of continuous compression on living articular cartilage: an experimental investigation. *J Bone Joint Surg* 42A:31-49, 1960.

29. Woo SL-Y, Matthews JV, Akeson WH, et al: Connective tissue response to immobility. Correlative study of biomechanical and biochemical measurements of normal and immobilized rabbit knees. *Arthritis Rheum* 18(3): 257-264, 1975.

30. Akeson WH, Amiel D, Woo SL-Y: Immobility effects on synovial joints: the pathomechanics of joint contracture. *Biorheology* 17(1-2):95-110, 1980.

31. Akeson WH, Woo SL, Amiel D, et al: The connective tissue response to immobility: biochemical changes in periarticular connective tissue of the immobilized rabbit knee. *Clin Orthop Relat Res* 93:356-362, 1973.

32. Laros GS, Tipton CM, Cooper RR: Influence of physical activity on ligament insertions in the knees of dogs. *J Bone Joint Surg Am* 53(2):275-286, 1971.

33. Newton PO, Woo SL, MacKenna DA, et al: Immobilization of the knee joint alters the mechanical and ultrastructural properties of the rabbit anterior cruciate ligament. *J Orthop Res* 13(2):191-200, 1995.

34. Woo SL, Inoue M, McGurk-Burleson E, et al: Treatment of the medial collateral ligament injury. II: Structure and function of canine knees in response to differing treatment regimens. *Am J Sports Med* 15(1):22-29, 1987.

35. Woo SL-Y, Gelberman RH, Cobb NG, et al: The importance of controlled passive mobilization on flexor tendon healing. A biomechanical study. *Acta Orthop Scand* 52(6): 615-622, 1981.

36. Woo SL-Y, Ritter MA, Amiel D, et al: The biomechanical and biochemical properties of swine tendons: long term effects of exercise on the digital extensors. *Connect Tissue Res* 7(3):177-183, 1980.

37. Dressler MR, Butler DL, Wenstrup R, et al: A potential mechanism for age-related declines in patellar tendon biomechanics. *J Orthop Res* 20(6):1315-1322, 2002.

38. Johnson GA, Tramaglini DM, Levine RE, et al: Tensile and viscoelastic properties of human patellar tendon. *J Orthop Res* 12(6):796-803, 1994.

39. Woo SL, Ohland KJ, Weiss JA: Aging and sex-related changes in the biomechanical properties of the rabbit medial collateral ligament. *Mech Ageing Dev* 56(2):129-142, 1990.

40. Flahiff CM, Brooks AT, Hollis JM, et al: Biomechanical analysis of patellar tendon allografts as a function of donor age. *Am J Sports Med* 23(3):354-358, 1995.

41. Weiss JA, Woo SL-Y, Ohland KJ, et al: Evaluation of a new injury model to study medial collateral ligament healing: primary repair versus nonoperative treatment. *J Orthop Res* 9(4):516-528, 1991.

42. Scheffler SU, Clineff TD, Papageorgiou CD, et al: Structure and function of the healing medial collateral ligament in a goat model. *Ann Biomed Eng* 29(2):173-180, 2001.

43. Frank C, Schachar N, Dittrich D: Natural history of healing in the repaired medial collateral ligament. *J Orthop Res*;1(2):179-188, 1983.

44. Niyibizi C, Kavalkovich K, Yamaji T, et al: Type V collagen is increased during rabbit medial collateral ligament healing. *Knee Surg Sports Traumatol Arthrosc* 8(5): 281-285, 2000.

45. Hart RA, Woo SL-Y, Newton PO: Ultrastructural morphometry of anterior cruciate and medial collateral ligaments: an experimental study in rabbits. *J Orthop Res* 10(1):96-103, 1992.

46. Bosch U, Decker B, Kasperczyk W, et al: The relationship of mechanical properties to morphology in patellar tendon autografts after posterior cruciate ligament replacement in sheep. *J Biomechics* 25(8):821-830, 1992.

47. Frank C, McDonald D, Wilson J, et al: Rabbit medial collateral ligament scar weakness is associated with decreased collagen pyridinoline crosslink density. *J Orthop Res* 13(2):157-165, 1995.

48. Werkmeister JA, Ramshaw JA, et al: Organization of fibrillar collagen in the human and bovine cornea: collagen types V and III. *Connect Tissue Res* 36(3):165-174, 1997.

49. Woo SL-Y, An KN, Arnoczky SP, et al: Anatomy, biology, and biomechanics of tendon, ligament, and meniscus. In Simon SR, editor: *Orthopaedic basic science*, pp. 45-87, Rosemont, IL, 1994, American Academy of Orthopaedic Surgery.

50. Frank C, McDonald D, Shrive N: Collagen fibril diameters in the rabbit medial collateral ligament scar: a longer term assessment. *Connect Tissue Res* 36(3):261-269, 1997.

51. Woo SL, Gomez MA, Inoue M, et al: New experimental procedures to evaluate the biomechanical properties of healing canine medial collateral ligaments, *J Orthop Res* 5(3):425-432, 1987.

52. Ohland KJ, Woo SL-Y, Weiss JA, et al: Healing of combined injuries of the rabbit medial collateral ligament and its insertions: a long term study on the effects of conservative vs. surgical treatment, *ASME Adv Bioeng*: 447-448, 1991.

53. Chimich D, Shrive N, Frank C, et al: Water content alters viscoelastic behaviour of the normal adolescent rabbit medial collateral ligament. *J Biomech* 25(8):831-837, 1992.

54. Abramowitch SD, Woo SL, Clineff TD, et al: An evaluation of the quasi-linear viscoelastic properties of the healing medial collateral ligament in a goat model. *Ann Biomed Eng* 32(3):329-335, 2004.

55. Indelicato PA: Isolated medial collateral ligament injuries in the knee. *J Am Acad Orthop Surg* 3(1):9-14, 1995.

56. Vailas AC, Tipton CM, Matthes RD, et al: Physical activity and its influence on the repair process of medial collateral ligaments. *Connect Tissue Res* 9(1):25-31, 1981.

57. Jokl P, Kaplan N, Stovell P, et al: Non-operative treatment of severe injuries to the medial and anterior cruciate ligaments of the knee. *J Bone Joint Surg Am* 66(5): 741-744, 1984.

58. Frolke JP, Oskam J, Vierhout PA: Primary reconstruction of the medial collateral ligament in combined injury of the medial collateral and anterior cruciate ligaments. Short-term results. *Knee Surg Sports Traumatol Arthrosc* 6(2): 103-106, 1998.

59. Hillard-Sembell D, Daniel DM, Stone ML, et al: Combined injuries of the anterior cruciate and medial

collateral ligaments of the knee. Effect of treatment on stability and function of the joint. *J Bone Joint Surg Am* 78(2):169-176, 1996.

60. Woo SL-Y, Young EP, Ohland KJ, et al: The effects of transection of the anterior cruciate ligament on healing of the medial collateral ligament. A biomechanical study of the knee in dogs. *J Bone Joint Surg Am* 72(3): 382-392, 1990.

61. Ohno K, Pomaybo AS, Schmidt CC, et al: Healing of the medial collateral ligament after a combined medial collateral and anterior cruciate ligament injury and reconstruction of the anterior cruciate ligament: comparison of repair and nonrepair of medial collateral ligament tears in rabbits, *J Orthop Res* 13(3):442-449, 1995.

62. Abramowitch SD, Yagi M, Tsuda E, et al: The healing medial collateral ligament following a combined anterior cruciate and medial collateral ligament injury—a biomechanical study in a goat model. *J Orthop Res* 21(6):1124-1130, 2003.

63. Ng GY, Oakes BW, Deacon OW, et al: Biomechanics of patellar tendon autograft for reconstruction of the anterior cruciate ligament in the goat: three-year study. *J Orthop Res* 13(4):602-608, 1995.

64. Papageorgiou CD, Ma CB, Abramowitch SD, Clineff TD, et al: A multidisciplinary study of the healing of an intraarticular anterior cruciate ligament graft in a goat model. *Am J Sports Med* 29(5):620-626, 2001.

65. Wilson TW, Zafuta MP, Zobitz M: A biomechanical analysis of matched bone-patellar tendon-bone and double-looped semitendinosus and gracilis tendon grafts. *Am J Sports Med* 27(2):202-207, 1999.

66. Hamner DL, Brown CH Jr, Steiner ME, et al: Hamstring tendon grafts for reconstruction of the anterior cruciate ligament: biomechanical evaluation of the use of multiple strands and tensioning techniques. *J Bone Joint Surg Am* 81(4):549-557, 1999.

67. Beynnon BD, Johnson RJ, Toyama H, et al: The relationship between anterior-posterior knee laxity and the structural properties of the patellar tendon graft. A study in canines. *Am J Sports Med* 22(6):812-820, 1994.

68. Rodeo SA, Arnoczky SP, Torzilli PA, et al: Tendon-healing in a bone tunnel. A biomechanical and histological study in the dog. *J Bone Joint Surg Am* 75(12): 1795-1803, 1993.

69. Grana WA, Egle DM, Mahnken R, et al: An analysis of autograft fixation after anterior cruciate ligament reconstruction in a rabbit model. *Am J Sports Med* 22(3): 344-351, 1994.

70. Anderson K, Seneviratne AM, Izawa K, et al: Augmentation of tendon healing in an intraarticular bone tunnel with use of a bone growth factor, *Am J Sports Med* 29(6):689-698, 2001.

71. Martinek V, Latterman C, Usas A, et al: Enhancement of tendon-bone integration of anterior cruciate ligament grafts with bone morphogenetic protein-2 gene transfer: a histological and biomechanical study. *J Bone Joint Surg Am* 84-A(7):1123-1131, 2002.

72. Schmidt CC, Georgescu HI, Kwoh CK, et al: Effect of growth factors on the proliferation of fibroblasts from the medial collateral and anterior cruciate ligaments. *J Orthop Res* 13(2):184-190, 1995.

73. Marui T, Niyibizi C, Georgescu HI, et al: Effect of growth factors on matrix synthesis by ligament fibroblasts. *J Orthop Res* 15(1):18-23, 1997.

74. Murphy PG, Loitz BJ, Frank CB, et al: Influence of exogenous growth factors on the synthesis and secretion of collagen types I and III by explants of normal and healing rabbit ligaments. *Biochem Cell Biol* 72(9-10):403-409, 1994.

75. Scherping SC Jr, Schmidt CC, Georgescu HI, et al: Effect of growth factors on the proliferation of ligament fibroblasts from skeletally mature rabbits. *Connect Tissue Res* 36(1):1-8, 1997.

76. Hildebrand KA, Woo SL-Y, Smith DW, et al: The effects of platelet-derived growth factor-BB on healing of the rabbit medial collateral ligament. An in vivo study. *Am J Sports Med* 26(4):549-554, 1998.

77. Celechovsky C, Niyibizi C, Watanabe N, et al: Analysis of collagens synthesized by cells harvested from MCL in the early stages of healing, Transactions of the Orthopaedic Research Society, San Francisco, CA, 2001.

78. Jia F, Shimomura T, Niyibizi C, et al: Regulating type III collagen gene expression using antisense gene therapy, 48th Annual Meeting of the Orthopaedic Research Society, Dallas, February 10-13, 2002.

79. Nakamura N, Shino K, Natsuume T, et al: Early biological effect of in vivo gene transfer of platelet-derived growth factor (PDGF)-B into healing patellar ligament. *Gene Ther* 5(9):1165-1170, 1998.

80. Hildebrand KA, Deie M, Allen CR, et al: Early expression of marker genes in the rabbit medial collateral and anterior cruciate ligaments: the use of different viral vectors and the effects of injury. *J Orthop Res* 17(1):37-42, 1999.

81. Nakamura N, Hart DA, Boorman RS, et al: Decorin antisense gene therapy improves functional healing of early rabbit ligament scar with enhanced collagen fibrillogenesis in vivo. *J Orthop Res* 18(4):517-523, 2000.

82. Shimomura T, Jia F, Niyibizi C, et al: Antisense oligonucleotides reduced type V collagen mRNA expression in human patellar tendon fibroblasts. Engineering Tissue Growth International Conference and Exposition, Pittsburgh, March 19-21, 2002.

83. Jia F, Shimomura T, Westcott A, et al: Effects of antisense oligonucleotides with different target sites on type III collagen gene expression in HPTFs in vitro. Midwest Connective Tissue Workshop, Chicago, Oct. 19-20, 2001.

84. Watanabe N, Woo SL, Papageorgiou C, et al: Fate of donor bone marrow cells in medial collateral ligament after simulated autologous transplantation. *Microsc Res Tech* 58(1):39-44, 2002.

85. Young RG, Butler DL, Weber W, et al: Use of mesenchymal stem cells in a collagen matrix for Achilles tendon repair. *J Orthop Res* 16(4):406-413, 1998.

86. Dressler MR, Butler DL, Boivin GP. Effects of age on the repair ability of mesenchymal stem cells in rabbit tendon. *J Orthop Res* 23(2):287-293, 2005.

87. Awad HA, Butler DL, Boivin GP, et al: Autologous mesenchymal stem cell-mediated repair of tendon. *Tissue Eng* 5(3):267-277, 1999.

88. Juncosa-Melvin N, Boivin GP, Gooch C, et al: The effect of autologous mesenchymal stem cells on the biomechanics and histology of gel-collagen sponge constructs used for rabbit patellar tendon repair. *Tissue Eng* 12(2):369-379, 2006.

89. Sacks MS, Gloeckner DC: Quantification of the fiber architecture and biaxial mechanical behavior of porcine intestinal submucosa. *J Biomed Mater Res* 46(1):1-10, 1999.

90. Badylak S, Arnoczky S, Plouhar P, et al: Naturally occurring extracellular matrix as a scaffold for musculoskeletal repair. *Clin Orthop* 367 Suppl:S333-343, 1999.

91. Badylak SF, Tullius R, Kokini K, et al: The use of xenogeneic small intestinal submucosa as a biomaterial for Achilles tendon repair in a dog model. *J Biomed Mater Res* 29(8):977-985, 1995.

92. Musahl V, Abramowitch SD, Gilbert TW, et al: The use of porcine small intestinal submucosa to enhance the healing of the medial collateral ligament—a functional tissue engineering study in rabbits. *J Orthop Res* 22(1): 214-220, 2004.

93. Woo S, Takakura Y, Liang R, et al: Treatment with bioscaffold enhances fibril morphology and the collagen composition of healing medial collateral ligament in rabbits. *Tissue Eng* 12(1):159-166, 2006.

94. Liang R, Moon DK, Takakura Y, et al: Functional tissue engineering can enhance the healing of the medial collateral ligament: a multidisciplinary study. Transactions Vol 30, Abstract 1731, Orthopaedic Research Society, Washington D.C., 2005.

CHAPTER

2

Denise Louise Smith
and Sharon Ann Plowman

Understanding Muscle Contraction*

LEARNING OBJECTIVES

After studying this chapter, the reader will be able to do the following:

1. Describe the functions of skeletal muscle tissue
2. Identify the characteristics of muscle tissue that make movement possible
3. Describe the macroscopic and microscopic organization of skeletal muscle tissue
4. Relate the molecular structure of the myofilaments to the sliding-filament theory of muscle contraction
5. Identify the regions of a sarcomere, and explain the changes that occur in these regions during contraction
6. Discuss the importance of specialized organelles, specifically the sarcoplasmic reticulum, the T tubules, and the myofibrils
7. Explain the events involved in excitation-contraction coupling
8. Describe the sequence of events involved in the generation of force within the contractile elements
9. Differentiate muscle fiber types on the basis of contractile and metabolic properties
10. Discuss the ramifications of fiber type distribution on the likelihood of success in a given athletic event
11. Describe the nerve supply to muscle
12. Describe the sequence of events at the neuromuscular junction
13. Describe the structure and innervation of the muscle spindle, and explain how the muscle spindle functions in the myotatic reflex
14. Differentiate between dynamic and static flexibility
15. Identify the anatomical factors that influence flexibility

MUSCULAR ASPECTS OF MOVEMENT

Muscle contractions provide the basis for all human movement. To understand how movement occurs requires an appreciation

of the interactions among the various systems of the body. For instance, the muscle cells (fibers) must be able to produce and utilize adenosine triphosphate (ATP) to provide the energy for contraction and force production. This process requires that the digestive, respiratory, endocrine, and cardiovascular systems operate effectively to provide muscle cells with the oxygen and nutrients they require to produce energy. For the purposes of this chapter, the assumption is that these other systems of the body are functioning properly.

Overview of Muscle Tissue

Muscle tissue produces force because of the interaction of its basic contractile elements (myofilaments), which are composed primarily of protein. The function of the muscle tissue ultimately depends on the type of muscle tissue involved: skeletal, smooth, or cardiac muscle. The force of contraction may be used for locomotion (skeletal muscle); the movement of materials through hollow tubes, such as the digestive tract or blood vessels (smooth muscle); or the pumping action of the heart (cardiac muscle). However, all muscle tissue has the ability to produce force because of certain basic characteristics common to all types.

Because skeletal muscles have various characteristics, physiologists refer to them by different names. On the one hand, skeletal muscles are under conscious control, so they are often referred to as *voluntary muscles.* On the other hand, skeletal muscles are sometimes referred to as *striated muscles* because of the repeating pattern of light and dark bands seen in the microscopic structure of the muscle. Additionally, in order to differentiate skeletal muscle fibers from intrafusal fibers found in sensory organs of the muscle, physiologists sometimes refer to skeletal muscle fibers as *extrafusal muscle fibers.*

Functions of Skeletal Muscle

Although locomotion is the primary function of skeletal muscle tissue, the muscular system also performs other important

---

*Based on Plowman SA, Smith DL: *Exercise physiology for health, fitness, and performance,* ed 2, San Francisco, 2003, Benjamin Cummings.

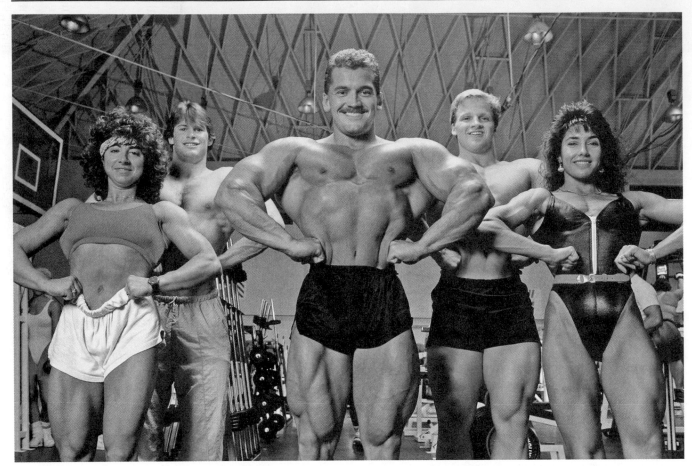

Figure 2-1 Bodybuilding poses demonstrate muscle hypertrophy and definition.

roles. In addition to locomotion and manipulation, skeletal muscles maintain body posture, assist in venous return of blood to the heart, and play an important role in thermogenesis (heat generation). Heat is a by-product of cellular respiration; and because muscles use a great deal of energy for movement, they also generate a great deal of heat. Additionally, muscles act as energy transducers by converting biochemical energy from ingested food into mechanical and thermal energy. Skeletal muscles also protect internal organs and make up most of the protein in the body. Because muscles represent such a large amount of protein, they constitute a potential but rarely used form of stored energy. The use of protein as an energy substrate is discussed in Chapter 3.

Characteristics of Muscle Tissue

Muscle tissue has unique characteristics that are specifically suited to its primary function, namely, converting an electrical signal (action potential [AP]) into a mechanical event (contraction of muscle fibers). The characteristics that allow a muscle to produce movement include irritability, contractility, extensibility, and elasticity. *Irritability* refers to the ability of a muscle to receive and respond to stimuli. The stimulus is generally in the form of a chemical message (from a neurotransmitter), and the response is the generation of an electrical current (AP) along the cell membrane. *Contractility* refers to the ability of a muscle to respond to a stimulus by shortening, which produces force. *Extensibility* refers to the ability of a muscle to be stretched or lengthened. Stretching occurs when a muscle is manipulated by external force. *Elasticity* refers to the ability of a muscle to return to its resting length after being stretched. These characteristics of muscles function together to allow for human movement.

Macroscopic Structure of Skeletal Muscles

The human body contains more than 400 skeletal muscles, and they account for 40% to 45% of the adult male body weight and 23% to 25% of the adult female body weight.[1,2] These muscles function together in a remarkable way to provide smooth, integrated movement for a wide variety of activities, many of which require little conscious thought. Muscle action also provides the basis for sport and fitness activities, and muscle definition itself, as seen in Figure 2-1, has become the goal of the sport of bodybuilding. To understand how muscles function in bodybuilding poses, or in any other activity, it is necessary to look beneath the skin.

Organization and Connective Tissue

Skeletal muscles are organized in a systematic fashion, as depicted in Figure 2-2. Some of this organization is apparent to

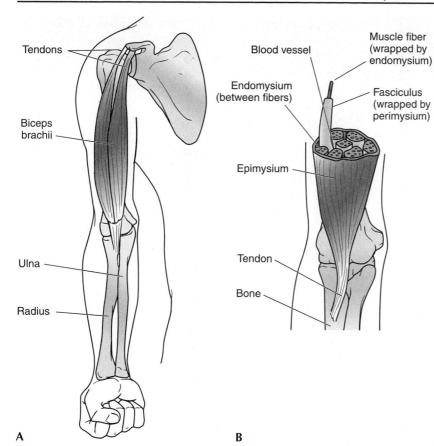

Figure 2-2 Organization of skeletal tissue. **A,** Intact skeletal muscle. Biceps brachii are attached to bones through tendons. **B,** Connective tissue. The entire muscle is surrounded by connective tissue called *epimysium*. The muscle is organized into bundles called fasciculi, which are surrounded by connective tissue called *perimysium*. Each fasciculus contains many individual fibers surrounded by connective tissue called *endomysium*. (From Plowman SA, Smith DL: *Exercise physiology for health, fitness, and performance*, ed 2, San Francisco, 2003, Benjamin Cummings.)

the naked eye, but other aspects are apparent only when muscle fibers are viewed through a simple or an electron microscope.

Skeletal muscles are attached to bones by tendons, an arrangement that allows the contraction of a muscle to move a bone. Each muscle is bound together by a thick layer (sheath) of connective tissue called *fascia*. Just beneath the fascia is a more delicate layer of connective tissue called *epimysium* that directly covers the muscle.

The interior of the muscle is subdivided into bundles of muscle fibers called *fasciculi* (the singular is fasciculus or fascicle), which are also surrounded by connective tissue. The sheath of connective tissue that separates the fasciculi within a skeletal muscle is called *perimysium*. The fasciculi are composed of many individual muscle fibers (cells), each of which is surrounded by its own sheath of connective tissue called *endomysium*. The three layers of connective tissue (epimysium, perimysium, and endomysium) provide the framework that holds the muscle together. These three layers of connective tissue come together at each end of the muscle to form the tendons that attach the muscle to bone. As a muscle contracts, it pulls on the connective tissue in which it is wrapped, causing the tendon to move the bone to which it is attached.

Architectural Organizations

Different arrangements of fasciculi within a muscle account for the different shapes that a muscle may take. Muscles can be described as longitudinal, fusiform, radiate, unipennate, bipen-

nate, or circular, as shown in Figure 2-3. The shape of the muscle determines its range of motion and influences its power production. The longer and more parallel muscle fibers, as found in longitudinal muscles, allow for greater muscle shortening. Bipennate and multipennate muscles, by contrast, shorten little but are more powerful.

Microscopic Structure of a Muscle Fiber

Individual muscle fibers are composed primarily of smaller units called myofibrils, which are in turn made up of myofilaments. This organization of skeletal muscle is shown in Figure 2-4.

Muscle fibers, also called *muscle cells,* are long, cylinder-shaped cells ranging from 10 to 100 μm in diameter and 1 to 400 mm in length.[2-5] The major structures of a muscle fiber and their functions are summarized in Table 2-1.

A skeletal muscle fiber contains many nuclei, which are located just below the cell membrane. The polarized plasma membrane of a muscle cell is referred to as the *sarcolemma,* and it is the properties of this membrane that account for the irritability of muscle. The sarcoplasm of a muscle cell is similar to the cytoplasm of other cells, but it has specific adaptations to serve the functional needs of muscle cells, namely, increased amounts of glycogen and the oxygen binding protein myoglobin.

The muscle fiber contains the organelles found in other cells (including a large number of mitochondria) along with some

Classification	Example	Diagram
Longitudinal	Sartorius	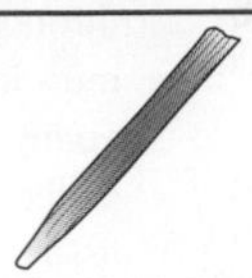
Fusiform	Biceps brachii	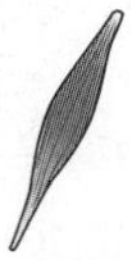
Radiate	Gluteus medius	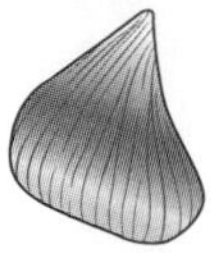
Unipennate	Tibalis posterior	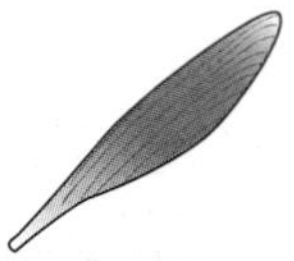
Bipennate	Gastrocnemius	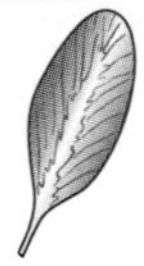
Circular	Orbicular oculi (and sphincters)	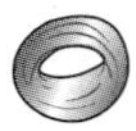

Figure 2-3 Arrangement of fasciculi. (From Plowman SA, Smith DL: *Exercise physiology for health, fitness, and performance*, ed 2, San Francisco, 2003, Benjamin Cummings.)

specialized organelles. The organelles of specific interest are the transverse tubules, sarcoplasmic reticulum, and myofibrils. The myofibrils are composed of the protein myofilaments and are responsible for the contractile properties of muscles.

Sarcoplasmic Reticulum and Transverse Tubules

Figure 2-4 illustrates the relationship among the myofibrils, sarcoplasmic reticulum, and transverse tubules. The sarcoplasmic reticulum (SR), a specialized organelle that stores and releases calcium, is an interconnecting network of tubules running parallel with and wrapped around the myofibrils. (Note: in the figure the sarcolemma has been partially removed in order to illustrate the SR and myofibrils.) The major significance of the sarcoplasmic reticulum is its ability to store, release, and take up calcium and thereby control muscle contraction. Calcium is stored in the portion of the sarcoplasmic reticulum called the *lateral sacs* or *cisterns.*

The transverse tubules (T tubules) are organelles that carry the electrical signal (AP) from the sarcolemma to the interior of the cell. T tubules are continuous with the sarcolemma and protrude into the sarcoplasm of the cell. Although the T tubules run in close proximity to the sarcoplasmic reticulum

and interact with it, they are anatomically separate organelles. As the name implies, the T tubules run perpendicular (transverse) to the myofibril. The spread of an electrical signal through the T tubules causes the release of calcium from the lateral sacs of the sarcoplasmic reticulum.

Myofibrils and Myofilaments

Each muscle fiber contains hundreds to thousands of smaller cylindrical units, or rodlike strands, called *myofibrils* (see Figure 2-4). Myofibrils are contractile structures composed of myofilaments. These myofibrils, or simply fibrils, typically lie parallel to the long axis of the muscle cell and extend the entire length of the cell. Myofibrils account for approximately 80% of the volume of a muscle fiber and are composed of two myofilaments (thick and thin myofilaments). Each repeating unit along the myofibril is referred to as a *sarcomere.*

Sarcomeres

A sarcomere is the functional unit (contractile unit) of a muscle fiber. As illustrated in Figure 2-5, each sarcomere contains two types of myofilaments: thick filaments, composed primarily of the contractile protein myosin, and thin filaments, composed primarily of the contractile protein actin. Thin filaments also contain the regulatory proteins, troponin and tropomyosin. When myofilaments are viewed under an electron microscope, their arrangement gives the appearance of alternating bands of light and dark striations. The light bands are called *I bands* and contain only thin filaments. The dark bands are called *A bands* and contain thick and thin filaments, with the thick filaments running the entire length of the A band. Thus the length of the thick filament determines the length of the A band.

The names for the various regions of the sarcomere are not arbitrary; they are derived from the first letter of the German word that describes their appearance. The names for the bands describe the refraction of light through the respective bands. The I band is abbreviated from the word *isotropic,* which means that this area appears lighter because more light can pass through it. The A band is so named because of its anisotropic properties, meaning that it appears darker because it does not allow as much light to pass through. These properties are directly related to the type of filament present.

Each A band is interrupted in the midsection by an H zone (from the German *Hellerscheibe,* for "clear disc"), where there is no overlap of thick and thin filaments. Running through the center of the H zone is a dense line called the *M line* (from the German *Mittelsclzeibe,* for "middle disc"). The I bands are also interrupted at the midline by a darker area called the Z disc (from the German Zwischenscheibe, for "between disc"). A sarcomere extends from one Z disc to the successive Z disc. The Z disc serves to anchor the thin filaments to adjacent sarcomeres.

Myofilaments occupy three-dimensional space. The arrangement of the myofilaments at different points in the sarcomere is shown in Figure 2-5, *D* and *F*. Notice that in regions where the thick and thin filaments overlap, each thick filament is

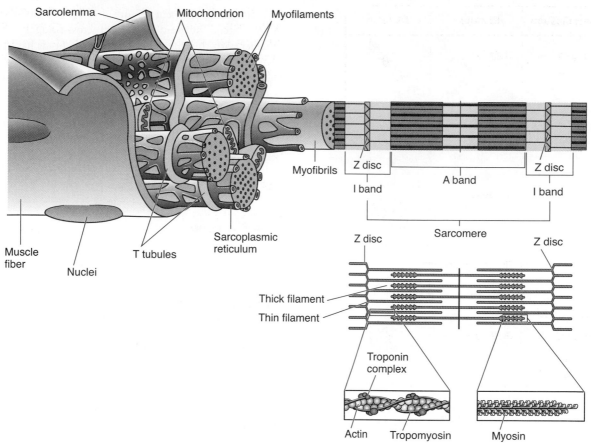

Figure 2-4 Organization of a muscle fiber. A close anatomical relationship exists among the organelles, specifically the myofibrils, T tubules, and sarcoplasmic reticulum. The repeating pattern of the myofibrils is due to the arrangement of the myofilaments. (From Plowman SA, Smith DL: *Exercise physiology for health, fitness, and performance*, ed 2, San Francisco, 2003, Benjamin Cummings.)

Table 2-1	Summary of Major Components of a Skeletal Muscle Cell	
Cell Part	**Description**	**Function**
Nucleus	Multinucleated	Is the control center for the cell
Sarcolemma	Polarized cell membrane	Is capable of receiving stimuli from the nervous system
Sarcoplasm	Intracellular material	Holds organelles and nutrients; provides the medium for glycolytic enzymatic reactions
Organelles		
Myofibrils	Rodlike structures composed of smaller units called *myofilaments:* account for 80% of muscle volume	Contain contractile proteins (myofilaments), which are responsible for muscle contraction
T tubules	Series of tubules that run perpendicular (transverse) to the cell and are open to the external part of the cell	Spread polarization from the cell membrane into the interior of cell, which triggers the sarcoplasmic reticulum to release calcium
Sarcoplasmic reticulum	Interconnecting network of tubules running parallel with and wrapped around the myofibrils	Stores and releases calcium
Mitochondria	Sausage or spherical-shaped organelles; numerous in a muscle cell	Are the major site of energy production

From Plowman SA, Smith DL: *Exercise physiology for health, fitness, and performance,* ed 2, San Francisco, 2003, Benjamin Cummings.

surrounded by six thin filaments and each thin filament is surrounded by three thick filaments.

A sarcomere consists of more than just contractile and regulatory proteins. Proteins of the cytoskeleton provide much of the internal structure of the muscle cell. Figure 2-6 diagrams the cytoskeleton of the sarcomere and its relationship to the contractile proteins.[6] The M line and the Z disc hold the thick and the thin filaments in place, respectively. The elastic filament helps keep the thick filament in the middle between the two Z discs during contraction.

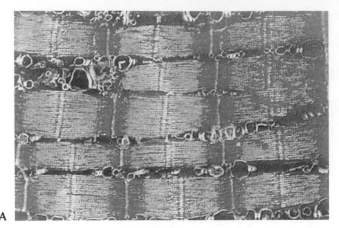

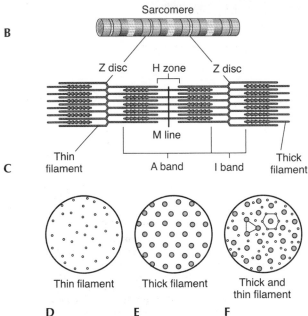

Figure 2-5 Arrangement of myofilaments in a sarcomere. **A,** Micrograph of sarcomeres. **B,** Model of sarcomeres. **C,** Relationship between thick and thin filaments. **D,** Cross-sectional view of thin filaments. **E,** Cross-sectional view of thick filaments. **F,** Cross-sectional view of thick and thin filaments. (From Plowman SA, Smith DL: *Exercise physiology for health, fitness, and performance*, ed 2, San Francisco, 2003, Benjamin Cummings.)

Molecular Structure of the Myofilaments

The sliding-filament theory of muscle contraction, which explains how muscles contract, is based on the sliding of the contractile proteins of the myofilaments over one another during muscular contraction. Therefore paying careful attention to the structure of the myofilaments is essential.

Thick Filaments

Thick filaments are composed primarily of myosin molecules (Figure 2-7). Each molecule of myosin has a rodlike tail and two globular heads (Figure 2-7, *A*). A typical thick filament contains approximately 200 myosin molecules.[4] These molecules are oriented so that the tails form the central rodlike

structure of the filament (Figure 2-7, *B*). The globular myosin heads extend outward and form cross-bridges when they interact with thin filaments. The myosin heads have two reactive sites: One allows it to bind with the actin filament, and one binds to ATP. Only when the myosin heads bind to the active sites on actin, forming a cross-bridge, does contraction occur.

The myosin subunits are oriented in opposite directions along the filament, forming a central section that lacks projecting heads (Figure 2-7, *C*). The result is a bare zone in the middle of the filament, which accounts for the H zone seen in the middle of the A band (Figure 2-7, *D*).

Thin Filaments

Thin filaments are composed primarily of the contractile protein actin. As illustrated in Figures 2-8, *A* and *B*, actin is composed of small globular subunits (G actin) that form long strands called *fibrous actin (F actin)*. A filament of actin is formed by two strands of F actin coiled about each other to form a double helical structure; it resembles two strands of pearls wound around each other and may be referred to as a *coiled coil* (Figure 2-8, *C*). The actin molecules contain active sites to which myosin heads will bind during contraction.

The thin filaments also contain the regulatory proteins called *tropomyosin* and *troponin,* which regulate the interaction of actin and myosin. Tropomyosin is a long, double-stranded, helical protein that is wrapped about the long axis of the actin backbone (Figure 2-8, *D*). Tropomyosin serves to block the active site on actin, thereby inhibiting actin and myosin from binding under resting conditions.

Troponin is a small, globular protein complex composed of three subunits that control the position of the tropomyosin (Figure 2-9). The three units of troponin are troponin C (Tn-C), troponin I (Tn-I), and troponin T (Tn-T). Tn-C contains the calcium-binding sites, Tn-T binds troponin to tropomyosin, and Tn-I inhibits the binding of actin and myosin in the resting state (Figure 2-9, *B*). When calcium binds to the Tn-C subunit, the troponin complex undergoes a configurational change. Because troponin is attached to tropomyosin, the change in the shape of troponin causes tropomyosin to be removed from its blocking position, thus exposing the active sites on actin.[3,4] Once the active sites are exposed, the myosin heads can bind to the actin, forming the cross-bridges (Figure 2-9, *C*). Thus calcium is the key to controlling the interaction of the filaments and therefore muscle contraction.

Contraction of a Muscle Fiber

In order for a muscle to contract, an AP must be generated in the motor neuron that innervates the muscle fibers that will contract. The message from the motor neuron must then be passed to the muscle fiber through the neuromuscular junction. Finally, the AP must be conducted along the sarcolemma and into the interior of the muscle fiber to initiate movement of the myofilaments. The process whereby electrical events in the

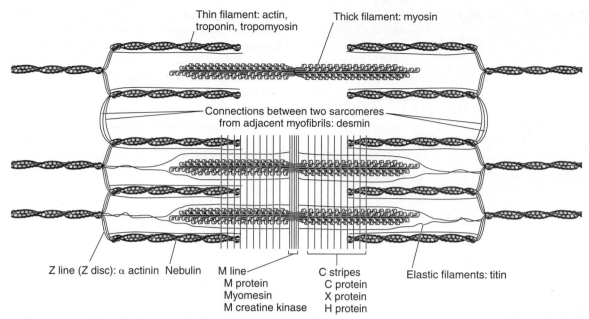

Thin filament: actin, troponin, tropomyosin

Thick filament: myosin

Connections between two sarcomeres from adjacent myofibrils: desmin

Z line (Z disc): α actinin   Nebulin   M line
M protein
Myomesin
M creatine kinase

C stripes
C protein
X protein
H protein

Elastic filaments: titin

Figure 2-6 Representation of auxiliary proteins in the sarcomere. (From Billeter R, Hoppeler H: Muscular basis of strength. In Komi PV, editor: *Strength and power in sport*, p. 45, Champaign, Ill, 1992, Human Kinetics.)

sarcolemma of the muscle fiber are linked to the movement of the myofilaments is called *excitation-contraction coupling*.

The description of the specific changes that occur during contraction requires careful attention to three factors: the position of the myofilaments, the location of calcium ions, and the role of ATP.

The Sliding-Filament Theory of Muscle Contraction

A great deal of data has been amassed since the 1950s on the basis of x-ray, light microscopic, and electron microscopic studies to support the sliding-filament theory of muscle contraction. The basic principles of this theory are summarized in three statements:

1. The force of contraction is generated by the process that slides the actin filament over the myosin filament.
2. The lengths of the thick and the thin filaments do not change during muscle contraction.
3. The length of the sarcomere decreases as the actin filaments slide over the myosin filaments and pull the Z discs toward the center of the sarcomere.

Excitation-Contraction Coupling

Excitation-contraction coupling refers to the sequence of events by which an AP (an electrical event) in the sarcolemma of the muscle cell initiates the sliding of the myofilaments, resulting in contraction (a mechanical event). Excitation-contraction coupling can be categorized into three phases:

1. The spread of depolarization
2. The binding of calcium to troponin
3. The generation of force

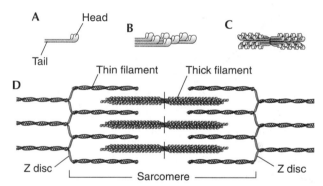

Figure 2-7 Molecular organization of thick filaments. **A,** Individual myosin molecules have a rodlike tail and two globular heads. **B,** Individual molecules are arranged so that the tails form a rodlike structure and the globular heads project outward to form crossbridges. **C,** Myosin subunits are oriented in opposite directions along the filament, forming a central bare zone in the middle of the filament (H zone). **D,** Thick filament (myosin) within a single sarcomere showing the myosin heads extending toward the thin filament. (From Plowman SA, Smith DL: *Exercise physiology for health, fitness, and performance*, ed 2, San Francisco, 2003, Benjamin Cummings.)

Figure 2-10 summarizes the events that occur during each phase of excitation-contraction coupling. Excitation-contraction coupling begins with depolarization and spread of an AP along the sarcolemma (point 2 in Figure 2-10) and continues with the propagation of the AP into the T tubules (point 2 in Figure 2-10). An AP in the T tubules causes the release of calcium from the lateral sacs of the sarcoplasmic reticulum (point 3 in Figure 2-10).

When calcium is released from the sarcoplasmic reticulum (the second phase), it binds to the troponin molecules on the thin filament. The binding of calcium to troponin causes

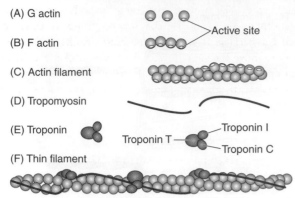

(A) G actin

(B) F actin

Active site

(C) Actin filament

(D) Tropomyosin

(E) Troponin

Troponin I

Troponin T —— —— Troponin C

(F) Thin filament

Figure 2-8 Molecular organization of thin filaments. **A,** Individual actin subunits (globular, G actin) shown with active site for binding to myosin heads. **B,** Fibrous actin (F actin). **C,** Actin filament with two strands of fibrous actin wound around itself to form a coiled coil. Active sites are exposed. **D,** Tropomyosin is a regulatory protein that covers the binding sites on actin. **E,** Troponin is a regulatory protein that, when bound to Ca^{2+}, removes tropomyosin from its blocking position on actin. **F,** The thin filament is composed of actin, tropomyosin, and troponin. (From Plowman SA, Smith DL: *Exercise physiology for health, fitness, and performance*, ed 2, San Francisco, 2003, Benjamin Cummings.)

troponin to undergo a configurational change, thereby removing tropomyosin from its blocking position on the actin filament (point 4 in Figure 2-10). The third phase of excitation-contraction coupling is the cross-bridging cycle (point 5 in Figure 2-10). The cross-bridging cycle describes the cyclic events that are necessary for the generation of force or tension within the myosin heads during muscle contraction. The generation of tension within the contractile elements results from the binding of the myosin heads to actin and the subsequent release of stored energy in the myosin heads. As shown in Figure 2-11, four individual steps are necessary for the cross-bridging cycle[3,4,7]:

1. Binding of myosin heads to actin (cross-bridge formation)
2. Power stroke
3. Dissociation of myosin and actin
4. Activation of myosin heads

The first step in the cross-bridge cycle is the binding of activated myosin heads (*M) with the active sites on actin, forming cross-bridges. In Figure 2-11 a centered dot (•) is used to indicate binding, and an asterisk (*) is used to indicate activated myosin heads. Thus A•*M indicates that the activated

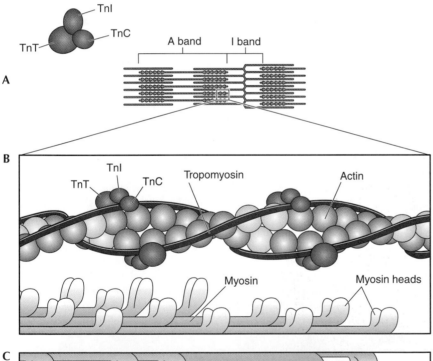

TnI

TnC

TnT

A band   I band

A

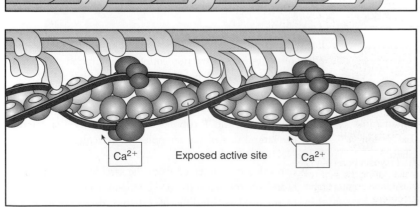

B

TnT   TnI   TnC   Tropomyosin   Actin

Myosin   Myosin heads

C

Ca²⁺   Exposed active site   Ca²⁺

Figure 2-9 Regulatory function of troponin and tropomyosin. **A,** Troponin is a small globular protein with three subunits. **B,** Resting condition: Tropomyosin blocks the active sites on actin, preventing actin and myosin from binding. **C,** Contraction: When troponin binds with Ca^{2+}, it undergoes a configurational change and *pulls* tropomyosin from the blocking position on the actin filament, following myosin heads to form cross-bridges with actin. (From Plowman SA, Smith DL: *Exercise physiology for health, fitness, and performance*, ed 2, San Francisco, 2003, Benjamin Cummings.)

myosin heads are bound to actin (A), whereas A + M indicates that actin and myosin are unbound.

The second step in the cross-bridging cycle is the power stroke. During this step, activated myosin heads swivel from their high-energy, activated position to a low-energy configuration (M with no *). This movement of the myosin cross-bridges results in a slight displacement (sliding) of the thin filament over the thick filament toward the center of the sarcomere. As shown in Figure 2-11, during the second step ADP and P$_i$ are released from the myosin heads, resulting in myosin bound only to actin (A•M).

The third step involves the binding of ATP to the myosin heads and subsequent dissociation (detachment) of the myosin cross-bridges from actin, which produces A + M•ATP. The binding of ATP molecules to the myosin heads allow the myosin heads to detach from actin. In the fourth step the

breakdown of ATP provides the energy to activate the myosin heads (*M). Activation of the myosin heads is extremely important because it provides the cross-bridges with stored energy to move the actin during the power stroke. The breakdown of ATP at this step depends on the presence of myosin ATPase (also known as *myofibrillar ATPase*), as depicted in the following reaction:

$$M•ATP \xrightarrow{\text{myosin ATPase}} *M•ADP + P_i$$

Notice that the products of ATP hydrolysis, ADP + P$_i$, remain bound to the myosin heads and that the myosin is now in its high-energy or activated state.

The cross-bridging cycle continues as long as ATP is available and calcium is bound to troponin (Tn-C), causing the

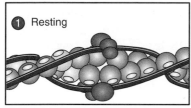

1 Resting

Figure 2-10 Phases of excitation-contraction coupling. (From Plowman SA, Smith DL: *Exercise physiology for health, fitness, and performance*, ed 2, San Francisco, 2003, Benjamin Cummings.)

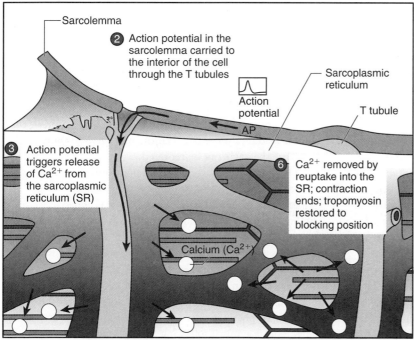

2 Action potential in the sarcolemma carried to the interior of the cell through the T tubules

3 Action potential triggers release of Ca^{2+} from the sarcoplasmic reticulum (SR)

6 Ca^{2+} removed by reuptake into the SR; contraction ends; tropomyosin restored to blocking position

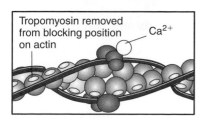

4 Calcium binds to Tn-C subunit of troponin, causing exposure of the actin active site

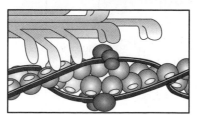

5 Activated myosin head binds to active site pulling the actin over the myosin and contracting the sarcomere

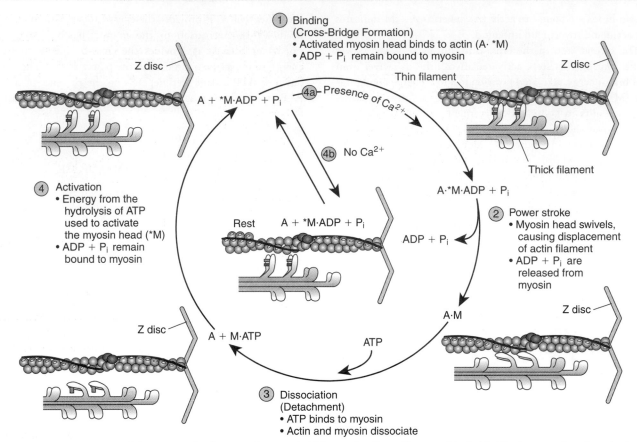

Figure 2-11 Force generation of the contractile elements: the cross-bridging cycle. (From Plowman SA, Smith DL: *Exercise physiology for health, fitness, and performance*, ed 2, San Francisco, 2003, Benjamin Cummings.)

active sites on actin to be exposed. On the other hand, activated myosin remains in the resting state awaiting the next stimulus if calcium is not available in sufficient concentration to remove tropomyosin from its blocking position on actin (see step 4b in Figure 2-11). Because each cycle of the myosin cross-bridges barely displaces the actin, the myosin heads must bind to the actin and be displaced many times for a single contraction to occur. Thus myosin makes and breaks its bond with actin hundreds or even thousands of times during a single muscle twitch. In order for this make-and-break cycle to occur, myosin heads must detach from actin and then be reactivated. This detaching and reactivating process requires the cycle to be repeated and requires the presence of ATP (see step 3).[4] The analogy of a spring-loaded mousetrap may be helpful for understanding the role of ATP in providing energy to activate the myosin head. It takes energy to set the trap, just as it takes the splitting of ATP to set or activate the myosin head. Once set, however, the trap releases energy when it is sprung. In a similar manner, the myosin head possesses stored energy, which is released when the myosin heads bind to actin and swivel.

A review of Figure 2-11 reveals that ATP plays several important roles in muscle contraction.

1. ATP breakdown provides the energy to activate and reactivate the myosin cross-bridge before binding with actin.

2. ATP binding to the myosin head is necessary to break the cross-bridge linkage between the myosin heads and actin so that the cycle can be repeated.

3. ATP is used for the return of calcium into the sarcoplasmic reticulum and restoration of the resting membrane potential once contraction has ended.

The final phase of muscular contraction is muscular relaxation (see point 6 in Figure 2-10 and step 4b in Figure 2-11). Relaxation occurs when the nerve impulse ceases and calcium is pumped back into the sarcoplasmic reticulum by active transport. In the absence of calcium, tropomyosin returns to its blocking position on actin, and myosin heads are not able to bind to actin. Although emphasis is often placed on muscle contraction, the ability to relax a muscle following contraction is just as important.

Changes in the Sarcomere during Contraction

Much of the evidence supporting the sliding-filament theory comes from observation of changes in the length of a sarcomere during muscular contraction. Diagrams of the sarcomere during rest and during contraction are shown in Figure 2-12, *A* and Figure 2-12, *B*, respectively. The following changes in a sarcomere result from contraction:

1. The A band does not change length, but the Z discs do move closer together. The length of the A band is

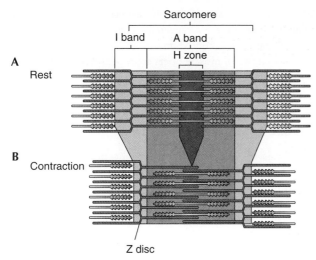

Figure 2-12 Changes in a sarcomere during contraction. **A,** Sarcomere at rest. **B,** During contraction of the sarcomere, the lengths of actin and myosin filaments are unchanged. Sarcomere shortens because actin slides over myosin, pulling Z discs toward the center of the sarcomere. The H zone disappears, the I band shortens, and the A band remains unchanged. (From Plowman SA, Smith DL: *Exercise physiology for health, fitness, and performance,* ed 2, San Francisco, 2003, Benjamin Cummings.)

Muscle Fibers			
Twitch properties	Slow	Fast	
Metabolic properties	Oxidative	Oxidative/ glycolytic	Glycolytic
Name based on twitch and metabolic properties	SO	FOG	FG
Other nomenclature	ST, Type I	FTa, FTA, Type IIA	FTb, FTB, Type IIB
Motor Neurons			
Neuron type	α_2	α_1	α_1
Neuron size	Small	Large	Large
Conduction velocity	Slow	Fast	Fast
Recruitment threshold	Low	High	High

Figure 2-13 Properties of motor units. (From Plowman SA, Smith DL: *Exercise physiology for health, fitness, and performance,* ed 2, San Francisco, 2003, Benjamin Cummings.)

preserved because the thick filament length does not change.

2. The I band shortens and may disappear. The I band shortens because the thin filaments are pulled over the thick filaments toward the center of the sarcomere. Thus there is little or no area where the thin filaments do not overlap the thick filaments.

3. The H zone shortens and may disappear because the thin filaments are pulled over the thick filaments toward the center of the sarcomere. If the thin filament overlaps the thick filament for the entire length of the thick filament, there is no H zone.

The shortening of the sarcomere is the result of the attachment of the myosin heads with the active site on actin and the subsequent release of stored energy that swivels the myosin crossbridges. This step causes the actin to pull the Z disc toward the center of the sarcomere, which, in turn, causes the sarcomere and hence the muscle fiber length to decrease.

All-or-None Principle

According to the *all-or-none principle,* when a motor neuron is stimulated, all of the muscle fibers in that motor unit contract to their fullest extent or they do not contract at all. The minimal amount of stimuli necessary to initiate that contraction is referred to as the *threshold stimulus;* that is, if the threshold of contraction is reached, a muscle fiber will contract to its fullest extent. This phenomenon is related to the electrical properties of the cell membrane and refers to the contractile properties of a motor unit or a single muscle fiber only, not to the entire muscle.

The analogy of turning on a light switch may help to elucidate this principle. If sufficient pressure is applied to the switch (to reach a threshold for flipping it on), the lights are turned on to their fullest extent. Expanding the analogy to a motor unit, when a light switch that controls a group of lights (such as the overhead lights in a classroom) is turned on, all of the lights connected to it will turn on to their fullest extent. The lights do not become brighter if the light switch is pulled (or pushed) harder. It is an all-or-none response. Either enough force is produced to turn the lights on, or it is not. The same is true for an individual muscle fiber or a motor unit: Either a threshold stimulus is reached and contraction occurs, or a threshold stimulus is not reached and contraction does not occur.

Muscle Fiber Types

Muscle fibers are typically described by two characteristics: their contractile, or twitch, properties and their metabolic properties (Figure 2-13).

Contractile (Twitch) Properties

On the basis of differences in contractile (twitch) properties, human muscle fibers can be divided into two types, slow-twitch (ST) and fast-twitch (FT) fibers. Slow-twitch fibers are sometimes called *Type I fibers;* fast-twitch fibers are correspondingly called *Type II fibers.* The difference between ST and FT fibers appears to be almost absolute—like the difference between black and white. Some FT fibers contract and relax slightly faster than other fast-twitch fibers, but both of them are clearly much faster than ST fibers. To understand the difference between twitch speeds, the integration of muscles and nerves must be considered.

Skeletal muscle fibers are innervated by alpha (α) motor neurons, which are subdivided into two categories, α_1 and α_2. The α_1 motor neurons innervate FT fibers, and the α_2 motor neurons innervate ST fibers. The α_2 motor neurons are the smaller of the two nerves and innervate the ST muscle fibers; the α_1 motor neurons are the larger nerves and innervate the FT muscle fibers. The size difference is important because small motor neurons have low excitation thresholds and slow conduction velocities and are thus recruited at low workloads. In contrast, larger motor neurons have a higher excitation threshold and are not recruited until high force output is necessary. Thus motor neurons are recruited according to the size principle. Smaller motor units (α_2 motor neurons innervating ST fibers) are recruited during activities that require low force output (i.e., maintaining posture). As the need for force production increases (e.g., lifting heavy weights), larger motor units (α_1 motor neurons innervating FT fibers) are recruited.

Figure 2-14 shows an experiment in which the innervation of muscle fibers was manipulated: The α_1 motor neuron was severed from the FT fibers and connected to the ST fibers, and the α_2 motor neuron was cut from the ST fibers and connected to the FT fibers. What conclusion can be drawn from this diagram regarding why a muscle fiber is either ST or FT? Because the ST fiber became an FT fiber when the α_1 motor neuron replaced the α_2 motor neuron and vice versa, it is logical to conclude that the contractile property of muscle depends on the type of motor neuron that innervates the muscle fiber.[8]

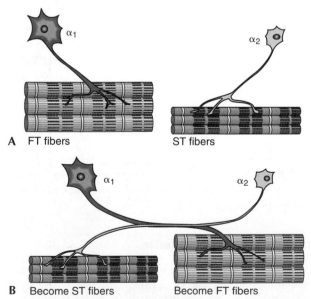

Figure 2-14 Results of cross-innervation. **A,** Under normal conditions α_2 motor neurons innervate ST fibers. **B,** If the neurons supplying the muscles are switched (cross-innervated), the muscle fibers acquire the properties of the new motor neuron. (Modified from Noth J: Motor units. In Komi PV, editor: *Strength and power in sport*, pp. 21-28, Oxford, 1992, Blackwell Scientific Publication.)

What cannot be seen from the experiment is that other elements in the muscle, especially the contractile enzyme myosin ATPase, also contribute to the variation in twitch speed.[9] Indeed, when muscle fibers are typed, often the amount of stain for myosin ATPase is used to distinguish twitch speed because the motor neurons are not typically biopsied.

Metabolic Properties

On the basis of differences in metabolic properties, human muscle fibers can be described as glycolytic, oxidative, or a combination of both, oxidative/glycolytic. All muscle fibers can produce energy both anaerobically (i.e., without oxygen, labeled as glycolytic) and aerobically (i.e., with oxygen, labeled as oxidative).

Despite the ability of all muscle fibers to produce energy by both glycolytic and oxidative processes, one or the other may predominate or the production may be balanced. Thus the metabolic properties of muscle fibers do not represent discrete entities as much as a continuum (oxidative to glycolytic), or shades of gray, as opposed to the black-and-white type of dichotomy seen for twitch speed (slow or fast twitch). The metabolic properties are determined by staining for key enzymes in the muscle specimen (often phosphofructokinase [PFK] for glycolytic processes and succinate dehydrogenase [SDH] for oxidative processes).[10]

Integrated Nomenclature

Slow-twitch fibers rely primarily on oxidative metabolism to produce energy and are therefore referred to as *slow oxidative (SO) fibers.* Fast-twitch fibers that have the ability to work under both oxidative and glycolytic conditions are called *fast oxidative glycolytic (FOG) fibers.* These fibers are also referred to as *fast-twitch A (FTa, FTA, or Type IIA) fibers.* Other fast-twitch fibers that perform predominantly under glycolytic conditions are called *fast glycolytic (FG) fibers.* These fibers are also called *fast-twitch B (FTb, FTB, or Type IIB) fibers.* A third type of fast-twitch fiber (between FTa and FTb, called *unclassified, undifferentiated, Type IIC, or FTc)* appears to represent a small percentage of total muscle fibers primarily in infants. By the end of the first year of life these Type IIC fibers have largely become differentiated, and by age 6 a normal adult pattern has been established.[11] Please refer to Figure 2-13 and Table 2-2 for a summary of the properties of motor units and muscle fibers.[12]

A motor unit is defined as a motor neuron (α_1 or α_2) and the muscle fibers it innervates. As described previously, the twitch speed of a muscle fiber depends largely on the motor neuron that innervates it. All muscle fibers within a motor unit will be either FT or ST. In addition, because all muscle fibers in a motor unit are recruited to contract together, they will require the same metabolic capabilities as well. Therefore a motor unit is composed exclusively of SO, FOG, or FG muscle fibers. Thus when reference is made to muscle fiber types, it also means motor unit types.

Table 2-2 further compares the different muscle fiber types in reference to important structural, neural, functional, and metabolic characteristics.[12] As the table indicates, the diameters of the individual muscle fibers differ between ST and FT fibers. The size of the muscle fiber is related to the size of the nerve fiber innervating it but primarily reflects the amount of contractile proteins within the muscle cell. ST fibers are smaller then FT fibers and have smaller motor neurons. The larger size of the FT fibers is the result of their having more contractile proteins, which, in turn, enables them to produce greater force. Figure 2-15 indicates differences in force production, twitch speed, and fatigue curves for the three types of muscle fibers.[13]

Other structural differences exist between fiber types that can be related directly to their predominant metabolic pathway for energy production. The SO fibers, which rely mainly on oxidative pathways for energy production, have a high number of mitochondria, high capillary density, high myoglobin content, and high oxidative enzyme activity. The FG fibers, which rely primarily on glycolytic pathways for energy production, have few mitochondria, low capillary density, low myoglobin content, and high glycolytic enzyme activity. The FOG fibers possess not only characteristics common to both SO and FG but also characteristics unique to themselves. Specifically, the FOG fibers have intermediate mitochondrial density, capillary density, myoglobin content, and oxidative enzyme activity and high PC stores, glycogen stores, and glycolytic enzyme activity.

The metabolic differences among muscle fibers both require and reflect differences in energy substrate availability. All muscles store and use glycogen, but because glycogen is the only substrate (along with its constituent parts-glucose) that can be used to fuel glycolysis, FOG and FG fibers have higher glycogen stores than SO fibers have. Conversely, because triglycerides can only be broken down and used oxidatively, SO fibers have more triglyceride storage than either FG or FOG fibers. Furthermore, FOG fibers have an intermediate amount of triglycerides—more than FG but less than SO fibers.

Table 2-2 Characteristics of Muscle Fibers

		Type I		Type II
Contractile (Twitch):	ST	FTa		FTb
Metabolic:	SO	FOG		FG
Structural Aspects				
Muscle fiber diameter	Small	Intermediate		Large
Mitochondrial density	High	Intermediate		Low
Capillary density	High	Intermediate		Low
Myoglobin content	High	Intermediate		Low
Functional Aspects				
Twitch (contraction) time	Slow	Fast		Fast
Relaxation time	Slow	Fast		Fast
Force production	Low	Intermediate		High
Fatigability	Low	Intermediate		High
Metabolic Aspects				
Phosphocreatine stores	Low	High		High
Glycogen stores	Low	High		High
Triglyceride stores	High	Intermediate		Low
Myosin-ATPase activity	Low	High		High
Glycolytic enzyme activity	Low	High		High
Oxidative enzyme activity	High	Intermediate		Low

From Plowman SA, Smith DL: *Exercise physiology for health, fitness, and performance,* ed 2, San Francisco, 2003, Benjamin Cummings.

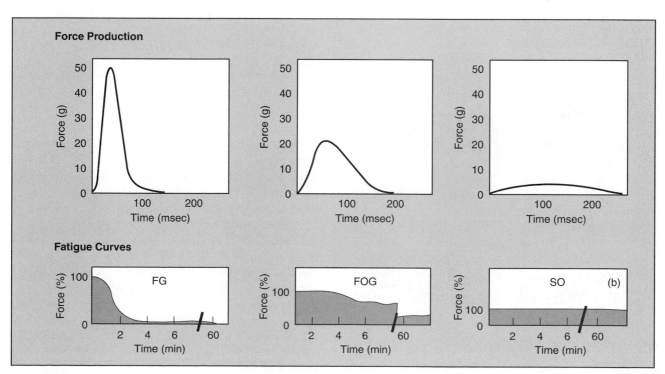

Figure 2-15 Force production and fatigue curves of fiber types. (From Edington DW, Edgerton VR: The biology of physical activity, Boston, 1986, Houghton Mifflin.)

Because SO fibers are so well supplied by the cardiovascular system and have ample fuel supplies (i.e., energy substrate), particularly from triglycerides, they are resistant to fatigue. Because FOG fibers have a substantial oxidative capability and FG fibers do not, FG fibers are the quickest to fatigue. FOG fibers are somewhat less resistant to fatigue than SO fibers and somewhat more resistant to fatigue than FG fibers.

Assessment of Muscle Fiber Type

Muscle fiber type is typically determined by an invasive procedure that involves collecting a small sample of skeletal muscle by a needle biopsy (Figure 2-16). Muscle biopsies are most commonly obtained from the gastrocnemius, vastus lateralis, or deltoid muscles. Before the collection of the muscle sample, the skin is thoroughly cleaned and a topical anesthetic is applied to numb the area. A small incision is made through the skin, subcutaneous tissue, and fascia. The biopsy needle is then inserted into the belly of the muscle to extract a small amount of skeletal muscle tissue ($\approx$20 to 40 mg). The small sample of muscle is frozen in liquid nitrogen and sliced into thin cross-sections. The cross-sections are then chemically stained so that the muscle fibers can be differentiated into categories. Muscle samples may be stained for the enzyme myosin ATPase and for glycolytic and oxidative enzymes. When the stained muscle fibers are viewed in cross-section under a microscope, the muscle fiber types appear a different color. Figure 2-17 is an example of skeletal muscle that has been histochemically stained, revealing ST and FT fibers. Notice that the different fiber types are intermingled, revealing a mosaic pattern. Counting the number of fibers of each category and dividing by the total number of fibers seen will indicate a percentage of each fiber type. In addition to counting the number of fibers and expressing them as a percentage, researchers often measure the diameter of the muscle fibers.

Muscle fibers also can be typed noninvasively by nuclear magnetic resonance spectroscopy (NMR), but this is still an expensive, little-used laboratory technique.[14] Attempts to use the vertical jump as a field measure of fiber type have proven unsuccessful.[15]

Knowledge about fiber types is important for at least three reasons:

1. Fiber type differences help explain individual differences in performance and response to training.
2. Fiber type differences help explain what training can and cannot do.
3. The relationship among fiber types, training, and performance in elite athletes helps in the design of training programs for others who wish to be successful in specific events even if they do not know their exact fiber type percentages or distribution.

Distribution of Fiber Types

All of the muscles of the human body are composed of a combination of slow-twitch and fast-twitch muscle fibers arranged in a mosaic pattern. This arrangement is thought to reflect the variety of tasks that human muscles must perform. The relative distribution, or percentage, of these fibers, however, may vary greatly from one muscle to another. For example, the soleus muscle may have as much as 85% ST fibers, and the triceps and ocular muscles may have as little as 30% ST fibers. The distribution may also vary considerably from one individual to another for the same muscle group.[10] In general the following statements describe the distribution of fiber types.

1. Although distribution of fiber type varies within and among individuals, most individuals possess between 45% and 55% ST fibers.
2. The distribution of fiber types is not different for males and females, although males tend to show greater extremes or variation than females.
3. After early childhood the fiber distribution does not change significantly as a function of age.
4. Muscles that are involved in sustained postural activity have the highest number of ST muscle fibers.

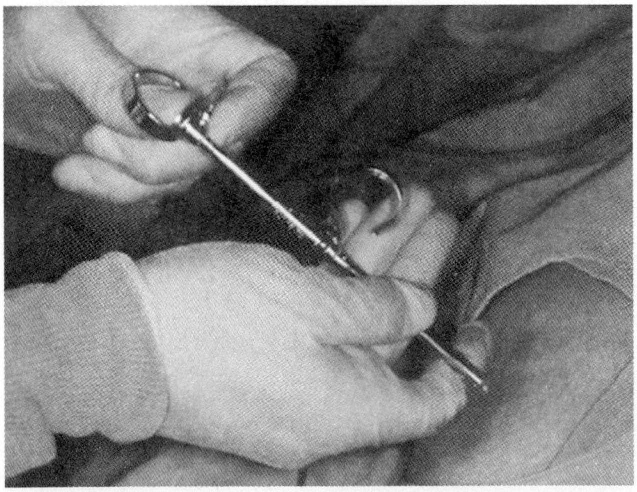

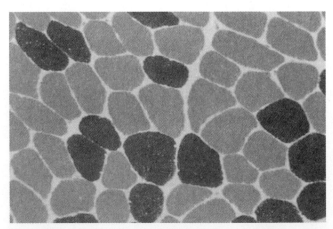

Figure 2-16 Muscle biopsy. (From Plowman SA, Smith DL: *Exercise physiology for health, fitness, and performance*, ed 2, San Francisco, 2003, Benjamin Cummings.)

Figure 2-17 Mosaic pattern of FT and ST muscle fibers. (From Plowman SA, Smith DL: *Exercise physiology for health, fitness, and performance*, ed 2, San Francisco, 2003, Benjamin Cummings.)

Fiber Type in Athletes

Few topics have caused as much interest and debate among exercise physiologists as the topic of fiber type in athletes. Figure 2-18 shows the distribution of fiber types for male and female athletes.[16] Athletes involved in endurance activities typically have a higher percentage of ST fibers; athletes involved in power activities have a higher percentage of FT muscle fibers. However, a large range of fiber type exists in each group, indicating that athletic success is not determined solely by fiber type.

Not only do endurance athletes differ in general fiber type from power or resistance athletes, but often these differences are site specific within athletic groups. The results of one study of fiber type distribution are reported in Figure 2-19.[17] According to the study, the vastus lateralis muscles of the legs possess a greater percentage of ST fibers in endurance athletes who rely heavily on the legs for their activity (such as runners). In contrast, athletes whose sport requires endurance of the upper body (e.g., kayakers) possess a greater percentage of ST fibers in the deltoid muscle.

An interesting question arises when looking at the fiber type distribution of various athletes: Did training for and participating in a given sport influence the fiber type, or did fiber type influence the type of athletic participation? Available evidence indicates that the distribution of fiber types based on contractile properties (ST or FT) is genetically determined and is not altered in humans by exercise training.[5,10,18] Evidence indicates, however, that training can alter the metabolic properties of the cell (e.g., enzyme concentration, substrate storage). These changes may lead to a conversion of FT fiber subdivisions. Indeed, with endurance training the oxidative potential of FOG and FG fibers can exceed that of SO fibers of sedentary individuals.[10]

In summary, the distribution of fiber types varies considerably within the muscle groups of an individual and among individuals. The basic distribution of fiber type appears to be genetically determined. Training may alter the metabolic capabilities of muscle fibers (but not the contractile properties), and there remains the possibility that this alteration could be significant enough to change the classification of the FT fibers.

NEURAL CONTROL OF MOVEMENT

Neural Control of Muscle Contraction

Nerve Supply

All skeletal muscles require nervous stimulation to produce the electrical excitation in the muscle cells that leads to contraction. The neurons that carry information from the central nervous system to the muscle are called *efferent neurons.* Efferent neurons that innervate skeletal muscles are referred to as *motor neurons.* Motor neurons may be classified as alpha (α) motor neurons or gamma (γ) motor neurons. Alpha motor neurons are relatively large motor neurons that innervate skeletal muscle fibers and result in contraction of muscles. Gamma motor neurons innervate proprioceptors.

As a nerve enters the connective tissue of the muscle, it divides into branches, with each branch ending near the surface of a muscle fiber. Because the axon of the motor neuron branches, each neuron is connected to several muscle fibers. A motor neuron and the muscle fibers it innervates is called a *motor unit* (Figure 2-20). The motor unit is the basic unit of contraction. Because each muscle fiber in a motor unit is connected to the same neuron, the electrical activity in that neuron controls the contractile activity of all the muscle fibers in that motor unit. The number of muscle fibers controlled by a single neuron (i.e., the number of muscle cells in a motor unit) varies tremendously, depending on the size and function of the muscle involved. Although a single neuron may innervate

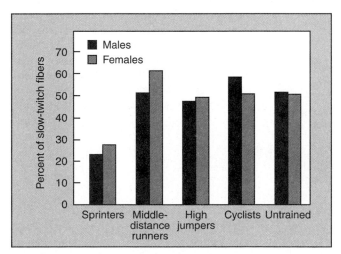

Figure 2-18 Fiber distribution among athletes. (From Plowman SA, Smith DL: *Exercise physiology for health, fitness, and performance*, ed 2, San Francisco, 2003, Benjamin Cummings. Based on data from Fox EL, Bowers RM, Foss ML: *Physiological basis for exercise and sport*, Dubuque, Iowa, 1993, Brown & Benchmark.)

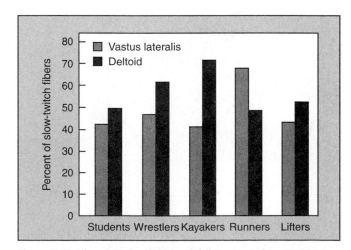

Figure 2-19 Fiber type distribution of different muscle groups among athletes. (From Plowman SA, Smith DL: *Exercise physiology for health, fitness, and performance*, ed 2, San Francisco, 2003, Benjamin Cummings. Based on data from Tesch PA, Karlsson J: *J Applied Physiol* 59:1716-1720, 1985.)

many muscle fibers, each muscle fiber is only innervated by a single neuron.

Figure 2-21 illustrates the relationship between the motor unit (originating in the central nervous system) and the muscle fibers. The cell body of the motor neuron is located within the gray matter of the spinal cord, and the axon extends through the ventral root of the spinal nerve to carry the electrical signal to the muscle fiber. Each branch of the motor neuron termi-

nates in a slight bulge called the *axon terminal*, which lies close to but does not touch the underlying muscle fiber.

The space between the membrane of the neuron and the muscle cell membrane at the motor end plate is called the *neuromuscular cleft*. The entire region is referred to as the *neuromuscular junction*. The neuromuscular junction is important because it is here that the electrical signal from the motor neuron is transmitted to the surface of the muscle cell that is to contract. Muscle cells are also supplied with afferent (sensory) nerve endings, which are sensitive to mechanical and chemical changes in the muscle tissue and which relay this information back to the central nervous system. The information carried by *afferent neurons* is used by the central nervous system to make adjustments in muscular contractions.

The Neuromuscular Junction

The neuromuscular junction is a specialized synapse formed between a terminal end of a motor neuron and a muscle fiber. Figure 2-22 summarizes the events that occur at the neuromuscular junction. When an AP reaches the axon terminal, the membrane of the neuron increases its permeability to calcium and calcium is taken up into the cell (Figure 2-22, *A*). The increased levels of calcium cause the synaptic vesicles to migrate to the cell membrane and release neurotransmitter (acetylcholine, ACh) into the neuromuscular cleft (by exocytosis) (Figure 2-22, *B*). The ACh then diffuses across the neuromuscular cleft and binds to receptors on the sarcolemma, causing changes in the ionic permeability and leading to the depolarization of the sarcolemma (Figure 2-22, *C*). This change in permeability and subsequent depolarization leads to the

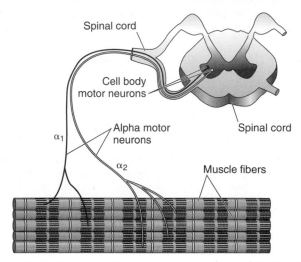

Figure 2-20 Motor units. Two motor units are depicted. Notice that the muscle fibers of the two motor units are intermingled. (From Plowman SA, Smith DL: *Exercise physiology for health, fitness, and performance*, ed 2, San Francisco, 2003, Benjamin Cummings.)

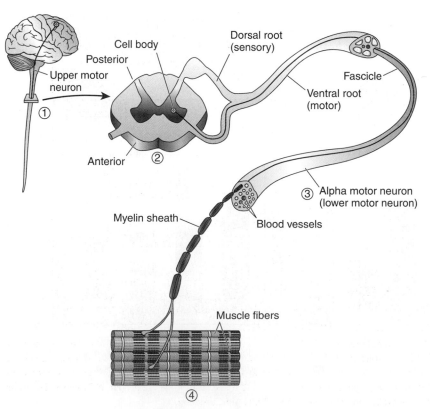

Figure 2-21 Functional relationship between motor (efferent) neurons and muscle cells. A motor neuron and the muscle cells it innervates is called a *motor unit*. *(1)* Schematic of central nervous system, *(2)* cross-sectional view of the spinal cord, *(3)* cross-sectional view of peripheral nerve emphasizing axon of motor neuron, and *(4)* the motor neuron branching near its terminal end where it forms the neuromuscular junction with the muscle fibers it innervates. (From Plowman SA, Smith DL: *Exercise physiology for health, fitness, and performance*, ed 2, San Francisco, 2003, Benjamin Cummings.)

generation of an AP in the sarcolemma of the muscle fiber. The AP spreads in all directions from the neuromuscular junction, depolarizing the entire sarcolemma. The AP is then spread into the interior of the cell through the T-tubules (Figure 2-22, *D*).

Although the neuromuscular junction functions much like other synapses, three important differences exist:
1. At a neuromuscular junction, a single presynaptic AP leads to a postsynaptic AP.
2. The synapse can only be excitatory.
3. A muscle fiber receives synaptic input from only one motor neuron.

Calcium plays two distinct roles in controlling muscular contraction. The first role is to assist the release of ACh from the synaptic vesicles in the motor neuron terminal. The second (and most often discussed) role of calcium is to control the position of the regulatory proteins troponin and tropomyosin on actin.

Reflex Control of Movement

Reflexes play an important role in maintaining an upright posture and in responding to movement in a coordinated fashion. A reflex is a rapid, involuntary response to stimuli in which a specific stimulus results in a specific motor response. Reflexes can be classified into two types: autonomic reflexes, which activate cardiac and smooth muscle and glands, and somatic reflexes, which result in skeletal muscle contraction.

Muscle Spindles

Muscle spindles (sometimes called *neuromuscular spindles,* NMS) are located in skeletal muscle; they lie parallel to and are embedded in the muscle fibers. Muscle spindles perform both sensory and motor functions. These receptors are stimulated by stretch, and they provide information to the central nervous system regarding the length and rate of length change in skeletal muscles. Stimulation of the muscle spindles results in reflex contraction of the stretched muscle via a myotatic reflex, also known as the *stretch reflex.*

Figure 2-23 represents a muscle spindle and its nerve supply. The muscle spindle consists of a fluid-filled capsule composed of connective tissue; it is long and cylindrical with tapered ends. The typical spindle is 4 to 7 mm long and approximately $\frac{1}{5}$ the diameter of the muscle fiber.[19] The capsule contains specialized muscle fibers called *intrafusal muscle fibers.* In contrast to intrafusal fibers, the muscle fibers that

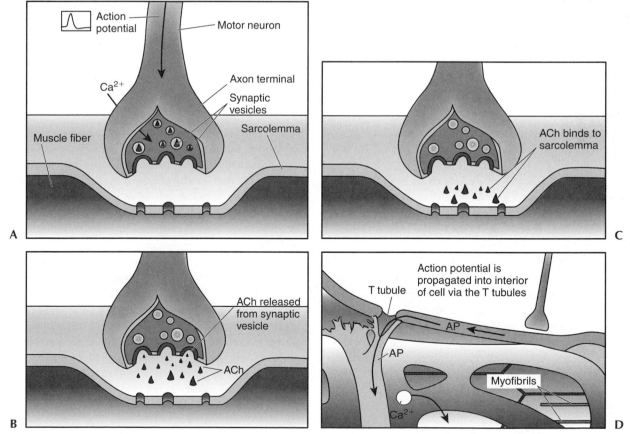

Figure 2-22 Events at the neuromuscular junction. **A,** An action potential (AP) in the axon terminal causes the uptake of Ca^{2+} into the axon terminal and the subsequent release of the neurotransmitter. **B,** The neurotransmitter (ACh) is released from the synaptic vesicles and diffuses across the synaptic cleft. **C,** Generation of action potential: The binding of the ACh to receptors of the sarcolemma causes a change in membrane permeability, causing the AP to be initiated in the sarcolemma. **D,** The AP is propagated into the interior of the cells via the T tubules. (From Plowman SA, Smith DL: *Exercise physiology for health, fitness, and performance,* ed 2, San Francisco, 2003, Benjamin Cummings.)

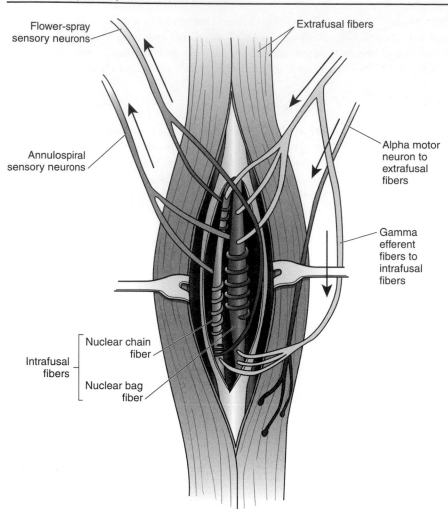

Flower-spray sensory neurons

Annulospiral sensory neurons

Intrafusal fibers
Nuclear chain fiber
Nuclear bag fiber

Extrafusal fibers

Alpha motor neuron to extrafusal fibers

Gamma efferent fibers to intrafusal fibers

Figure 2-23 Muscle spindle and its nerve supply. (From Plowman SA, Smith DL: *Exercise physiology for health, fitness, and performance,* ed 2, San Francisco, 2003, Benjamin Cummings.)

produce muscular movement are sometimes called *extrafusal fibers.* Each end of the spindle is attached to extrafusal muscle fibers.

Two types of intrafusal fibers are located within the muscle spindle: nuclear bag fibers and nuclear chain fibers. Nuclear bag fibers are thicker and contain many nuclei that are centrally located. These fibers extend beyond the spindle capsule and attach to the connective tissue of the extrafusal fibers. Nuclear chain fibers are shorter and thinner and have fewer nuclei in the central area of the fiber. Both types of intrafusal fibers contain contractile elements at their distal poles. The central region of the fibers does not contain contractile elements; this represents the sensory receptor area of the spindle.

A typical muscle spindle contains two nuclear bag fibers and approximately five nuclear chain fibers. The intrafusal fibers of the spindle are innervated by sensory nerves called *annulospiral* and *flower-spray neurons.* The branches of the large, myelinated annulospiral neurons wrap around the center of both types of intrafusal fibers.[7]

The branches of the flower-spray neurons are located on either side of the annulospiral neurons and wrap around only the nuclear chain fibers. The flower-spray fibers are smaller than and conduct impulses more slowly than the annulospiral fibers. Both types of afferent fibers are stimulated when the central portion of the spindle is stretched. Because the intrafusal fibers are arranged in parallel with the extrafusal fibers, they are stretched or shortened with the whole muscle. The flower-spray nerve endings have a higher threshold of excitation than the annulospiral nerve endings. The flower-spray nerve endings provide information about the relative muscle length; the annulospiral nerve endings are concerned primarily with the rate of length change.

The contractile intrafusal fibers also receive motor innervation from the central nervous system. The efferent fibers that terminate on the intrafusal fibers are called gamma efferents (γ motor neurons) or fusimotor neurons. The axons of γ motor neurons travel in the spinal nerve and terminate on the distal ends of the intrafusal fibers. Stimulation of the γ motor neurons produces contraction of the intrafusal fiber, which causes the central region of the spindle to be stretched. Gamma motor neurons are important enough to comprise almost one third of all motor neurons in the body.

Myotatic Reflex

The myotatic or stretch reflex comprises two separate components: a dynamic reaction and a static reaction. The dynamic reaction occurs in response to a sudden change in length of the

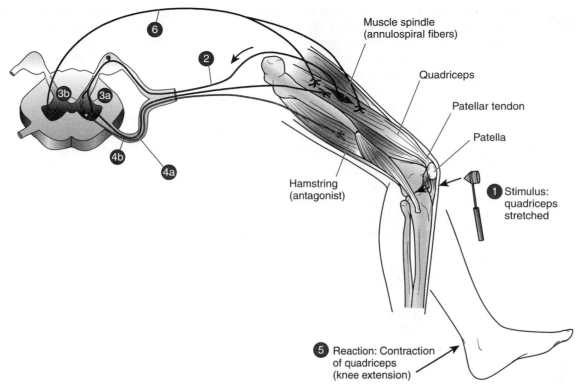

Figure 2-24 Myotatic (stretch) reflex. (From Plowman SA, Smith DL: *Exercise physiology for health, fitness, and performance*, ed 2, San Francisco, 2003, Benjamin Cummings.)

muscle. When a muscle is quickly stretched, the annulospiral nerve endings transmit an impulse to the spinal cord, which results in an immediate strong reflex contraction of the same muscle from which the signal originated.[20] This is what happens in the knee jerk response, diagrammed in Figure 2-24.

Stretching of the skeletal muscle results in the stimulation of the muscle spindle fibers, which monitor changes in muscle length. In this example the stretch is initiated by tapping on the patellar tendon, thereby causing a deformation that causes the quadriceps muscle group to be stretched (Figure 2-24, 1). Sudden stretching of the muscle spindle causes an impulse to be sent to the spinal cord by way of the annulospiral nerve fibers (Figure 2-24, 2). In the gray matter of the spinal cord this sensory fiber bifurcates, with one branch synapsing with an α motor neuron (Figure 2-24, 3a). The other branch synapses with an association neuron (Figure 2-24, 3b). The α motor neuron exits the spinal cord and synapses with the skeletal muscle, which was originally stretched (Figure 2-24, 4a), resulting in a contraction that is roughly equal in force and distance to the original stretch (Figure 2-24, 5). The inhibitory association neuron synapses with another efferent neuron, which innervates the antagonist muscle (hamstring group in this example), where it causes inhibition; this reflex relaxation of the antagonist muscle in response to the contraction of the agonist is called *reciprocal inhibition.* This response assists contraction of the agonist muscle that was stimulated; the inhibited antagonist cannot resist the contraction of the agonist (Figure 2-24, 4b). The muscle spindle is also supplied with a γ

efferent neuron; for clarity, this neuron is shown on the opposite side of the spinal cord (Figure 2-24, 6).

As soon as the lengthening of the muscle has ceased to increase, the rate of impulse discharge returns to its original level, except for a small static response that is maintained as long as the muscle is longer than the normal length. The static response is elicited by both the annulospiral and flower-spray nerve endings. The resultant low-level muscle contractions oppose the force that is causing the excess length, with the ultimate goal of returning to the resting length. A static response is also invoked if the sensory receptor portion of the neuromuscular spindle is stretched slowly.

Normally, the muscle spindles emit low-level sensory nerve signals that assist in the maintenance of muscle tonus and postural adjustments. Muscle tonus is a state of low-level muscle contraction at rest. Muscle spindles also respond to stretch by an antagonistic muscle, to gravity, or to a load being applied to the muscle. The head jerk is an example of the response to gravity, but other muscles such as the back extensors and quadriceps function the same way for unconscious postural adjustments. An example for the load stimulus is when a person standing with elbows at 90 degrees, palms up has a 10-lb weight placed in his or her hands. Before the person can consciously adjust to this weight, and because the weight stretches the biceps, the muscle spindles will have caused a reflex contraction to stop the person's hands from dropping too far.

In addition to providing maintenance of muscle tone and adjustments for posture and load, the neuromuscular spindles serve as a damping mechanism that assists smooth muscle contractions. This is accomplished by a γ loop, in which the stretch reflex is activated by the γ motor neuron. As noted previously, the γ motor neurons originate in the spinal cord and innervate the distal contractile portions of the intrafusal fibers. Gamma motor neurons stimulate contractions at both ends of the intrafusal fibers. The central, noncontractile portion of the fibers is stretched, deforming the sensory nerve endings and eliciting the myotatic stretch response. The questions then are what stimulates the γ motor neurons and why are they stimulated. When signals are transmitted to the α motor neurons from the motor cortex or other areas of the brain, the γ motor neurons are almost always simultaneously stimulated. This action is called *coactivation*, and it serves several purposes. First, it provides damping, as mentioned earlier. Sometimes the α and γ neural signals to contract arrive asynchronously. But because the response to the γ motor neuron stimulation is contraction anyway, the gaps can be filled in by reflex contractions—that smooth out the force of contraction. Second, coactivation maintains proper load responsiveness regardless of the muscle length. If, for example, the extrafusal fibers contract less than the intrafusal fibers owing to a heavy external load, the mismatch would elicit the stretch reflex and the additional extrafusal fiber excitation would cause more shortening.[20] Similarly, because the intrafusal and extrafusal lengths are adjusted to each other, the neuromuscular spindle may be able to help compensate for fatigue by recruiting additional extrafusal fibers by reflex action. Finally, sensory information from the neuromuscular spindles is always carried to the higher brain centers, where it is unconsciously integrated with other sensory information. If the muscle spindles were not adjusted to the length of the extrafusal fibers during contraction, information on muscle length and the rate of change of that length could not be transmitted.[3] Because the γ fibers do adjust the muscle spindle fibers, the γ loop can assist voluntary motor activity but it does not actually control voluntary motor activity.

Plyometrics

Plyometrics, also known as *depth jumping* or *rebound training,* is a training exercise that involves eccentric-concentric sequences of muscle activity. It involves such activities as jumping off a box with both feet together and then immediately performing a maximal jump back onto the box. Whereas the training has proven effective in increasing jumping performance, the mechanisms responsible for the improved performance have not been fully elucidated, although the stretch-shortening cycle, which relies on the elastic properties of the muscle, is thought to be involved. It is also thought that the myotatic reflex plays a role. During the eccentric phase (lengthening) muscle spindles are believed to be activated, thus enhancing the contraction of the muscle during the concentric phase.

Golgi Tendon Organ

Golgi tendon organs (GTOs) are receptors that are activated by stretch or active contraction of a muscle and that transmit

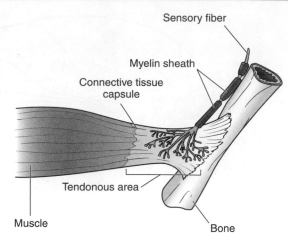

Figure 2-25 Golgi tendon organ. (From Plowman SA, Smith DL: *Exercise physiology for health, fitness, and performance,* ed 2, San Francisco, 2003, Benjamin Cummings.)

information about muscle tension. Activation of these receptors results in a reflex inhibition of the muscle via the inverse myotatic reflex.[7] GTOs are located in the tendons, close to the point of muscular attachment. As shown in Figure 2-25, each Golgi tendon organ consists of a thin capsule of connective tissue that encloses collagenous fibers. The collagenous fibers within the capsule are penetrated by fibers of sensory neurons, the terminal branches of which intertwine with the collagenous fibers. This afferent neuron relays information about muscle tension to the spinal cord. The information is then transmitted to higher brain centers, particularly the cerebellum or muscle efferents, or both.

The GTO is in series with the muscle. Thus the GTO can be stimulated by either stretch or contraction of the muscle. Because of elongation properties of the muscle during stretch, however, active contraction of a muscle is more effective in initiating APs within the GTO.

Inverse Myotatic Reflex

As with the myotatic reflex, the inverse myotatic reflex has both static and dynamic components. When tension increases abruptly and intensely, the dynamic response is invoked. Within milliseconds this dynamic response becomes a lower-level static response within the GTO that is proportional to the muscle tension. The sequence of events in the inverse myotatic reflex is diagrammed in Figure 2-26.

Contraction of a skeletal muscle (or stretching) results in tension that stimulates the GTOs in the tendon attached to the skeletal muscle (Figure 2-26, *1*). Stimulation of the GTO results in the transmission of impulses to the spinal cord by afferent neurons (Figure 2-26, *2*). In the spinal cord the afferent neuron synapses with an inhibitory association neuron and an excitatory motor neuron (Figure 2-26, *3*). In turn, the inhibitory association neuron synapses with a motor neuron that innervates the muscle attached to the tendon; the inhibitory impulses lead to the relaxation of the contracted

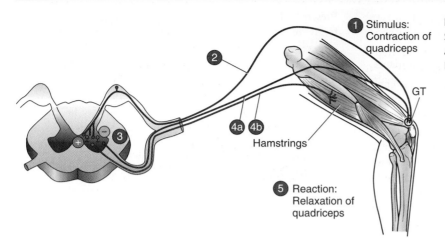

Figure 2-26 Inverse myotatic reflex. (From Plowman SA, Smith DL: *Exercise physiology for health, fitness, and performance*, ed 2, San Francisco, 2003, Benjamin Cummings.)

muscle (Figure 2-26, *4a*). The excitatory association neuron synapses with a motor neuron that innervates the antagonist muscle (Figure 2-26, *4b*).

Note that as the muscle group originally exhibiting the tension (the agonist) is relaxed, the opposing muscle group (or antagonist) is reciprocally activated. The relaxing action of the GTO serves several important functions.[20] First, excessive tension that might cause muscle and tendons to be torn or pulled away from their attachments is avoided. For example, a weight lifter who manages to get a heavier barbell off the ground than he or she can really handle may suddenly find that his or her muscles give out. The GTOs are responsible for the muscles giving out. Increases in the amount of weight that can be lifted following resistance training are believed to be partly due to an inhibition of the GTO, allowing for a more forceful muscle contraction.[20]

The second important advantage of GTO-mediated relaxation is that muscle fibers that are relaxed can be stretched further without damage. This response is useful in the development of flexibility. Third, the sensory information regarding tension, which is provided to the cerebellum, allows for muscle adjustment so that only the amount of tension necessary to complete the movement is produced. This feature ensures both a smooth beginning and a smooth ending to a movement and is particularly important in movements such as running that involve a rapid cycling between flexion and extension.[21]

Flexibility

Flexibility is defined as the range of motion (ROM) in a joint or series of joints that reflects the ability of the musculotendon structures to elongate within the physical limitations of the joint.[22] Two basic types of flexibility exist: static and dynamic. Static flexibility refers to the range of motion about a joint with no consideration of how easily or quickly the ROM is achieved. Dynamic flexibility refers to the resistance to motion in a joint that will affect how easily and quickly a joint can move through the ROM and, more recently, as the rate of increase in tension in a contracted or relaxed muscle as it is stretched. Thus dynamic flexibility accounts for the resistance to stretch.[23] Dynamic flexibility is undoubtedly the more important of the two when one considers athletic performances (especially speed event) and the health or diseased condition of the joints (such as arthritis). Dynamic flexibility is measured as stiffness. The opposite of stiffness is compliance (alteration in response to force). Stiffness is determined by the slope of a curve that plots the load (torque) against elongation (ROM) for each individual tested. The steeper the line, the stiffer the muscle. This testing requires specialized laboratory equipment.[24] No standardized measurement technique exists that can be used in practical settings for evaluating dynamic flexibility,[25] so little information on dynamic flexibility is available.[26] Therefore unless specifically stated otherwise, the discussion that follows is limited to static flexibility.

Several anatomical factors affect the ROM in any given joint. The first is the actual structural arrangement of the joint (i.e., the way the bones articulate). Each joint has a specific bony configuration that, in general, cannot and should not be altered. The soft tissue surrounding the joint including the skin, ligaments, fascia, muscles, and tendons also affects joint ROM. The skin has little influence on ROM under normal circumstances. The ligaments provide joint stability, and whatever restriction to the ROM they provide is generally considered to be both necessary and beneficial. Thus the muscles and their connective tissues are the critical factors that determine flexibility and that are altered by flexibility training.

Muscles actively resist elongation through contraction and passively resist elongation owing to the noncontractile elements of elasticity and plasticity. What one is attempting to do in flexibility training is to influence the plastic deformation so that a degree of elongation remains when the force causing the stretch is removed.[25] Neuromuscular disorders characterized by spasticity and rigidity, any injuries resulting in scar tissue, or adaptive muscle shortening from casting will affect flexibility.

Flexibility and stretching are important for everyday living (putting on shoes, reaching the top shelf), muscle relaxation and proper posture, and relief of muscle soreness. In relation to exercise, stretching is advocated for two primary reasons: (1) as preparation for activity because it enhances the performance of that activity and (2) as a means of decreasing the likelihood of injury during physical activity.

Undoubtedly, flexibility is important in sport performance. The degree of importance differs, of course, with the sport. Box 2-1 provides a partial listing of popular sport and fitness activities according to the degree of flexibility required. The three degrees of flexibility listed are a normal ROM, a slightly above average ROM in one or more joints, and an extreme ROM in specific joints.

Gymnasts obviously need to be more flexible than long-distance runners and cyclists. However, no scientific studies directly link selected flexibility values with performance if the athletes can move through the required ROM.[24,25] For example, a bicyclist with normal ROM in the ankle, knee, hip, and trunk will not become a better cyclist just by increasing his or her flexibility in those joints. But what about preventing injury?

Muscles, tendons, and ligaments are the tissues injured most frequently in work and in fitness and sports participation.

Presently, however, there is no conclusive evidence that high levels of flexibility or improvements in flexibility either protect against injury or reduce the severity of injury[25,26] including low-back pain. Indeed, some data indicate that hypermobility, or loose ligamentous structure, may predispose some individuals to injury or low-back pain.[24,25]

Nevertheless, individuals with poor flexibility for the task they are expected to perform probably have an increased risk of exceeding the extensibility limits of the musculotendon unit. Such individuals should work on improving their flexibility. Likewise, individuals whose sports may cause maladaptive shortening in certain muscles should perform stretching exercises to counteract this tendency. Individuals who are shown to be hypermobile need to concentrate on strengthening the musculature around those joints.

BOX 2-1   Flexibility in Sport and Fitness Activities

Activities requiring extreme range of motion in specific joints:
- Figure skating
- Gymnastics
- Diving
- Hurdles
- Pitching
- Dancing (ballet, modern)
- Karate
- Yoga

Activities requiring greater-than-normal range of motion in one or more joints:
- Jumping
- Swimming
- Wrestling
- Sprinting
- Racquet sports
- Most team sports

Activities requiring only normal range of motion in involved joints:
- Boxing
- Long distance jogging or running
- Archery
- Shooting
- Curling
- Basketball
- Bicycling
- Stair stepping
- Skating (in-line, roller)
- Horseback riding
- Resistance training

Modified from Plowman SA, Smith DL: *Exercise physiology: for health, fitness, and performance*, ed 2, San Francisco, 2003, Benjamin Cummings. Based on data from Hubley-Kozey CL: Testing flexibility. In MacDougall JD, Weuger HA, Green HJ, editors: *Physiological testing of the high-performance athlete*, Champaign Ill, 1991, Human Kinetics.

Evidence-Based Clinical Application: Increasing Protein Synthesis—Interaction of Training and Nutrition

Many athletes, especially those engaged in resistance training, are interested in increasing protein synthesis. Increased protein synthesis increases the amount of contractile proteins and hence makes the muscles larger and stronger. Protein synthesis is enhanced in several circumstances: (a) following resistance exercise, (b) when amino acid availability is increased, and (c) when blood insulin levels are high. Recent research by Rasmussen et al[27] suggests that when these three conditions occur together, the effect on protein synthesis is additive. These researchers had participants ingest a drink containing six essential amino acids and 35 g of sucrose following a bout of resistance training. The participants consumed the drink at either 1 hour or 3 hours posttraining, and the results were compared with a control group that consumed a flavored placebo drink. The ingestion of sucrose caused an elevation in blood insulin levels.

The combination of essential amino acids, elevated insulin levels, and resistance training stimulated protein synthesis approximately 400% above predrink levels when the drink was consumed 1 hour or 3 hours after resistance exercise. This increase in protein synthesis is greater than that reported following resistance training alone (≈100% increase in protein synthesis), increased amino acid availability alone (≈150% increase in protein synthesis), and the combination of resistance training and increased amino acid availability (≈200% increase in protein synthesis). On the basis of these results, fitness professionals may recommend that exercise participants who are interested in increasing muscle size consider consuming a drink containing essential amino acids and carbohydrates following resistance training workouts. The supplement is equally effective if consumed 1 hour or 3 hours after a workout.

From Rosmussen BB, Tipton KD, Miller SL, Wolf SE, Wolfe RR. *J Appl Physiol* 88:386-392, 2000.

APPLYING SCIENCE TO PRACTICE: DOES FIBER-TYPE DISTRIBUTION AFFECT MAXIMAL OXYGEN UPTAKE?

Researchers have long been interested in the fiber-type distribution of athletes. At the time that Bergh and et al[28] undertook this study, researchers knew that aerobically trained individuals were characterized by a high percentage of ST fibers (and hence a lower percentage of FT fibers) and that anaerobically trained individuals (e.g., sprinters) were more likely to have a high percentage of FT fibers. Researchers also knew that aerobic training was associated with a high $\dot{V}O_2$max, which is the greatest amount of oxygen an individual can take in, transport, and use during strenuous work; it is considered the best measure of an individual's aerobic (or cardiovascular) fitness. Thus Bergh et al proposed that there would be a relationship between the percentage of ST fibers and a person's $\dot{V}O_2$max. The results in the graph support their hypothesis.

Two important points emerge from these data:
1. There is a strong linear relationship between VO_2max and %ST fibers. This makes sense because ST fibers have the greatest oxidative ability (i.e., the ability to use oxygen to produce large amounts of ATP to support long-duration activities).
2. At any given %ST ($> \approx 40\%$), an athlete has a greater $\dot{V}O_2$max than does a nonathlete. This is consistent with what we know about the trainability of muscle fibers. Endurance training increases the oxidative capacity of muscle, thereby allowing the muscle to use more oxygen and thus achieve a higher $\dot{V}O_2$max.

In addition to specific points mentioned earlier, this research also reinforces the tremendous amount of interaction among the various systems of the body.

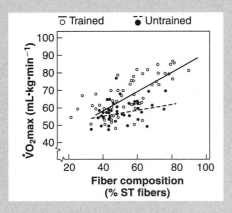

REFERENCES

1. Fox S: *Human physiology*, Dubuque, Iowa, 1987, WC Brown.
2. Hunter GR: Muscle physiology. In Baechle TR, Earle RW, editors: *Essentials of strength training and conditioning*, pp. 3-13, Champaign, Ill, 2000, Human Kinetics.
3. Marieb E: *Human anatomy and physiology*, ed 6, Redwood, Calif, 2004, Benjamin/Cummings Publishing.
4. Vander AJ, Sherman JH, Luciano DS: *Human physiology: the mechanisms of body function*, ed 7, New York, 1998, McGraw-Hill.
5. Williams J: Normal musculoskeletal and neuromuscular anatomy, physiology, and responses to training. In Hasson SM, editor: *Clinical exercise physiology*, St Louis, 1994, Mosby-Year Book Publishers.
6. Billeter R, Hoppler H: Muscular basis of strength. In Komi PV, editor: *Strength and power in sport*, pp. 39-63, Oxford, 1992, Blackwell Scientific Publications.
7. Berne RB, Levy MN: *Physiology*, ed 5, pp. 315-342, St Louis, 2004, Mosby.
8. Noth J: Motor units. In Komi PV, editor: *Strength and power in sport*, pp. 21-28, Oxford, 1992, Blackwell Scientific Publications.
9. Van deGraaff KM, Fox SI: *Concepts of human anatomy and physiology*, ed 4, pp. 291-355, Dubuque, Iowa, 1995, WC Brown Publishers.
10. Saltin B, Henriksson J, Nygaard E, et al: Fiber types and metabolic potentials of skeletal muscles in sedentary man and endurance runners, *Ann N Y Acad Sci* 301:3-29, 1977.
11. Baldwin KM: Muscle development: neonatal to adult. In Terjung RL, editor: *Exercise and sport sciences reviews*, 12:1-19, Baltimore, 1984, Williams & Wilkins.
12. Harris RT, Dudley G: Neuromuscular anatomy and physiology. In Baechle TR, Earle RW, editors: *Essentials of strength and conditioning*, pp. 15-23, Champaign, Ill, 2000, Human Kinetics.
13. Edington DW, Edgerton VR: *The biology of physical activity*, Boston, 1986, Houghton Mifflin.
14. Boicelli CA, Baldassarri AM, Borsetto C, et al: An approach to non-invasive fiber type distribution by nuclear magnetic resonance, *Int J Sports Med* 10:53-54, 1989.
15. Costill DL: *Muscle biopsy research: application of fiber composition to swimming*, Proceedings from Annual Clinic of American Swimming Coaches Association, Fort Lauderdale, Fla, 1978, ASCA.
16. Fox EL, Bowers RM, Foss ML: *Physiological basis for exercise and sport*, Dubuque, Iowa, 1993, Brown & Benchmark.
17. Tesch PA, Karlsson J: Muscle fiber types and size in trained and untrained muscles of elite athletes, *J Applied Physiol* 59:1716-1720, 1985.
18. Kraemer WJ: Physiological adaptations to anaerobic and aerobic training programs. In Baechle TR, Earle RW, editors: *Essentials of strength and conditioning*, pp. 137-168, Champaign, Ill, 2000, Human Kinetics.

19. Sage G: *Introduction to motor behavior: a neurophysiological approach,* Reading, Mass, 1971, Addison-Wesley.

20. Guyton AC: *Textbook of medical physiology,* Philadelphia, 1986, Saunders.

21. Biering-Sorenseu F: Physical measurements as risk indicators for low-back trouble over a one year period, *Spine* 9(2):106-119, 1984.

22. Hubley-Kozey CL: Testing flexibility. In MacDougall JD, Weuger HA, Green HJ, editors: *Physiological testing of the high-performance athlete,* Champaign, Ill, 1991, Human Kinetics.

23. Knudson DV, Magnusson P, McHugh M: Current issues in flexibility fitness, *President's Council on Physical Fitness and Sports Research Digest Series* 3(10):1-8, 2000.

24. Gleim GW, McHugh MP: Flexibility and its effects on sports injury and performance, *Sports Med* 24(5):289-299, 1997.

25. Plowman SA: Physical activity, physical fitness and low back pain. *Exerc Sport Sci Rev* 20:221-242 (1992).

26. Shellock FG, Prentice WE: Warming-up and stretching for improved physical performance and prevention of sports-related injuries, *Sports Med* 2(4):267-278, 1985.

27. Rasmussen BB, Tipton KD, Miller SL, et al: An oral essential amino acid–carbohydrate supplement enhances muscle protein anabolism after resistance exercise, *J Applied Physiol* 88:386-392, 2000.

28. Bergh U, Thorstensson A, Sjodin B, et al: Maximal oxygen uptake and muscle fiber types in trained and untrained humans, *Med Sci Sports Exercise* 10(3):151-154, 1978.

3

Sharon Ann Plowman
and Denise Louise Smith

Anaerobic Metabolism during Exercise*

LEARNING OBJECTIVES

After studying this chapter, the reader will be able to do the following:

1. Describe the energy continuum as it relates to varying durations of maximal exercise
2. Provide examples of sports or events within sports in which the adenosine triphosphate–phosphocreatine (ATP-PC), lactic acid, or oxygen system predominates
3. List the major variables that are typically measured to describe the anaerobic response to exercise
4. Explain the physiological reasons why lactate may accumulate in the blood
5. Distinguish between the power and the capacity of the ATP-PC, lactic acid, and oxygen systems
6. Identify the oxygen deficit and excess postexercise oxygen consumption, and explain the causes of each
7. Describe the changes in ATP and PC that occur during constant-load, heavy exercise lasting 3 minutes or less
8. Describe the changes in lactate accumulation that occur during constant-load, high-intensity, anaerobic exercise lasting 3 minutes or less; short-term, light to moderate, and moderate to heavy submaximal aerobic exercise; long-term moderate to heavy submaximal aerobic exercise; incremental exercise to maximum; and dynamic resistance exercise
9. Differentiate among the terms anaerobic threshold, ventilatory threshold, and lactate threshold, and explain why anaerobic threshold is a misnomer
10. Discuss why the accumulation of lactate is a physiological and performance problem
11. Explain the fate of lactate during exercise and recovery
12. Compare anaerobic metabolism during exercise for children and adolescents versus young and middle-age adults; males versus females; and the elderly versus young and middle-aged adults, and cite possible reasons for these differences

*Based on Plowman SA, Smith DL: *Exercise physiology for health, fitness, and performance*, ed 2, San Francisco, 2003, Benjamin Cummings.

THE ENERGY CONTINUUM

Adenosine triphosphate (ATP), the ultimate energy source for all human work, is produced by the metabolic pathways. This chapter and the next discuss ATP production and utilization on the basis of the need for oxygen. Anaerobic metabolism does not require oxygen to produce ATP, but aerobic metabolism does. Critical to understanding anaerobic and aerobic exercise metabolism is the fact that these processes are not mutually exclusive (i.e., anaerobic metabolism and aerobic metabolism are not either/or situations in terms of how ATP is provided). Both systems can and usually do work concurrently. When describing muscular exercise, the terms *aerobic* or *anaerobic* refer to which system predominates.

Figure 3-1 reviews the three sources of ATP production. Figure 3-1, *A* describes alactic anaerobic metabolism, sometimes called the *phosphagen* or *adenosine triphosphate–phosphocreatine (ATP-PC) system*. Once ATP has been produced, it is stored in the muscle. This amount is relatively small and can provide energy for only 1 to 2 seconds of maximal effort. However, another high-energy compound, PC, also known as *creatinephosphate* (CP), can be utilized to resynthesize ATP from ADP instantaneously. The amount of PC in muscle is about three times that of ATP.[1] Muscles differ in the amount of stored PC by fiber type. Muscle fibers that produce energy predominantly by anaerobic glycolysis are called *glycolytic* (G); those that produce energy predominantly aerobically are called *oxidative* (O). In terms of contraction speed, muscle fibers are either fast-twitch (FT) or slow-twitch (ST). When contractile and metabolic characteristics are combined, three fiber types are generally described: fast-twitch glycolytic (FG), fast-twitch oxidative glycolytic (FOG), and slow-twitch oxidative (SO). Fast-twitch fibers have proportionally more PC and ATP compared with slow-twitch oxidative fibers. Any time the energy demand is increased, whether the activity is simply turning a page of this book, coming out of the blocks for a sprint, or starting out on a long bicycle ride, at least part of the immediate need for energy is supplied by these stored forms, which must ultimately be replenished. These sources are also utilized preferentially in high-intensity, very short duration activity.

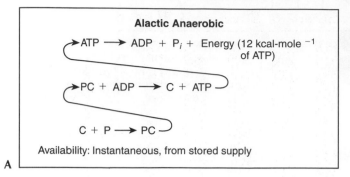

Alactic Anaerobic

$$ATP \longrightarrow ADP + P_i + Energy\ (12\ kcal\text{-}mole^{-1}\ of\ ATP)$$

$$PC + ADP \longrightarrow C + ATP$$

$$C + P \longrightarrow PC$$

Availability: Instantaneous, from stored supply

A

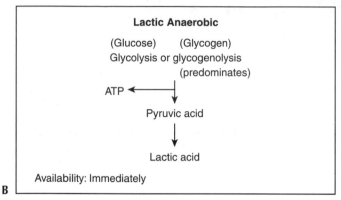

Lactic Anaerobic

(Glucose)   (Glycogen)
Glycolysis or glycogenolysis
(predominates)

ATP ◄——

Pyruvic acid

↓

Lactic acid

Availability: Immediately

B

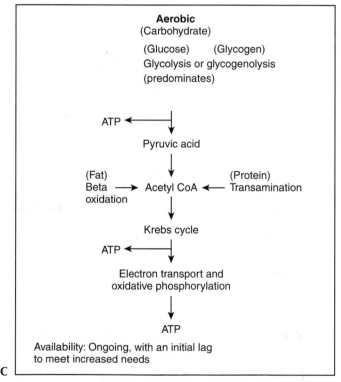

Aerobic
(Carbohydrate)

(Glucose)   (Glycogen)
Glycolysis or glycogenolysis
(predominates)

ATP ◄——

Pyruvic acid

↓

(Fat)   (Protein)
Beta ——► Acetyl CoA ◄—— Transamination
oxidation

↓

Krebs cycle

ATP ◄——

↓

Electron transport and
oxidative phosphorylation

↓

ATP

Availability: Ongoing, with an initial lag
to meet increased needs

C

Figure 3-1 Anaerobic and aerobic sources of adenosine triphosphate. (From Plowman SA, Smith DL: *Exercise physiology for health, fitness, and performance,* ed 2, San Francisco, 2003, Benjamin Cummings.)

Representative sports activities with a heavy reliance on the ATP-PC system include most football plays; sprints (e.g., track 100 and 200 m; swimming 50 m, softball/baseball base stealing, gymnastic vaults); shot put and javelin throwing; racquet, club, or limb swings (e.g., badminton, tennis, golf,

volleyball, kicking); goalie reactions; and specific mountain biking moves. Together, the ATP-PC supply can support slightly less than 10 seconds of maximal activity. This ATP-PC system neither uses oxygen nor produces lactic acid (LA) and is thus said to be *alactic anaerobic.*

Figure 3-1, *B* represents anaerobic glycolysis, also called the *lactic acid system.* When the demands for ATP exceed the capacity of the phosphagen system and the aerobic system (either at the initiation of any activity or during high-intensity, short-duration exercise), fast (anaerobic) glycolysis is utilized. This is like "calling in the reserves" because glycolysis can produce supplemental energy quickly. This system makes such activities as a 1500-m speed skating event possible. Other sport activities with a heavy reliance on the LA system include middle distances (e.g., track 200 to 800 m, swimming 100 m, slalom and downhill skiing); gymnastic floor exercise; parallel bars; a round of boxing; and a period of wrestling. The benefit is the ability to perform events with speed and power. The cost is that the production of lactic acid often exceeds clearance, resulting in lactate accumulation. Because this system does not involve the utilization of oxygen but does result in the production of lactic acid, it is said to be *lactic anaerobic.*

Figure 3-1, *C* shows aerobic oxidation, also called the *O_2 system.* The generation of ATP from slow (aerobic) glycolysis, the Krebs cycle, and electron transport-oxidative phosphorylation is constantly in operation at some level. Under resting conditions this system provides basically all of the energy necessary. When activity begins or occurs at moderate levels of intensity, oxidation increases quickly and proceeds at a rate that supplies the necessary ATP. If the workload is continuously incremented, aerobic oxidation proceeds at a correspondingly higher rate until its maximal limit is reached. The highest amount of oxygen the body can consume during heavy dynamic exercise for the aerobic production of ATP is called *maximal oxygen uptake* ($\dot{V}O_2$max). $\dot{V}O_2$max is primarily an index of cardiorespiratory capacity and as such is often used as a measure of cardiovascular-respiratory fitness. However, because $\dot{V}O_2$max reflects the amount of oxygen available for the aerobic production of ATP, it is also an important metabolic measure. Both aerobic and anaerobic exercises are often described in terms of a given percentage of $\dot{V}O_2$max (either < or > 100% $\dot{V}O_2$max). Anaerobic metabolic processes are important at the onset of all aerobic exercise, contribute significantly at submaximal levels, and increase their contribution as the exercise intensity gets progressively higher. Depending on an individual's fitness level, lactic anaerobic metabolism begins to make a significant contribution to dynamic activity at approximately 40% to 60% $\dot{V}O_2$max. Even then the ability to process oxygen is most important. Because the aerobic system involves the use of oxygen and proceeds completely to oxidative phosphorylation, it is said to be *aerobic* or *oxidative.* Sport activities that rely predominantly on the O_2 system include long distances (e.g., track 5000 m and 10,000 m, marathons, swimming 1500 m); cross-country (running, skiing, orienteering); field hockey; soccer and lacrosse; and race walking.

These three sources of ATP—the phosphagen system (ATP-PC), the glycolytic system (LA), and the oxidative system

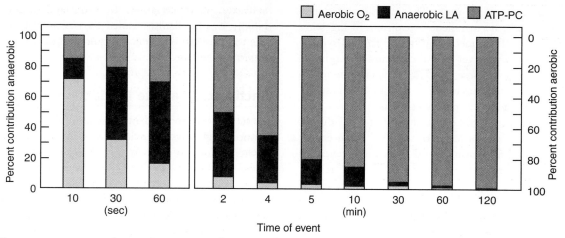

Figure 3-2 Time energy system continuum. Approximate relative contributions of aerobic and anaerobic energy production at maximal maintainable intensity for varying durations. The graphs assume 100% maximal oxygen uptake ($\dot{V}O_2$max) at 10 minutes; 95% $\dot{V}O_2$max at 30 minutes; 85% of $\dot{V}O_2$max at 60 minutes; and 80% $\dot{V}O_2$max at 120 minutes. Adenosine triphosphate–phosphocreatine ≤10 seconds. (From Plowman SA, Smith DL: *Exercise physiology for health, fitness, and performance,* ed 2, San Francisco, 2003, Benjamin Cummings. Based on data from Astrand P-O, Rodahl K, Dahl HA, et al: *Textbook of work physiology: physiological bases of exercise,* ed 4, Champaign, Ill, 2003, Human Kinetics; Gollnick PD, Hermansen L: Biochemical adaptations to exercise: anaerobic metabolism. In Wilmore JH, editor: *Exercise and sport sciences reviews,* pp. 1-43, New York, 1973, Academic Press.)

(O_2)—are recruited in a specific sequence called the *time-energy continuum.* This continuum assumes that the individual is working at a maximal maintainable intensity for a continuous duration. This means it is assumed that an individual can go all out for 5 minutes or less or can work at 100% $\dot{V}O_2$max for 10 minutes, at 95% $\dot{V}O_2$max for 30 minutes, at 85% $\dot{V}O_2$max for 60 minutes, and at 80% $\dot{V}O_2$max for 120 minutes. Although there are individual differences, these assumptions are reasonable in general.

Figure 3-2 indicates the relative contributions of each energy system to the total energy requirement under these conditions. These values are estimates that sometimes overlap but provide general trends, as well as some specific values.[2,3] For example, during an all-out event that lasts 30 seconds, the dominant metabolism is anaerobic (80%), with approximately 33% being provided by the ATP-PC system and 47% by the LA system. Which system predominates during an event that takes 5 minutes, and what are the percentages? If you take time to analyze the graph, you should discover that the breakdown at 5 minutes is a mirror image of what occurs at 30 seconds. Now 80% of the energy is provided by aerobic oxidative metabolism and only 20% by anaerobic metabolism, split 3% ATP-PC and 17% LA.

Four basic patterns can be discerned from this continuum. Understanding these patterns is helpful when developing training programs:

1. All three energy systems (ATP-PC, LA, O_2) are involved in providing energy for all durations of exercise.
2. The ATP-PC system predominates in activities lasting 10 seconds or less and still contributes at least 8% of the energy supply for maximal activities up to 2 minutes in length. Because the ATP-PC system is involved primarily at the onset of longer activities, it becomes a smaller

portion of the total energy supply as the duration gets longer.
3. Anaerobic metabolism (ATP-PC and LA) predominates in supplying energy for exercises lasting less than 2 minutes. However, even exercises lasting as long as 10 minutes use at least 15% anaerobic sources. Within the anaerobic component, the longer the duration, the greater the relative importance of the lactic acid system in comparison with the phosphagen system.
4. By 5 minutes of exercise, the O_2 system is clearly the dominant system. The longer the duration, the more important it becomes.

The rest of this chapter concentrates on the anaerobic contribution to energy metabolism. Chapter 4 concentrates on the aerobic contribution to energy metabolism, although it must be emphasized that the two systems work together, with one or the other predominating primarily on the basis of the duration and intensity of the activity.

ANAEROBIC ENERGY PRODUCTION

Alactic Anaerobic Phosphocreatine Production

As previously described, alactic anaerobic production of ATP involves the use of PC, which is simply creatine bound to inorganic phosphate. An adult human has a creatine level of approximately 120 to 125 mmol·kg^{-1} of dry muscle, although there is considerable individual variation from a low of 90 to 100 mmol·kg^{-1} to a high of about 150 to 160 mmol·kg^{-1}. Each day approximately 2 g of creatine are degraded in a non-reversible reaction to creatinine. This creatinine is ultimately excreted by the kidneys in urine. The individual counterbalances this loss under normal dietary conditions by ingesting about 1 g of creatine from meat, poultry, or fish and synthesizing another gram in the liver from the amino acids arginine, glycine, and methionine. Close to 95% of the creatine in the body is stored in skeletal muscle. From 30% to 40% is stored as free creatine, and the rest as phosphocreatine.

Figure 3-3 shows the breakdown of ATP and PC during heavy exercise. It also shows restoration of ATP from energy substrate sources and restoration of PC from the regenerated ATP. The process continues until both the PC and ATP resting levels are regained. Specifically, when ATP is hydrolyzed by the contractile proteins in muscle (large inner circle), the resulting ADP is rephosphorylated in the cytoplasm by the PC that is available there (small inner circle). In turn, the now free creatine is rephosphorylated at the inner mitochondrial membrane from ATP produced at that site (large outside oval). The remnant ADP is then free, in turn, to be phosphorylated again by

oxidative phosphorylation. In addition to providing ATP rapidly, this mechanism, called the *creatine phosphate shuttle,* is one way in which electron transport and oxidative phosphorylation are regulated.[4]

Lactic Acid/Lactate Production

Lactic acid is produced in muscle cells when NADH + H$^+$ formed in glycolysis is oxidized to NAD$^+$ by a transfer of the hydrogen ions to pyruvic acid ($C_3H_4O_3$), which, in turn, is reduced to lactic acid ($C_3H_6O_3$).[9,10] In muscle tissue, lactic acid is produced in amounts that are in equilibrium with pyruvic acid under normal resting conditions. In addition, lactic acid is always produced by red blood cells, portions of the kidneys, and certain tissues within the eye. Both resting and exercise values depend on the balance between lactic acid production (appearance) and removal (disappearance, or clearance). This balance of appearance and disappearance is called *turnover.*

Evidence-Based Clinical Application: Creatine as an Ergogenic Aid

Because of its role in the rephosphorylation of adenosine triphosphate from adenosine diphosphate and the theoretical impact this might have on performance and fatigue resistance, creatine (primarily in the form of creatine monohydrate) has enjoyed unprecedented popularity as an ergogenic aid. Oral creatine supplementation can reportedly increase muscle phosphocreatine content by approximately 20%, depending on an individual's starting level. An upper limit for storage exists, so if an individual is already at that point ($\approx$160 mmol·kg^{-1} of dry muscle), supplementation will not further increase storage. Excess ingested creatine is excreted in the urine.[5,6] This can explain why one individual might respond to creatine monohydrate supplementation and another might be a "nonresponder."

Despite numerous studies, the effectiveness of creatine supplementation has not been established. An American College of Sports Medicine Roundtable consensus statement concluded that the majority (approximately two thirds) of the studies reviewed that measured muscular force or power output, or both, during short bouts of maximal exercise in healthy, young (18 to 35 years old) adults (almost exclusively males) showed an enhancement. The greatest improvement in performance seemed to be found in the later bouts of a repetitive series of exercises in which the high power output lasted only a matter of seconds separated by rest periods of 20 to 60 seconds.[5] These increases have been seen largely in average power outputs, however, not in peak power outputs.[6] A number of studies have also indicated that creatine supplementation, along with heavy resistance training, enhances the normal training adaptation.[5] However, when a mathematical analysis (called a *meta-analysis*) was conducted of studies that tested anaerobic performance, creatine supplementation showed no significant improvements for fatigue resistance, power, speed, strength, or total work.[7]

As with any supplement, concerns have been expressed regarding the safety of creatine ingestion. Two credible reviews have concluded that although there have been numerous anecdotal reports of gastrointestinal disturbances (nausea/vomiting/diarrhea), liver and kidney dysfunction, cardiovascular/thermal impairment, and muscular damage (cramps/strains), the supporting evidence, with a few notable exceptions, is not definitive. The most notable exceptions involved documented medical case reports of individuals with preexisting kidney problems that were aggravated with creatine supplementation and resolved when the supplementation was stopped. The following precautions are advised[8]:

1. Individuals with preexisting kidney dysfunction or those at high risk for kidney disease (e.g., diabetics and individuals with a family history of kidney disease) should either avoid creatine supplementation or undergo regular medical monitoring. Regular checkups are recommended for everyone taking creatine because any individual may react adversely to any substance, and excess creatine is a burden that must be eliminated by the kidneys.
2. Individuals wishing to maintain or decrease body weight while participating in strenuous exercise should avoid creatine supplementation.
3. High-dose creatine supplementation should be avoided during periods of physical activity under high thermal stress.
4. Adequate fluid and electrolytes should always be ingested.
5. Individuals younger than the age of 18 should not supplement with creatine.
6. Pregnant or lactating females should not supplement with creatine.
7. The ingestion of creatine during exercise should be avoided.

At normal pH levels lactic acid almost completely (≈99%) dissociates into hydrogen ions (H^+) and lactate ($C_3H_5O_3^-$, designated as La^-). Thus technically, lactic acid is formed, but lactate is what is measured in the bloodstream. Despite this distinction, the terms *lactic acid* and *lactate* are often used synonymously.[9] When production exceeds removal, lactate is said to accumulate. The questions, then, especially during exercise, are what conditions result in lactic acid production and what processes lead to lactic acid/lactate removal? This section deals with the first of these questions.

In general, the relative rates of glycolytic activity and oxidative activity determine the production of lactic acid/lactate. Specifically, five factors play important roles: muscle contraction, enzyme activity, muscle fiber type, sympathetic nervous system activation, and insufficient oxygen (anaerobiosis, the onset of anaerobic metabolism).

1. Muscle contraction. During exercise, muscle activity obviously increases. The process of muscle contraction requires the release of calcium (Ca^{++}) from the sarcoplasmic reticulum. In addition to its role in the coupling process of actin and myosin, calcium also causes glycogenolysis by activating the enzyme glycogen phosphorylase. Glycogen is processed by fast glycolysis and results in the production of lactic acid whether oxygen levels are sufficient or not.[4,11]

2. Enzyme activity. The conversion of pyruvate and NADH + H^+ to lactate and NAD^+ is catalyzed by specific isozymes of the enzyme lactic dehydrogenase (LDH), whereas the conversion of pyruvate to acetyl CoA before entry into the Krebs cycle is catalyzed by the enzyme pyruvate dehydrogenase (PDH). LDH has the highest rate of functioning of any of the glycolytic enzymes and is much more active than the enzymes that provide alternate pathways for pyruvate metabolism including PDH and the rate-limiting enzymes in the Krebs cycle. Any increase in pyruvate and NADH + H^+ further increases the activity of LDH and results in the production of lactic acid.[12] Therefore lactic acid production is an inevitable consequence of glycolysis.[12-14] The more pyruvate provided, the more lactate produced. The shifting of the hydrogen atoms from NADH + H^+ to pyruvate forming lactate serves to maintain the redox potential of the cell. The redox, or oxidation-reduction, potential is the ratio of NADH + H^+ to NAD^+. A finite amount of NAD^+ is available in the cytoplasm to accept hydrogen atoms and keep glycolysis going. To maintain this supply, NADH + H^+ must either transfer the hydrogen atoms into the mitochondria to the electron transport chain or give them up to pyruvate.

3. Muscle fiber type. During high-intensity, short-duration activities, FG muscle fibers are preferentially recruited. These fast-contracting glycolytic fibers produce lactic acid when they contract whether oxygen is present in sufficient amounts or not. This response appears to be a function of the low mitochondrial density and the specific lactic dehydrogenase isozymes found in these fibers.[15] LDH isozymes 4 and 5 predominate in fast twitch fibers and

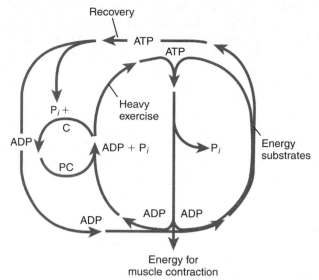

Figure 3-3 Use and regeneration of ATP-PC. ATP → ADP + P_i + energy for muscle contraction *(large inner circle)*. During heavy exercise the ADP is regenerated to ATP by the breakdown of CP (CP + ADP → C + ATP) *(small inner circle)*. Only in recovery will the nearly depleted CP stores be restored from the breakdown of ATP resulting from aerobic metabolic production *(large outside oval)*. *ATP,* Adenosine triphosphate; *ADP,* adenosine diphospate; *CP,* creatine phosphate; *Pi,* organic phosphate. (From Plowman SA, Smith DL: *Exercise physiology for health, fitness, and performance,* ed 2, San Francisco, 2003, Benjamin Cummings.)

facilitate the conversion of pyruvate to lactate. Conversely, LDH isozymes 1 and 2 predominate in cardiac, slow-twitch oxidative and fast-twitch mitochondria and catalyze the conversion of lactate to pyruvate.[16]

4. Sympathetic neural/hormonal activation. During heavy exercise, activity of the sympathetic nervous system stimulates the release of epinephrine and glucagon and suppression of insulin. The result is an increased breakdown of glycogen, leading ultimately to high levels of glucose-6-phosphate (G6P). High levels of G6P increase the rate of glycolysis and hence the production of pyruvic acid.[13] As previously described, any increase in pyruvate and NADH + H^+ ultimately results in an increase in lactic acid. In addition, late in prolonged endurance activity, epinephrine-mediated glycogen breakdown may bring about the release of lactate from resting muscle when an increased lactate release is no longer occurring in contracting muscle.[17]

5. Insufficient oxygen (anaerobiosis, onset of anaerobic metabolism). Finally, during high-intensity, short-duration, or near-maximal exercise or during static contractions when blood flow is impaired,[17] the delivery of oxygen to the mitochondria and hence the availability of oxygen as the final oxygen acceptor at the end of the respiratory chain can become deficient. Under these circumstances glycolysis proceeds at a rate that produces larger quantities of NADH + H^+ than the mitochondria has oxygen to accept. Again, "something" must be done

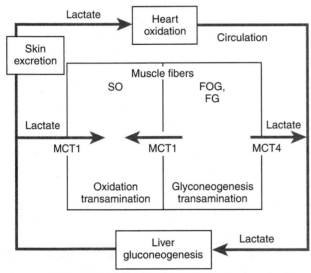

Intracellular Lactate Shuttle

Stage I glycolysis

Glucose/glycogen

A   Cytoplasm

Extracellular Lactate Shuttle

B

Figure 3-4 Intracellular and extracellular lactate shuttles. **A,** The intracellular lactate shuttle transports lactate from the cytoplasm into the mitochondria by MTC1 transporters, where it is reconverted to pyruvate and proceeds through oxidative metabolism. **B,** The extracellular lactate shuttle moves lactate directly between lactic acid–producing fast-twitch glycolytic fibers (FOG and FG) and lactate-consuming slow-twitch oxidative fibers. The extracellular lactate shuttle also transports lactate through the circulation to the liver, skin, and heart, where it is cleared by oxidation, transamination, gluconeogenesis, or excretion. Most lactate remaining in fast-twitch glycolytic fibers is reconverted to glycogen by glyconeogenesis. (From Plowman SA, Smith DL: *Exercise physiology for health, fitness, and performance,* ed 2, San Francisco, 2003, Benjamin Cummings.)

with the hydrogen atoms so that the NAD^+ can be regenerated. That "something" is the transfer of the hydrogen atoms to pyruvic acid and the formation of lactic acid.

Thus although lactic acid is associated with high-intensity, short-duration exercise, it is not the only exercise condition that results in the production of lactic acid. In addition, although a lack of oxygen can contribute to the production of lactic acid, the presence of lactic acid does not absolutely indicate a lack of oxygen. The presence of lactic acid simply reflects the use of the fast (anaerobic) glycolytic pathway for ATP production and the balance between glycolytic and mitochondrial activity. Furthermore, rather than lactic acid being a "waste product," lactate provides a means of coordinating carbohydrate metabolism in diverse tissues.[4] The formation, distribution, and utilization of lactate is a way for glycogen reserves to be mobilized and utilized either within the original cell or other cells. In the process, blood glucose is spared for use by other tissues.[18,19] The use or reconversion, or both, of lactate comprise lactate clearance.

Lactate Clearance

Lactate clearance during rest and exercise occurs primarily by three processes: oxidation (50% to 80%), gluconeogenesis/glyconeogenesis (10% to 25%), and transamination (5% to 10%). All three processes involve the movement of lactate.[18]

As stated previously, at physiological pH more than 99% of the lactic acid produced quickly dissociates into lactate (La^-) anions and protons (H^+). Lactate moves readily between cytoplasm and mitochondria, muscle and blood, blood and muscle, active and inactive muscle, glycolytic and oxidative muscle, blood and heart, blood and liver, and blood and skin.[20] Lactate moves between lactate-producing and lactate-consuming sites by means of intracellular and extracellular lactate shuttles.[18] Transport across cellular and mitochondrial membranes occurs by facilitated exchange down concentration and hydrogen ion (pH) gradients using lactate transport proteins known as *monocarboxylate transporters* (MCTs).[20]

As of 1999, nine monocarboxylate transporters had been reported in the literature. MCT1 is abundant in oxidative skeletal and cardiac muscle fibers and mitochondrial membranes. MCT4 is most prevalent in the cell membranes of glycolytic skeletal fibers.

The intracellular lactate shuttle (Figure 3-4, *A*) involves the movement of lactate by MCT1 transporters between the cytoplasm, where it is produced, and the mitochondria. Once inside the mitochondria, lactate is oxidized to pyruvate and NAD^+ is reduced to $NADH + H^+$. The pyruvate and $NADH + H^+$ proceed through aerobic metabolism/oxidation. This is a relatively new, and somewhat controversial, concept[20-23] indicating that muscle cells can both produce and consume lactate at the same time.

Extracellular lactate shuttles act to move lactate among tissues (Figure 3-4, *B*). Muscle cell membrane lactate proteins (MCT1 and MCT4) move the lactate out of and into tissues. Intermuscularly, most lactate moves out of active fast-twitch glycolytic skeletal muscle cells (FOG and FG) and into active SO skeletal muscle cells. This can occur either by a direct shuttle between the skeletal muscle cells or through the circulation. Once lactate is in the bloodstream, it can also circulate to cardiac cells. During heavy exercise, lactate becomes the preferred fuel of the heart. In this manner glycogenolysis in one cell can supply fuel for another cell. In each case the ultimate fate of the lactate is oxidation to ATP, CO_2, and H_2O by aerobic metabolism.[13,20,24]

Lactate circulating in the bloodstream can also be transported to the liver, where it is reconverted by the processes of gluconeogenesis/glyconeogenesis into glucose or glycogen, respectively. Indeed, the liver appears to preferentially make glycogen from lactate as opposed to glucose. In human glycolytic muscle fibers (both FOG and FG) some of the lactate produced during high-intensity exercise is retained, and in the postexercise recovery period it is reconverted to glycogen in that muscle cell.[4,25,26]

Both oxidative and glycolytic fibers can also clear lactate by transamination. Transamination forms keto acids (including some Krebs cycle intermediates) and amino acids. The predominant amino acid produced is alanine. In turn, alanine can undergo gluconeogenesis in the liver.[13,14]

A small amount of lactate in the circulation moves from the blood to the skin and exits the body in sweat. Finally, some lactate remains as lactate circulating in the blood. This comprises the resting lactate level.

Oxidation is by far the predominant process of lactate clearance both during and after exercise. As stated previously, the accumulation of lactate in the blood depends on the relative rate of appearance (production) and disappearance (clearance), which in turn is directly related to the intensity and duration of the exercise being done.

THE ANAEROBIC EXERCISE RESPONSE

Oxygen Deficit and Excess Postexercise Oxygen Consumption

When exercise begins, no matter how light or heavy it is, there is an immediate need for additional energy. Thus the most obvious exercise response is an increase in metabolism. All three energy systems are involved in this response, with their relative contributions being proportional to the intensity and duration of the activity.

Figure 3-5 shows two scenarios for going from rest to different intensities of exercise. In Figure 3-5, *A*, the activity is a moderate submaximal bout. The oxygen requirement for this particular exercise is 1.4 $L\cdot min^{-1}$. The individual has a $\dot{V}O_2max$ of 2.5 $L\cdot min^{-1}$. Therefore this individual is working at 56% $\dot{V}O_2max$. The area under the smoothed curve during both exercise and recovery represents oxygen utilized. Notice, however, that there is an initial lag during which the oxygen supplied and utilized is below the oxygen requirement for providing energy. This difference between the oxygen required during exercise and the oxygen supplied and utilized is called the

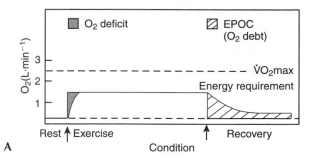

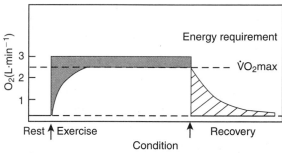

Figure 3-5 Oxygen deficit and excess postexercise oxygen consumption (EPOC) during submaximal exercise and supramaximal exercise. **A,** During light to moderate submaximal exercise, both the oxygen deficit, indicated by the convex curve at the start of exercise, and the excess postexercise oxygen consumption, indicated by the concave curve during the recovery time period, are small. **B,** During heavy or supramaximal exercise, both the O_2 deficit and the EPOC are large. Under both conditions energy is supplied during the O_2 deficit period by using stored adenosine triphophosphate–phosphocreatine (ATP-PC), anaerobic glycolysis, and oxygen stores in capillary blood and bound to myoglobin. The heavier the exercise, the more the reliance on anaerobic glycolysis. The EPOC is a result of the restoration of ATP-PC; removal of lactate; restoration of O_2 stores; elevated cardiovascular and respiratory function; elevated hormone levels; and, especially, the elevated body temperature. (From Plowman SA, Smith DL: *Exercise physiology for health, fitness, and performance*, ed 2, San Francisco, 2003, Benjamin Cummings.)

oxygen deficit. Because of this supply and demand discrepancy, anaerobic sources must be involved in providing energy at the onset of all activity.

The O_2 deficit has traditionally been explained as the inability of the circulatory and respiratory systems to respond quickly enough to the increased energy demands. More modern evidence, however, indicates that the O_2 deficit is probably due to limited cellular utilization of O_2 as a result of metabolic adjustments.[27] That is, the increasing levels of ADP, organic phospate (P_i), and NADH + H^+, brought about by the suddenly elevated energy demands, stimulate both aerobic and anaerobic energy processes, not just one or the other. Thus it is not that the aerobic system cannot supply all of the necessary energy but that the regulatory system does not allow it to. Therefore during the transition from rest to work, energy is supplied by the following:

1. O_2 transport and utilization
2. Utilization of O_2 stores in capillary blood and bound to myoglobin

3. The splitting of stored ATP-PC
4. Anaerobic glycolysis, with the concomitant production of lactic acid

Eventually, as long as the exercise intensity is low enough (as in the example in Figure 3-5, *A*), the aerobic system will predominate and the oxygen supply will equal the oxygen demand. This condition is called *steady-state, steady-rate,* or *steady-level exercise.*

Figure 3-5, *B*, shows a smoothed plot of O_2 consumption at rest and during and after an exercise bout in which the energy requirement is greater than $\dot{V}O_2$max, sometimes called *supramaximal exercise.* The initial period of lag between O_2 supply and demand is once again evident and, as in the first example, the added energy is provided by stored ATP-PC, anaerobic glycolysis, and stored O_2. However, in this case, when the O_2 consumption plateaus or levels off, it is at $\dot{V}O_2$max and more energy is still necessary if exercise is to continue.

This plateau is not considered to be a steady state because the energy demands are not being totally met aerobically. The supplemental energy is provided by anaerobic glycolysis. Exactly what the energy demand is in this situation is difficult to determine precisely. However, in a practical application of oxygen deficit theory, a measurement called *maximal accumulated oxygen deficit* (MAOD), expressed as O_2 $mL\cdot kg^{-1}$, is sometimes calculated. This requires a controlled testing session with a duration of 2 to 3 minutes at an intensity of 110% to 125% $\dot{V}O_2$max. The resulting difference between a computed oxygen requirement and the measured oxygen consumption is taken as an indication of anaerobic capacity.[28] Not surprisingly, sprinters and middle distance runners have been shown to have higher MAOD values than endurance distance runners.[29] Although experimental results are promising, the validity of this technique is still a matter of debate.[30] Without the anaerobic energy contribution, activity could not continue at this intensity.

The recovery from exercise represented by the concave curves following the cessation of exercise in Figure 3-5 shows that oxygen consumption drops quickly (a fast component lasting 2 to 3 minutes) and then tapers off (a slow component lasting 3 to 60 minutes). The magnitude and duration of this elevated oxygen consumption depend primarily on the intensity of the preceding exercise. In the case of light submaximal work (see Figure 3-5, *A*) recovery takes place quickly; after heavy exercise (see Figure 3-5, *B*) recovery takes much longer.

Historically, this period of elevated metabolism after exercise has been called the *O_2 debt,* the assumption being that the "extra" O_2 consumed during the "debt" period was being utilized to "pay back" the deficit incurred in the early part of exercise.[31,32] More recently, the terms *O_2 recovery* or *excess postexercise oxygen consumption* (EPOC) have come into favor. EPOC is defined as the oxygen consumption during recovery that is above normal resting values.

A critical question is what causes this elevated metabolism in recovery. Although no complete explanation of EPOC exists, six factors have been suggested:
1. Restoration of ATP-PC stores: About 10% of the EPOC is utilized to rephosphorylate creatine and ADP to PC and

ATP, respectively, thus restoring these substances to resting levels.[14,31] Approximately 50% of the ATP-PC is restored in 30 seconds.[33] This time is called the *half-life restoration of ATP-PC.* Full recovery requires slightly more than 2 minutes.[11]

2. Restoration of O_2 stores: Although the amount of O_2 stored in the blood (bound to hemoglobin) and muscle (bound to myoglobin) is not large, it does need to be replenished at the cessation of exercise. Replenishment probably occurs completely within 2 to 3 minutes.[31,32]

3. Elevated cardiovascular-respiratory function: Both the respiratory system and the cardiovascular system remain elevated postexercise; that is, neither the breathing rate and depth nor heart rate recover instantaneously. Although this circumstance enables the extra amounts of oxygen to be processed, the actual energy cost of these cardiovascular-respiratory processes probably accounts for only 1% to 2% of the excess oxygen.[31,32]

4. Elevated hormonal levels: During exercise the circulating levels of the catecholamines (epinephrine and norepinephrine), thyroxine, and cortisol are all increased. In addition to their fuel mobilization and utilization effects, these hormones increase Na^+-K^+ pump activity in muscles and nerves by changing cell membrane permeability to Na^+ and K^+. As an active transport process, the Na^+-K^+ pump requires ATP. The increased need for ATP means an increased need for O_2. Until the hormones are cleared from the bloodstream, the additional O_2 and ATP use is a significant contributor to EPOC.[14,31]

5. Elevated body temperature: When ATP is broken down to supply the energy for chemical, electrical, or mechanical work, heat is produced as a by-product. During exercise, heat production may exceed heat dissipation, causing a rise in body core temperature. For each degree Celsius that body temperature rises, the metabolic rate increases approximately 13% to 15%.[34] Thus in recovery, although the need for high levels of energy to support the exercise has ceased, the influence of the elevated temperature has not because cooling takes some time to occur. This temperature effect is by far the most important reason for EPOC, accounting for as much as 60% to 70% of the slow component after exercise at 50% to 80% $\dot{V}O_2$max.[14,31]

6. Lactate removal: The lactate that has accumulated must be removed. Historically, it was thought that the majority of this lactate was converted to glycogen and that this conversion was the primary cause of the slow component of EPOC. As previously described, the fate of lactic acid is now seen as more complex and its contribution as a causative factor for EPOC is minimal.[14,32]

Energy Power and Capacity

Energy system capacity is defined as the total amount of energy that can be produced by the energy system. Energy system power is defined as the maximal amount of energy that can be produced per unit of time. Table 3-1 clearly shows that the phosphagen (ATP-PC) system is predominantly a power

Table 3-1	Estimated Maximal Power and Capacity in Untrained Males				
Energy System	Power		Time	Capacity	
	kcal.min^{-1}	kJ.min^{-1}	hr:min:sec	kcal	kJ
ATP-PC (phosphagen)	72	300	:09-:10	11	45
LA (anaerobic glycolysis)	36	150	1:19.8	48	200
O$_2$ (aerobic glycolysis + Krebs cycle + ETS-OP; fuel = CHO)	7.2-19.1	30-80	2:21:00*	359-1268	1500-5300

From Plowman SA, Smith DL: *Exercise physiology for health, fitness, and performance*, ed 2. San Francisco, 2003, Benjamin Cummings.
ATP-PC, Adenosine triphosphate phosphocreatine; *CHO,* carbohydrate; *ETS-OP,* electron transport system–oxidative phosphorylation; *LA,* lactic acid.
*When all fuels are considered, the time is unlimited.

system with very little capacity. The lactic anaerobic glycolytic system has almost equal power and capacity, just slightly favoring capacity. The anaerobic capacity is the total amount of energy available from nonaerobic sources. The information on the aerobic (O$_2$) system is included here just to show how truly high in power and low in capacity the anaerobic systems are.

Although the ATP-PC system can put out energy at the rate of 72 kcal·min^{-1}, it can only sustain that value when working maximally for 9 to 10 sec, for a total output of only 11 kcal. The LA system has a lower power (36 kcal·min^{-1}) but can sustain it for almost 1 minute and 20 seconds. By comparison, if the O$_2$ system worked at a power output of 9 kcal·min^{-1}, exercise could be sustained for more than 2 hours just using carbohydrate fuel sources. In fact, when all fuel supplies are included, the capacity of the aerobic system is, for all intents and purposes, unlimited.

Unfortunately, there is still no generally accepted means by which to directly measure the anaerobic contribution during whole body exercise.[30] However, there are two general approaches to describe the anaerobic exercise response. One approach describes changes in the chemical substances either utilized in alactic anaerobic metabolism (specifically, ATP and PC levels) or produced as a result of lactic anaerobic metabolism (lactic acid or lactate). The second approach quantifies the amount of work performed or the power generated during short-duration, high-intensity activity. The assumption is that such activity could not be done without anaerobic energy; therefore measuring such work or power indirectly measures anaerobic energy utilization.

ATP-PC Changes

The measurement of ATP and PC can be done by chemical analysis of muscle biopsy specimens. Figure 3-6 indicates what happens to ATP and PC levels in muscle during constant-load, supramaximal exercise (105% to 110% $\dot{V}O_2$max) lasting 3 minutes or less. As shown in the figure, the ATP level decreases only slightly. In fact, the maximum ATP depletion observed in skeletal muscle after heavy exercise is only about 30% to 40% in both males and females. Thus even after exhaustive work, 60% to 70% of the resting amount of ATP is still present.[1,37]

Conversely, the level of PC changes dramatically such that it is nearly depleted. The greatest depletion of PC occurs in the initial 20 sec of exercise, with the result that ATP is almost

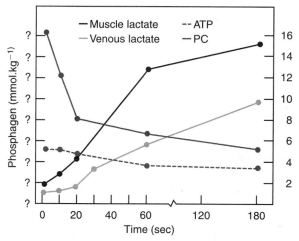

Figure 3-6 Time course for the depletion of phosphocreatine (PC) and adenosine triphosphate (ATP) and the accumulation of lactate in muscle and veins. Muscle levels of ATP are maintained relatively constant during high-intensity, short-duration exercise at the expense of PC. Muscle lactate levels rise sooner and higher than venous levels owing to the diffusion time lag and dilution. (From Plowman SA, Smith DL: *Exercise physiology for health, fitness, and performance*, ed 2, San Francisco, 2003, Benjamin Cummings. Modified from Gollnick PD, Hermansen L: Biochemical adaptation to exercise: anaerobic metabolism. In Wilmore JH, editor: *Exercise and sports sciences reviews*, New York, 1973, Academic Press.)

maintained at resting levels during that time span. From 20 to 180 seconds the decline in PC and ATP is both gradual and parallel.[3] Obviously, the ATP level is maintained at the expense of the PC. However, some ATP is also being provided from glycolysis, as indicated by the rise in lactate. As the activity continues, ATP is provided increasingly by oxidation.

Lactate Changes

Lactate is the most frequently measured anaerobic metabolic variable, in part because it can also be measured from blood samples. The blood sample may be obtained by venipuncture, ear, or finger prick, all of which are less invasive than a muscle biopsy. As previously mentioned, lactate is a small molecule that moves easily from the muscles to the blood and most other fluid compartments. However, much of the lactate that is produced does not get into the bloodstream. It takes time for the portion that does get into the bloodstream to reach equilibrium between muscle and blood. This equilibrium and the achievement of peak blood values may take as long as 5 to 10 minutes. Until equilibrium occurs, muscle lactate values are higher than blood lactate values. This also means that the highest blood lactate values are typically seen after several minutes of recovery, not during high-intensity work.[3]

Lactate levels are reported using a variety of units. The two most common are millimoles per liter (mmol·L^{-1}, sometimes designated as mM) or milligrams per 100 milliliters of blood (mg·100 mL^{-1}, sometimes designated as mg% or mg·dL^{-1}). One mmol·L^{-1} of lactate is equal to 9 mg·100 mL^{-1}. Resting levels of lactate of 1 to 2 mmol·L^{-1} or 9 to 18 mg·100 mL^{-1} are typical. A value of 8 mmol·L^{-1} or 72 mg·100 mL^{-1} is usually taken to indicate that an individual has worked maximally.[2] Peak values as high as 32 mmol·L^{-1} or 288 mg·100 mL^{-1} have been reported.[2]

Lactate levels in response to exercise depend primarily on the intensity of the exercise. Acute exercise does not result in any meaningful enhancement of lactate transporters. Instead, transmembrane lactate and hydrogen ion gradients increase. Lactate transport is faster in oxidative fibers than in glycolytic ones. The fast transport of lactate by oxidative fibers may reflect lactate's role as an energy substrate, while the slower transport in glycolytic fibers may contribute to a greater retention of lactate during recovery for reconversion into glycogen.[26]

Short-Term, High-Intensity Supramaximal Exercise

Figure 3-6 includes muscle and blood lactate response to high-intensity, short-duration (≤3 minutes), supramaximal exercise. As indicated, muscle lactate levels rise immediately with the onset of such hard work (105% to 110% V̇O$_2$max) and continue to rise throughout the length of the task. The blood lactate values show a similar pattern, if the lag for diffusion time is taken into account. This lactate response (a rapid and consistent accumulation) is representative of what occurs when the exercise bout is greater than 90% V̇O$_2$max.[3]

Short- and Long-Term, Low-Intensity Submaximal Aerobic Exercise

Figure 3-7 depicts what occurs in both short-term and long-term low-intensity submaximal aerobic activity. During the first 3 minutes of such steady-state work the lactate (La$^-$) level rises. This increase reflects the lactate accumulated during the oxygen deficit.[3] When a similar workload is continued for 60 minutes, the lactate level remains unchanged after the initial rise. The reason for this result lies in the balance between lactate production (the rate of lactate appearance) and lactate clearance (the rate of lactate disappearance).

Figure 3-8 shows the results from a study that directly measured the rate of lactate appearance (R$_a$) and the rate of lactate disappearance (R$_d$) by radioactive tracers, as well as the blood levels of lactate concentration ([La$^-$]).[9] In the transition from rest to steady-state submaximal exercise, the rate of both lactate appearance and lactate disappearance increased. During the next 30 minutes of exercise, the turnover rate was higher than at rest. The result was an initial increase in [La$^-$], which

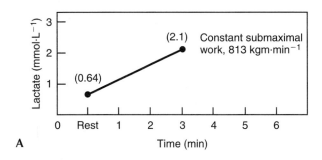

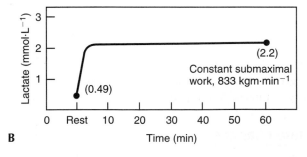

Figure 3-7 Lactate accumulation during short- and long-term dynamic, aerobic, constant, submaximal work. After an initial rise in accumulation during the oxygen deficit period **(A),** lactate levels off and remains relatively constant during long duration submaximal aerobic work **(B).** (From Plowman SA, Smith DL: *Exercise physiology for health, fitness, and performance,* ed 2, San Francisco, 2003, Benjamin Cummings. Based on data from Freund H, Oyono-Enguelle S, Heitz A, et al: *Int J Sports Med* 11:284-288, 1990.)

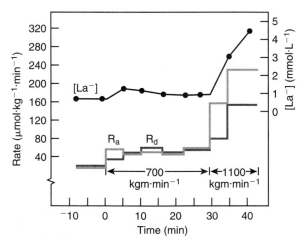

Figure 3-8 The impact of the rates of lactate appearance and disappearance on lactate accumulation during light and heavy submaximal aerobic exercise. During light (700 kgm·min^{-1}) submaximal aerobic exercise, the rate of lactate disappearance (R$_d$) *(left y-axis)* lags behind the rate of lactate appearance (R$_a$) *(left y-axis)* so that the 30-minute lactate concentration [La$^-$] value *(right y-axis)* approximates rest. During heavy submaximal exercise (minutes 30 to 45), the R$_d$ lags behind the R$_a$ and [La$^-$] increases. (From Brooks GA: *Med Sci Sports Exerc* 17:22-31, 1985.)

declined after 5 minutes of activity to almost resting levels by 30 minutes. When the workload was increased, the rate of clearance (R_d) was no longer able to keep up with the rate of production (R_a) and the lactate concentration in the blood [La⁻] showed a sharp increase.

Figure 3-9 shows how lactate level varies with competitive distance (and hence duration) in highly trained male runners.[39] At the shorter distances the predominant energy source is anaerobic, and the anticipated high lactate values are seen. As the distance increases and more of the energy is supplied aerobically, the intensity that can be maintained decreases. As a result, lactate also decreases, doing so in a negative exponential curvilinear pattern. By approximately 30 km (18 miles) the lactate levels are little different from what they are at rest.

Long-Term, Moderate to Heavy Submaximal Aerobic Exercise

The importance of the intensity of exercise, even at the marathon distance, is illustrated in Figure 3-10. Two groups of runners were matched according to their $\dot{V}O_2$max. One group ran a simulated marathon on the treadmill at 73.3% $\dot{V}O_2$max (in ≤ 2 hours and 45 minutes); the other group ran the same distance but at 64.5% $\dot{V}O_2$max (in 3 hours and 45 minutes or slightly less). Within the slow group blood lactate values remained relatively stable and at a level considered to be within normal resting amounts. The blood lactate levels in the fast group were statistically significantly higher throughout the marathon than those of the slow group. As absolutes, however, both sets of values were low, with the slow group being within a normal resting range and the fast group barely above normal resting range.[40]

In general, during light to moderate work (i.e., <50% to 60% of $\dot{V}O_2$max), the blood lactate level is likely to rise slightly at first. Then it either remains the same or decreases slightly, even if the exercise lasts 30 to 60 minutes.

At moderate to heavy intensities between 50% and 85% $\dot{V}O_2$max (depending on the genetic characteristics and training

status of the individual), lactate levels increase rapidly during the first 5 to 10 minutes of exercise. If the workload continues for more than 10 minutes, the lactate level may continue to rise, stabilize, or decline, depending on the individual and other conditions.

One of these "other conditions" may be the exercise intensity in relation to the individual's maximal lactate steady state. Maximal lactate steady state (MLSS) is the highest workload that can be maintained over time without a continual rise in blood lactate; it indicates an exercise intensity above which lactate production exceeds clearance. MLSS is determined by a series of workloads performed on different days. Each succeeding workload gets progressively more difficult until the blood lactate accumulation increases more or less steadily throughout the test or increases more than 1 mmol·L⁻¹ after the initial rise and establishment of a plateau in the early minutes. Thus in a 30-minute test this means that changes in the first 10 minutes are ignored, and only the last 20 minutes are utilized to determine if the change is less than or greater than 1 mmol·L⁻¹. When the blood concentration meets the criterion, the previous workload that exhibited a plateau in lactate throughout the duration (after the initial rise) is labeled as the *MLSS workload.* Often the MLSS workload is compared with the individual's maximal workload and expressed as a percentage known as *MLSS intensity.*[41] Performances at the MLSS intensity result in a steady state for lactate; performances below this intensity show declining lactate values, and performances above this level exhibit progressively increasing lactate values. Extensive endurance performance cannot be completed above the MLSS, but portions of the event certainly may be.

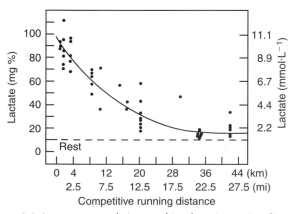

Figure 3-9 Lactate accumulation resulting from increasing distances of competitive running races. Blood lactate accumulation shows an inverse curvilinear relationship with distance in running races. (From Costill DL: *J Applied Physiol* 28(3):251-255, 1970.)

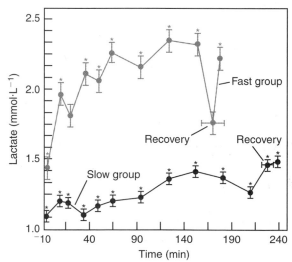

Figure 3-10 Blood lactate accumulation during the marathon. Blood lactate accumulation during a fast marathon (≤2 hours and 45 minutes) was greater than the accumulation during a slow marathon (≤3 hours and 45 minutes). The lactate levels for slow marathoners never exceeded normal resting levels, and the lactate levels for the fast marathoners barely exceeded normal resting levels. (From O'Brien MJ, Viguie CA, Mazzeo RS, et al: *Med Sci Sports Exercise* 25(9):1009-1017, 1993.)

Incremental Exercise to Maximum

Figure 3-11 depicts the accumulation of lactate during incremental exercise to maximum. The oxygen consumption (Figure 3-11, *A*) increases in a rectilinear pattern to meet the increasing demands for energy, but blood lactate (Figure 3-11, *B*) shows little initial change and then increases continuously.[42,43] These particular results are below the 8 mmol·L^{-1} generally considered to indicate a maximal test, however. As depicted, this pattern is best described as a positively accelerating exponential curve. Alternatively, the accumulation of lactate during incremental exercise can be depicted, as in Figure 3-12, as a rectilinear rise with two breakpoints or thresholds.

Since the early 1970s a great deal of attention has been paid to a concept that has been labeled variously as the *anaerobic threshold, ventilatory threshold(s),* or *lactate threshold(s).* The original concept of an anaerobic threshold is based on the lactate response to incremental exercise, as depicted in Figure 3-12, and the relationship of the lactate response to minute ventilation (the volume of air breathed each minute).

As espoused by Wasserman and colleagues,[44] the anaerobic threshold is defined as the exercise intensity, usually described as a percentage of V̇O$_2$max or workload, above which blood lactate levels rise and minute ventilation increases disproportionately in relation to oxygen consumption. The onset of anaerobic metabolism (or anaerobiosis), which is assumed to lead to the lactate accumulation, is attributed to the failure of the cardiovascular system to supply the oxygen required to the muscle tissue. The disproportionate rise in ventilation is attributed to excess carbon dioxide resulting from the buffering of the lactic acid.[45,46]

Theoretically, these interactions can occur as follows: Lactic acid is a strong acid and, as noted earlier, it readily dissociates into hydrogen ions (H$^+$) and lactate (La$^-$). Because an excess

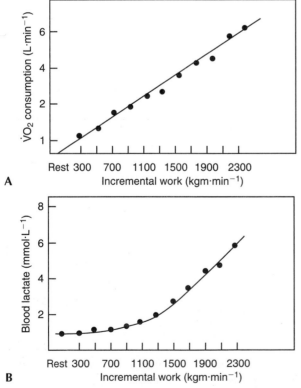

Figure 3-11 Changes in oxygen consumption and blood lactate as a function of a work rate. The rise in O$_2$ consumption is directly proportional to the increase in workload. Blood lactate levels show little change at low work rates and then increase continuously in a curvilinear pattern. (Modified from Hughes EF, Turner SC, Brooks GA: *J Applied Physiol* 52(6):1598-1607, 1982.)

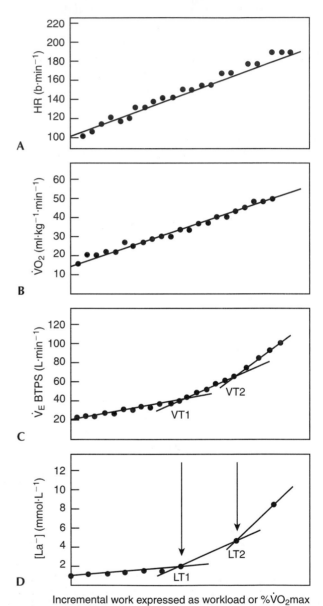

Figure 3-12 Ventilatory and lactate thresholds during incremental work to maximum. Both heart rate (**A**) and O$_2$ consumption (**B**) increase in direct rectilinear patterns during an incremental work task whether the work is expressed in terms of absolute workload or percentage of V̇O$_2$max. In contrast, both ventilation (**C**) and lactate (**D**) appear to exhibit two distinct breakpoints as they rise. The circumstance of VT$_1$ occurring at the same time as LT$_1$ and VT$_2$ occurring at the same time as LT$_2$ is coincidental. (From Plowman SA, Smith DL: *Exercise physiology for health, fitness, and performance,* ed 2, San Francisco, 2003, Benjamin Cummings.)

of hydrogen ions would change the pH (or acid-base balance) of the muscles and blood, the body attempts to bind these hydrogen ions to a chemical buffer. For example, sodium bicarbonate (a weak base) may be used as a buffer in the reaction:

$$NaHCO_3 + HLa \rightleftharpoons NaLa + H_2CO_3$$

sodium bicarbonate + lactic acid $\rightleftharpoons$ sodium lactate
+ carbonic acid

Carbonic acid is a much weaker acid than lactic acid and can be further dissociated into water and carbon dioxide:

$$H_2CO_3 \rightleftharpoons H_2O + CO_2$$

Carbon dioxide is a potent stimulant for respiration and can easily be removed from the body through respiration, thereby facilitating in the maintenance of pH.[47] The carbon dioxide thus formed is said to be nonmetabolic carbon dioxide because it does not result from the immediate breakdown of an energy substrate (carbohydrate, fat, or protein).

Figure 3-12 clearly shows that despite a continuous rectilinear rise in heart rate (Figure 3-12, *B*) during incremental work to maximum, there are distinct breaks from linearity in respiration (Figure 3-12, *C*). These breakpoints (Figure 3-12, *C*) have been labeled as *VT1* (the first ventilatory threshold) and *VT2* (the second ventilatory threshold). They were originally thought to result from corresponding lactate thresholds (labeled in Figure 3-12, *D*, as *LT1* and *LT2*, the first lactate threshold and the second lactate threshold) as a result of the buffering of lactic acid. The original work by Wasserman and others[44,45] postulated only one anaerobic threshold (which would

have been VT1 in Figure 3-12, *C*), but later work identified at least two thresholds, which were given various names.[48-50] The designations VT1, VT2, LT1, and LT2 are used here for simplicity and because no causal mechanism is implied.

The idea that the point of lactate accumulation can be determined noninvasively by respiratory values typically measured during laboratory exercise testing of oxygen consumption is appealing because few people truly enjoy having multiple blood samples taken. However, the terminology, determination, and mechanistic explanations are not without controversy.[52] Four concerns are discussed.

The primary concern is that the presence of lactate does not automatically mean that the oxygen supply is inadequate.[19,42] This fact was discussed at length earlier in this chapter. Lactate accumulation does not occur at the time of increased production; rather, it occurs when the turnover rate (or balance between production and removal) cannot keep up and appearance exceeds clearance.

Figure 3-13, *A*, shows this concept graphically for incremental exercise. That is, as the exercise and oxygen consumption increases, the rate of lactate appearance (R_a) in the muscle also increases (Figure 3-13, *B*). At low-intensity exercise the rate of lactate disappearance (R_d) does not differ much from R_a. However, as the intensity increases, the gap between R_a and R_d grows progressively wider. The result is the blood lactate

 NEW RESEARCH TRENDS

Seven collegiate female rowers participated in two incremental exercise bouts to maximum on a cycle ergometer. One trial (hydrated state-H) was preceded the night before by a 45-minute submaximal ride at a heart rate of 130 to 150 b·min⁻¹, during which the participants were allowed unlimited access to fluid. The other trial (dehydrated state-D) consisted of the same submaximal exercise, but the participants performed in a full sweat suit and were denied fluid until after the incremental test the next morning. Despite mild dehydration—associated with a net drop of 1.5% in body weight—a statistically significant shift occurred in the lactate threshold, defined as *LT1*, to a lower percentage of peak oxygen consumption (H = 72.2% vs. D = 65.5%). This was accompanied by a significant decrease in work performance both in terms of power output (H = 250 W vs. D = 235 W) and time to exhaustion (H = 17.3 minutes vs. D = 16.3 minutes). However, similar values were attained for maximal HR, oxygen consumption, and lactate. Thus it appears that dehydration (or failure to rehydrate adequately after exercise) alters the relative contributions of aerobic and anaerobic metabolism to an external workload and negatively affects performance.[51]

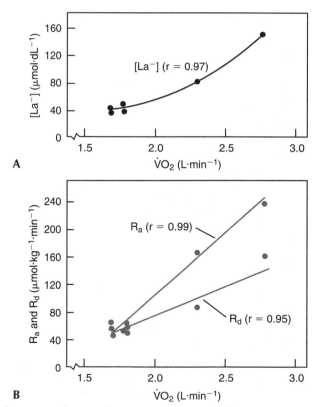

Figure 3-13 The rate of appearance (R_a), rate of disappearance (R_d), and resultant accumulation of lactate as a consequence of incremental exercise. The measured change in lactate concentration [La⁻] **(A)** is a result of a growing imbalance between the rate of appearance (R_a) and the rate of disappearance (R_d) **(B)** as exercise intensity increases. (From Brooks GA: *Med Sci Sports Exercise* 17(1):22-31, 1985.)

concentration [La⁻] depicted in Figure 3-13, *A*. Thus it is incorrect to label the appearance of elevated levels of lactic acid in the blood as representing an anaerobic threshold.

A second concern is exactly how to interpret the lactate response to incremental work. Look closely at the lactate patterns in Figures 3-11 and 3-12. Basically, the circles representing individual data points are the same. However, in Figure 3-12, lines are imposed on the data points that clearly indicate two breaks in the linearity, or two thresholds.[50] The same data points are described as an exponential curve in Figure 3-11. Experimental evidence and mathematical models[43] support the curvilinear interpretation. Nevertheless, the term *lactate threshold* continues to be used to indicate marked increases in the accumulation of lactate. The ventilatory thresholds are always considered to be true breakpoints.

A third concern involves carbon dioxide, which is involved in the control of respiration. An excess of hydrogen ions from a source such as lactic acid can cause an increase in the amount of carbon dioxide through the bicarbonate buffering system just described. However, the presence of lactic acid is not the only mechanism that can account for an increase in carbon dioxide or the concomitant increase in minute ventilation.[53] Evidence is particularly strong in McArdle's syndrome patients. McArdle's syndrome patients are deficient in the enzyme glycogen phosphorylase, which is necessary to convert glycogen to lactic acid. Thus no matter how hard these patients exercise, their lactic acid values remain negligible. On the other hand, their minute ventilation values have the same distinctive breakpoints shown by anyone not deficient in glycogen phosphorylase.[54] Thus something other than the accumulation of lactic acid must be operating to explain the ventilatory response.

Fourth, the lactate thresholds and the ventilatory thresholds do not change to the same extent in the same individuals as a result of training, glycogen depletion, caffeine ingestion, or varying pedaling rates.[42,55] If they were causally linked, they should change together.

Current theory therefore says that although lactic acid increases and ventilatory breaks or threshold often occur simultaneously, these responses are due to coincidence, not cause and effect.[9,52] Exactly what these various thresholds mean is still unknown.

Despite a lack of complete understanding of the lactate threshold, the amount of work an athlete can do before accumulating large amounts of lactate has a definite bearing on performance. Distance running performance, for example, depends to a large extent on some combination of $\dot{V}O_2$max, the oxygen cost of running at a given submaximal speed (called *economy*), and the ability to run at a high percentage of $\dot{V}O_2$max without a large accumulation of lactic acid.[56-58] An indication of the running speed that represents the optimal percentage of $\dot{V}O_2$max can be achieved by determining the lactate thresholds. The first lactate threshold (LT1) generally occurs between 40% and 60% of $\dot{V}O_2$max; the second (LT2) is generally more than 80% of $\dot{V}O_2$max and possibly as high as 95% of $\dot{V}O_2$max. LT1 is sometimes equated with a lactate concentration of 2 mmol·L^{-1} and LT2 with a lactate concentration of 4 mmol·L^{-1}. This 4 mmol·L^{-1} level, also called the *onset of blood lactate accumulation* (OBLA), is frequently used to decide both training loads and racing strategies.[48,59] Running at a pace that results in a continual accumulation of lactate has a detrimental effect on endurance time that is directly related to changes brought about by the lactate.

Dynamic Resistance Exercise

Lactate responses to dynamic resistance exercise vary greatly because the possible combination of exercises, repetitions, sets, and rest periods is almost endless. In addition, values are generally not taken repeatedly during the workout; instead, the most frequently reported values are simply postexercise ones. In general, postexercise lactate values have been shown to range from approximately 4 to 21 mmol·L^{-1}. The higher values result from high-volume, moderate-load, short rest period sequences and circuit-type exercise bouts.[60-64]

Table 3-2 summarizes the anaerobic metabolic exercise responses discussed in this section.

Why Is Lactic Acid Accumulation a Problem?

Hydrogen ions (H^+) that dissociate from lactic acid, rather than undissociated lactic acid or lactate (La⁻), present the primary problems to the body. This distinction is important because of the almost complete and immediate dissociation of lactic acid

Table 3-2	Lactic Anaerobic Exercise Response				
Short-Term, Light to Moderate, Submaximal Exercise	Short-Term, Moderate to Heavy, Submaximal Exercise	Long-Term, Moderate to Heavy, Submaximal Exercise	Short-Term, High-Intensity, Supramaximal Exercise	Incremental Exercise to Maximum	Dynamic Resistance Exercise
≤ 2 mmol·L^{-1}	≈4-6 mmol·L^{-1}	Depends on relationship to MLSS	Large increase; interval may to go 32 mmol·L^{-1}	Positive exponential curve; LT1 ≈2 mmol·L^{-1}; LT2 ≈4 mmol·L^{-1}; max = >8 mmol·L^{-1}	4-21 mmol·L^{-1}; greatest with high volume and circuit type

LT1, Lactate threshold 1; *MLSS,* maximal lactate steady state.

to H^+ and La^- $(C_3H_5O_3^-)$.[9,19] As long as the amount of free H^+ does not exceed the ability of the chemical and physiological mechanisms to buffer them and maintain the pH at a relatively stable level, there are few problems. Most problems arise when the amount of lactic acid—and hence H^+—exceeds the body's immediate buffering capacity and pH decreases.[19] The blood has become more acidic. At that point pain is perceived and performance suffers. The mechanisms of these results are described in the following subsections.

Pain

Anyone who has raced or run the 400-m distance all out understands the pain associated with lactic acid. Such an event takes between approximately 45 seconds and 3 minutes (depending on the ability of the runner) and relies heavily on the ATP-PC and LA systems to supply the needed energy. The resultant hydrogen ions accumulate and stimulate pain nerve endings located in the muscle.[65]

Performance Decrement

The decrement in performance associated with lactic acid is brought about by fatigue that is both metabolic and muscular in origin.

1. Metabolic fatigue results from reduced production of ATP linked to enzyme changes, changes in membrane transport mechanisms, and changes in substrate availability.

    Enzymes, particularly the rate-limiting enzymes in the metabolic pathways, can be inactivated by high hydrogen ion concentrations (low pH). The hydrogen ion attaches to these enzyme molecules and in so doing changes their size, shape, and hence ability to function. Phosphofructokinase (PFK) is thought to be particularly sensitive, although oxidative enzymes can also be affected.[66]

    At the same time, changes occur in membrane transport mechanisms (either to the carriers in the membrane or to the permeability channels). These changes affect the movement of molecules across the cell membrane and between the cytoplasm and organelles such as the mitochondria.[66]

    Energy substrate availability can be inhibited by a high concentration of hydrogen ions. Glycogen breakdown is slowed by the inactivation of the enzyme glycogen phosphorylase. Fatty acid utilization is decreased because lactic acid inhibits mobilization. Thus a double-jeopardy situation is evident. With fatty acid availability low, a greater reliance is placed on carbohydrate sources at the time when glycogen breakdown is inhibited. At the same time, phosphocreatine (PC) breakdown is accelerated, leading to a faster depletion of substrate for ATP regeneration.[2,66,67]

    Thus both the inactivation of enzymes and the decrement in substrate availability lead to a reduction in the production of ATP and, ultimately, a decrement in performance.

2. Muscular fatigue is evidenced by reduced force and velocity of muscle contraction. A lowered pH can have two major effects on muscle contraction. The first is an inhibition of actomyosin ATPase, the enzyme responsible for the breakdown of ATP to provide the immediate energy for muscle contraction. The second is an interference of H^+ with the actions and uptake of calcium (Ca^{++}) that is necessary for the excitation-contraction coupling and relaxation of the protein crossbridges within the muscle fiber. High levels of lactate ions (La^-) may also interfere with crossbridging.[19,68] The result of these actions is a decrease in both the force a muscle can exert and the velocity of muscle contraction.

Time Frame for Lactate Removal

Lactate is removed from the bloodstream relatively rapidly following exercise.[69] However, removal does not occur at a constant rate. If it did, then higher levels of lactate would take proportionately longer to dissipate than lower levels. For example, if a person could do one pushup in 2 seconds and could not change that rate or speed, then 10 pushups would take twice as long to do as 5 pushups (20 versus 10 seconds). On the other hand, if the person could change that rate, he or she might be able to do 10 pushups in the same time as 5 were done (in 10 seconds). Many chemical reactions have this ability to change the rate or speed at which they occur. That is, the rate is proportional to the amount of substrate and product present. The more substrate available and the less product, the faster the reaction proceeds, and vice versa. This characteristic is called the mass action effect. Lactate appears to be one of those substrates whose utilization and conversion is linked with the amount of substrate present.[70]

Thus despite wide interindividual differences (which may be related to muscle fiber type), in a resting recovery situation approximately half of the lactate is removed in about 15 to 25 minutes no matter what the starting level is. This time is called the *half-life of lactate*. Near-resting levels are achieved in about 30 to 60 minutes, regardless of the starting level. Thus the initial postexercise concentration of lactate is the first factor that influences the rate of removal. The higher the concentration, the faster the rate of removal is.[68,70,71]

Figure 3-14 shows typical resting recovery curves from cycling and running studies. Note that in each case the value close to 50% (shown in parentheses) of the initial postexercise lactate levels occurs between 15 and 25 minutes of recovery.

The second factor that determines the rate of lactate removal is whether the individual follows a rest (passive) recovery or an exercise (active) recovery regimen. Third, if an exercise recovery is employed, the intensity of the exercise (expressed as a percentage of $\dot{V}O_2max$) makes a difference. Fourth, the modality of the exercise employed in the recovery phase may influence the optimal percentage of $\dot{V}O_2max$ at which removal occurs. Finally, whether the recovery exercise is continuous or intermittent seems to make a difference.

Evidence suggests that lactate removal occurs more quickly when an individual exercises during recovery than when he or she rests by sitting quietly.[60] Figure 3-15 shows the results of a study conducted by Bonen and Belcastro[73] in which six

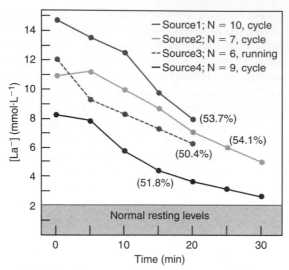

Figure 3-14 The time course of lactate removal during resting recovery from exercise. During resting recovery from exercise, lactate exhibits a half-life of 15 to 25 minutes. (From Plowman SA, Smith DL: *Exercise physiology for health, fitness, and performance*, ed 2, San Francisco, 2003, Benjamin Cummings. Based on data from Bonen A, Campbell CJ, Kirby RL, et al: *Pflugers Arch* 380:205-210, 1979; Belcastro AN, Bonen A: *J Appl Physiol* 39:932-936, 1975; Bonen A, Belcastro AN: *Med Sci Sports Exerc* 8:176-178, 1976; McGrail JC, Bonen A, Belcastro AN: *Eur J Appl Physiol* 39:87-97, 1978.)

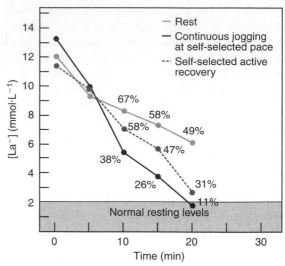

Figure 3-15 Lactate removal in active versus passive recovery. Lactate removal is faster under active than passive conditions, although the magnitude of the benefit of active recovery depends on the type and intensity of the activity. In this study, continuous jogging at 61.4% maximal oxygen uptake was more effective than a mixture of walking, jogging, and calisthenics. (From Plowman SA, Smith DL: *Exercise physiology for health, fitness, and performance*, ed 2, San Francisco, 2003, Benjamin Cummings. Based on data from Bonen A, Campbell CJ, Kirby RL, et al: *Pflugers Arch* 380:205-210, 1979.)

trained runners completed a mile run on three different occasions. In randomized order they then performed three different 20-minute recoveries: (1) seated rest, (2) continuous jogging at a self-selected pace, and (3) self-selected active recovery. During self-selected active recovery the subjects did calisthenics, walked, jogged, and rested for variable portions of the total time.

As shown in Figure 3-15, after 5 minutes there is no appreciable difference in the level of lactate between the different recovery protocols. However, over the next 15 minutes the level of lactate removal was significantly faster for the jogging recovery than for either the self-selected active recovery or the rest recovery. The self-selected activity (which is what you would typically see athletes doing at a track meet), although not as good as continuous jogging (in part because it was intermittent), was still significantly better than resting recovery.

After 20 minutes of jogging recovery, the lactate that remained was within the normal resting levels of 1 to 2 mmol·L^{-1}. The self-selected active recovery had removed 70% of the lactate, but the resting recovery had only removed 50% of the lactate. Thus full recovery was, and generally is, delayed if a seated rest is employed. Because athletes who run the distances from 400 to 1500 m (440 yards to 1 mile) often double at track meets, such a delay could impair their performances in the second event. On the basis of these results, an athlete competing or training at distances that are likely to cause large accumulations of lactic acid should cool down with an active continuous recovery.

Why does activity increase the rate of lactate removal? The rate of lactate removal by the liver appears to be the same

whether an individual is resting or exercising. However, during exercise blood flow is increased, as is the oxidation of lactate by skeletal and cardiac muscles.[3,60,68,72,74] These changes appear to be primarily responsible for the beneficial effects of an active recovery.

At what intensity should an active recovery be performed? Studies that have attempted to answer this question have found an inverted U-shaped response.[68,72] That is, up to a point, a higher intensity of exercise (as measured by percentage of $\dot{V}O_2$max) during recovery is better. But after that point, as the intensity continues to rise, the removal rate decreases. This pattern is depicted in Figure 3-16, where the curve is both an inverted U-shape and skewed toward the lower $\dot{V}O_2$max percentage values, with the optimal rate being between 29% and 45% of $\dot{V}O_2$max. These data were collected after cycle ergometer rides. Data collected for track and treadmill exercises show the same type of inverted U-shaped curve response, but in the 55% to 70% $\dot{V}O_2$max range.[68,72] This difference in optimal intensity may be a function of the modality (there is a higher static component for the cycle ergometer than for running) or of the training status of the subjects tested.

The actual value of these optimal percentages should not be surprising. The first lactate threshold has been shown to occur between 40% and 60% of $\dot{V}O_2$max and may be higher in trained individuals. Thus it appears that the optimal intensity for recovery would be just below an individual's lactate threshold, where lactate production is minimal but clearance is maximized.

A cautionary note is that although an active recovery is best for lactate removal, it can delay glycogen resynthesis by further depleting glycogen stores.[75] This has more relevance for an

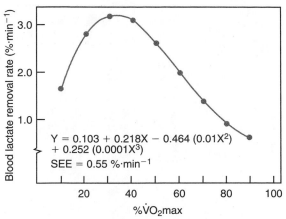

$$Y = 0.103 + 0.218X - 0.464 (0.01X^2) + 0.252 (0.0001X^3)$$
$$SEE = 0.55 \%\cdot min^{-1}$$

Figure 3-16 Lactate removal rate as a function of the percentage of maximal oxygen uptake in recovery exercise for cycling. Lactic acid removal rates during controlled and uncontrolled recovery exercise. (From Plowman SA, Smith DL: *Exercise physiology for health, fitness, and performance,* ed 2, San Francisco, 2003, Benjamin Cummings. Modified from Belcastro AN, Bonen A: *J Applied Physiol* 39(6):932-936, 1975.)

individual attempting to recover from a hard interval-training session than for someone just completing a middle-distance race and preparing for another. Glycogen depletion is likely to be more severe in the former case, and getting rid of the lactate quickly is more of an immediate concern in the latter case. For athletes recovering from an interval training session or competing in heats on successive days, the best procedure may be to combine an initial dynamic active recovery (just to the point of regaining a near-resting heart rate) with stretching and then engage in a passive recovery during which carbohydrates are consumed.

Tests of Anaerobic Power and Capacity

When measuring the anaerobic systems, one would ideally have a test that could distinctly evaluate alactic anaerobic power, alactic anaerobic capacity, lactic anaerobic power, and lactic anaerobic capacity. Because no such tests exist, attempts have been made to get this information indirectly by measuring (1) the total mechanical power generated during high-intensity, short-duration work; (2) the amount of mechanical work done in a specific period of time; or (3) the time required to perform a given amount of presumably anaerobic work.[76] The most commonly used laboratory test is the Wingate Anaerobic Test (WAT).[36,76,77] The WAT is an all-out cycle ergometer ride for 30 seconds against a resistance based on body weight. Both arm and leg versions are available, although the leg test is most frequently used. Three variables are typically calculated: peak power (PP), mean power, and fatigue. PP is defined as the maximal power (force times distance divided by time) exerted during very short-duration (≤5 seconds) work. Originally, peak power was thought to reflect only alactic processes—alactic anaerobic capacity, in particular. However, subsequent research has shown that muscle lactate levels rise to high values as early as 10 seconds into such high-intensity work. This result indicates that glycolytic processes are occur-

ring almost immediately with ATP-PC breakdown. Therefore peak power cannot be interpreted as being only alactic.[77] Mean power (MP) is defined as the average power exerted during short-duration (typically 30 seconds) work. It can be expressed in both absolute (Watts; W) and relative (Watts per body weight; $W\cdot kg^{-1}$) units. Mean power is sometimes said to represent lactic anaerobic capacity, although this has not been substantiated.[78] The fatigue index (FI) is the percentage of peak power drop-off during high-intensity, short-duration work.

Stair climb tests[36,78] and sprint and middle distance runs are also often used to test the anaerobic systems. For example, dashes of 40, 50, or 60 yards or m take approximately 4 to 15 seconds and can be used as an indication of alactic anaerobic power or capacity, or both. Longer runs, probably between 200 and 800 m (or 220 and 880 yards) and lasting 40 to 120 seconds, can be used as an indication of lactic anaerobic power and capacity. Faster speeds in covering a given distance would indicate higher anaerobic power or capacity, or both.

ANAEROBIC EXERCISE CHARACTERISTICS OF CHILDREN

The anaerobic characteristics of children are not as well developed as those of adults. Furthermore, children do not tend to be the metabolic specialists that adults are. For example, one would not expect Asafa Powell (world record holder in the 100-m dash, with a time of 9.77 set in 2005) to do well at the marathon distance or Paula Radcliffe (who set the women's marathon record at 2:15:25 in 2003) to be successful at the sprint distances. Yet when children are at play, more often than not, the fastest at short distances or strength-type events also do well at long distances or in aerobic-type games such as soccer. Although much research is still necessary to explain the anaerobic differences between children and adults, some patterns are apparent.[79]

The Availability and Utilization of ATP-PC

Local resting stores of ATP per kilogram of wet muscle weight appear to be the same for children and adults.[30] Levels of resting PC per kilogram of wet muscle weight have been reported as slightly lower in children[79,80] or no different from adult levels.[80,81] The rate of utilization of these reserves during exercise does not differ. However, because children are smaller in stature than adults, the total amount of energy that can be generated from this source is lower.

The Accumulation of Lactate

On average, blood lactate values obtained during submaximal exercise and after maximal exercise are lower in children than in adults.[79,81,82] Furthermore, peak lactate values after maximal exercise exhibit a relatively positive rectilinear increase with age until adulthood. Figure 3-17 depicts this relationship and shows that there is no meaningful sex difference in children in the ability to accumulate lactate, although the girls' values are

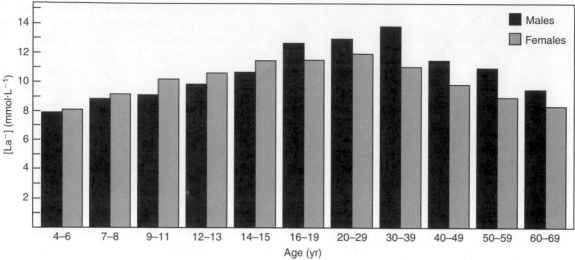

Figure 3-17 Lactate values after maximal exercise as a function of age and sex. (From Plowman SA, Smith DL: *Exercise physiology for health, fitness, and performance*, ed 2, San Francisco, 2003, Benjamin Cummings. Computed mean value data for 4 to 20 year olds from Eriksson BO: *Acta Physiol Scand (Suppl)* 384:1-48,1972. Cumming GR, Hastman L, McCort J: Treadmill endurance times, blood lactate, and exercise blood pressures in normal children In Binkhorst RA, Kemper HCG, Saris WHM, editors: *Children and exercise XI*, pp. 140-150, Champaign, Ill, 1985, Human Kinetics; Saris WHM, Noordeloos AM, Ringnalda BEM, et al: Reference values for aerobic power of healthy 4 to 18 year old Dutch children: preliminary results. In Binkhorst RA, Kemper HCG, Saris WHM, editors: *Children and exercise XI*, pp. 151-160, Champaign, Ill, 1985, Human Kinetics; Astrand P-O, Engstrom BO, Eriksson O, et al: *Acta Paediatr (Suppl)* 147:1-73, 1963. Computed mean data for 20 to 60 year olds from Bouhuys A, Pool J, Binkhorst RA, et al: *J Appl Physiol* 21:1040-1046, 1966; Sidney KH, Shephard RJ: *J Appl Physiol Resp Environ Exerc Physiol* 43:280-287, 1977; Astrand I: *Acta Physiol Scand (Suppl)* 169:1-92, 1960; Robinson S: *Arbeitsphysiol* 10:251-323, 1938; Astrand P-O: *Experimental studies of physical working capacity in relation to sex and age*, Copenhagen, 1952, Munksgaard.)

slightly higher than the boys' values throughout the growth period.

The Lactate Threshold(s)

The phenomenon of ventilatory breakpoints and lactate accumulation is seen in children, as well as in adults.[91] Because children do not use anaerobic metabolism as early in work as adults do, the work level of children at the fixed lactate level of 4 mmol·L⁻¹ is relatively higher than that of adults.[92,93] Williams et al[94] report a value of almost 92% of $\dot{V}O_2$max for 4 mmol·L⁻¹ of lactate in 11- to 13-year-old boys and girls. Values for adults tend to be about 15% below this value. Thus the child is working relatively harder (at a higher %$\dot{V}O_2$max) than the adult at the same lactate level. Consequently, the assessment of exercise capacity and the monitoring of training by a 4 mmol·L⁻¹ value is inappropriate in prepubertal children.

Mechanical Power and Capacity

Peak power and peak power per kilogram of body weight have consistently been shown to be lower in prepubertal boys and girls than in adolescents or young adults when evaluated by a stair climb test. The results are similar to those for the WAT, although there is a lack of information on females for the WAT except for isolated ages (10 to 13 years).[95-97] In boys peak power and mean power increase consistently from age 10 to adulthood (Figure 3-18). This is true whether the values are expressed in absolute terms (watts) or are corrected for body weight (watts per kilogram). The absolute differences between children and adults, however, are much greater (children can achieve only about 30% of adult values) than the relative differences (children can achieve about 60% to 85% of the adult values). Peak values seem to occur in the late 30s for the legs and the late 20s for the arms.[43,98]

Data are available to compare boys and girls on peak power from a variation of an all-out cycle ergometer test called the *force-velocity test*.[99-101] The results of the most comprehensive study in terms of age range are shown in Figure 3-19. These results indicate that from ages 7 to 16 girls increased peak power by 273% and then plateaued between ages 16 and 17. Boys' results increased by 375% between ages 7 and 17. Sex differences were not apparent in peak power until age 14.[99]

Mechanisms

Several theories have been postulated to explain children's inability to function at a high level anaerobically. All of these ideas are based on two assumptions: the children tested put forth a maximal effort, and there is a physiological cause for the observed differences.

Muscle Enzymes

Eriksson et al[81] have shown that resting phosphofructokinase (PFK) activity in 11- to 13-year-old boys is considerably lower than in trained or sedentary adult men. Because PFK is a rate-limiting enzyme of glycolysis, this lowered activity may be

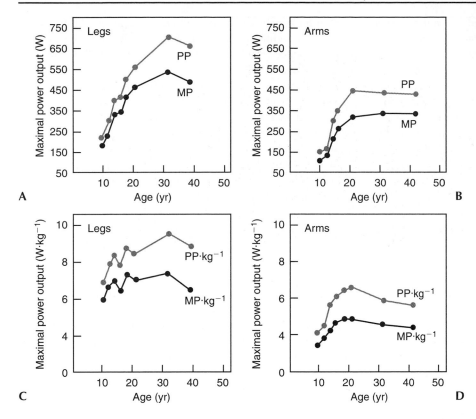

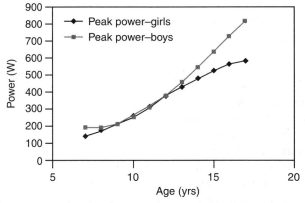

Figure 3-18 The effect of age on anaerobic performance. Cross-sectional data on 306 males who performed both arm and leg Wingate Anaerobic Tests. The pattern of increase in values from childhood to young adulthood is similar for leg (**A** and **C**) and arm (**B** and **D**) cycling whether the unit of measurement is absolute (**A** and **B**) or relative (**C** and **D**). (From Inbar O, Bar-Or O: *Med Sci Sports Exercise* 19(3):264-269, 1986.)

indicative of a decreased ability to produce lactic acid. In addition, the availability and the utilization of glycogen as a substrate are both lower in children than in adults. However, other glycolytic enzymes, such as lactic dehydrogenase (the enzyme involved in the conversion of pyruvic acid to lactic acid), have just the opposite response; that is, the highest level of activity has been seen in 12- to 14-year-old boys.[102] Therefore no definitive conclusion can be made about the role of the glycolytic enzymes.

In general, the oxidative enzymes show higher activity in young children than in older individuals.[94,103] This result, along with higher mitochondrial density and intracellular lipids, means that lipid utilization is greater in the child. Thus it may be that children have a finer balance between aerobic and anaerobic metabolism than adults. Additional evidence for this observation comes from the fact that children show a lower oxygen deficit and reach a steady state faster than adults.[80,90,93]

Muscle Characteristics

Several muscle characteristics have been suggested as explaining the lower anaerobic function in children and adolescents than adults. These include muscle fiber differentiation, contractile properties, muscle fiber size, muscle size, and muscle mass.[30]

The development of muscle fiber type distribution continues from birth to approximately 6 years old, when the individual achieves his or her profile of ST and FT fibers. However, the relative proportion of FOG and FG fibers continues to change through late adolescence. Typically there is a greater predominance of FOG than FG fibers during childhood and

Figure 3-19 Peak power by age in boys and girls. Force-velocity test results indicate that both boys and girls increase the production of peak power from 7 to approximately 17 years of age. Sex differences are not apparent until age 14, when boys' peak power production increased more than girls'. (Based on data from Martin RJF, Dore E, Twisk J, et al: *Med Sci Sports Exerc* 36:498-503, 2004.)

adolescence, and boys develop greater FG area than girls as they mature. The contractile properties of FG fibers favor force and power expression.

Muscle fiber size, measured as diameter, and muscle size, measured as cross-sectional area, both increase rectilinearly with age from birth to young adulthood. Assuming a parallel neural adaptation to recruit and activate more motor units, muscle force changes closely parallel changes in cross-sectional area, and these power changes during growth favor boys over girls after puberty. However, when normalized for muscle cross-sectional area, age and sex differences in force disappear.

Finally, total muscle mass is directly related to the ability to generate force/power. As the child grows, obviously so does his or her total muscle mass. However, even normalized for muscle mass, force production is lower in children and adolescents than adults.[30] Body composition changes (more total muscle mass, less fat for boys) favor males in force production.[95]

Sexual Maturation

Limited evidence suggests that the increase in glycolytic capacity (and hence the production of lactate) in children is related to the hormonal changes that occur to bring about sexual maturation.[30,94] In particular, testosterone is thought to have a role.

Neurohormonal Regulation

Sympathetic nervous system activity is significantly lower in children than in adults at maximal exercise. One result of sympathetic stimulation during exercise is hepatic vasoconstriction. The liver plays a major role in the clearance of lactate. If blood flow to the liver is reduced, not as much lactate is cleared. Thus because the child maintains a higher liver blood flow, more lactate can be cleared. This implies that children are not deficient in the production of lactate but can better remove or reconvert it than can adults.[82,103,104]

Which of these theories—muscle enzymes, muscle characteristics, sexual maturation, neurohormonal regulation, or a combination—is correct remains to be shown.

MALE VERSUS FEMALE ANAEROBIC EXERCISE CHARACTERISTICS

The anaerobic characteristics of females are in general lower than those of males during the young and middle-aged adult years. Much of the difference is undoubtedly related to the smaller overall muscle mass of the average female compared with that of the average male.[105]

The Availability and Utilization of Adenosine Triphosphate–Phosphocreatine

Neither the local resting stores of ATP per kilogram of muscle nor the utilization of ATP-PC during exercise varies between the sexes.[13,69] However, in terms of total energy available from these phosphagen sources, males exceed females because of muscle mass differences.

Accumulation of Lactate

Resting levels of lactate are the same for males and females. Lactate thresholds, when expressed as a percentage of $\dot{V}O_2$max, are also the same for both sexes, although the absolute workload at which the lactate thresholds occur is higher for males

than for females. Thus at any given absolute workload that is still submaximal but above LT1 or LT2, females have a higher lactate value than males. Consequently, the workload is more stressful for females and requires a greater anaerobic contribution. However, at a given relative workload or percentage of $\dot{V}O_2$max above the lactate thresholds, lactate concentrations are equal for both sexes.[105]

Lactate values at maximal exercise from ages 16 through 50 are higher by approximately 0.5 to 2 $mmol\cdot L^{-1}$ for males than for females (see Figure 3-17). Once again, females are generally doing less in terms of an absolute workload than males at maximum.

The accumulation of lactate during maximal exercise presents a special dilemma for nursing mothers. A portion of the lactate present in blood diffuses into breast milk and remains present for at least 90 minutes.[106,107] Infants have fully developed taste buds at birth and can detect sour tastes such as that produced by lactic acid. In fact, some infants have reportedly rejected postexercise milk that contained lactic acid.[106] If a nursing mother finds that her infant fusses or refuses to nurse after she has exercised, she can try one of several things. The first option is to feed the baby just before exercising or collect the milk at that time and store it for later feeding. The second possibility is to discard postexercise milk and implement supplemental feeding. The third possibility is to experiment with lower-intensity workouts that may not lead to a substantial lactate accumulation. Indeed, lactating women participating in a moderate submaximal aerobic exercise program (60% to 70% heart rate reserve, progressing from 20 to 45 $min\cdot d^{-1}$, 5 $d\cdot wk^{-1}$ for 12 weeks) did not report any difficulties nursing after exercise.[108] A later study that investigated maximal exercise and 30-minute exercise sessions at LT1 and 20% below LT1 confirmed that the appearance of lactate in breast milk is a function of exercise intensity. Milk lactate levels were significantly higher following maximal and LT1 threshold intensity exercise, but not the LT1-20% intensity sessions, when compared with nonexercise control values. LT1-20% represents moderate exercise that was performed at a rate of perceived exertion of 12. Infant acceptance of postexercise milk was not directly reported in this study, but the role of lactate in infant rejection of milk in the previously described study was questioned.[109]

Mechanical Power and Capacity

As previously mentioned, on average males produce higher absolute work output than females. Data available from the WAT show that values for peak power for women are approximately 65% of values for men if expressed in watts, improve to 83% if expressed in watts per kilogram of body weight, and come close to 94% when expressed in watts per kilogram of lean body mass. The corresponding comparisons for mean power are 68%, 87%, and 98%, respectively. The peak power of women (in watts per kilogram of body weight) is similar to the mean power of men. The fatigue index does not show a significant sex difference, indicating that both sexes tire at the same rate.[110]

Mechanisms

The key to these male-female anaerobic differences lies in the muscle. The same factors implicated in the mechanisms for differences between maturing boys and girls operate between adult males and females. The young male adds muscle during maturation under the influence of testosterone, whereas the young female is adding fat under the influence of estrogen. Therefore both absolutely and relatively, the male has greater muscle mass than the female.[111] In addition, muscle fiber size (especially FT) is typically larger in males than in females.

ANAEROBIC EXERCISE CHARACTERISTICS OF OLDER ADULTS

Evidence detailing anaerobic characteristics in the elderly is scarce. The reason is undoubtedly a combination of caution on the part of researchers and uncertain motivation on the part of subjects when faced with the necessarily high-intensity exercise. What data are available indicate that anaerobic variables show a common aging pattern; that is, there is typically a peak in the second or third decade and then a gradual decline into the sixth decade. Despite this, the elderly can still participate successfully in basically anaerobic activities. One must always remember when interpreting aging results, however, that no one knows how much of the reduction is a direct result of aging, how much is the result of detraining that accompanies the reduced activity level of the elderly, and how much is the result of disease.

Availability and Utilization of Adenosine Triphosphate–Phosphocreatine

Local resting stores of ATP-PC are reduced and levels of creatine and ADP are elevated in muscles of the elderly.[92] Results from a stair climb test have shown a reduction in ATP-PC power of as much as 45% and a reduction in ATP-PC capacity of 32% from youth to old age.[80] This means that ATP-PC stores are both reduced and unable to be utilized as quickly. The result is a decrease in alactic anaerobic power.

Accumulation of Lactate

On average, resting levels of blood lactate are remarkably consistent across the entire age span, varying only from 1 to 2 $mmol \cdot L^{-1}$.

Lactate values during the same absolute submaximal work tend to be higher for individuals older than the age of 50.[88-90,112] However, this generalization is confounded by the fact that at any given absolute load of work, the older individual is working at a higher percentage of his or her maximal aerobic power, which would be expected to involve anaerobic metabolism more.[87] When younger and older individuals work at the same relative workload (%$\dot{V}O_2$max), lactate concentrations are lower in older people than in the young, probably because the elderly are using less muscle mass to do less

work.[113] Maximal lactate levels reach a peak between 16 and 39 years of age and then show a gradual decline (see Figure 3-17). Both males and females exhibit the same pattern, with the absolute values of females being considerable lower than those of males.

Lactate Threshold(s)

Although individuals continue to exhibit at least one lactate threshold as they age, the point at which this is evident, expressed as %$\dot{V}O_2$max, appears to shift to a higher value in both sexes. In a study of 111 male and 57 female runners from 40 to 70 years of age, the lactate threshold increased from approximately 65% to 75% across the decades. In addition, there is some controversy about the value of the LT to predict endurance performance in this age group.[114]

Mechanical Power and Capacity

The average peak power value obtained on a stair climb test declines precipitously over the 20- to 70-year-old age range.[35] Published results are unavailable for the WAT for individuals older than the age of 40 and for females except in the 18- to 28-year-old range.[115] However, Makrides et al[110] have presented data on 50 male and 50 female subjects from 15 to 70 years old on a test similar to the WAT (Figure 3-20). In this case peak power represents an instantaneous value rather than a 5-second value. Mean power is still the average of 30 seconds of pedaling but at a controlled rate of 60 $rev \cdot min^{-1}$. The results from this study show a decline of approximately 6% for each decade of age for sedentary individuals of both sexes. However, the absolute values for the females are consistently lower than those for the males. Indeed, in the Makrides et al study the peak power of the females coincides with the mean power of the males. For both sexes lean thigh volume was found to be closely related to peak power and mean power, but it did not account for all the variation in the values or in the decline with age.

An analysis of weight lifting (e.g., snatch, clean and jerk) and power lifting (e.g., dead lift, squat, bench press) records for males and females from 40 to 70 years old showed declines in anaerobic muscular performance. The decline was greatest (and curvilinear) in the weight lifting tasks that required not only explosive coordinated movements but also high-balance skills. The decline in weight lifting was higher in females ($\approx-70\%$) than males ($\approx-50\%$). The overall decline in the power lifts was rectilinear and similar in males ($\approx-40\%$) and females ($\approx-50\%$).[116]

Mechanisms

Undoubtedly, muscle mass is lost with age. Between the ages of 30 and 70 years almost 25% of muscle mass is lost in both males and females.[117] Obviously, the loss of muscle mass leads to a concomitant loss in force and power production. In addition, as individuals age the percentage of FT muscle fibers, particularly FG fibers, decreases. With this shift there is a decline

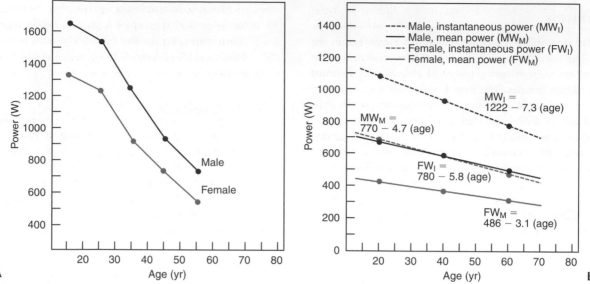

Figure 3-20 Mechanical power changes with age in males and females. **A,** Average peak power ratings determined from the Margaria-Kalamen stair climb test are higher for males than females across the age span from adolescence to middle adulthood. Males and females show steady and parallel declines in peak power during the adult years. **B,** Instantaneous peak power and mean power measured during a 30-second cycle test are higher for males (MW_1 and MW_M, respectively) than for females (FW_1 and FW_M, respectively) across the age span from late adolescence to older adulthood. Female instantaneous peak power (FW_1) is equal to male mean power (MW_M). Instantaneous peak power and mean power show rectilinear and parallel declines with age in males and females. Each line was calculated from the experimentally determined equations associated with that line on the graph. (From Plowman SA, Smith DL: *Exercise physiology for health, fitness, and performance*, ed 2, San Francisco, 2003, Benjamin Cummings. **A,** Based on data from Bouchard C, Taylor AW, Simoneau JA, et al: Testing anaerobic power and capacity. In MacDougall JD, Wenger HW, Green HJ, editors: *Physiological testing of the high-performance athlete*, pp. 61-73, Hamilton, Ontario, 1982, Canadian Association of Sports Sciences Mutual Press Limited. **B,** Based on data from Makrides L, Heigenhauser GJF, McCartney N, et al: *Clin Sci* 69:197-205, 1985.)

in potential glycolytic function and force production. Finally, neural activation and integration declines with age. Thus moves requiring high levels of coordination are at risk.[116,118]

REFERENCES

1. Gollnick PD, King DW: Energy release in the muscle cell, *Med Sci Sport Exerc* 1:23-31, 1969.

2. Astrand P-O, Rodahl K, Dahl HA, et al: *Textbook of work physiology: physiological bases of exercise*, ed 4, Champaign, Ill, 2003, Human Kinetics.

3. Gollnick PD, Hermansen L: Biochemical adaptations to exercise: anaerobic metabolism. In Wilmore JH, editor: *Exercise and sport sciences reviews*, pp. 1-43, New York, 1973, Academic Press.

4. Brooks GA, Fahey TD, White TP, et al: *Exercise physiology: human bioenergetics and its applications*, ed 3, Mountain View, Calif, 1999, Mayfield.

5. American College of Sports Medicine Roundtable: The physiological and health effects of oral creatine supplementation, *Med Sci Sports Exerc* 32:706-717, 2000.

6. Zoller RF, Angelopoulou TJ: Creatine supplementation and exercise performance, *ACSM's Certified News* 8(2): 1-4, 1998.

7. Misic MM, Kelley GA: The impact of creatine supplementation on anaerobic performance: a meta-analysis, *Am J Med Sports* 4:116-124, 2002.

8. Poortmans JR, Francaux M: Adverse effects of creatine supplementation: fact or fiction? *Sports Med* 30:155-170, 2000.

9. Brooks GA: Anaerobic threshold: review of the concept and directions for future research, *Med Sci Sports Exerc* 17:22-31, 1985.

10. Newsholm EA, Leech AR: *Biochemistry for the medical sciences*, New York, 1983, Wiley.

11. Fox EL: Measurement of the maximal lactic (phosphagen) capacity in man, *Med Sci Sports Exerc* (abstract) 5:66,1973.

12. Spriet LL, Howlett RA, Heigenhauser GJF: An enzymatic approach to lactate production in human skeletal muscle during exercise, *Med Sci Sports Exerc* 32:756-763, 2000.

13. Brooks GA: The lactate shuttle during exercise and recovery, *Med Sci Sports Exerc* 18:360-368, 1986.

14. Gaesser GA, Brooks GA: Muscular efficiency during steady-rate exercise: effects of speed and work rate, *J Appl Physiol* 38:1132-1139, 1975.

15. Green HJ: Muscle power: fiber type recruitment, metabolism and fatigue. In Jones NL, McCartney M, McComas AJ, editors: *Human muscle power*, pp. 65-79, Champaign, Ill, 1986, Human Kinetics.

16. Houston ME: *Biochemistry primer for exercise science*, Champaign, Ill, 1995, Human Kinetics.

17. Stallknecht B, Vissing J, Galbo H: Lactate production and clearance in exercise: effects of training. A mini-review, *Scand J Med Sci Sports* 8:127-131, 1998.

18. Brooks GA: Lactate shuttles in nature, *Biochem Soc Trans* 30:258-264, 2000.

19. Gladden LB: Lactate metabolism: a new paradigm for the third millennium, *J Physiol* 558:5-30, 2004.

20. Brooks GA: Intra-and extra-cellular lactate shuttles, *Med Sci Sports Exerc* 32:790-799, 2000.

21. Brooks GA: Lactate shuttle—between but not within cells? *J Physiol* 541:333-334, 2000.

22. Rasmussen HN, van Hall G, Rasmussen UF: Lactate dehydrogenase is not a mitochondrial enzyme in human and mouse vastus lateralis muscle, *J Physiol* 541:575-580, 2002.

23. Sahlin K, Fernstrom M, Svensson M, et al: No evidence of an intracellular lactate shuttle in rat skeletal muscle, *J Physiol* 541:569-574, 2002.

24. Chatham JC: Lactate—the forgotten fuel! *J Physiol* 542:333, 2002.

25. Donovan CM, Pagliasotti MJ: Quantitative assessment of pathways for lactate disposal in skeletal muscle fiber types, *Med Sci Sports Exerc* 32:772-777, 2000.

26. Gladden LB: Muscle as a consumer of lactate, *Med Sci Sports Exerc* 32:764-771, 2000.

27. Sahlin K, Ren JM, Broberg S: Oxygen deficit at the onset of submaximal exercise is not due to a delayed oxygen transport, *Acta Physiol Scand* 134:175-180, 1988.

28. Finn J, Gastin P, Withers R, et al: Estimation of peak power and anaerobic capacity of athletes In Gore CJ, editor: *Physiological tests for elite athletes: Australian Sports Commission,* pp. 37-49, Champaign, Ill, 2000, Human Kinetics.

29. Scott CB, Roby FB, Lohman TG, et al: The maximally accumulated oxygen deficit as an indicator of anaerobic capacity, *Med Sci Sports Exerc* 23:618-624, 1991.

30. Van Praagh E: Development of anaerobic function during childhood and adolescence, *Pediatr Exerc Sci* 12:150-173, 2000.

31. Bahr R: Excess postexercise oxygen consumption—Magnitude, mechanisms and practical implications, *Acta Physiol Scand (Suppl)* 32:396-402, 2000.

32. Stainsby WN, Barclay JK: Exercise metabolism: O_2 deficit, steady level O_2 level and O_2 uptake for recovery, *Med Sci Sports Exerc* 2:177-181, 1970.

33. Margaria R, Edwards MT, Dill DB: The possible mechanisms of contracting and paying the oxygen debt and the role of lactic acid in muscular contraction, *Am J Physiol* 106:689-715, 1933.

34. Kapit W, Macey RI, Meisami E: *The physiology coloring book,* ed 2, San Francisco, 2000, Addison Wesley Longman.

35. Bouchard C, Taylor AW, Dulac S: Testing maximal anaerobic power and capacity. In MacDougall JD, Wenger HW, Green HJ, editors: *Physiological testing of the high-performance athlete,* ed 2, pp. 175-221, Champaign, Ill, 1991, Human Kinetics.

36. Bouchard C, Taylor AW, Simoneau JA, et al: Testing anaerobic power and capacity. In MacDougall JD, Wenger HW, Green HJ, editors: *Physiological testing of the high-performance athlete,* pp. 61-73, Hamilton, Ontario, 1982, Canadian Association of Sports Sciences Mutual Press Limited.

37. Cheetham ME, Boobis LH, Brooks, et al: Human muscle metabolism during sprint running, *J Appl Physiol* 61:54-60, 1986.

38. Freund H, Oyono-Enguelle S, Heitz A, et al: Comparative lactate kinetics after short and prolonged submaximal exercise, *Int J Sports Med* 11:284-288, 1990.

39. Costill DL: Metabolic responses during distance running, *J Appl Physiol* 28:251-255, 1970.

40. O'Brien MJ, Viguie CA, Mazzeo RS, et al: Carbohydrate dependence during marathon running, *Med Sci Sports Exerc* 25:1009-1017, 1993.

41. Beneke R, Hutler M, Leithauser RM: Maximal lactate-steady-state independent of performance, *Med Sci Sports Exerc* 32:1135-1139, 2000.

42. Hughes EF, Turner SC, Brooks GA: Effect of glycogen depletion and pedaling speed on anaerobic threshold, *J Appl Physiol* 52:1598-1607, 1982.

43. Hughson RL, Weisiger KH, Swanson GD: Blood lactate concentration increases as a continuous function in progressive exercise, *J Appl Physiol* 62:1975-1981, 1987.

44. Wasserman K, Whipp BJ, Koyal SN, et al: Anaerobic threshold and respiratory gas exchange during exercise, *J Appl Physiol* 35:236-243, 1973.

45. Jones NL, Ehrsam RE: The anaerobic threshold. In Terjung RL, editor: *Exercise and sport sciences reviews,* pp. 49-83, Philadelphia, 1982, The Franklin Institute.

46. Wasserman K, McIlroy: Detecting the threshold of anaerobic metabolism in cardiac patients during exercise, *Am J Cardiol* 14:844-852, 1964.

47. Pitts RF: *Physiology of the kidney and body fluids,* ed 3, Chicago, 1974, Year Book Medical.

48. Jacobs I: Blood lactate: implications for training and sports performance, *Sports Med* 3:10-25, 1986.

49. Reinhard V, Muller PH, Schmulling RM: Determination of anaerobic threshold by the ventilation equivalent in normal individuals, *Respiration* 38:36-42, 1979.

50. Skinner JS, McLellan TH: The transition from aerobic to anaerobic metabolism, *Res Q Exerc Sport* 51:234-248, 1980.

51. Moquin A, Mazzeo RS: Effect of mild dehydration on the lactate threshold in women, *Med Sci Sports Exerc* 32:396-402, 2000.

52. Walsh ML, Banister EW: Possible mechanisms of the anaerobic threshold: a review, *Sports Med* 5:269-302, 1988.

53. Inbar O, Bar-Or O: Anaerobic characteristics in male children and adolescents, *Med Sci Sports Exerc* 18:264-269, 1986.

54. Hagberg JM, Coyle EF, Carroll JE, et al: Exercise hyperventilation in patients with McArdle's disease, *J Appl Physiol* 52:991-994, 1982.

55. Poole DC, Gaesser GA: Response of ventilatory and lactate threshold to continuous and interval training, *J Appl Physiol* 58:1115-1121, 1985.

56. Costill DL, Thomason H, Roberts E: Fractional utilization of the aerobic capacity during distance running, *Med Sci Sports Exerc* 5:248-252, 1973.

57. Farrell PA, Wilmore JH, Coyle EF, et al: Plasma lactate accumulation and distance running performance, *Med Sci Sports Exerc* 11:338-344, 1979.

58. Kinderman W, Simon G, Keul J: The significance of the aerobic-anaerobic transition for the determination of workload intensities during endurance training, *Eur J Appl Physiol* 42:25-34, 1979.

59. Hermansen L, Maehlum S, Pruett EDR, et al: Lactate removal at rest and during exercise. In Howald H, Poortmans JR, editors: *Metabolic adaptation to prolonged exercise*, pp. 101-105, Basel, 1975, Birkhauser.

60. Bangsbo J, Graham T, Johansen L, et al: Muscle lactate metabolism in recovery from intense exhaustive exercise: impact of light exercise, *J Appl Physiol* 77:1890-1895, 1994.

61. Burleson MA Jr, O'Bryant HS, Stone MH, et al: Effect of weight training exercise and treadmill exercise on post-exercise oxygen consumption, *Med Sci Sports Exerc* 30:518-522, 1998.

62. Keul J, Haralambie G, Bruder M, et al: The effect of weight lifting exercise on heart rate and metabolism in experienced weight lifters, *Med Sci Sports Exerc* 10:13-15, 1978.

63. Reynolds TH IV, Frye PA, Sforzo GA: Resistance training and the blood lactate response to resistance exercise in women, *J Strength Cond Res* 11:77-81, 1997.

64. Tesch PA: Short-and long-term histochemical and biochemical adaptation in muscle. In Komi PV, editor: *Strength and power in sports*, pp. 239-248, Oxford, England, 1992, Blackwell Scientific.

65. Guyton AC: *Textbook of medical physiology*, ed 7, Philadelphia, 1986, Saunders.

66. Hultman E, Sahlin K: Acid-base balance during exercise. In Hutton RS, Miller DI, editors: *Exercise and sport sciences reviews*, pp. 41-128, Philadelphia, 1980, The Franklin Institute.

67. Davis JA: Response to Brooks' manuscript, *Med Sci Sports Exerc* 17:32-34, 1985.

68. Hogan MC, Gladden LB, Kurdak SS, et al: Increased [lactate] in working dog muscle reduces tension development independent of pH, *Med Sci Sports Exerc* 27:371-377, 1995.

69. Gollnick PD, Bayly WM, Hodgson DR: Exercise intensity, training, diet, and lactate concentration in muscle and blood, *Med Sci Sports Exerc* 18:334-340, 1986.

70. Bonen A, Campbell CJ, Kirby RL, et al: A multiple regression model for blood lactate removal in man, *Pflugers Arch* 380:205-210, 1979.

71. Hermansen L, Svensvold I: Production and removal of lactate during exercise in man, *Acta Physiol Scand* 86:191-201, 1972.

72. Belcastro AN, Bonen A: Lactic acid removal rates during controlled and uncontrolled recovery exercise, *J Appl Physiol* 39:932-936, 1975.

73. Bonen A, Belcastro AN: Comparison of self-selected recovery methods on lactic acid removal rates, *Med Sci Sports Exerc* 8:176-178, 1976.

74. McGrail JC, Bonen A, Belcastro AN: Dependence of lactate removal on muscle metabolism in man, *Eur J Appl Physiol* 39:87-97, 1978.

75. Choi D, Cole KJ, Goodpaster BH, et al: Effect of passive and active recovery on the resynthesis of muscle glycogen, *Med Sci Sports Exerc* 26:992-996, 1994.

76. Green S: Measurement of anaerobic work capacity in humans, *Sports Med* 19:32-42, 1995.

77. Bar-Or O: The Wingate Anaerobic Test: an update on methodology, reliability and validity, *Sports Med* 4:381-394, 1987.

78. Vandewalle H, Peres G, Monod H: Standard anaerobic exercise tests, *Sports Med* 4:268-289, 1987.

79. Bar-Or O: *Pediatric sports medicine for the practitioner: from physiological principles to clinical applications*, New York, 1983, Springer-Verlag.

80. Shephard RJ: *Physical activity and growth*, Chicago, 1982, Year Book Medical.

81. Eriksson BO: Physical training, oxygen supply and muscle metabolism in 11-13 year old boys, *Acta Physiol Scand (Suppl)* 384:1-48, 1972.

82. Rowland TW: *Exercise and children's health*, Champaign, Ill, 1990, Human Kinetics.

83. Cumming GR, Hastman L, McCort J: Treadmill endurance times, blood lactate, and exercise blood pressures in normal children In Binkhorst RA, Kemper HCG, Saris WHM, editors: *Children and exercise XI*, pp. 140-150, Champaign, Ill, 1985, Human Kinetics.

84. Saris WHM, Noordeloos AM, Ringnalda BEM, et al: Reference values for aerobic power of healthy 4 to 18 year old Dutch children: preliminary results. In Binkhorst RA, Kemper HCG, Saris WHM, editors: *Children and exercise XI*, pp. 151-160, Champaign, Ill, 1985, Human Kinetics.

85. Astrand P-O, Engstrom BO, Eriksson O, et al: Girl swimmers: with special reference to respiratory and circulatory adaptation and gynecological and psychiatric aspects, *Acta Paediatr (Suppl)* 147:1-73, 1963.

86. Bouhuys A, Pool J, Binkhorst RA, et al: Metabolic acidosis of exercise in healthy males, *J Appl Physiol* 21:1040-1046, 1966.

87. Sidney KH, Shephard RJ: Maximum and submaximum exercise tests in men and women in the seventh, eighth, and ninth decade of life, *J Appl Physiol Resp Environ Exerc Physiol* 43:280-287, 1977.

88. Astrand I: Aerobic work capacity in men and women with special reference to age, *Acta Physiol Scand (Suppl)* 169:1-92, 1960.

89. Robinson S: Experimental studies of physical fitness in relation to age, *Arbeitsphysiol* 10:251-323, 1938.

90. Astrand P-O: *Experimental studies of physical working capacity in relation to sex and age*, Copenhagen, 1952, Munksgaard.

91. Gaisl G, Buchberger J: Determination of the aerobic and anaerobic thresholds of 10-11 year old boys using blood-

gas analysis. In *Children and exercise IX*, pp. 93-98, Baltimore, 1979, University Park Press.

92. Kanaly JA, Boileau RA: The onset of the anaerobic threshold at three stages of physical maturity, *J Sports Med and Phys Fit* 28:367-374, 1988.

93. Reybrouck TM: The use of the anaerobic threshold in pediatric exercise testing. In Bar-Or O, editor: *Advances in pediatric sport sciences*, pp. 131-150, Champaign, Ill, 1989, Human Kinetics.

94. Williams JR, Armstrong N, Kirby BJ: The 4 mM blood lactate level as an index of exercise performance in 11-13 year old children, *J Sport Sci* 8:139-147, 1990.

95. Armstrong N, Welsman JR, Kirby BJ: Performance on the Wingate Anaerobic Test and maturation, *Pediatr Exerc Sci* 9:253-261, 1997.

96. Armstrong N, Welsman JR, Williams CA, et al: Longitudinal changes in young people's short-term power output, *Med Sci Sports Exerc* 32:1140-1145, 2000.

97. Chia MYH, Armstrong N, De Ste Croix MBA, et al: Longitudinal changes in Wingate Anaerobic Test determined peak and mean power in 10 to 12 year olds, *Pediatr Exerc Sci* 11:272, 1999.

98. Bar-Or O: The prepubescent female. In Shangold MM, Mirkin G, editors: *Women and exercise: physiology and sports medicine*, pp. 109-119, Philadelphia, 1988, Davis.

99. Martin RJF, Dore E, Twisk J, et al: Longitudinal changes of maximal short-term peak power in girls and boys during growth, *Med Sci Sports Exerc* 36:498-503, 2004.

100. Santos AMC, Armstrong N, De Ste Croix MBA, et al: Optimal peak power in relation to age, body size, gender, and thigh volume, *Pediatr Exerc Sci* 15:406-418, 2003.

101. Santos AMC, Welsman JR, De Ste Croix MBA, et al: Age-and sex-related differences in optimal peak power, *Pediatr Exerc Sci* 14: 202-212, 2002.

102. Berg A, Kim SS, Keul J: Skeletal muscle enzyme activities in healthy young subjects, *Int J of Sports Med* 7: 236-239, 1986.

103. Berg A, Keul J: Biochemical changes during exercise in children. In Malina RM, editor: *Young athletes: biological, psychological, and educational perspectives*, pp. 61-77, Champaign, Ill, 1988, Human Kinetics.

104. Macek M, Vavra J: Anaerobic threshold in children. In Binkhorst RA, Kemper CG, Saris WHM, editors: *Children and exercise XI*, pp. 110-113, Champaign, Ill, 1985, Human Kinetics.

105. Wells CL: *Women, sport and performance: a physiological perspective,* ed 2, Champaign, Ill, 1991, Human Kinetics.

106. Wallace JP, Inbar G, Ernsthausen K: Infant acceptance of postexercise breast milk, *Pediatr* 89:1245-1247, 1992.

107. Wallace JP, Rabin J: The concentration of lactic acid in breast mild following maximal exercise, *Int J Sports Med* 12:328-331, 1991.

108. Dewey KG, Lovelady CA, Nommsen-Rivers LA, et al: A randomized study of the effects of aerobic exercise by lactating women on breast-milk volume and composition, *N Engl J Med* 330:449-453, 1994.

109. Quinn TJ, Carey GB: Does exercise intensity or diet influence lactic acid accumulation in breast mild? *Med Sci Sports Exerc* 31:105-110, 1999.

110. Makrides L, Heigenhauser GJF, McCartney N, et al: Maximal short term exercise capacity in healthy subjects aged 15-70 years, *Clin Sci* 69:197-205, 1985.

111. Malina RM, Bouchard C: *Growth, maturation, and physical activity*, Champaign, Ill, 1991, Human Kinetics.

112. Astrand P-O: Human physical fitness with special reference to sex and age, *Physiol Rev* 36:307-335, 1956.

113. Kohrt WM, Spina RJ, Ehsani A, et al: Effects of age, adiposity, and fitness level on plasma catecholamine responses to standing and exercise, *J Appl Physiol* 75: 1828-1835, 1993.

114. Wiswell RA, Jaque SV, Marcell TJ, et al: Maximal aerobic power, lactate threshold, and running performance in master athletes, *Med Sci Sports Exerc* 32:1165-1170, 2000.

115. Maud PJ, Shultz BB: Norms for the Wingate Anaerobic Test with comparison to another similar test, *Res Q Exerc Sport* 60:144-151, 1989.

116. Anton MM, Spirduso WW, Tanaka H: Age-related declines in anaerobic muscular performance: weightlifting and powerlifting, *Med Sci Sports Exerc* 36:143-147, 2004.

117. Rogers MA, Evans WJ: Changes in skeletal muscle with aging: effects of exercise training In Holloszy JO, editor: *Exercise and sport sciences reviews*, pp. 65-102, Baltimore, 1993, Williams & Wilkins.

118. Larsson L, Yu F, Hook P, et al: Effects of aging on regulation of muscle contraction at the motor unit, muscle cell, and molecular levels, *Int J Sport Nutr Exerc Metab* 11(Suppl):S28-S43, 2001.

Stephanie Petterson,
Christopher Kuchta,
and Lynn Snyder-Mackler

CHAPTER 4

Aerobic Metabolism during Exercise

LEARNING OBJECTIVES

After studying this chapter, the reader will be able to do the following:

1. Describe cardiovascular and respiratory anatomy and physiology, as well as describe the physiological processes of aerobic metabolism
2. Identify the acute cardiovascular and respiratory responses resulting from aerobic and resistive exercise, as well as describe the long-term cardiorespiratory adaptations that occur with both aerobic and resistive training
3. Discriminate age- and sex-related differences in acute exercise responses and long-term training adaptations
4. Design an appropriate age-, sex-, and task-specific training program to enhance cardiorespiratory function

This chapter summarizes aerobic responses to exercise, both acutely and in the long term, in order for the health care professional to develop a physiologically based aerobic training program. The chapter focuses on the cardiovascular and respiratory systems and aerobic metabolism. Oxidative energy pathways are essential to cardiovascular health and improvements in aerobic and sport performance. Aerobic metabolic pathways are the most efficient and predominant mechanisms responsible for producing sufficient adenosine triphosphate (ATP) supplies to perform even the most basic daily activities. The respiratory system brings oxygen into the body via the lungs, combines with hemoglobin in the blood, is propelled through the circulatory system by the heart, and provides energy for movement through aerobic metabolic pathways. A fundamental understanding of the cardiovascular and respiratory systems and the physiology of aerobic metabolism is necessary to comprehend acute and long-term adaptations to aerobic training.

CARDIOVASCULAR ANATOMY AND PHYSIOLOGY

The cardiovascular (CV) system is composed of the heart and a matrix of blood vessels carrying blood away from the heart (arteries) and blood vessels returning blood to the heart (veins).

Arteries and veins differ functionally in their muscular composition. Arterial walls are thick and muscular to withstand the pressure necessary to pump blood through the body. In contrast, veins function on the basis of low pressure regulation and therefore their walls are much thinner. Veins rely on surrounding muscle to assist in pumping blood back to the heart. Capillaries are a third type of vessel connecting the arterial and venous systems and making the CV system a closed-circuit system. Capillaries provide the site for exchange of oxygen (O_2), carbon dioxide (CO_2), nutrients, and fluids between blood and body tissues and are therefore the thinnest vessels.

The heart is composed of four chambers: two halves, right and left, each consisting of two chambers, an atria and a ventricle. The right side of the heart receives deoxygenated blood from the body and pumps blood to the lungs to be oxygenated. The left side of the heart receives oxygenated blood returning from the lungs and pumps the blood to the head, trunk, and extremities. The atria function as reservoirs for blood received from the periphery. The ventricles are pumping chambers responsible for pumping deoxygenated blood to the lungs and maintaining adequate circulation to meet the regional demands of physical activity. Similar to the vasculature, muscle composition of each chamber differs on the basis of its primary functions. The walls of the left ventricle are thicker compared with the right ventricle. Increased left ventricular wall thickness and muscle mass increase the force-generating capacity of this chamber, enabling blood to be pumped to the most distal extremities. On the other hand, the walls of the right ventricle are much thinner because blood only has to be pumped a short distance to the lungs.

Valves are present between the heart chambers, as well as within the heart and blood vessels. They function to control the volume of blood ejected from the heart and prevent the backflow of blood with each contraction. The right and left atrioventricular (AV) valves prevent the backflow of blood from the ventricles to the atria during ventricular contraction. The right AV valve is a tricuspid valve because it is composed of three cusps. The left AV valve only has two cusps and is therefore bicuspid. Two semilunar valves regulate the flow of blood from the ventricles. The right semilunar valve, also known as the *pulmonary semilunar valve,* is positioned between the right ventricle and pulmonary arteries. The left semilunar valve positioned between the left ventricle and the aorta is referred to as the *aortic valve.* The AV valves and semilunar valves have opposing functions; AV valves control ventricular filling during ventricular relaxation, called diastole, and semilunar valves control ventricular emptying during ventricular contraction, called systole.

Myocardial muscle is composed of striated skeletal muscle supporting both the mechanical and electrical fundamentals of circulation. The intricate network of specialized muscle connects the chambers of the heart with the rest of the body to allow for easy propagation of electrical impulses, depolarize myocardial muscle, and induce muscular contraction to sustain circulatory processes. This specialized electrical conduction system initiates and controls myocardial contraction and heart rate (HR). The sinoatrial (SA) node, located in the right atrial wall, is the origin of each electrical impulse, or heartbeat. The SA node is referred to as the heart's pacemaker because it regulates the rhythmicity of each heartbeat. At rest the SA node has an intrinsic firing rate of approximately 70 bpm. Following depolarization by the SA node, the electrical signal depolarizes both atria and travels to the AV node, located between the right atria and ventricle. The conduction velocity of the electrical impulse generated by the SA node is slowed as it travels through the AV node. Slowed conduction velocity through the AV node functions to separate atrial contraction and ventricular depolarization. At rest the intrinsic rate of the AV node is 50 to 60 bpm. Following depolarization of the AV node, the action potential then proceeds down a specialized

conduction system known as the *bundle of His* into the right and left bundle branches before terminating in the Purkinje fibers.

The autonomic nervous system (ANS) is the central command center responsible for stimulating the SA and AV nodes, ultimately regulating the firing rate and rhythmicity of the heart. The ANS consists of two branches—the sympathetic and parasympathetic branches—with opposing functions. Parasympathetic input slows the firing rate of the SA node, and sympathetic input increases the firing rate by accelerating depolarization of the SA node, which increases HR. The conduction system of the ANS enables rapid responses to exercise-imposed demands. Normal resting heart rate (RHR) in an average adult ranges from 60 to 100 bpm. An HR less than 60 bpm is referred to as *bradycardia,* and an HR greater than 100 bpm is referred to as *tachycardia.*

Evidence-Based Clinical Application: Electrocardiogram

An electrocardiogram (ECG) is a clinical test that records the electrical activity of the heart. A normal ECG is composed of three primary distinctions: P wave, QRS complex, and T wave. The P wave represents atrial depolarization. The QRS complex represents ventricular depolarization. The QRS complex consists of a Q wave (septal depolarization, first downward deflection), R wave (depolarization of apex, upward deflection), and S wave (ventricular depolarization, downward deflection following R wave). The T wave represents ventricular repolarization. The PR interval (range = 0.12 to 0.2 second) is the time it takes for the electrical impulse to travel from the SA node to the AV node. The QT interval (from the beginning of the QRS complex to the return of the T wave to baseline) varies as a function of HR. The ST segment (from the end of the S wave to the beginning of the T wave) is most important to observe on an ECG during exercise stress testing because it is indicative of ischemia. The J-point is the junction of the S wave to the ST segment.

Normal ECG changes that occur with exercise include: shortening of the PR and QT intervals, decrease in the distance between R waves, decrease in the amplitude of R waves, increase in the amplitude Q and T waves, and progressive upslope from J-point with return to baseline within 60 to 80 milliseconds.

Evidence-Based Clinical Application: Blood Pressure

BP is a good indicator of CV health and the demand imposed on the heart at rest and with physical activity. The cardiac cycle is composed of two main events, systole and diastole. Systole is a period of ventricular contraction. Ventricular pressure increases until the aortic and pulmonary valves close. SBP is a measure of the pressure exerted by the blood against the arterial walls during ventricular contraction indicating the work performed by the heart. Diastole is a period of ventricular relaxation allowing the ventricles to fill with blood in preparation for the next cardiac cycle. DBP is a measure of the pressure imposed by the blood against the arterial walls during ventricular relaxation. The pressure gradient arising from blood flow during systole and diastole gives rise to BP. During systole, the left ventricular pressure is approximately 120 mmHg. During diastole, aortic pressure drops to 80 mmHg, giving rise to a BP of 120/80.

Obtaining BP measurement is a quick clinical measure to monitor CV work rate. A sphygmomanometer, or BP cuff, and stethoscope are the necessary instruments. The most commonly used site to measure BP is in the arm, but the leg can be used. To measure BP, the sphygmomanometer is placed around the upper arm just proximal to the antecubital fossa. The brachial pulse is then palpated in the antecubital fossa before placing the head of the stethoscope over the pulse site. The sphygmomanometer is then inflated until the pressure in the cuff exceeds the pressure in the brachial artery. The cuff is then deflated by turning the nose of the valve. The first pulse sound heard is the point at which pressure in the brachial artery exceeds cuff pressure. The number on the gauge is equivalent to the SBP. The last sound heard is equivalent to DBP. The unit of measurement for both SBP and DBP is millimeters of mercury, or mmHg.

A normal BP in an average adult is 120/80 mmHg (SBP/DBP). Hypertension, or high BP, is characterized by SBP > 140 mmHg and DBP > 90 mmHg. Hypotension, or low BP, is characterized by SBP < 70 mmHg.[1]

RESPIRATORY ANATOMY AND PHYSIOLOGY

The function of the respiratory system is to supply O_2 and remove CO_2 from blood in order to maintain a state of homeostasis. The respiratory system consists of a network of many airway branches or generations. The trachea is the first-generation and largest airway opening. The trachea divides into two main branches, the right and left bronchi (second-generation passages), which further subdivide into bronchioles that branch approximately 23 times before terminating in the smallest passageway, the alveoli. Alveoli are minute sacs that make up the lungs and provide the site for gas exchange.

Respiratory airways can be classified as part of the conducting zone or the respiratory zone. The conducting zone is the part of the respiratory system that purifies, humidifies, and transports air to the lower respiratory system. No gas exchange occurs in these regions. The conducting zone originates at the nasal passages, travels through the pharynx and trachea (first-generation passageway), and terminates at the terminal bronchioles (generation 16). The respiratory zone is the zone of gas exchange. Generation 17, or the first generation of the respiratory zone, is known as the *respiratory bronchioles*. The respiratory zone terminates at the alveoli.

In the alveoli the movement of O_2 and CO_2 occurs by the process of simple diffusion. O_2 and CO_2 move along pressure gradients, from areas of high pressure to areas of low pressure between the alveoli and capillaries. At the site of gas exchange, O_2 is taken up by the capillaries and CO_2 is removed from the blood to be excreted during exhalation. The gas exchange process is known as *respiration*. As O_2 is used to create energy, CO_2 is given off as a by-product (as demonstrated in the following equation).

$$glucose + O_2 \rightarrow H_2O + CO_2 + ATP$$

As CO_2 is taken up by the blood to be excreted by the body, blood pH rises, making the blood more acidic (as demonstrated in the following equation).

$$H^+ + HCO_3^- \rightleftharpoons H_2CO_3 \rightleftharpoons H_2O + CO_2$$

Ventilation is a dynamic, time-dependent process involving the mechanical movement of air based on the passive elastic properties of the lungs and the function of accessory muscles of inspiration and exhalation. The diaphragm is the primary muscle of respiration, separating the thoracic and abdominal cavities. In its resting position the diaphragm is dome shaped. Contraction of the diaphragm within the chest cavity during inspiration creates a negative pressure, causing the thorax and lungs to expand and air to flow into the lungs. During exhalation the diaphragm relaxes and air is expelled by the elastic recoil of the lungs, chest wall, and abdomen. During exercise and heavy breathing, forces of elastic recoil are not sufficient to inhale the necessary amount of air. Accessory muscles must be recruited to assist in the processes of inhalation and exhalation to enhance O_2 delivery and CO_2 removal. The muscles of inspiration, external intercostals, sternocleidomastoid, serratus anterior, and scalenes assist in lung expansion by contracting and raising the rib cage. The muscles of expiration—rectus abdominis, internal obliques, external obliques, transverse abdominis, and internal intercostals—depress the rib cage and assist with exhalation.

Lower brain centers, specifically the medulla oblongata and the pons, assist in breath initiation and regulate the volume of each breath. Therefore the nervous system is responsible for controlling the rate and depth of ventilation to meet the demand of the body maintaining relatively constant concentrations of O_2 and CO_2. If the respiratory rate is too slow, O_2 delivery is inadequate to meet the metabolic requirements of the body. This breathing state, referred to as *hypoventilation,* is characterized by slow, shallow breathing leading to increased levels of CO_2 in the blood. Conversely, increased depth and rate of breathing is referred to as *hyperventilation.* Hyperventilation results in abnormally low levels of CO_2 in the blood, disrupting blood homeostasis. As a result, blood pressure (BP) significantly drops and individuals may experience symptoms of dizziness, tingling, and possible fainting spells.

Lungs differ in both size and capacity, significantly contributing to the overall functional capacity of the respiratory system. Normative values of static, anatomical measurements of the respiratory system have been recorded in healthy adults (see the following box). Functional measurements have also been determined for dynamic components of respiration. These values are important determinants of aerobic capacity determining the efficiency of the cardiorespiratory system. Pulmonary

---

Evidence-Based Clinical Application: Lung Volumes

Tidal volume (TV)	The amount of air inspired or expired in a normal breath at rest (0.5 L)
Inspiratory reserve volume (IRV)	The maximal amount of air that can be inspired beyond the TV (3 L)
Expiratory reserve volume (ERV)	The maximal amount of air that can be expired beyond the normal TV expiration (1L)
Residual volume (RV)	The volume of air that remains in the lungs after a forced, maximal expiration (1.2 L)
Inspiratory capacity (IC)	The maximal amount of air that can be inspired; equivalent to TV + IRV
Functional residual capacity (FRC)	The amount of air remaining in the lungs after normal exhalation; equivalent to ERV + RV
Vital capacity (VC)	The volume of air exhaled during a forced exhalation; IRV + TV + ERV
Total lung capacity (TLC)	TV + IRV + ERV + RV (4 L in females; 5.7 L in males)

minute volume (V_E) is the amount of air moved in 1 minute. Minute alveolar ventilation (V_A) is the amount of air capable of participating in gas exchange or the volume of air breathed each minute. During exercise, V_A increases with increases in metabolic rate and CO_2 production. V_E increases with the onset of exercise to meet the demands of V_A to remove excess CO_2. When exercise intensity reaches a particular level, blood flow to the exercising muscles becomes inadequate to provide the necessary O_2. This is termed the *anaerobic threshold* and is the point at which anaerobic pathways become the primary source of energy production.

AEROBIC METABOLISM

Aerobic metabolism is the most efficient mechanism used by the body to convert food energy into energy easily used by the body for fuel. ATP is the primary energy source at rest and during low-intensity exercise. It is composed of a ribose sugar backbone, a nitrogen and carbon chain, adenine, and three phosphate molecules. Aerobic metabolic pathways are also referred to as *oxidative* because of their dependence on O_2 to generate ATP. Aerobic metabolism is therefore limited by the function of the cardiovascular, respiratory, and musculoskeletal systems, in addition to readily available supplies of O_2. If one of these systems is deficient or unable to generate enough ATP rapidly through oxidative means, the body must rely on less efficient anaerobic systems. Although submaximal activity performed for an extended period primarily taxes the aerobic system, greater-intensity activity performed for a shorter period taxes both aerobic and anaerobic pathways, and near-maximal activity for an even shorter period relies almost solely on anaerobic means for fuel.

The primary sources of fuel driving the aerobic system are carbohydrates and fats. Fat molecules, or triglycerides, are composed of one glycerol molecule and three fatty acid chains.

Because the body cannot store triglycerides in their ingested form, they are broken down during a process known as *lipolysis* into glycerol and fatty acid chains. Fatty acid chains, composed predominantly of hydrogen and carbon atoms, are stored either in fat cells or released into the bloodstream to be oxidized for energy. When taken up by mitochondria, free fatty acid chains undergo beta oxidation, a process that produces acetyl CoA and hydrogen. Acetyl CoA enters the Krebs cycle, and H^+ is carried by nicotinamide adenine dinucleotide (NADH) and flavin adenine dinucleotide ($FADH_2$) to the electron transport chain (ETC). For every two carbons in a fatty acid, oxidation yields five ATPs generating acetyl CoA and 12 more ATPs oxidizing the coenzyme, producing a net 17 ATP (Figure 4-1).

Carbohydrates are composed of carbon, hydrogen, and oxygen and classified on the basis of the number of sugar molecules that compose the compound (monosaccharide, disaccharide, or polysaccharide). Aerobic glycolysis is the process by which glucose is broken down into pyruvate. The Krebs cycle begins with pyruvate, the end product of glycolysis. The Krebs cycle produces two ATP molecules from guanine triphosphate (GTP) per molecule of glucose consumed. In addition, six molecules of NADH and two molecules of $FADH_2$ are produced and enter the ETC. The ETC uses these molecules to produce ATP from ADP. The process ATP formation from aerobic pathways is referred to as *oxidative phosphorylation.* The resultant energy production in a net of 38 ATP0 molecules generated from one molecule of glucose is shown in Figures 4-2 and 4-3.

Efficiency is the proportion of total available energy that is used for work or is stored for future use. Fat is a more efficient fuel source during low-level activities because it is more readily available through fat stores and lipolysis. Energy produced from 1 g of fatty acids is 9 kcal compared with 4 kcal/g from carbohydrate or protein. The individual's nutritional intake, as well as the intensity and duration of exercise performed, dictates whether fats or carbohydrates are the primary or secondary fuel source in aerobic metabolic pathways. Fats are

Figure 4-1 Energy stores.

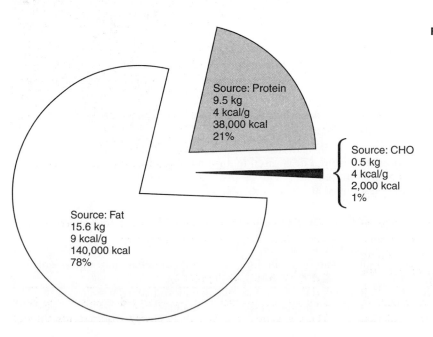

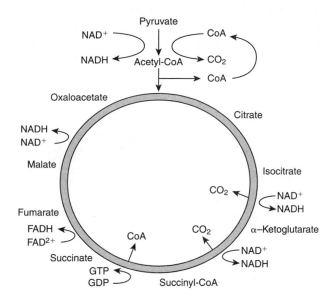

Figure 4-2 Krebs cycle.

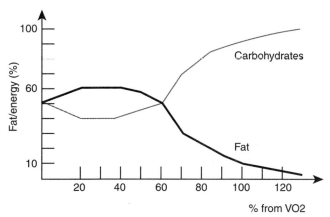

Figure 4-3 Fuel source as a function of exercise intensity.

primarily used during lower-intensity activities over a long duration. Carbohydrates are primarily used during more intense activities of shorter duration activities. At rest, more fats than carbohydrates are typically burned for fuel. As activity level increases, a shift from the utilization of fats to more carbohydrates occurs to meet the increasing energy demands (Figure 4-4).

ACUTE CHANGES IN AEROBIC METABOLISM WITH EXERCISE

Exercise-imposed demands on the cardiovascular and respiratory systems alter O_2 availability via circulation, respiration, ventilation, and aerobic metabolic pathways while maintaining O_2 saturation. If the CV system is not up-regulated with the initiation of exercise, adequate O_2 supplies will not reach working muscles and CO_2 will accumulate in the blood. In addition, if the respiratory system fails to increase ventilation

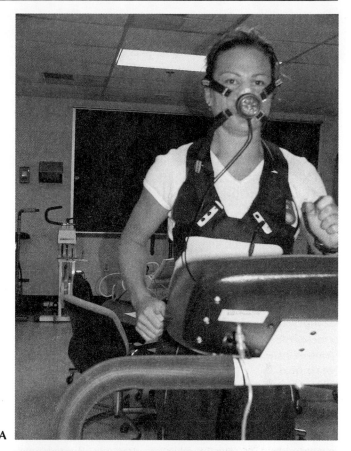

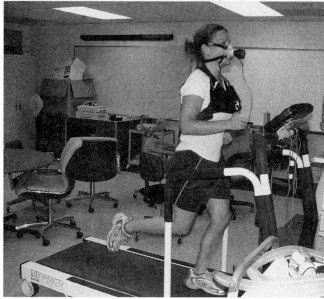

Figure 4-4 **A** and **B,** Maximal oxygen consumption ($\dot{V}O_2$max) testing.

rate, inadequate O_2 supplies will cause a shift to less efficient anaerobic metabolic pathways for energy.

Cardiovascular System

Exercise rapidly increases the energy demands of the body. The CV system matches these energy requirements through the regulation of blood flow to working muscles. Increasing circulation ensures adequate O_2 supplies for aerobic energy pathways and removal of waste products to prevent the accumulation of CO_2, lactic acid, and heat. Changes in both central and peripheral centers aid in the regulation of O_2 delivery and CO_2 removal.

Central Mechanisms

HR is one of the most commonly used means to determine exercise intensity. As mentioned earlier, the number of times the heart contracts per minute in a resting state is referred to as the RHR. With the onset of both aerobic and resistance exercise, RHR rapidly rises.[2] The rapid increase in HR is a function of parasympathetic stimulation by the ANS. Older, sedentary adults may have a more rapid increase in HR in response to low-intensity exercise compared with more active older adults or even sedentary, younger adults. HR continues to rise in a positive, linear fashion with an increase in exercise intensity. Maximal heart rate (MHR) is the maximum number of times the heart can beat in 1 minute. Prediction models have generated simple mathematical equations that easily predict MHR from age.

$$\text{Females: MHR} = 226 - \text{age}$$

$$\text{Males: MHR} = 220 - \text{age}$$

For example, a 29-year-old male, based on age-adjusted equations, would have an MHR of 191 beats/min. The heart's response to exercise depends on age, gender, body mass, fitness level of the individual, and disease presence. More sophisticated means of determining MHR, such as treadmill stress testing, are more accurate determinants of MHR; however, these tests must be performed by trained health care professionals and are expensive to perform.

Stroke volume (SV) is the volume of blood ejected from the left ventricle with each beat. SV is the difference in volumes between the end diastolic volume (EDV), or amount of blood available in the left ventricle after diastole, and end systolic volume (ESV), or volume of blood available after systole. Initiation of aerobic exercise results in increased SV[2] explained by the Frank-Starling mechanism. The Frank-Starling mechanism is a mechanical property of cardiac muscle stating that

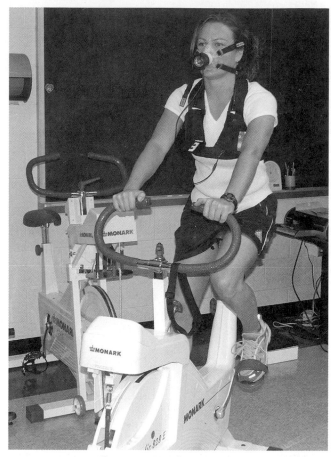

Figure 4-5 Bicycle ergometer.

Evidence-Based Clinical Application: Assessing Aerobic Capacity

Aerobic capacity is the ability of the cardiovascular system to deliver and use O_2. Assessment of aerobic capacity can be determined via direct, maximal test measures or indirect, submaximal testing. The "gold standard" for determining aerobic capacity is $\dot{V}O_2$max testing. $\dot{V}O_2$max testing measures the amount of O_2 consumed per unit of time. These values are derived from inspiratory and expiratory volume measures, as well as inspired O_2 and expired CO_2 concentrations. Treadmills, stationary bicycles, and upper body ergometers are the main methods used to determine aerobic capacity. During $\dot{V}O_2$max testing individuals are asked to perform an activity while workload is progressively increased until an increase in workload does not elicit a further increase in O_2 consumption (Figure 4-5).

Gold standard methods are not always easy to administer and are often time consuming, making them impractical clinical tests. Submaximal tests, although less accurate, have been validated through correlation of $\dot{V}O_2$max and physiological measures of submaximal exercise such as HR. Predictive equations have been derived on the basis of the linear relationships between HR and O_2 consumption. Examples of submaximal assessments of aerobic capacity include the YMCA cycle ergometer test, 3-minute Step Test, Cooper 12-minute walk/run test, and the Rockport One-Mile Fitness Test (Figure 4-6).

Older adults have reduced exercise capacity; therefore when measuring O_2 uptake, a longer warm-up, smaller increments of speed/slope per stage, and lower work peak rate should be used. As a result of reduced exercise capacity with age, some health care professionals prefer to predict aerobic capacity on the basis of submaximal exercise intensity.

Classification of Intensity of Exercise (based on 30-60 minutes of endurance training)				
Intensity	MHR	V̇O₂max	RPE level	MET
Very light	<35%	<30%	<10	
Light	35%-59%	30%-49%	10-11	<3
Moderate	60%-79%	50%-74%	12-13	3-6
Heavy	80%-89%	75%-84%	14-16	>6
Very heavy	≥90%	≥85%	>16	

Figure 4-6 Borg Rate of Perceived Exertion Scale. (© Gunnar Borg.)

muscle contraction force is directly proportional to a muscle's length. With exercise, there is an increase in left ventricular filling during diastole. The rise in circulatory blood volume increases the stretch, or length, on ventricular myocardial muscle. The greater muscle stretch yields a more forceful contraction during systole, ejecting a greater volume of blood with each heart beat. The volume of blood or fraction of EDV ejected from the heart with each beat is called the *ejection fraction.*

Although SV rapidly rises with the onset of aerobic exercise,[2,3] it reaches a plateau at which SV remains at a specific volume despite increasing exercise intensity. At 40% of maximal oxygen consumption (V̇O₂max), SV approaches near maximum levels.[3] The early increase in SV is a function of increased venous return. Heavy resistance training does not induce similar changes in SV. SV does not change or changes little in response to resistance exercise. During resistance training, individuals often hold their breath to generate greater force. This results in increased intra-abdominal and intrathoracic pressures, which limits venous return and subsequently does not significantly alter EDV. This mechanism of enhancing force-generating capacity is referred to as the *Valsalva maneuver.*

Cardiac output (CO) is the amount of blood ejected from the heart per minute. CO is directly related to HR and SV and is expressed in liters or milliliters per minute. This is demonstrated in the following equation:

$$CO = HR \times SV$$

At rest, SV is approximately 80 ml and resting HR is about 70 beats/min, giving rise to a CO of approximately 5.6 L/min at rest.

At the onset of aerobic exercise there is a concomitant rapid increase in CO as a function of increased HR and SV.[2,3] As exercise intensity and exertion increase continue to rise, HR and SV and therefore CO continue to increase. As O₂ uptake values approach maximum, CO reaches a steady-state or plateau at which CO remains constant despite increasing intensity.[3] Increased myocardial contractility, increased blood flow to working muscles, constriction of venous blood vessels, and decreased total peripheral resistance also influence CO during exercise. CO can increase from 5.6 L/min at rest to 35 to 40 L/min with strenuous exercise in young adults. This represents a sevenfold to eightfold increase in CO.

Heavy resistance training does not appear to significantly alter CO. Small increases may be visible secondary to a rise in

Evidence-Based Clinical Application: The Valsalva Maneuver

The Valsalva maneuver, a natural response to lifting heavy loads, is characterized by a forced exhalation against a closed glottis. During forced exhalation, a sudden increase in intra-abdominal and intrathoracic pressures is produced by the contractions of the abdominal and respiratory muscles. Elevated pressures compress the blood vessels within the chest cavity, leading to a decrease in venous return and CO. In addition, compression of the aorta leads to stimulation of the baroreceptors, producing a reflex-induced bradycardia to compensate for the increased pressures. Aortic pressure subsequently rises, stimulating sympathetic activity. HR and BP rise in response to maintain CO and perfusion. At the cessation of the forced exhalation, venous return rapidly increases, intra-abdominal pressures drop, and CO is increased, dramatically increasing the mechanical load on the heart.[4]

The Valsalva maneuver can be dangerous due to the sudden and abrupt changes in BP. These dramatic changes in HR, BP, and CO may produce symptoms including dizziness, lightheadedness, and syncope. However, the Valsalva technique can help protect against injury during heavy weight lifting. The supporting ligaments of the spine can only support 4 to 5 lb of pressure before failing.[5] Therefore performing the Valsalva maneuver during heavy lifts, such as the Roman dead lift, squats, bench press, and clean and jerk, assists core musculature in supporting the spine and decreases the compressive load on the intervertebral disks.[6]

Strength and conditioning coaches often recommend the Valsalva maneuver during weight-lifting exercises requiring a stable core. Individuals are coached to perform the maneuver during the work phase of the lift. Individuals should inhale before the exercise, hold their breath through the most difficult phase of the lift, and exhale to complete the lift. Because the consequences of improper breathing with weight lifting can be severe, proper education is essential.

HR with heavy resistance training. Modification of resistance training parameters to stress more aerobic energy pathways may produce more substantial changes in CO. This can be achieved by increasing the number of repetitions and lowering the resistance.

BP is a function of CO and resistance to blood flow or total peripheral resistance (TPR). Increases in systolic blood pressure (SBP) are also evident at the onset of aerobic exercise, whereas small decreases, if any, are noted in diastolic blood pressure (DBP).[2] SBP continues to increase in a positive, linear fashion as exercise intensity progressively increases. A 10- to 20-mmHg increase in SBP can be expected during dynamic exercise. DBP, on the other hand, has been observed to slightly decrease during dynamic treadmill exercise. Resistance training results in increased central/carotid SBP, although BP returns to pre-exercise levels within 30 minutes of the exercise bout.[7]

$\dot{V}O_2$max is a measure of the body's utilization of O_2 and is the greatest amount of O_2 consumed per minute at maximum effort. $\dot{V}O_2$max is a major determinant of cardiopulmonary fitness and is often expressed relative to body weight (ml/kg/min). The rate of extraction of O_2 in the tissues of an individual at rest is 4 to 5 ml of O_2 per 100 ml of blood. The amount of O_2 consumed and the percent of $\dot{V}O_2$max used depend on body mass, exercise intensity, and mode of exercise. At the onset of aerobic exercise, O_2 uptake increases progressively. As intensity increases and nears $\dot{V}O_2$max, O_2 extraction rate increases to approximately 13 to 16 ml of blood during maximal aerobic exercise intensity. As a general rule, the greater the percentage of muscle mass used during aerobic exercise, the greater the rate of O_2 extraction. Activities such as running, swimming, and cycling use a large percentage of $\dot{V}O_2$max because larger muscle groups (i.e., quadriceps femoris, gluteal muscles, latissimus dorsi) are the prime workers.

Resistance training often takes the form of short bursts of physical activity and therefore does not significantly alter $\dot{V}O_2$max. However, programs consisting of low resistance and high numbers of repetitions model trends in O_2 uptake similar to aerobic modes of training. For example, a continuous circuit resistance training exercise consisting of 10 exercises at 40% of 1 repetition max (RM) allows individuals to sustain O_2 uptake at approximately 50% of $\dot{V}O_2$max for more than a 15-minute period, although VO_2 increases more rapidly with treadmill exercise. In addition, continuous circuit resistance training can result in higher exercise HRs of up to 10 beats/min faster than can be achieved during similar-intensity treadmill exercise.[8] These changes are much less than typical aerobic endurance training protocols and are also not evidenced with traditional strength training programs.[9,10] In addition, no further CV benefit is achieved as a result of combining strength training with endurance training.[11,12]

Peripheral Mechanisms

Aerobic exercise increases the metabolic requirements of working muscles, which in turn induces changes in local blood circulation and perfusion. Sufficient supplies of O_2 must be readily available for oxidative processes to generate ATP. At rest, blood is relatively evenly distributed throughout the body. At the onset of exercise, blood is shunted away from the less involved muscles and organs (i.e., kidneys and digestive tract) via vasoconstriction to ensure adequate perfusion to working muscles. Vasoconstriction of peripheral blood vessels occurs as a function of contraction of smooth muscles of the blood vessel wall, which decreases blood vessel diameter and in turn increases TPR. In addition, vasodilation occurs in the blood vessels supplying the working muscles. Vasodilation results in increased blood vessel diameter and decreased TPR to improve blood flow to the working area. Together the mechanisms of vasoconstriction and vasodilation ensure adequate perfusion and O_2 supply.

The percentage of blood diverted to working muscles depends on the intensity of exercise. The more intense the physical activity is, the larger the percentage of total blood supply diverted to working muscles. As submaximal work intensities approach maximum levels, a greater percentage of muscle mass is recruited, raising O_2 demand substantially. When O_2 demand exceeds O_2 supply, insufficient O_2 delivery inhibits the efficiency of oxidative processes. When this occurs, anaerobic mechanisms supplement aerobic pathways to generate sufficient ATP supplies.

Resistance training consisting of low weight and high repetitions produces similar changes in local circulation to high-resistance, low-repetition resistance programs. More aggressive resistance exercise, however, increases the amount of blood shunted, supplying working muscles with even greater blood flow to support the metabolic cost of the increased workload.

Respiratory System

Respiratory changes in response to aerobic exercise match the O_2 uptake required for a particular activity level. A notable increase in gas exchange rate occurs within the first one to two breaths. This sudden response in gas exchange rate is triggered by altered levels of O_2 saturation. O_2 uptake continues to increase for the first few minutes until a steady-state is reached.[13,14] During steady-state exercise, O_2 demand equals O_2 consumption. Increases in alveolar ventilation rate can be as high as 10 to 20 times the resting rate in response to heavy exercise in order to match the additional O_2 demand and excrete excess CO_2 imposed by increased physiological demand. Increased CO_2 production also results from aerobic exercise as a function of increased O_2 utilization. Increased blood CO_2 levels cause a decrease in blood P_{O_2}, an increase in blood P_{CO_2}, an increase in blood H^+ (more acidic), and an increase in core body temperature.

During high levels of exertion, O_2 demand exceeds O_2 supply, resulting in a state in which the breakdown of pyruvic acid under aerobic conditions is not sufficient to generate a sufficient amount of ATP to perform the activity. Therefore anaerobic mechanisms are necessary to supplement ATP formation. These processes lead to an accumulation of lactic acid in muscle tissue resulting in fatigue and pain during repeated muscle contractions. Once the high-demand exercise has ceased, the additional O_2 necessary to return the body to its normal, homeostatic state is called *oxygen debt*. Oxygen debt is the total O_2 consumed in excess of preexercise levels. The greater an individual's $\dot{V}O_2$max, the greater degree of exertion that can be exhibited before reaching oxygen debt. In addition, oxygen debt in individuals with large $\dot{V}O_2$max is less than in individuals with smaller $\dot{V}O_2$max.

In response to states of O_2 deficiency, the respiratory system is triggered to increase the frequency of breathing (respiratory rate) or depth of each breath (tidal volume [TV]), or both. Both an increase in respiratory rate and an increase in TV lead to an increase in minute ventilation. In addition, more O_2 is extracted from each liter of blood to meet the O_2 demand of working muscles. The resultant pressure gradient set up by a decreased P_{O_2} and increased P_{CO_2} assists this process. Larger diffusion gradients increase the amount of O_2 unloaded from hemoglobin.

After the completion of a bout of exercise, O_2 uptake, respiratory rate, Po_2, and Pco_2 return to normal preexercise levels. The duration to which these measures return to their normal state depends on exercise intensity and duration of the exercise. The function of increased postexercise O_2 uptake is to replenish deficient stores of ATP, remove lactic acid accumulation in muscle tissues, replace myoglobin O_2 content, and replenish glycogen stores. Within 30 seconds of low-intensity aerobic exercise, approximately one half of the oxygen debt is replenished and return to baseline occurs within several minutes. With greater levels of exertion and longer duration of exercise, there is a more substantial increase in blood lactate levels, which may require up to 24 hours before returning to baseline.

LONG-TERM ADAPTATIONS OF AEROBIC METABOLISM WITH EXERCISE

Long-term endurance and resistance training enhance cardiorespiratory function. Improved utilization of O_2 leads to enhanced energy efficiency and improved economy of movement during physical activity. Central adaptations to long-term exercise programs contribute minimally to enhanced aerobic capacity because myocardial O_2 consumption is similar at rest and with exercise.[15] Peripheral adaptations discriminate the novice exerciser from the highly trained exerciser. The magnitude of change over the course of a prolonged exercise program varies on the basis of an individual's fitness level, CV health, exercise intensity, and duration. Individuals with low fitness levels often exhibit the most dramatic improvement because they have the greatest potential for gain. Highly trained individuals do exhibit improvements in cardiorespiratory function, although to a lesser degree. These individuals have a higher threshold for change, and therefore a greater stimulus (i.e., exercise intensity) is necessary to elicit change. Regardless, exercise training intensity must exceed current CV performance[16] in order to evoke change. Moderate-intensity training for at least 3 months is sufficient to show significant improvements. Higher-intensity or prolonged training programs above moderate levels do not result in significantly greater CV improvement.[17] On the contrary, reversal of CV adaptations occurs rapidly after only 2 to 3 weeks of no aerobic training. Improvements in SBP, DBP, CO, and TPR return to pretraining levels following the cessation of training.[17]

Although both endurance and resistance training induce positive CV changes, the nature and degree of change vary substantially between the two types of exercise. Decreases in RHR of up to 20 beats/min are evident following 2 to 3 weeks of aerobic training. The amount of blood ejected from the heart with each beat is increased and can reach up to 5 to 6 L/min. HR $_{submax}$ at a prescribed exercise intensity has been shown to be reduced by 21 beats/min following 16 weeks of exercise, and individuals exhibit lower HR at maximal workloads.[15] In addition, individuals recover more quickly and return to baseline levels following an exercise bout.

Rate pressure product (RPP), a function of HR × SBP, becomes reduced both at rest and during simulated activities as a result of reductions in both HR and SBP with both resistance and endurance training.[12,17] Improved RPP lowers the myocardial demand and therefore the economy of movement during submaximal exercise. Other improvements from long-term resistance and aerobic exercise programs include reduced DBP and improved SV, CO, and TPR.[15,17]

As a function of aerobic training, O_2 carrying capacity increases as a result of increased numbers of red blood cells. Red blood cells contain hemoglobin, which bind and carry O_2 throughout the body. In conjunction with a greater number of capillaries from long-term training, O_2 delivery to working muscles is improved. Not only is O_2 delivery enhanced with training, but the ability to use available O_2 is also improved as evidenced by improvements in $\dot{V}O_2max$.[15,18,19] Improvements in $\dot{V}O_2max$ allow individuals to increase exercise duration and intensity. Small increases in $\dot{V}O_2max$ are seen as early as 2 to 3 weeks following the commencement of an aerobic training program. Substantial increases in $\dot{V}O_2max$ are notable after 16 weeks of endurance training. Similar changes in $\dot{V}O_2max$ are not evident with resistance training.[12]

Larger mitochondrial size and number are evident in response to training. This training adaptation increases the ability for cells to produce energy for muscular work because the process of oxidative phosphorylation occurs in the mitochondria.

Long-term CV changes that occur at rest include the following: (1) decreased resting HR, (2) decreased SBP, (3) decreased peripheral vascular resistance, and (4) increased blood volume and hemoglobin. Long-term CV changes seen during exercise include the following: (1) decreased exercise HR, (2) increased SV, (3) increased CO, (4) increased extraction of oxygen by working muscles, (5) increased $\dot{V}O_2max$, (6) decreased blood flow per kilogram of working muscle, and (7) decreased myocardial O_2 consumption for any given exercise intensity.

In long-term CV changes with aerobic training, local adaptations include (1) increased mitochondrial size and number; (2) improved O_2 extraction; (3) increased muscle strength; (4) increased aerobic, mitochondrial enzyme activity; (5) increased perfusion of working muscles; (6) decreased peripheral vascular resistance; (7) increased arteriovenous oxygen (A-VO_2) difference; (8) increased parasympathetic nervous system activity; and (9) increased peak O_2 intake. Central adaptations include (1) increased SV; (2) increased CO; (3) increased parasympathetic nervous system activity (improves RHR and working HR); (4) improved myocardial metabolic response; (5) decreased myocardial oxygen consumption during submaximal exercise; (6) decreased SBP; (7) increased venous tone; and (8) improved myocardial contractility.

Long-term respiratory changes at rest include larger lung volume and larger diffusion of capillaries. Long-term respiratory changes during exercise include larger diffusion capacity, lower amount of air ventilated at the same O_2 consumption, increased maximal minute ventilation, increased ventilatory efficiency, and lowered O_2 uptake at submaximal workloads.

Long-term metabolic changes at rest include muscle hypertrophy, increased capillary density, increased number of mitochondria, and increased concentration of muscle myoglobin. Long-term metabolic changes with exercise include decreased

Evidence-Based Clinical Application: Left Ventricular Hypertrophy[20,21]

Left ventricular hypertrophy is a result of normal physiological responses to prolonged strenuous exercise and is also known as an *enlarged heart* or *athlete's heart*. Common characteristics of left ventricular hypertrophy include enlarged ventricles,[22] low RHR, lower than normal exercise HRs, increased SV, ventricular dilation with preserved fractional shortening, and faster myocardial relaxation.[23] Enlargement of the left ventricle is a function of dynamic, aerobic exercise rather than static, resistance exercise. Ventricular hypertrophy results in greater CO and a larger ejection fraction. In addition, because more blood is being pumped from the heart with each beat, resting HR is lowered. Regular exercise training at appropriate intensity, duration, and frequency increases the number and size of myocardial cells, resulting in an increased size of the heart. This results in an increased force of myocardial contraction, subsequently increasing SV and CO.

Changes characterizing an athlete's heart are not necessarily negative adaptations, but they can mask other underlying CV problems such as hypertrophic cardiomyopathy (HCM). Similar to athlete's heart, HCM is characterized by ventricular hypertrophy. In these individuals exercise-induced changes can be symptomatic and result in sudden death either at rest or during exercise as a function of reduced myocardial efficiency and increased myocardial demand. Careful diagnosis and management is critical to prevent adverse events.

rate of depletion of muscle glycogen at submaximal work levels, lower blood lactate levels at submaximal work, less reliance on PC and ATP in skeletal muscle, and increased capability to oxidize carbohydrates.

AGE- AND SEX-RELATED CHANGES IN AEROBIC CAPACITY

Developmental changes of both the CV and respiratory systems occur through adolescence, altering aerobic capacity as a function of age. Developmental changes of the cardiorespiratory system often parallel changes in the musculoskeletal system as the body develops and matures. Therefore some changes during early childhood and throughout adolescence are a function of increased body mass and body size. In turn, these changes affect aerobic metabolic processes that affect the efficiency of movement and functional performance.

Throughout adulthood, changes in cardiorespiratory function are mediated by physical activity level, in addition to disease processes. In general, CV performance decreases with aging beginning around the sixth decade of life. Older adults usually adopt more sedentary lifestyles, and therefore it is difficult to ascertain whether the primary cause of age-related changes in cardiorespiratory function is solely a function of

aging, a result of physical inactivity, or both. Individuals of all ages with sedentary lifestyles have reduced myocardial function (i.e., difficulty maintaining SV at maximum aerobic effort). Therefore age-related declines may be magnified as a function of lifestyle and failure to stress the CV system at high intensities of aerobic effort.

Early Developmental Changes

Cardiovascular changes during growth and development often mimic changes in the body's musculoskeletal composition. As children grow, increases in body weight, muscle mass, lung volume, and heart volume lead to increased $\dot{V}O_2$max, especially between the ages of 5 and 15 years.[24,25] $\dot{V}O_2$max in boys aged 16 to 18 is almost double that of boys aged 7 to 9 years.[26] Before puberty, no sex-related differences are evident, although large differences are noted in adults. Sex-related differences in $\dot{V}O_2$max are a function of lean body mass; when controlling for lean body mass in adults, sex-related differences in $\dot{V}O_2$max are minimal.

Performance on timed measures, such as a 1-mile walk/run time, depend on the percentage of $\dot{V}O_2$max used.[25,27] During growth and development, VO_2submax decreases[25,27] and less O_2 consumption is necessary at similar intensities of submaximal walking and running.[28] These changes lead to a lowered aerobic demand for a specific activity.[24,25] The greatest variability in walking economy is seen among 6- to 10-year-old children despite the fact that mature gait patterns emerge at ages 4 to 5.[29] Differences in young children may be apparent due to differences in step frequency, ventilatory efficiency, or body surface area–to–body mass ratio.[29] During puberty, both running and walking economy improve up to 10% and 24%, respectively.[30] The greatest improvement in running appears during puberty (5 ml/kg/min decrease in VO_2 from ages 13 to 16 years old) with small changes occurring after puberty (2 ml/kg/min decrease in VO_2 from ages 16 to 27 years old).[28]

Although increased muscle mass and body size contribute to the overall decrease in energy expenditure, differences in exercise O_2 consumption still exist between adolescents and adults independent of body composition.[31] Factors such as biomechanical gait characteristics (i.e., stride variability, muscle cocontraction),[32,33] and behavioral and psychological variables (i.e., effort, race strategy, pacing strategies) must be considered in addition to biological factors (i.e., $\dot{V}O_2$max, HR_{max}, muscle fiber composition, aerobic capacity) when assessing children. For example, Allor et al[31] demonstrated that younger body-size–matched females (mean age = 13.3 ± 0.9 years) had a 14 beats/min higher HR during walking and 17 beats/min higher HR during running compared with older females (mean age = 21 ± 1.5 years), as well as an 18% increase in O_2 consumption, a 6 breath/min increase in respiratory rate during walking, and a 9 breath/min increase during running.[31]

SV is also related to body size, and therefore a concomitant increase in SV is apparent during the growing period. As the body increases in size, the heart changes in size proportionally to meet increasing O_2 demands. Children between the ages of 5 and 16 years old have an average SV of 30 to 40 ml compared with adults whose average SV is 60 to 80 ml at rest and 100 ml during maximal exercise. As compensation for smaller SV, children exhibit a greater tolerance to large A-V O_2 differences, allowing them to play or exercise at higher intensities.

At birth, RHR on average is typically greater than 125 beats/min (126 beats/min in girls, 135 beats/min in boys). Throughout development RHR gradually decreases to average RHR levels of 60 to 65 beats/min at around 17 to 18 years of age, matching adult RHR. CO in children is similar to that in adults for any given O_2 consumption and remains similar throughout life. However, endurance increases with age until approximately the second decade of life as a function of improved O_2 extraction. In a mature adult, 25% to 30% of O_2 is extracted from blood by muscles, organs, and other tissues at rest and increases twofold to threefold during exercise. Additionally, SBP increases from 40 mmHg at birth to 80 mmHg at 1 month and to 100 mmHg just before puberty, matching adult levels. DBP models trends in SBP increase from 55 to 70 mmHg between 4 and 14 years of age, with little change during adolescence.

Infants have a rapid respiratory rate at birth secondary to incomplete lung maturation. Respiratory rate (RR) in infants is approximately 30 breaths/min and decreases throughout childhood and late adolescence (17 to 18 years) to levels similar to those of adults, 16 breaths per minute. As the lungs mature and increase in volume, breathing capacity increases, changing the rate and depth of breathing. Sex differences are also evident as a function of body size and lung volume. Vital capacity and maximal voluntary ventilation are greater in males compared with females. Therefore the greatest difference in respiratory capacities between males and females occurs during puberty and continues throughout adulthood.

Exercise in prepubescent children appears to influence CV function. Children who participate in regular physical fitness have a higher $\dot{V}O_2$max and CO compared with children who do not. Physically active children have larger SV despite no differences in HR. Therefore improved $\dot{V}O_2$max appears to be a function of ventricular size.[34]

Changes in Late Adulthood

Cardiorespiratory function decreases with age and is influenced by lifestyle with greater declines evident among more sedentary adults. $\dot{V}O_2$max decreases approximately 10% per decade among sedentary individuals and is approximately 36% to 62% lower in older adults compared with younger adults.[35] A longitudinal study by Astrand et al[36] demonstrated declines in $\dot{V}O_2$max as high as 20% over an 11-year period in individuals 20- to 33 years old. An average 25-year-old has a $\dot{V}O_2$max of 47.7 ml/kg/min compared with a $\dot{V}O_2$max of 25.5 ml/kg/min in an average 75-year-old adult. Age-related declines in $\dot{V}O_2$max are influenced by activity level, and engaging in exercise and vigorous physical activity buffers age-associated losses.[37-39]

In addition, older adults have a lowered tolerance to large A-V O_2 differences. Reductions in tolerance are associated with increases in fat mass or decreases in fat-free mass. These reduc-

tions result in a smaller O_2-carrying capacity and decreases in peak work rate capacity by up to 20%.

Age-related declines in SV adversely affect CO. Declines in CO range from 3.4 to 7 L/min per year beginning during the second decade of life. CO in an adult at rest is 75 beats/min times 75 ml, or 6.5 L/min. With maximal exercise, CO is 190 beats/min times 100 ml, or 19 L/min.

Increases in BP are also evident with age.[35,38] In the average adult, SBP at rest is approximately 120 mmHg and 190 to 240 mmHg during peak exercise. SBP can increase by 50 mmHg in older adults. Similarly, increases in DBP from 80 mmHg to 90 mmHg can result during the aging process, although DBP responses to exercise do not appear to change. SBP and DBP increase during exercise in older adulthood.[35] These decreases in SV, CO, and BP lead to decreased TPR, especially among sedentary older adults.[38]

HR response to exercise decreases as a result of aging. RHR remains stable throughout adulthood and late life despite significant reductions in MHR.[36,40] As reflected in prediction models, MHR is an age-dependent function (MHR = 220 − age). Decreases of up to 14% are evident. Prediction models indicate the average MHR at 20 to 29 years old is approximately 190 beats/min compared with an adult 60 to 69 years old, who exhibits an average MHR of 164 beats/min. HR response is elevated during bouts of submaximal exercise intensities, negatively influencing peak exercise capacity.[35,36] Peak HR during exercise decreases about 25% in older adults, lowering exercise capacity and tolerance.

Respiratory rate slightly increases at rest in older adults from 12 to 15 breaths/min as a function of changes in vital capacity. Vital capacity in an average 20- to 30-year-old adult male is approximately 4800 ml. Progressive declines of up to 25% are evident, resulting from aging processes.

Although changes in cardiorespiratory function may be inevitable, exercise and more active lifestyles may minimize or even prevent age-associated declines. Reductions in HR variability are less among older adults who participate in strenuous exercise (18%) compared with adults who participate in moderately strenuous exercise (38%) and sedentary older adults (64%).[37,38,40] Masters athletes, competitive athletes older than the age of 40, have a $\dot{V}O_2$max similar to younger individuals.[38]

Comorbidities and chronic health issues are important to consider when assessing cardiorespiratory function because disease states substantially alter an individual's ability to participate in physical activity. Alterations in aerobic exercise prescription may be necessary to accommodate for baseline aerobic fitness or disease states; however, all older adults should be encouraged to participate in some form of physical activity. Older adults achieve cardiorespiratory benefit as a result of aerobic endurance training similar to younger cohorts.[41,42] These benefits include increased blood volume, peripheral vascular tone, end-diastolic filling, increased SV at rest and with submaximal exercise, decreased RHR and HR during submaximal exercise, and increased ventricular muscle size.[37,43] Older adults who participate in a long-term, moderately intense exercise program (>75% of peak HR) demonstrate significant improvement in $\dot{V}O_2$max, as well as significant improvements in peak exercise HR that improve peak VO_2 and CO during submaximal exercise.[44-46] Older adults after 9 months of endurance training also exhibit lowered HR during submaximal exercise at similar exercise training, indicating significant improvement in aerobic fitness.[44,46]

Research indicating the optimal dose (frequency, intensity, duration) is not clear. Notable changes are evident within 3 months, and more substantial changes occur in the long term over a 6- to 12-month period.[38] Optimal intensity of aerobic training should be between 60% and 80% of $\dot{V}O_2$max, with higher-intensity exercise eliciting changes.[38] No visible change in $\dot{V}O_2$max and RHR is noticeable following 3 months of walking at 65% to 80% of MHR; however, older adults do exhibit decreased HR during submaximal work intensities, as well as improved exercise tolerance.[40] Longer-term changes, following 6 months of aerobic training, include decreased RHR and increased $\dot{V}O_2$max, peak work rate, and HR variability both at rest and during submaximal exercise intensities[37] with continued improvement in $\dot{V}O_2$max as a result of prolonged aerobic exercise over a 12-month period.[38]

Sex-Related Differences in Aerobic Capacity

Differences in aerobic power between males and females at all ages may be attributed to higher percentages of body fat, lower hemoglobin levels, smaller hearts, and lower blood volumes in females compared with males. Males have a larger inspiratory capacity compared with females as a function of increased body size,[47] which influences breathing patterns during exercise. As a result of smaller inspiratory capacity and TV, females exhibit greater respiratory rates compared with males at similar exercise intensities.[47]

EXERCISE PROGRAM DESIGN

Hasson[48] described endurance as follows: "Endurance is the most important component of training. Endurance is the ability of the heart, lungs, and circulatory system to take oxygen from the air and deliver it throughout the body. The body undergoes an adaptive response to the demands of repeated exercise. The heart pumps faster, and the arteries become dilated so that more blood can be carried to the working muscles. The muscles become more efficient at absorbing oxygen from the blood and converting stored carbohydrates and fats into energy. These effects are referred to as training effects."

All individuals and athletes need a minimum level of CV fitness for optimal performance. In designing an aerobic endurance program, health professionals must consider an individual's age, health status, physical condition and fitness level, and current training regimen. No single program is sufficient for all individuals or even for athletes of the same sport. Each training program must be individualized on the basis of strengths, weaknesses, sport-specific demands, and goals. Numerous principles, modes of training, and training parameters can be manipulated to tailor an exercise program

for each individual. Regardless, HR must be elevated to at least 60% of HR reserve to improve cardiorespiratory fitness (see following equation).[49]

$$(HR_{max} - rest \times 60\% + HR_{rest})$$

Principles of Exercise Prescription

Cardiovascular adaptations occur with almost any regular exercise program, independent of the mode of exercise, although adaptations are task specific. The Specific Adaptation to Imposed Demands (SAID) principle, or principle of specificity, implies that adaptations resulting from a training program are specific to the energy system and muscles used or stressed. A runner who is participating in a running program to improve CV fitness will demonstrate improved aerobic capacity with minimal to no changes in muscle strength and little carry-over to sports such as cycling or swimmer. Furthermore, a swimmer must engage in a swimmer endurance training program in order to enhance aerobic capacity and economy for swimming in order to achieve improved swimming endurance. A land program consisting of running and cycling will not be sufficient to achieve improved performance during swimming.

Although cross-training is important to minimize the effects of overtraining and occurrence of musculoskeletal overuse-related injuries, in order to excel in a sport or activity an individual's training program must incorporate that sport or activity to stressing the primary aerobic and physiological systems used during that sport. Different programs must be designed for the endurance athlete than for the strength and power athlete. An upper extremity weight-lifting program stresses anaerobic systems but does not enhance $\dot{V}O_2$max. Although benefits of upper extremity strengthening are carried over to sports such as climbing and rowing, training must include climbing and rowing simulations to improve the economy of the sport-specific demands.

Exercise intensity also influences the magnitude of cardiorespiratory benefit. Jogging or walking programs at light intensities of less than 50% $\dot{V}O_2$max are not likely to enhance cardiorespiratory endurance. Physiological systems must be stressed beyond their typical demand in order to achieve improved performance. This is known as the *overload principle.* Just as overloading the musculoskeletal system increases muscle strength, overloading aerobic systems enhances aerobic capacity. The rate of physiological improvement depends on the amount of stress or overload placed on the system.

The longer individuals participate in a regular exercise program and a higher baseline at the initiation of an exercise program warrant adjustments to elicit further gains. Manipulation of program variables (i.e., frequency of training, intensity of exercise, and duration of exercise) is necessary to alter the stress induced on metabolic systems and to increase the demand of the activity. The variables and degree to which they are regulated vary on the basis of the desired training adaptations. As a general rule, alteration of rest periods adjusts the metabolic demand of the activity. Shorter rest periods between exercise bouts tend to increase exercise intensity and can reach levels closer to the anaerobic threshold.[50] A second variable that can be adjusted to raise or lower exercise demand is resistance, often defined by repetition maximum (RM). RM is the maximal amount of resistance/weight that can be performed during a specific task or exercise. A 1 RM is the amount of weight that can be performed once, whereas an 8 RM is the maximal amount of weight that can be performed 8 times repeatedly before failure or fatigue. Activities defined by higher RM place more stress on aerobic systems. This can be achieved by lowering the resistance and increasing the number of repetitions. Intensity levels greater than 8 RM have a greater impact on aerobic endurance.[51] Such programs are beneficial to endurance athletes because they allow individuals to maintain strength to minimize or prevent other musculoskeletal injuries while still taxing the aerobic system.

Variation is also important for continued benefit with long-term exercise programs. Performing the same exercise program over a prolonged period leads to a reduction in peak heart work rate and O_2 demand, lowering the physiological demand placed on the CV system. This negative phenomenon as a result of a repetitive training program is referred to as *habituation*. When these changes occur, the CV system has difficulty adapting to altered CV demands. Therefore by varying training programs regularly every 4 to 6 weeks, the CV can adjust more favorably to different stresses it may encounter. Cross-training is an ideal means to vary the CV demand and minimize habituation. Cross-training often stresses both aerobic and anaerobic energy systems. By varying metabolic and CV demands, cross-training exposes these systems to various training stimuli, training the systems to adapt to altered physiological demands.

Components of Exercise Program

Although these principles can be applied to any exercise program, this section specifically addresses programs to enhance cardiorespiratory and aerobic performance.

Warm-Up

The warm-up period prepares the body and working muscles for upcoming physiological demands by directly accessing the working muscles. The warm-up period should consist of movements that mimic those of the muscles about to be used. This phase of the exercise program increases circulation and dilation of local blood vessels. The warm-up period also increases muscle temperature, improves the efficiency of muscle contraction, augments O_2 delivery to meet increasing energy demands, and improves venous return to offset the increased production of CO_2.

Work/Aerobic Period

The aerobic period is the core segment of the training program. This phase is the bulk of the program that will elicit both short- and long-term adaptations and improvements. The mode, intensity, and duration of the work performed will influence overall outcomes. The goals of the individual and

sport-specific skills will ultimately dictate and govern the development of an appropriate program. For example, a soccer player needs to train both aerobically and anaerobically based on the demands of the game (i.e., springing over distance, jumping to head a ball, leg power to shoot) and would benefit from both endurance and strength training. Therefore interval- or circuit-type training may best achieve the desired results for this athlete.

Considering the environment (i.e., temperature, terrain, wind, rain, etc.) is important when designing the work phase of the program. These factors may dictate the work-to-rest ratio or type of program prescribed.

Cool Down and Stretch

Lastly, an exercise program should be completed with a cool-down phase or a period of recovery. This phase consists of two parts. First, an active recovery period slowly returns the CV and pulmonary systems to baseline levels. Typically, movements incorporating the working muscles of the training period are worked at gradually lowered intensities. Second, stretching of the worked muscles helps to improve and maintain flexibility.

Types of Aerobic Endurance Programs

The mode and implementation of exercise allow individuals to vary the intensity of the program by increasing or decreasing the work time and altering the demand on different energy systems. A continuous bout of exercise is characterized by a program usually about 20 to 60 minutes in duration. During this type of exercise, muscle obtains its energy through aerobic mechanisms minimizing the use of anaerobic metabolic means. In contrast, circuit training consists of a series of activities involving an array of large and small muscle groups through a range of exercises. Circuit training can equally tax both the aerobic and anaerobic systems depending on the duration, intensity, and type of exercise employed.

Long, Slow Distance

Long, slow distance programs are a form of continuous exercise. Exercise intensity is approximately 70% of $\dot{V}O_2$max or 80% of MHR, or both. This type of training is referred to as *conversation exercise* because the individual should be able to easily maintain a conversation during the exercise. Duration of long, slow distance programs can vary from 30 minutes to 3 hours, and therefore this type of activity primarily stresses aerobic fuel sources. For the athlete, training distances in a long, slow distance program are typically longer than race distances.

Benefits of long, slow distance training include enhanced CV and thermoregulatory function, improved mitochondrial efficiency for energy production, and increased utilization of fat stores for energy. A drawback to long, slow distance program is that training intensity must often be below competition intensity in order to work for an extended period of time.

Evidence-Based Clinical Application: Dangers of Aerobic Exercise in the Heat

Heat illness is most commonly described and best understood in three degrees of severity: heat cramping, heat exhaustion, and heat stroke. Importantly, these levels of severity do not necessarily occur in progression and each should be taken seriously.

Muscle cramping that occurs during aerobic exercise in the heat is not completely understood and in fact may be the result of a number of factors, such as dehydration and electrolyte loss. In addition, a low-sodium diet, excessive sweating, poor hydration, and poor acclimation to an environmental condition (i.e., heat and humidity) have also been considered as predisposing factors. As such, the treatment for general muscle cramps for this individual should include stretching, replacement of fluids and electrolytes, and rest.

Improper aerobic training in the heat can result in inadequate thermoregulatory performance by the CV system. Signs of heat exhaustion can be highly variable but most commonly include fatigue; faintness; dizziness; chills; and cool, clammy skin. Heat exhaustion can quickly become life-threatening heat stroke without early, proper treatment. The individual displaying any one or combination of symptoms of heat exhaustion should move to a cool, shaded area; rest; and drink plenty of fluids to rehydrate and restore electrolyte balance.

The most severe form of heat-related illness is heat stroke. In the most extreme cases heat stroke can result in death without quick, adequate treatment. Heat stroke results from a failure of the central nervous system to maintain thermoregulation. Early warning signs of heat stroke include signs similar to heat exhaustion—weakness, nausea, dizziness, and drowsiness—in addition to more extreme behavioral changes, such as confusion, disorientation, and irrational behavior. These symptoms may be transient and may not occur at all in some individuals at risk for heat stroke, making identification and diagnosis difficult in some situations. Continued exertion in the heat in the presence of early warning signs may lead to collapse. On collapse of the exercising individual, heat stroke can be identified by confusion or agitation, or both; coma; convulsions; vomiting; diarrhea; hypotension (systolic < 90 mmHg); or dry skin.[52] Treatment needs to be immediate and aggressive at this point. The ultimate goal of treatment is to lower the individual's core body temperature via packing the individual with ice packs or submersion in an ice water bath. Death is imminent if body temperature reaches a level of hyperthermia (about 104° F), a point of severe organ damage or failure.

Case Study: Heat Stroke

The patient is a 17-year-old, healthy lacrosse player. The season is about to start, and he is highly motivated to perform well at practice. The day is hot and humid, marking the start of a heat wave, with the temperature being 92° F with 60% humidity. The medical staff is not aware of any problems until the player collapses on the field. When they reach the athlete, they see that his mental state is altered because he is confused and incoherent. He is wet with sweat, and his respiration is fast. After removing him from the sun and off the artificial turf, his equipment including helmet, gloves, shirt, and pads is removed and he is packed with ice bags around his neck, groin, and under his armpits. His BP is 132/60, and his HR is 130 beats/min. He loses consciousness while having his vital signs taken. His rectal temperature is taken and is found to be 106° F. He is then transported to the emergency department and suffers cardiac arrest en route. He is declared dead on arrival at the hospital.

This is an example of exertional heat stroke. Of the risk factors for serious heat illness, those that the athlete can control to a degree are lack of acclimatization, overzealous performance or "competing above one's head,"[53-56] and dehydration. When and where possible, athletes should be made aware of the need to acclimatize,[57] maintain an athletic pace that is within their limits, and maintain adequate fluid intake. Considering that the event occurred during a heat wave, the athlete was most likely not acclimated to the environment. Further, a highly motivated athlete may "play through" early warning signs of heat illness, such as dizziness, weakness, or cramping. Although lack of sweating may be a sign of classic heat-stroke, athletes with exertional heatstroke may continue to sweat. Correct diagnosis must then be based on mental status and core (rectal) temperature. Mental status changes associated with exertional heat stroke include coma, confusion and disorientation, and psychotic behavior.[53] The hallmark sign of heat stroke is rectal temperature greater than 104° F and thus should be taken if the collapsed athlete has these mental status changes. This method of measuring temperature must be used because oral, axillary, and aural temperature measurements are all believed to reflect peripheral or shell temperatures, which may not correlate to core temperature.[58] Initial treatment should then be to remove the athlete from the hot environment, remove equipment, and make every attempt to decrease core temperature. The most effective cooling method is ice water immersion[59]; however, this may not be practical. Other methods include wrapping with cool wet towels, packing the athlete with ice, and dousing with cold water. Despite efforts of decreasing core temperature and maintaining an airway, internal hemorrhaging may lead to irreversible internal bleeding and organ failure, as in this case.

Pace/Tempo

Pace/tempo training is referred to as *threshold training* because it is performed at an intensity just below the anaerobic/lactic acid threshold. Intensities for this type of training regimen are equivalent and oftentimes greater than competition intensity. Duration of a pace/tempo program is typically 20 to 30 minutes and stresses primarily aerobic mechanisms. Pace/tempo

Evidence-Based Clinical Application: Dehydration

The means that the body dissipates heat to regulate body temperature are radiation, conduction, convection, and evaporation. Radiation is the transfer of heat through electromagnetic waves projected or absorbed by the body. Heat loss to decrease body temperature through the process of radiation is only effective when the skin temperature is greater than the environment around the body. The second method of temperature regulation, conduction, is a mechanism by which energy is transferred between two mediums. An example is the use of a cool towel placed around the body to lower body temperature on a hot day. Thirdly, convection is the transfer of heat to air currents moving around the body. Two examples are the cooling effect of the wind while running on a windy day and cold water passing around a swimmer. Finally, the primary mechanism of heat dissipation used by the body is evaporation of sweat from the outer skin's surface. During exercise, the body produces sweat on the skin's surface. Heat is removed from the body as the sweat evaporates, providing a cooling effect. Evaporation of sweat to lower body temperature depends on environmental conditions, accounting for up to 80% of heat loss. The amount of sweat produced by an athlete varies according to a person's size, fitness level, environmental climate, clothing, equipment, hydration, exercise duration and intensity, acclimatization to the environment, and heredity. Although generalization is difficult, professional athletes have been known to lose up to 2 or more quarts of sweat per hour of competition.[60]

Muscles, blood, and vital organs are composed of up to 80% fluid. Therefore it is imperative to keep the body in a hydrated state in order to maintain homeostasis and normal physiological function. Consequences of dehydration include increased core body temperature, impaired skin blood flow, and delayed sweat response.[61] These effects are precursors to heat illness including heat exhaustion and heat stroke, which can be deadly. Loss of 3% or more of body weight via sweating increases the risk of developing heat illness.[62] In addition, losing up to 2% of body weight through sweating results in increased CV strain as a result of elevated HR. Therefore maintaining a hydrated state during exercise or athletic events

not only serves to maintain performance, but also to prevent heat-related illness.

The following are hydration recommendations from different organizations:

1. *American College of Sports Medicine* (1996): "It is recommended that individuals drink about 500 ml (about 17 oz) of fluid about 2 hours before exercise to promote adequate hydration and allow time for the excretion of excess ingested water. During exercise, athletes should start drinking early and at regular intervals in an attempt to consume fluids at a rate sufficient to replace all the water lost through sweating (i.e., body weight loss), or consume the maximal amount that can be tolerated."[63]

2. *American Academy of Pediatrics* (2000): "Before prolonged physical activity, the child should be well hydrated. During the activity, periodic drinking should be enforced (e.g., each 20 minutes 150 ml [5 oz] of cold tap water or a flavored salted beverage for a child weighing 40 kg (88 lb) and 250 ml [9 oz] for an adolescent weighing 60 kg [132 lb]), even if the child does not feel thirsty. Weighing before and after a training session can verify hydration status if the child is wearing little to no clothing."[64]

3. *American Dietetics Association, Dietitians of Canada, and American College of Sports Medicine* (2000): "Athletes should drink enough fluid to balance their fluid losses. Two hours before exercise, 400 to 600 ml (14 to 22 oz) of fluid should be consumed, and during exercise, 150 to 350 ml (6 to 12 oz) of fluid should be consumed every 15 to 20 minutes depending on tolerance."[65]

4. *National Athletic Training Association* (2000): "To ensure proper preexercise hydration, the athletes should consume approximately 500 to 600 ml (17 to 20 oz) of water or a sports drink 2 to 3 hours before exercise and 200 to 300 ml (7 to 10 oz) of water or a sports drink 10 to 20 minutes before exercise. Fluid replacement should approximate sweat and urine losses and at least maintain hydration at less than 2% bodyweight reduction. This generally requires 200 to 300 ml (7 to 10 oz) every 10 to 20 minutes."[61]

---

training can either take the form of continuous or circuit training.

Interval

Intermittent or interval training is a method of exercise characterized by alternating intervals of work and rest (work-to-rest). A series of short work intervals are performed at a high intensity interspersed with brief rest periods stressing both aerobic and anaerobic systems. Similar to pace/tempo training, the purpose of interval training is to allow the individual to

exercise at near $\dot{V}O_2max$ intensities. However, interspersing rest allows individuals to train for longer periods than with continuous exercise. A major benefit of interval training is to improve race pace.

Typically, interval programs have work-to-rest ratios of 1:1 or 1:1.5 at near $\dot{V}O_2max$ intensities for 3 to 5 minutes. Although gains in strength and power are greater than gains in endurance, the longer the work interval, the more the aerobic system is taxed and results in increased $\dot{V}O_2max$. As exercise capacity improves, work intervals should be increased while decreasing rest intervals.

Repetition

Repetition training involves performance at high intensities for brief bursts of time. Traditional weight-lifting programs are a common example. Intensity is often greater than $\dot{V}O_2$max, and therefore a large demand is placed on the anaerobic system. Exercise is performed in 30- to 90-second bouts with long recovery periods. A typical work-to-rest ratio is 1:5. Benefits of repetition training include increased power and strength and therefore improved running speed, enhanced running economy, and increased capacity of anaerobic metabolism.

Fartlek

Fartlek training was designed by the Swedish. It means "speed play." Fartlek training involves a combination of continuous and interval training within one workout. The primary goal is to enhance endurance. Typically, low-intensity running at approximately 70% of $\dot{V}O_2$max is interspersed with either hill running or short, fast bursts of higher intensity at approximately 85% to 90% $\dot{V}O_2$max.

Variables of an Exercise Program

Frequency

Frequency of an exercise program refers to how often the exercise program is performed (i.e., twice a day, three times a week). The optimal frequency and duration of an exercise program should be based on the acute response to exercise, recovery process, and the short- and long-term goals of the individual. Individuals should perform moderate intensity exercise 3 to 4 days per week. Programs of lower intensity may require individuals to exercise more frequently to achieve cardiovascular benefit.

Rest is essential for the recovery process to take place. The rest period is time for the body to rebuild to a higher level of function. Replenishment of glycogen stores and repair of the musculoskeletal system can take up to 2 days to complete and therefore should be considered during program design. Resistance training should allow at least a 24- to 48-hour rest period before engaging in a resistance program using the same muscle groups. Endurance training can occur more frequently because endurance programs often have a lower intensity. However, speed or hill workouts and long training runs should not be performed on consecutive days but rather alternated for adequate recovery.

Exercise Intensity

Exercise intensity refers to the level of exertion during an exercise program. It can be quantified by power output, or work performed per unit of time. Aerobic endurance programs are often considered to be lower-intensity workouts because they are performed over much longer intervals, requiring larger aerobic energy reserves. Resistance training programs are characterized as high intensity because a large amount of work is

Evidence-Based Clinical Application: Continuous versus Intermittent Exercise

With the rise of obesity and other health-related consequences in the United States, it is important that individuals participate in regular physical activity. The Centers for Disease Control recommends individuals participate in 30 minutes of moderately intense physical activity on most, if not all, days of the week to attain cardiovascular health benefits and optimum health.[66]

Do individuals attain the same cardiovascular benefit from three smaller bouts of moderately intense physical activity compared with one longer-duration exercise session? A study by Peterson et al demonstrated no significant difference in caloric energy expenditure when individuals partook in 30 minutes of continuous exercise compared with three 10-minute bouts of exercise.[67]

Therefore when prescribing exercise programs, it is important to consider the needs of the patient. Sedentary older adults may not be able to tolerate 30 minutes of continuous aerobic exercise. If an individual is unable to sustain an exercise intensity level of approximately 70% of $\dot{V}O_2$max, breaking up the exercise into smaller bouts may be more beneficial. The goal of the shorter exercise program is to allow the individual to sustain higher exercise intensities approaching levels of 70% of $\dot{V}O_2$max in order to reap some CV benefit.

performed in a short time. As a general rule, activities of low intensity and long duration require energy from aerobic systems, whereas activities characterized by high intensity and short duration require energy from anaerobic means.

Similar to other training variables, the intensity of a given training program must be prescribed on the basis of an individual's fitness level, training level, and goals of exercise. Training threshold is the minimal level at which a patient should exercise in order to achieve optimal benefit from a training program. The optimal intensity of endurance training lies at or just below a work rate at which lactic acid begins to accumulate. Interval training allows individuals to train at higher levels of effort for longer periods. Conditioning responses typically occur when performing exercise at 60% to 80% of $\dot{V}O_2$max or 70% to 85% of MHR, with healthy young adults seeing adaptations at the lower end of this range and athletes at the upper end of the range. On the basis of the guidelines from the American College of Sports Medicine, an individual should participate in an aerobic program at a minimum of 60% to 75% of MHR in order to achieve long-term improvements.[68]

The rate of perceived exertion (RPE) scale is a subjective means to obtain an individual's training intensity on the basis of the physical sensations a person experiences during physical activity including HR, respiration rate, sweating, and fatigue.[69] RPE is a reliable indicator of perceived exertion during exercise and is strongly correlated with HR and $\dot{V}O_2$max.[70,71] RPE levels of 12 to 14, somewhat hard, have been correlated with moderate-intensity physical activity (Figure 4-7). On the basis of these ratings, a person becomes accustomed to physical sensations correlated with exertion, allowing him or her to increase or decrease exercise effort to achieve a desired training intensity.

Metabolic equivalent of the task (MET) is a measure used to estimate the amount of O_2 consumed by the body during physical activity.[72] The harder the body works, the more O_2 is consumed, and the higher the MET. 1 MET is equivalent to the amount of O_2 consumed while at rest, approximately 3.5 ml of O_2 per kilogram of body weight per minute (1.2 kcal/min for a 70-kg or 154-lb individual). A 5 MET activity requires 5 times more metabolic energy expenditure than sitting at rest. Activities characterized as 3 to 6 MET are considered to be of moderate intensity, and activities characterized as greater than 6 MET are considered to of vigorous intensity (Figure 4-7).

Other means to determine exercise intensity include pulse rate, onset of sweating, and ability to carry a normal conversation.

Calculation of the time necessary to accumulate a certain energy expenditure can be derived from the MET of the activity. Dividing the number of kcal, or energy expenditure, by the MET level gives the time necessary to perform the activity. For example, to determine the time necessary to perform the same 6 MET activity and accumulate 300 kcal, the activity would have to be at least 50 minutes in duration.

Exercising at a higher intensity for a shorter duration appears to elicit greater improvement in $\dot{V}O_2$max than exercising at a moderate intensity for a longer period. Karvonen et al[49] suggest initiating an exercise program at an intensity of 60% to 70% of the individual's $\dot{V}O_2$max and progressing to intensities of 70% to 80% $\dot{V}O_2$max. Ideally, a 20- to 30-minute session at 70% of MHR is sufficient.

Mode

The specificity principle is important when determining the mode of exercise. Activities involving large muscle groups in a rhythmic, aerobic manner best maintain or improve overall cardiovascular fitness. CV benefit depends on the amount of muscle mass incorporated in the activity. The rise in BP during exercise is generally proportional to the fraction of maximal muscle force that is exerted. Activities involving smaller active muscles (i.e., hand muscles) impart fewer changes in systemic BP than activities engaging larger muscles (i.e., quadriceps and hamstring muscles). In addition, peak HR is generally lower during arm exercise compared with leg exercise because effort with upper extremity exercise is limited to peripheral muscular fatigue rather than cardiovascular performance.

Special Considerations

Children

Similar to adults, children achieve benefit from regular, formal exercise training. Formal exercise is becoming increasingly

---

Instructions to the Borg–RPE–Scale®

During the work we want you to rate your perception of exertion, i.e., how heavy and strenuous the exercise feels to you and how tired you are. The perception of exertion is mainly felt as strain and fatigue in your muscles and as breathlessness, or aches in the chest. All work requires some effort, even if this is only minimal. This is true also if you only move a little, e.g., walking slowly.

Use this scale from 6 to 20, with **6** meaning "No exertion at all" and **20** meaning "maximal exertion".

6 "No exertion at all", means that you don't feel any exertion whatsoever, e.g. no muscle fatigue, no breathlessness or difficulties breathing.

9 "Very light" exertion, as taking a shorter walk at your own pace.

13 A "Somewhat hard" work, but it still feels OK to continue.

15 It is "hard" and tiring, but continuing isn't terribly difficult.

17 "Very hard". This is very strenuous work. You can still go on, but you really have to push yourself and you are very tired.

19 An "extremely" strenuous level. For most people this is the most strenuous work they have ever experienced.

Try to appraise your feeling of exertion and fatigue as spontaneously and as honestly as possible, without thinking about what the actual physical load is. Try not to underestimate and not to overestimate your exertion. It's your own feeling of effort and exertion that is important, not how this compares with other people's. Look at the scale and the expressions and then give a number. Use any number you like on the scale, not just one of those with an explanation behind it.

Any questions?

Figure 4-7 Classification of exercise intensity related to MHR, $\dot{V}O_2$max, rate of perceived exertion, and metabolic equivalent of the task. (©GunnarBorg.)

---

indicated in children as a result of the growing epidemic of childhood obesity. Special considerations are necessary especially during the years of optimal growth to prevent injury. Exertion is rarely detrimental to a child's health; however, children have difficulty pacing themselves during physical activities. Typically, children go at maximal capacity at the onset of exercise, which prevents them from being able to perform exercise at a sustained intensity, such as 75% of their maximal speed. This challenges the health professional to communicate on an appropriate age level to the exercise participant.

Other considerations include goals of the exercise program; risks and contraindications of exercise in children; and expectations of the children, parents, and health care professionals. Parents are among the most important components of training programs because they oversee the daily implementation of the exercise program. Goals must be attainable; clearly understood by children; and, most importantly, fun. Children often do not understand goals focused on physiological demand. Implementation of token systems leads children to increase adherence and attain goals while making the physical activity fun.

The American Heart Association recommends that (1) all children aged 2 and older should participate in at least 30 minutes of enjoyable, moderate-intensity activities each day;

Evidence-Based Clinical Application: Do You Burn More Calories Running or Walking a Mile?

The short answer is that you burn more calories running a given distance rather than walking. However, if you can walk 4 hours and only run 4 minutes, this becomes a nonissue. Analyses of the biomechanics of walking versus running suggest that walking is a more efficient gait except at higher speeds. At the cross-over speed, walking and running are equally efficient. Below the cross-over point, running is less efficient. Above the cross-over speed, walking becomes less efficient, even among race-walkers.

Economy of mobility is a speed-dependent, sub-maximal measure of O_2 uptake.[73,74] This measure is often expressed as VO_2submax per unit of body mass (ml/kg/min). Activities that are less economical require more physical work to perform the task, and greater fatigue will be exhibited during a task. A more efficient or economical individual would use less O_2 to perform a specified activity. Running and walking are two commonly studied movement patterns to determine VO_2submax. With increasing velocities of movement, there is a cross-over point based on HR at which running becomes more economical than walking. This occurs at approximately 8 to 9 km/hr or 2.5 m/sec.[75,76] Typically individuals choose a preferred running or walking speed-dependent on the basis of its efficiency. Thirty-percent more energy is required to walk at 3.5 m/sec than to run at the same speed.[74] Walking at 2 to 3 mph costs approximately 70 to 80 kcal/mile, whereas running at 5 to 7 mph costs approximately 120 to 130 kcal/mile.[77] The biomechanics of normal walking occur up to speeds approximately 3 m/sec, and race walking can occur at speeds of approximately 4 m/sec; however, the mechanics of movement are significantly altered, increasing the energy demands. The most efficient speed occurs at approximately 1.4 m/sec. Community ambulation speeds in young adults approximate this at average speeds of approximately 1.5 m/sec. The caloric cost of running at 5, 6, or 7 mph is significantly greater than walking at 2, 3, or 4 mph. When ankle and hand weights are added to walking at 2 to 4 mph, the caloric cost exceeds that of running at 5 to 7 mph.[77]

The use of fatty acids and glucose is duration- and intensity-dependent during exercise. Fatty acids are used as the primary fuel source because more ATP can be produced by oxidation of a fat molecule than by oxidation of a glucose molecule. When O_2 supplies are scarce, glucose becomes the preferential fuel source because oxidation of glucose requires less O_2 per mole than the oxidation of fatty acids. Low-intensity exercise of long duration (<50% $\dot{V}O_2$max) is characterized by oxidation of both FFA and glucose. Increased exercise duration or lowered intensity activities, or both, rely on a greater percentage of FFA oxidation for ATP production. Conversely, when exercise is performed at workloads of moderate to heavy intensity (>50% $\dot{V}O_2$ max), glucose becomes the predominant fuel source. At high-intensity workloads (75% to 90% of $\dot{V}O_2$max), FFA oxidation accounts for approximately 25% of the fuel, and during maximal and supermaximal exercising conditions (>100% $\dot{V}O_2$max), little if any energy is derived from FFA metabolism.

$$V_{O_2} = 1.866 + (speed \times 0.177) + (run = 4.855 \text{ or walk} = 0)$$

Several researchers have tried to develop models to estimate the energy cost of walking and running.

$$MET_{walking} = 75 \times (mile/min)$$

$$MET_{running} = 100 \times (mile/min)$$

Training significantly influences running economy; trained individuals are more economical than untrained individuals.[78,79] Age-related differences are also evident in running economy. Young children are less efficient than older, prepubescent children and adults, and older adults become less economical during running with increased age.[80] Although the research is not conclusive, it appears that men may be more economical than women.[78] Running surface must be considered when determining energy expenditure of walking and running. Treadmill running compared with over-ground running both on level surface and inclined surfaces requires similar O_2 uptakes.[81] Walking or running on dry sand is 1.5 to 2.5 times more costly than walking or running on hard surfaces,[82,83] walking in deep snow is 5 times more costly than walking on a treadmill,[84] and walking on soft surfaces is more costly than walking on firm surfaces. When walking or running at extreme slopes of 0.45, the economy of movement becomes similar.[85] Although running is more efficient than walking at speeds above 2.5 m/sec, walking becomes more economical than running when traversing terrains with greater than 10% to 15% inclines.[86]

(2) children should perform at least 30 minutes of vigorous physical activities at least 3 to 4 days each week to achieve and maintain a good level of cardiorespiratory (heart and lung) fitness; and (3) if children do not have a full 30-minute activity break each day, at least two 15-minute periods or three 10-minute periods of vigorous activities appropriate to age, gender, and stage of physical and emotional development should be provided.

Older Adults

Training and the potential for gains in strength and endurance depend on compliance and the regular upward adjustments in training programs independent of the age of the participant. Similar to younger adults, gains made with regular training programs are lost after 2 to 3 weeks of detraining. However, the more sedentary the individual at the onset of an exercise program, the lesser the magnitude of the training effects.[44,87] In addition, although older adults achieve benefit from low-intensity exercise programs, more intense programs yield more substantial improvement in CV function.[87]

Conventional thought has led to increased concern regarding elevated BP among older individuals. However, rise in BP at any given fraction of maximal volitional force is not greater in elderly individuals compared with younger adults. Therefore this should be of minimal concern when prescribing exercise to older adults. Rather, it is more important to remember that in older adults the slowed physiological processes should be considered in exercise prescription.

SUMMARY

The cardiovascular system, consisting of the heart and the network of blood vessels, is responsible for supplying O_2 and removing CO_2 and waste products to ensure adequate perfusion of working muscle during exercise. The primary function of the respiratory system is to bring O_2 into the lungs to supply the cardiovascular system through the processes of respiration and ventilation.

Aerobic metabolism is the oxidative process of the generation of ATP or energy that occurs in the body to provide the body with fuel during both resting and exercise states. Aerobic activities impart significant changes in cardiorespiratory function. Long-term participation in aerobic exercise programs leads to favorable adaptations in CV health. These adaptations occur independent of age and sex, although the magnitude of change varies according to lean muscle mass, baseline cardiorespiratory function, and training parameters.

Manipulation of training variables is necessary to develop individualized programs to meet goals and achieve desired training effects. Programs should be sport specific, and modifications should be made at appropriate intervals to allow the body to adjust favorably to altered physiological loads.

REFERENCES

1. Chobanian AV, Bakris GL, Black HR, et al: The Seventh Report of the Joint National Committee on Prevention, Detection, Evaluation, and Treatment of High Blood Pressure, *JAMA* 289(19):2560-2572, 2003.
2. MacKnight J: Hypertension in athletes and active patients, *Physician Sportsmedicine* 27(4):35-44, 1999.
3. Astrand I, Hedman R: Muscular strength and aerobic capacity in men 50-64 years old, *Int Z Angew Physiol* 19:425-429, 1963.
4. Childs JD: The impact of the Valsalva maneuver during resistance exercise, *J Strength Cond Res* 21(2):54-55, 1999.
5. Morris J, Lucas D, Bresler B: Role of the trunk in stability of the spine, *J Bone Joint Surg* 43-A:327-351, 1961.
6. Findley BW: Is the Valsalva maneuver a proper breathing technique? *J Strength Cond Res* 25(4):52-53, 2003.
7. DeVan AE, Anton MM, Cook JN, et al: Acute effects of resistance exercise on arterial compliance, *J Appl Physiol* 98(6):2287-2291, 2005.
8. Gotshalk LA, Berger RA, Kraemer WJ: Cardiovascular responses to a high-volume continuous circuit resistance training protocol, *J Strength Cond Res* 18(4):760-764, 2004.
9. Keeler LK, Finkelstein LH, Miller W, et al: Early-phase adaptations of traditional-speed vs. superslow resistance training on strength and aerobic capacity in sedentary individuals, *J Strength Cond Res* 15(3):309-314, 2001.
10. Frontera WR, Meredith CN, O'Reilly KP, et al: Strength training and determinants of {Vdot}O_2max in older men, *J Appl Physiol* 68(1):329-333, 1990.
11. Ferketich AK, Kirby TE, Alway SE: Cardiovascular and muscular adaptations to combined endurance and strength training in elderly women, *Acta Physiol Scand* 164(3):259-267, 1998.
12. Goldberg L, Elliot DL, Kuehl KS: A comparison of the cardiovascular effects of running and weight training, *J Strength Cond Res* 8(4):219-224, 1994.
13. Weissman ML, Jones PW, Oren A, et al: Cardiac output increase and gas exchange at start of exercise, *J Appl Physiol* 52(1):236-244, 1982.
14. Askanazi J, Milic-Emili J, Broell JR, et al: Influence of exercise and CO_2 on breathing pattern of normal man, *J Appl Physiol* 47(1):192-196, 1979.
15. Ekblom B, Astrand PO, Saltin B, et al: Effect of training on circulatory response to exercise, *J Appl Physiol* 24(4):518-528, 1968.
16. Banister EW, Morton RH, Fitz-Clarke J: Dose/response effects of exercise modeled from training: physical and biochemical measures, *Ann Physiol Anthropol* 11(3):345-356, 1992.
17. Iwasaki K, Zhang R, Zuckerman JH, et al: Dose-response relationship of the cardiovascular adaptation to endurance training in healthy adults: how much training for what benefit? *J Appl Physiol* 95(4):1575-1583, 2003.
18. Ekblom B: Effect of physical training in adolescent boys, *J Appl Physiol* 27(3):350-355, 1969.
19. Morris CK, Froelicher VF: Cardiovascular benefits of improved exercise capacity, *Sports Med* 16(4):225-236, 1993.
20. Kokkinos PF, Narayan P, Colleran JA, et al: Effects of regular exercise on blood pressure and left ventricular hypertrophy in African-American men with severe hypertension, *N Engl J Med* 333(22):1462-1467, 1995.
21. Raskoff WJ, Goldman S, Cohn K: The "athletic heart." Prevalence and physiological significance of left ventricular enlargement in distance runners, *JAMA* 236(2):158-162, 1976.
22. Turpeinen AK, Kuikka JT, Vanninen E, et al: Athletic heart: a metabolic, anatomical, and functional study, *Med Sci Sports Exerc* 28(1):33-40, 1996.
23. Puffer JC: The athletic heart syndrome, *Physician Sportsmed* 30(7):41-47, 2002.

24. Daniels J, Oldridge N, Nagle F, et al: Differences and changes in VO_2 among young runners 10 to 18 years of age, *Med Sci Sports* 10(3):200-203, 1978.

25. McCormack WP, Cureton KJ, Bullock TA, et al: Metabolic determinants of 1-mile run/walk performance in children, *Med Sci Sports Exerc* 23(5):611-617, 1991.

26. Daniels JT, Yarbrough RA, Foster C: Changes in VO_2 max and running performance with training, *Eur J Appl Physiol Occup Physiol* 39(4):249-254, 1978.

27. Cureton KJ, Sloniger MA, Black DM, et al: Metabolic determinants of the age-related improvement in one-mile run/walk performance in youth, *Med Sci Sports Exerc* 29(2):259-267, 1997.

28. Ariens GA, van Mechelen W, Kemper HC, et al: The longitudinal development of running economy in males and females aged between 13 and 27 years: the Amsterdam Growth and Health Study, *Eur J Appl Physiol Occup Physiol* 76(3):214-220, 1997.

29. Morgan DW, Tseh W, Caputo JL, et al: Longitudinal profiles of oxygen uptake during treadmill walking in able-bodied children: the locomotion energy and growth study, *Gait Posture* 15(3):230-235, 2002.

30. Morgan DW, Tseh W, Caputo JL, et al: Longitudinal stratification of gait economy in young boys and girls: the locomotion energy and growth study, *Eur J Appl Physiol* 91(1):30-34, 2004.

31. Allor KM, Pivarnik JM, Sam LJ, et al: Treadmill economy in girls and women matched for height and weight, *J Appl Physiol* 89(2):512-516, 2000.

32. Hausdorff JM, Zemany L, Peng C, et al: Maturation of gait dynamics: stride-to-stride variability and its temporal organization in children, *J Appl Physiol* 86(3):1040-1047, 1999.

33. Frost G, Bar-Or O, Dowling J, et al: Explaining differences in the metabolic cost and efficiency of treadmill locomotion in children, *J Sports Sci* 20(6):451-461, 2002.

34. Nottin S, Vinet A, Stecken F, et al: Central and peripheral cardiovascular adaptations to exercise in endurance-trained children, *Acta Physiol Scand* 175(2):85-92, 2002.

35. Fleg JL, O'Connor F, Gerstenblith G, et al: Impact of age on the cardiovascular response to dynamic upright exercise in healthy men and women, *J Appl Physiol* 78(3):890-900, 1995.

36. Astrand I, Astrand PO, Hallback I, et al: Reduction in maximal oxygen uptake with age, *J Appl Physiol* 35(5):649-654, 1973.

37. Levy WC, Cerqueira MD, Harp GD, et al: Effect of endurance exercise training on heart rate variability at rest in healthy young and older men, *Am J Cardiol* 82(10):1236-1241, 1998.

38. Okazaki K, Iwasaki KI, Prasad A, et al: Dose-response relationship of endurance training for autonomic circulatory control in healthy seniors, *J Appl Physiol* 99(3):1041-1049, 2005.

39. Dehn MM, Bruce RA: Longitudinal variations in maximal oxygen intake with age and activity, *J Appl Physiol* 33(6):805-807, 1972.

40. Monahan KD, Dinenno FA, Tanaka H, et al: Regular aerobic exercise modulates age-associated declines in cardiovagal baroreflex sensitivity in healthy men, *J Physiol* 529 (Pt 1):263-271, 2000.

41. Pescatello LS, Franklin BA, Fagard R, et al: American College of Sports Medicine position stand. Exercise and hypertension, *Med Sci Sports Exerc* 36(3):533-553, 2004.

42. Hagberg JM, Montain SJ, Martin WH III, et al: Effect of exercise training in 60- to 69-year-old persons with essential hypertension, *Am J Cardiol* 64(5):348-353, 1989.

43. De Vito G, Hernandez R, Gonzalez V, et al: Low intensity physical training in older subjects, *J Sports Med Phys Fitness* 37(1):72-77, 1997.

44. Ehsani AA, Spina RJ, Peterson LR, et al: Attenuation of cardiovascular adaptations to exercise in frail octogenarians, *J Appl Physiol* 95(5):1781-1788, 2003.

45. Evans EM, Racette SB, Peterson LR, et al: Aerobic power and insulin action improve in response to endurance exercise training in healthy 77-87 yr olds, *J Appl Physiol* 98(1):40-45, 2005.

46. Spina RJ, Meyer TE, Peterson LR, et al: Absence of left ventricular and arterial adaptations to exercise in octogenarians, *J Appl Physiol* 97(5):1654-1659, 2004.

47. Neder JA, Dal Corso S, Malaguti C, et al: The pattern and timing of breathing during incremental exercise: a normative study, *Eur Respir J* 21(3):530-538, 2003.

48. Hasson SM: *Clinical exercise physiology,* St Louis, 1994, Mosby-Year Book.

49. Karvonen MJ, Kentala E, Mustala O: The effects of training on heart rate; a longitudinal study, *Ann Med Exp Biol Fenn* 35(3):307-315, 1957.

50. Kraemer WJ: Exercise prescription in weight training: a needs analysis, *NSCA J* (February-March):64-65, 1983.

51. Anderson T, Kearney JT: Effects of three resistance training programs on muscular strength and absolute and relative endurance, *Res Q Exerc Sport* 53(1):1-7, 1982.

52. Armstrong LE, Epstein Y: Fluid-electrolyte balance during labor and exercise: concepts and misconceptions, *Int J Sport Nutr* 9(1):1-12, 1999.

53. Costrini AM, Pitt HA, Gustafson AB, et al: Cardiovascular and metabolic manifestations of heat stroke and severe heat exhaustion, *Am J Med* 66(2):296-302, 1979.

54. England AC III, Fraser DW, Hightower AW, et al: Preventing severe heat injury in runners: suggestions from the 1979 Peachtree Road Race experience, *Ann Intern Med* 97(2):196-201, 1982.

55. Hanson PG, Zimmerman SW: Exertional heatstroke in novice runners, *JAMA* 242(2):154-157, 1979.

56. Bartley JD: Heat stroke: is total prevention possible? *Mil Med* 142(7):528-535, 1977.

57. Armstrong LE, Maresh CM: The induction and decay of heat acclimatization in trained athletes, *Sports Med* 12(5):302-312, 1991.

58. Roberts WO: Assessing core temperature in collapsed athletes: what's the best method? *Phys Sportsmed* 22(8):49-55, 1994.

59. Armstrong LE, Crago AE, Adams R, et al: Whole-body cooling of hyperthermic runners: comparison of two field therapies, *Am J Emerg Med* 14(4):355-358, 1996.

60. Armstrong LE, Maresh CM: Fluid replacement during exercise and recovery from exercise. In Buskirk ER, Puhl SM, editors: *Body fluid balance: exercise and sport,* pp. 259-281, New York, 1996, CRC Press.

61. Casa DJ, Armstrong LE, Hillman S, et al: National Athletic Trainers' Association position statement: fluid replacement for athletes, *J Athl Trn* 35(2):212-224, 2000.

62. Montain SJ, Coyle EF: Influence of graded dehydration on hyperthermia and cardiovascular drift during exercise, *J Appl Physiol* 73:1340-1350, 1992.

63. Convertino VA, Armstrong LE, Coyle EF, et al: American College of Sports Medicine position stand. Exercise and fluid replacement, *Med Sci Sports Exerc* 28(1):i-vii, 1996.

64. Climatic heat stress and the exercising child and adolescent. American Academy of Pediatrics. Committee on Sports Medicine and Fitness, *Pediatrics* 106(1 Pt 1): 158-159, 2000.

65. Manore MM, Barr SI, Butterfield GE: Nutrition and athletic performance: position of the American Dietetic Association, Dietitians of Canada, and the American College of Sports Medicine, *J Am Diet Assoc* 100:1543-1556, 2000.

66. Pate RR, Pratt M, Blair SN, et al: Physical activity and public health. A recommendation from the Centers for Disease Control and Prevention and the American College of Sports Medicine, *JAMA* 273(5):402-407, 1995.

67. Peterson MJ, Palmer DR, Laubach LL: Comparison of caloric expenditure in intermittent and continuous walking bouts, *J Strength Cond Res* 18(2):373-376, 2004.

68. American College of Sports Medicine Position Stand. The recommended quantity and quality of exercise for developing and maintaining cardiorespiratory and muscular fitness, and flexibility in healthy adults, *Med Sci Sports Exerc* 30(6):975-991, 1998.

69. Borg GA: Psychophysical bases of perceived exertion, *Med Sci Sports Exerc* 14(5):377-381, 1982.

70. Prevention CfDCa: *Physical activity for everyone: measuring physical activity intensity: perceived exertion (Borg Rating of Perceived Exertion Scale)*, vol 2005, 2005.

71. Eston RG, Williams JG: Reliability of ratings of perceived effort regulation of exercise intensity, *Br J Sports Med* 22(4):153-155, 1988.

72. Ainsworth BE, Haskell WL, Leon AS, et al: Compendium of physical activities: classification of energy costs of human physical activities, *Med Sci Sports Exerc* 25(1): 71-80, 1993.

73. Martin PE, Rothstein DE, Larish DD: Effects of age and physical activity status on the speed-aerobic demand relationship of walking, *J Appl Physiol* 73(1):200-206, 1992.

74. di Prampero PE: The energy cost of human locomotion on land and in water, *Int J Sports Med* 7(2):55-72, 1986.

75. Ljunggren G, Hassmen P: Perceived exertion and physiological economy of competition walking, ordinary walking and running, *J Sports Sci* 9(3):273-283, 1991.

76. Ardigo LP, Saibene F, Minetti AE: The optimal locomotion on gradients: walking, running or cycling? *Eur J Appl Physiol* 90(3-4):365-371, 2003.

77. Miller JF, Stamford BA: Intensity and energy cost of weighted walking vs. running for men and women, *J Appl Physiol* 62(4):1497-1501, 1987.

78. Bransford DR, Howley ET: Oxygen cost of running in trained and untrained men and women, *Med Sci Sports* 9(1):41-44, 1977.

79. Margaria R, Cerretelli P, Aghemo P, et al: Energy cost of running, *J Appl Physiol* 18:367-370, 1963.

80. Morgan DW, Martin PE, Krahenbuhl GS: Factors affecting running economy, *Sports Med* 7(5):310-330, 1989.

81. Bassett DR Jr, Giese MD, Nagle FJ, et al: Aerobic requirements of overground versus treadmill running, *Med Sci Sports Exerc* 17(4):477-481, 1985.

82. Zamparo P, Perini R, Orizio C, et al: The energy cost of walking or running on sand, *Eur J Appl Physiol Occup Physiol* 65(2):183-187, 1992.

83. Pinnington HC, Dawson B: The energy cost of running on grass compared to soft dry beach sand, *J Sci Med Sport* 4(4):416-430, 2001.

84. Pandolf KB, Haisman MF, Goldman RF: Metabolic energy expenditure and terrain coefficients for walking on snow, *Ergonomics* 19(6):683-690, 1976.

85. Minetti AE, Moia C, Roi GS, et al: Energy cost of walking and running at extreme uphill and downhill slopes, *J Appl Physiol* 93(3):1039-1046, 2002.

86. Association AH: Exercise (physical activity) and children, vol 2005, Dallas, 2005, American Heart Association.

87. Binder EF, Schechtman KB, Ehsani AA, et al: Effects of exercise training on frailty in community-dwelling older adults: results of a randomized, controlled trial, *J Am Geriatr Soc* 50(12):1921-1928, 2002.

Suggested Readings

Conley M: Bioenergetics of exercise training. In Baechle TR, Earle RW, editors: *Essentials of strength training and conditioning,* pp. 73-90, Champaign, Ill, 2000, Human Kinetics.

Heyward VH: *Designing cardiorespiratory exercise programs.* In *Advanced fitness assessment and exercise prescription,* pp. 83-104, Champaign, Ill, 1998, Human Kinetics.

Heyward VH: *Assessing cardiorespiratory fitness.* In *Advanced fitness assessment and exercise prescription,* Champaign, Ill, 1998, Human Kinetics.

Kraemer WJ: Physiological adaptations to anaerobic and aerobic endurance training programs. In Baechle TR, Earle RW, editors: *Essentials of strength training and conditioning,* pp. 137-168, Champaign, Ill, 2000, Human Kinetics.

CHAPTER

5

Harvey W. Wallmann

Muscle Fatigue

LEARNING OBJECTIVES

After studying this chapter, the reader will be able to do the following:

1. Discuss the underlying causes of muscle fatigue
2. Describe the use of in vitro and in vivo models for examining different mechanisms of muscle fatigue
3. Identify and discuss the different peripheral mechanisms involved in muscle fatigue
4. Describe the interaction of the various energy systems to the onset of muscle fatigue
5. Discuss how accumulation of metabolic by-products can induce muscle fatigue
6. Discuss central nervous system involvement in muscle fatigue
7. Describe how task dependency influences muscle fatigue

Muscles are capable of generating tremendous forces and power outputs during physical activities. In many types of sprint sports, the effort required is maximal-intensity, intermittent exercise. As such, repeated attempts at producing equivalent outputs may quickly lead to muscle fatigue, which can be observed as a reduction in the ability to maintain a given force. This is also true of other athletic endeavors in which sustained repetitive submaximal forces during prolonged or endurance exercise may result in fatigue.

A strict definition of muscle fatigue has been difficult to establish but may be defined as the inability of muscle to maintain the expected force or power output, resulting in a decline of maximum force-generating capacity.[1-4] Although it may be easy to loosely define fatigue, the question "What causes muscle fatigue?" is infinitely more difficult to answer. Due to the complexity, intensity, and repetitive nature of activities and tasks in general, many components can potentially influence both the onset and progress of fatigue. For example, fatigue may depend on a person's state of fitness, diet, sex, age, health status, overall body composition, fiber type composition, muscle

groups involved, the type of sport being performed, the specific task at hand, or the physical and chemical composition of the environment in which the task is performed.[5,6] Fatigue during voluntary muscle contractions can be a complex and multifaceted phenomenon, and researchers are just beginning to understand some of the specific mechanisms involved. Consequently, identification of a single definitive mechanism may be somewhat unrealistic.[7] In addition, motivation can be a crucial factor, allowing the individual to push beyond the discomforts of fatiguing exercise. Motivational factors are undoubtedly more difficult to categorize or quantify but play a major role when attempting to achieve superior performance. An in-depth discussion of motivational factors is not discussed here.

This chapter explores mechanisms involved in examining fatigue, as well as several factors that may contribute to fatigue, some of which include the following: mechanical manifestations, central and peripheral components to include specific fatigue sites, task dependency, and metabolic and nonmetabolic factors. However, in order to understand the onset and progression of fatigue, it is first necessary to investigate some of the models used to examine muscle fatigue mechanisms.

EXAMINATION OF MUSCLE FATIGUE MECHANISMS

Several different approaches have been used to advance the understanding of how and why the neuromuscular system fatigues. This understanding has occurred primarily through the use of in vitro and in vivo models.

In vitro investigations attempt to study function by simulating various intracellular environments using test tubes. This allows researchers to address mechanisms, such as metabolite accumulation, activation failure, substrate depletion, impairment of calcium (Ca^{2+}) kinetics, and disruption of the myofibrillar complex.[8] For example, when studying muscle fatigue, researchers may use fractionated muscle tissue to examine the function of specific organelles, such as the sarcolemma, the sarcoplasmic reticulum (SR), or the myofibrillar complex (i.e., actin-myosin cross-bridge dynamics) and their role in energy metabolism. With this approach, fatigued muscle is compared with fresh muscle in order to determine differences between the two as a result of exercise.[9] Of course, caution must be observed when interpreting the results because it is quite possible that the organelles may be disrupted by the preparation or possibly only partially recovered.

Additionally, researchers may study the muscle tissue itself, without disruption, using in vitro techniques. In this case, either the whole muscle, a bundle of muscle, or single muscle fibers dissected from an experimental animal are placed in a physiological medium and connected to a force transducer.[8,9] Moreover, single fibers may be examined with an intact sarcolemma or with the sarcolemma removed. Examining the fiber with the sarcolemma removed, known as the *skinned fiber technique,* allows the researcher to directly manipulate the intracellular environment.[9] In other words, the researcher can put holes in the membrane and directly add ions to the fiber to observe force changes. Although these experiments do help researchers understand muscle fiber physiology, they may not necessarily identify those rate-limiting mechanisms that occur with human performance.

In vivo experiments, using whole animal preparations, may be advantageous because these experiments use intact tissue and presumably do not disturb the intracellular organization of the fiber. Induced or imposed contractile patterns are used with these preparations, resulting in an earlier and more pronounced fatigue than when using voluntary activity at the same mechanical demands.[9,10] In these preparations, the stabilized, anesthetized limb is isolated and prepared for mechanical simulation using different protocols. Measurement of fatigue manifestations can then be characterized. Because experiments may take several hours, the main concern with these studies is the physiological viability of the preparations while waiting for the experimental protocol to take place.

Fatigue studies can also be performed using single motor units, in which the motor units can be isolated using dorsal root dissection; this may allow the researcher to relate specific alterations in motor unit function with changes at the level of the single fiber.[9]

MECHANICAL MANIFESTATIONS OF MUSCLE FATIGUE

Before changes in specific intracellular processes can be determined to contribute to fatigue, the mechanical parameters must first be defined. When discussing fatigue, identifying the underlying mechanical basis is crucial. Determining what type of exercise or task is performed is important because fatigue may develop secondary to failure at one particular site or at a combination of sites along the pathway of force production.[1]

A common complicating factor when studying human fatigue concerns the motor unit activation pattern. Motor unit recruitment simply means adding motor units to increase

muscle force. For example, low-force muscle activity requires only a few motor units to be activated, whereas a higher-force activity requires progressively more motor unit enlistment. Additionally, as motor force increases, motor neurons with progressively larger axons are recruited.[11] Most muscles are composed of a mixture of different fiber types. However, all motor units in a muscle do not fire at the same time; this allows a smooth control of muscle force output.

Evidence-Based Clinical Application: Motor Unit Recruitment

Because muscles are composed of motor units and each motor unit is essentially recruited in an orderly fashion (depending on the task), fatigability may be enhanced in some motor units more than others with all fiber types being recruited during intense activity.[12,13]

The recruitment sequence reflects the order of threshold for activation. In this case the slow-twitch Type I fiber (lowest threshold for activation) is more fatigue resistant than Type IIA, which is more fatigue resistant than Type IIX (intermediate fiber), which is more fatigue resistant than Type IIB (fast-twitch fatigable).[14,15] Performance of submaximal contractions usually involves recruitment of Type I (and possibly Type IIA) fibers from the onset of the activity. Exercise progression results in an increasing number of Type II fibers being recruited until exhaustion, when all motor units have been brought into play.

As can be observed, the fiber type composition of the individual may be one component of fatigue. Consequently, different levels of investigation may be necessary to determine the interplay of other factors. For example, the mechanical complexity of the task performed may determine the rate at which fatigue occurs. Even under the best of conditions, identification of a primary failing muscle may not be possible. The task demands may be such that several muscle groups may come into play, thereby making it difficult to definitively identify the absolute contribution from a single muscle because muscles generally work together synergistically and therefore may compensate for each other.

In using the simple model of isometric activity, if the contraction is intense, a tetanus or fused contraction is produced, allowing the site of fatigue to be easily identified because only one mechanical parameter is involved.[9] However, at lower intensities of contraction (oscillatory nonfused contractions), other factors that might impair performance, such as contraction time and relaxation time, become involved.

UNDERLYING CAUSES AND SITES OF MUSCLE FATIGUE

Muscle fatigue can be broken down essentially into two main components: central (neural) and peripheral (muscular). *Peripheral fatigue* refers to the motor units and involves processes associated with mechanical and cellular changes in the muscular system.[11] *Central fatigue* refers to the physiological processes that occur within the central nervous system (CNS). Although many researchers would agree that both peripheral and central factors play a role in muscle fatigue, the relative contribution of both may vary and remains poorly understood. Following is a brief discussion of the various aspects of neuromuscular fatigue and the mechanisms involved.

PERIPHERAL FATIGUE

When examining peripheral fatigue, the goal is to specify what process in excitation and contraction of the muscle represents the primary site(s) of failure. As such, peripheral fatigue may involve the following sites and pathways: (1) neuromuscular junction, (2) the *excitation-contraction (E-C) coupling process*, and (3) the activation of the contractile elements involved in force and power generation.[14] Contractile force can decrease with interruption of any one of these processes.

With voluntary activity, processes involved in force production can be located outside the muscle (central processes) or in the muscle. Because the nerve ending terminates at the neuromuscular junction and further invaginates into the muscle fiber, the neuromuscular junction is considered for this discussion as part of the peripheral mechanism, although it may be argued that it is under the control of central processes. These outside processes may include events leading to muscle fiber recruitment involving the alpha motoneuron, potentially altering its excitability. In this case motor nerve impulses may be distorted because of branch point fatigue or inhibition at the neuromuscular junction.[16] In other words, fatigue can occur at the neuromuscular junction if an action potential (AP) fails to adequately reach the muscle fiber from the motor neuron.

Fatigue may also come about with nerve fiber stimulation at rates greater than 100 times per second. In this case there is a decreased number of acetylcholine vesicles released with each impulse that ultimately fails to pass into the muscle fiber, leading to fatigue of the neuromuscular junction.[17] Of course, this would probably only occur at extreme levels of muscular exhaustion.

The E-C coupling process can be broadly defined as the complex signaling process from nerve depolarization to muscle contraction.[18] Basically, excitation sites include the sarcolemma and the transverse tubule (t tubule) system, which are specialized to conduct the electrical signals into the muscle fiber's interior. In order for a contraction to take place, the signal must result in the opening of the Ca^{2+} channels in the SR, leading to a release of the stored Ca^{2+} into the cytosol. But to do this, the signal in the t tubule membrane must communicate with the Ca^{2+} channels in the terminal cisternae of the SR (traversing an approximate 10 to 15 nm gap).[9]

The E-C coupling process begins with transmission of APs down the motor neuron axon, thereby activating the surface membrane. Then the alpha motoneuron releases acetylcholine at the neuromuscular junction, resulting in binding of acetylcholine to its receptor and depolarization at the end-plate, which opens the voltage-gated Na^+ channels. This leads to depolarization of the sarcolemma, resulting in propagation down the t-tubules (within the sarcolemma) and subsequent release of Ca^{2+} from the SR (the terminal cisternae) into the cytosol. Here Ca^{2+} can bind to troponin C (on the thin filament) and initiate cross-bridge cycling.[19] Consequently, muscle relaxation occurs by reuptake of Ca^{2+} into the SR and subsequent deactivation of the actin-myosin cross-bridges. Disruptions in E-C coupling would involve events affecting the level of Ca^{2+} in the cytosol. Alterations in either the release of Ca^{2+} into the cytosol or its subsequent sequestration back into the SR may affect the myofibrillar complex, resulting in fatigue.

Another potential fatigue site involves the myofibrillar complex. This complex, representing the contractile apparatus, includes the regulatory proteins troponin and tropomyosin, as well as the contractile proteins actin and myosin and their cross-bridge interaction. Revisiting the E-C coupling process, if the amount of Ca^{2+} released from the SR into the cytosol is diminished, the binding of Ca^{2+} to troponin C will be attenuated. The inability of the regulatory proteins to respond to the Ca^{2+} signal or the inability of the actin and myosin to transition to different binding states could cause a decrease in force to occur. Consequently, fewer cross-bridges will be formed, resulting in a lower force or power generation.[15] Additionally, cross-bridge cycling depends on an adequate supply of adenosine triphosphate (ATP) through aerobic and anaerobic metabolic pathways.

The Sarcoplasmic Reticulum, the Sarcolemma-T-Tubule System, and Muscle Fatigue

As a brief review, the SR is a membranous network, structurally divided into regions, that covers each myofibril in a muscle fiber. These regions consist of longitudinal tubules that terminate in large chambers called the *terminal cisternae* (TC) and run parallel to the myofibrils; these TCs subsequently abut the t-tubules. One t-tubule and two TCs form a structure referred to as a *triad* and represent the site of E-C coupling. The t-tubules penetrate all the way from one side of the muscle fiber to the opposite side and originate from the cell membrane (sarcolemma), thereby leaving them open to communicate with the cell's exterior. Simply put, the t-tubules are invaginations of the sarcolemma that connect with the interior of the fiber, specifically the TC (the storage site for Ca^{2+}).

The sarcolemma and the t-tubules both contain resting membrane potentials and are capable of being depolarized and conducting an AP. In essence, they represent an electrical pathway whereby motor nerve excitation via the neuromuscular junction and motor end plate is transported to specific intracellular sites.[9] Thus when an AP occurs, it spreads over the sarcolemma and courses deep into the interior of the muscle fiber via the t-tubules causing a change in the permeability of the TC and permitting Ca^{2+} to escape, thereby eliciting a muscle contraction.[20] As such, the force developed by a muscle fiber is closely dependent on the frequency with which APs can be regenerated in the sarcolemma and t-tubules.

The generation of an AP depends on the opening of the Na^+ and K^+ channels (Na^+ to the interior of the cell and K^+ to the interstitial space) and the ability to quickly reestablish the Na^+ and K^+ gradients along the membrane. The reestablishment of these ionic gradients is controlled primarily by the ATPase pump, which is triggered by the Na^+ and K^+ concentrations on the interior and exterior of the cell, respectively, resulting in increased cycling.[9] This process depends on the use of energy generated by the hydrolysis of ATP.[21,22] However, it should be noted that a suppression in ATPase activity could be a result of increased by-products of ATP hydrolysis (i.e., phosphate and hydrogen ions). These ions would alter the ATPase activity once certain levels were attained.[23] If the sarcolemma and t-tubules are to conduct APs at a rate necessary to maximally activate the fiber, then the ATPase pump must have high ATPase activity and an increased capacity for rapid ATP hydrolysis.[7]

An inability to repeatedly generate APs at high frequency for maximal force generation by the fiber may result in excitation failure, referred to as *high-frequency fatigue*.[24] This fatigue seems to occur due to an inability to restore NA^+ and K^+ gradients across the sarcolemma before the next AP. An inability to reestablish these gradients could alter the membrane potential and compromise force production secondary to potentially impairing the ability of the t-tubule to signal the SR.

Three key issues are of importance involving the SR, which may possibly determine its vulnerability to fatigue. The first issue concerns the storage capability of the SR for Ca^{2+}, which is sequestered when the muscle is quiet. Secondly, the SR must be able to release the stored Ca^{2+} into the cytoplasm on excitation, which occurs primarily at the TC (the Ca^{2+} storage site). Thirdly, the SR must be able to sequester the Ca^{2+} via the transporting enzyme Ca^{2+}-ATPase back into the SR against an electrochemical gradient, which requires energy. Sequestration is necessary for relaxation of the muscle fiber following excitation.[9]

Skeletal muscle displays wide variability in mechanical function. Research has shown differences in the ability of fast- and slow-twitch muscles to activate the Na^+-K^+ pump.[25] Consequently, the speed which with a fiber responds to different excitation patterns varies. For example, fast-twitch fibers contract and relax much faster than slow-twitch fibers because the SR in fast-twitch fibers is more extensive and they have a higher density of both Ca^{2+} channels and Ca^{2+}-ATPase enzymes. This may help to explain some of the differences noted in fatigability.[9]

The Myofibrillar Complex and Muscle Fatigue

As previously alluded to, loss of force may also be subsequent to some process or entity more distal to the SR, such as the myofibrillar complex. In this case, fatigue would result from an inability of the complex to trigger an expected force from the Ca^{2+} signal. Alterations in several sites, such as the regulatory proteins (troponin and tropomyosin), may be implicated in myofibrillar complex failure, resulting in problems with actin

and myosin and cross-bridge interaction.[9] For example, a problem may occur secondary to a change in the sensitivity of troponin C for Ca^{2+}, resulting in a different conformational change within the thin filament, thereby affecting the binding of actin and myosin and therefore force generation. Moreover, failure to activate the thin filament may also contribute to fatigue.

Unfortunately, isolating myofibrillar failure from E-C coupling or excitation failure is practically impossible in the intact muscle fiber secondary to the lack of knowledge regarding what is happening to the free cytosolic calcium concentration $(Ca^{2+})_i$. However, research with frog and mouse fibers has shown that, with high-frequency stimulation, fatigue appears to be a result of disturbances in excitation, whereas, with lower frequencies, myofibrillar failure is observed.[26] Basically, studies have shown that with certain types of fatigue, the myofibrils are unable to translate the Ca^{2+} signal into an expected force.[9]

The rate at which actomyosin cycles between states depends heavily on the activity of myosin ATPase, as well as the rate at which free energy is made available from ATPase hydrolysis.[27] As such, decreased myosin ATPase activity may have profound effects on fiber force and velocity characteristics.

Components of Muscle Fatigue

Nonmetabolic

The peripheral mechanisms underlying muscle fatigue observed during high, repetitive force–generating activities seem to have both nonmetabolic and metabolic components.[28,29] The nonmetabolic component appears to stem from the high-repetition forces that are generated, resulting in muscle damage. Although concentric activity may produce muscle damage, it usually involves eccentric exercise; this is believed to be due to the higher force levels that are generated with eccentric activity. As such, the damage seems to result in weakness, thereby impairing performance, particularly if exercise is attempted before recovery can take place. This can especially hinder performance at maximal levels because there may remain only a limited ability to recruit other motor units and hence increase firing frequency.[7]

Metabolic

Prolonged exercise performance depends on an available supply of energy. Metabolic fatigue is fatigue associated with the energetic changes in the muscle and involves the ability to sustain high-intensity exercise; in other words, it involves the metabolic pathways used for ATP supply. Submaximal effort and single movements at maximal force levels can be performed without depleting ATP levels by using phosphocreatine to regenerate ATP. As repetition increases, alongside intensity, activation of both glycolysis and oxidative phosphorylation is necessary to maintain adequate ATP levels to sustain activity. As such, glycolysis assumes increasing importance with the increased number of repetitions. In fact, after a period of repetitive, high-intensity activity, muscles can display reductions in ATP up to 40%, with almost complete reductions in phosphocreatine.[30-32] During the recovery phase, replenishment of phosphocreatine stores depends on ATP regenerated from aerobic processes.[33]

Essentially, three pathways are responsible for supplying energy to the body during skeletal muscle contraction: the ATP–creatine phosphate (CP) (phosphagen) system, the glycolytic (glycolysis or glycogen-lactic acid) system, and the oxidative (aerobic) system. The ATP-CP system is not considered a metabolic pathway because it consists of only a single reaction. However, the glycolytic and oxidative pathways are considered metabolic pathways and involve a sequence of reactions. Several factors come into play when attempting to determine the relative contribution of each system to ATP production; these factors include exercise parameters, such as intensity, duration, and rest intervals.[34] Moreover, anaerobic metabolism primarily involves the phosphagen system and glycolysis (or anaerobic glycolysis), whereas aerobic metabolism involves the oxidative system.

Adenosine Triphosphate–Creatine Phosphate System

ATP is the immediate energy source for all exercise. However, due to the limited amount of ATP stored in the muscle (about 2 to 3 seconds' worth of energy), another readily accessible source of energy is necessary for short-duration exercises of high intensity that is not dependent on the availability of O_2 to function. The phosphagen system answers the body's need for energy and uses CP, a high-energy phosphate compound found in skeletal muscle. To illustrate, the energy released from the breakdown of ATP into adenosine diphosphate (ADP) and phosphate (inorganic phosphate) is used for muscle contraction. However, it is necessary to convert ADP back to ATP. In order to do this, a secondary energy source must be provided. This secondary energy source is CP. Consequently, ATP is resynthesized from energy stored in the bonds of ADP and CP, allowing maintenance of high levels of ATP in the working muscle for short periods of time. The duration of maximal ATP production in this system is the shortest ($\approx$10 seconds) of the three pathways.[35] However, the availability of this energy source is crucial during periods of rapid conversion from low to high-energy demand in which a maximal effort during performance is required. As such, success in several types of activities requiring brief bursts of power output by the muscles relies heavily on this system for energy transfer (i.e., sprinting, football, wrestling).

Glycolysis

For maximal intensity exercises to continue beyond a brief period in the absence of O_2 (lasting about 30 seconds to 2 minutes), ATP must be rapidly resynthesized. This task is the responsibility of the glycolytic system. Anaerobic glycolysis involves the breakdown of glucose to pyruvic acid (pyruvate) and, subsequently, to lactic acid (lactate). The energy production from glycolysis is small, but when combined with the phosphagen system, it allows muscle contraction to take place

without O_2 present. (See Chapter 3 for a more detailed discussion.) Thus it is a crucial aspect of energy production and is relied on heavily at the beginning of exercise, as well as during exercise of high intensity.[36] Bear in mind that the energy supplied for high-intensity exercise is limited, not by the unavailability of fuel sources, but by the inability of the body to tolerate lactate buildup. If exercise is continued in the absence of O_2, accumulating lactate levels in the muscles begin to affect muscle contraction, thus causing fatigue.

Oxidative System

Aerobic exercise involves the use of O_2 to produce the necessary energy for sustained periods of submaximal physical activity. The oxidative system involves the Krebs cycle and electron transport chain, as well as other oxidative pathways that donate hydrogen atoms to the electron transport chain. The oxidative system extracts ATP from CHO (glucose), fat (fatty acids), and protein (amino acids), as opposed to the glycolytic system, which only uses glucose as a fuel.[35] With O_2 present, pyruvate is converted to acetyl-CoA and is oxidized completely to carbon dioxide (CO_2) and water. The longer the bout of exercise, the more the body relies on aerobic metabolism for energy production. The duration of maximal ATP production is the longest of all the systems and is the major source of fuel for continuous submaximal endurance activities, provided a continuous supply of fuel and O_2 is present.[35] (See Chapter 4 for a more detailed discussion.) This also enables the individual to sustain longer periods of work without lactate accumulation impeding muscular contraction.

Muscle ATP concentration reflects a balance between ATP synthesis rates and ATP utilization rates.[9] Increases in activity increase ATP utilization rates dramatically. As such, the ATP regenerative pathways must help to offset this reduction in ATP levels. As previously mentioned, the CP, glycolytic, and oxidative systems are rapidly activated to protect ATP levels. Theoretically, fatigue can be construed as a mechanism necessary to protect ATP levels when demand for energy cannot be met.

Baldwin et al[37] showed that a substantial reduction in intramuscular glycogen content was related to fatigue in both endurance-trained and untrained individuals during prolonged high-intensity cycling exercise. Their data demonstrated that fatiguing submaximal exercise was associated with a similar low level of intramuscular glycogen in both trained and untrained men, but a mismatch between ATP supply and demand only occurred in the untrained individuals. This research suggests that fatigue occurs with decreased glycogen levels even when sufficient O_2 is present to generate energy through the metabolic pathways.

 Evidence-Based Clinical Application: Adenosine Triphosphate Concentration

A reduction in ATP may not be the primary cause of failure leading to fatigue because ATP concentration remains in excess of that needed to saturate the ATPase enzymes.[38]

Other researchers suggest instead that the accumulation of specific metabolic by-products are responsible for causing fatigue. Previous experiments have extended the understanding of how specific metabolites selectively alter different mechanical parameters.[9]

Metabolic By-products

The absence of O_2 coupled with an increased level of blood and muscle lactate is associated with muscle fatigue in short-term, maximal exercise. The high-energy phosphate reactions generate metabolic by-products, resulting in large increases in inorganic phosphate, creatine, free ADP, and free AMP, in addition to large increases in lactic acid. These increases in lactic acid, combined with hydrogen ions generated from ATP hydrolysis, produce muscle acidosis, thereby decreasing pH levels, which ultimately disrupts the intracellular environment.[7]

Evidence-Based Clinical Application: Metabolic By-products

Of all the metabolic end-products examined, inorganic phosphate (P_i) and hydrogen (H^+) have been shown to have the most profound effect on mechanical function.

During activity, P_i increases as CP decreases. Research has shown that increases in P_i result in a rightward shift in the isometric force–calcium concentration relationship, thereby depressing force.[39,40] These changes are thought to occur directly at the level of the contractile proteins, actin and myosin.[9]

Increases in H^+ concentration also appear to modulate myofibrillar behavior. As previously mentioned, the H^+ generated from ATP hydrolysis can dramatically lower pH levels. Low pH values can substantially depress both the peak isometric force and the maximal velocity of shortening. Although the actual mechanism is unknown, both the regulatory and contractile proteins are thought to be involved. Consider the following two examples to illustrate this point. A decrease in Ca^{2+} binding to troponin C (regulatory protein) could occur because H^+ ions compete for the Ca^{2+} binding sites on this protein. Alternatively, H^+ could affect actomyosin behavior by reducing the weak to strong bonding complexes, thereby reducing the cross-bridge force generation, or H+ could affect the association of actin and myosin.[9] When actin initially binds to myosin, there is a low force bridge. In other words, not much force is generated. As the force transitions from a low-force to a high-force state, a liberation of P_i and H^+ occur, driving the reaction backward to prevent the production of the high-force state.[5] Thus an increase in these metabolic by-products directly produces fatigue by preventing the transition from low to high force.

ADP also increases in fatigue. As ADP increases, velocity appears to be inhibited, alongside a reduction in power. Additionally, there is a decrease in free energy that may contribute to the slowing down of the SR reuptake of Ca^{2+}.[5]

CENTRAL FATIGUE

Processes involved in force production that occur outside the muscle within the CNS are collectively referred to as *central processes* and include events leading to fiber recruitment. This includes the ability to generate an appropriate central command for the task, transmission of the command to the involved motor pools, and sustained muscle activation by the motor neurons.[8]

Generally speaking, fatiguing contractions seem to be associated with a gradual increase in cortical activity. For one to sustain a fatiguing contraction, the motor cortex and other suprasegmental centers need to sustain a central command signal in order to allow continued use of the muscles involved in the task. In studying muscular-fatiguing and nonfatiguing rhythmical hand contractions, Freude and Ullsperger[41] discovered that fatigue was associated with an increase in the readiness potential (an electroencephalographic signal thought to originate in cerebral cortical structures). Furthermore, they showed that muscular-fatiguing contractions at 80% maximal voluntary contraction (MVC) were accompanied by an increased potential. This was suggested to be the result of an increase in the central nervous activation required when preparing for motor activity with fatigued muscles.[41] Duchateau and Hainaut[42] observed an increased amplitude of the long latency reflex in the abductor pollicis brevis muscle when the first dorsal interosseous (a synergist) performed a fatiguing contraction. They concluded that the muscle fatigue induced an enhanced central drive to the fatiguing muscle, which spread to the cortical area associated with the neighboring muscle.[42]

As alluded to earlier, the concept of orderly recruitment maintains that motor units are recruited in a relatively fixed order for a particular muscle. However, it seems fatigue can affect motor unit behavior, which, in turn, may influence orderly recruitment. For example, Enoka et al[43] noted that both recruitment order and modulation of discharge rate during submaximal contractions are affected by fatigue. They found that the net force contributed by the motor units for a ramp-and-hold contraction that is performed to the same absolute target force before and after a fatiguing contraction can vary, as can the discharge rate of the activated motor units.[43]

Many would argue that the greatest manifestation of fatigue resides in the muscle. Although this may be true, a central process failure may also play a role with intense activity. Central failure may result in compromised motor unit and fiber activation, thereby leading to fatigue. In fact, it has become apparent through research that the mechanisms responsible for fatigue can vary, depending on the task.[8]

Evidence-Based Clinical Application: Task Failure

Central fatigue can be illustrated by examining fatigue when a task cannot be continued (task failure). In this case the subject is unable to continue the task, but the muscles can produce the necessary force when stimulated electrically.[2]

Using research conducted by Loscher et al[44] to illustrate, they found that when subjects could no longer voluntarily plantarflex the ankle at 30% maximum, the force could be maintained by electrically stimulating the innervation to the plantarflexors. Consequently, the response produced by muscle under these circumstances is used as evidence for central command failure.

Much research has also been conducted examining the motor cortex and other suprasegmental centers. Although an in-depth discussion of central command signals is beyond the scope of this chapter, it appears that fatiguing contractions are associated with a gradual increase in the level of cortical activity.[42,45]

STUDIES DIFFERENTIATING PERIPHERAL VERSUS CENTRAL FATIGUE

As previously mentioned, many factors come into play when attempting to determine the causes of peripheral versus central fatigue. As such, it is necessary to be able to differentiate between central and peripheral failure in the neuromuscular system.

This differentiation can be accomplished using a number of techniques. One such approach, using voluntary activity, compares the differences between the generation of an MVC with the force that can be induced via electrical stimulation.[46] MVC is defined as the maximal force recorded during an isometric contraction with the subject giving a maximal effort.[47] MVCs progressively decline as a muscle fatigues. Differences between the force generated by electrical stimulation and the MVC resulting in fatigue, if the electrical stimulation exceeds the MVC, are recognized as having a central component.

Another application of this technique is the use of an interpolated twitch, which is an impulse superimposed on an MVC.[48] The absence of a further increase in force from the muscle would indicate peripheral fatigue, whereas an increase in the electrically induced superimposed contraction (i.e., the impulse) would suggest that the reduced voluntary force resulted from decreased muscle activation by the CNS and would thus be indicative of central fatigue.[49]

Electromyography (EMG) can also be used to help differentiate between central and peripheral fatigue. Decreases in the integrated EMG (iEMG) alongside decreases in force may suggest a weakened central drive. However, in order for these decreases in EMG to be viable indicators, one must be able to establish the integrity of the neuromuscular junction and the sarcolemma. This may be possible by stimulating the motor nerve of the muscle and recording a compound muscle AP (M-wave).[9] A change in the amplitude of the M-wave may be suggestive of a sarcolemma problem, or it may be due to an impaired neuromuscular activation. However, if the M-wave is not compromised, sites peripheral to the sarcolemma might underlie the loss of force. Some research has shown that the M-wave amplitude is depressed after 1 or 2 hours of exercise.[50,51] Moreover, it has been shown that a slowed impulse conduction in the sarcolemma is apparent when the M-wave becomes broader and its peak amplitude declines.[52] Some researchers

would agree that changes in M-wave and EMG during fatiguing contractions reveal two different mechanisms of fatigue.[53,54] The problem is that research has not definitively shown whether decreases in iEMG are entirely explained by changes in M-wave amplitude after long-term exercise or if central fatigue is occurring.[55]

Further differentiation, although difficult, involves elucidating the cellular and molecular mechanisms by which the T-tubular AP leads to Ca^{2+} release from the SR. Force measurements combined with direct monitoring of cytosolic Ca^{2+} via use of fluorescent dyes have allowed associations to be made between declines in force generation and the reduction in cytosolic Ca^{2+} concentration.[9] The difficulty lies in being able to determine whether or not changes have also occurred in the Ca^{2+} sensitivity of the contractile apparatus and troponin C.

Pharmacological agents, such as methylxanthines (i.e., caffeine), have also been used in trying to isolate the role of the SR. These agents bind to the Ca^{2+} channel, thereby stimulating the release of sequestered Ca^{2+} in the SR. For example, caffeine is capable of holding the channel open, thereby eliciting large releases of Ca^{2+} into the cytoplasm. The advantage, of course, is that this type of approach provides the opportunity to examine the role of the SR in an exercising human.[9]

NEW RESEARCH TRENDS: INVESTIGATING IMPLICATIONS FOR FATIGUE

Current research involves investigations of P_i at physiological temperatures that more closely simulate normal body temperatures than did previous work. Data suggest that at near physiological temperatures and at saturating levels of intracellular Ca^{2+}, elevated levels of P_i were shown to contribute less to fatigue than might be expected from data derived from lower-temperature studies.[56]

TASK DEPENDENCY AND MUSCLE FATIGUE

As previously mentioned, fatigue is a multifaceted phenomenon. In fact, mechanisms involved in limiting performance secondary to fatigue vary according to the details of the specific task. This is known as *task dependency* of muscle fatigue and is probably caused by many different mechanisms that act concurrently, but with different time courses.[8,57] Identifying the parameters for the different mechanisms involved with muscle fatigue has been a recent focus of attention and involves the following variables: subject motivation, flexibility in the central command, the intensity and duration of the activity, the speed and type of contraction, and the extent to which the activity is continuously sustained.[8] However, to date, little evidence substantiates the role these variables play in contributing to fatigue.

CONCLUSIONS

Despite more than a century of research and scientific inquiry into muscle fatigue and its mechanisms, many issues are unresolved. Yet considerable progress has been made in the past few years toward understanding the fatigue process. The topic is challenging due to the difficulty in isolating the various mechanisms involved and the multiple potential sites that may play a role. For example, the cellular cause of skeletal muscle fatigue may involve multiple agents acting at different sites within the cell. Other factors also come into play, such as the type of exercise, a person's state of fitness, diet, sex, age, health status, and overall body composition. Additionally, the degree of fatigue may vary with muscle fiber type composition, as well as the number of muscle groups involved.

Prolonged exercise performance depends on an available supply of energy. Muscle ATP concentration represents a balance between ATP synthesis rates and ATP utilization rates. The ATP regenerative pathways must help to offset a reduction in ATP levels as a result of increases in ATP utilization. This occurs via the CP, glycolytic, and oxidative systems, which are rapidly activated to protect ATP levels. As such, fatigue acts as a mechanism to protect ATP levels when demand for energy cannot be met.

Most muscle fatigue research has focused on static contractions of well-defined muscle groups. Muscle fatigue is evidently a multifactorial phenomenon that may be caused by the impairment of many different peripheral and central physiological processes. However, the feasibility of measuring progressively impaired muscle function during complex, multijoint movements is difficult. Thus the degree of fatigue among specific muscles is likely to differ widely.[58] Consequently, it is also apparent that the mechanisms involved may vary depending on the details of the task being performed. Future areas of research should concentrate on studies that establish conditions for which these mechanisms can contribute to muscle fatigue.

REFERENCES

1. Paasuke M, Ereline J, Gapeyeva H: Neuromuscular fatigue during repeated exhaustive submaximal static contractions of knee extensor muscles in endurance-trained, power-trained and untrained men, *Acta Physiol Scand* 166(4):319-326, 1999.
2. Gandevia SC: Neural control in human muscle fatigue: changes in muscle afferents, motoneurons and motor cortical drive, *Acta Physiol Scand* 162(3):275-283, 1998.
3. Allman BL, Rice CL: Neuromuscular fatigue and aging: central and peripheral factors, *Muscle Nerve* 25(6):785-796, 2002.
4. Hill CA, Thompson MW, Ruell PA, et al: Sarcoplasmic reticulum function and muscle contractile character following fatiguing exercise in humans, *J Physiol* 531 (Pt 3):871-878, 2001.
5. Fitts RH: Muscle fatigue: the cellular aspects, *Am J Sports Med* 24(6):S9-13, 1996.
6. Hunter SK, Duchateau J, Enoka RM: Muscle fatigue and the mechanisms of task failure, *Exerc Sport Sci Rev* 32(2):44-49, 2004.
7. Green HJ: Mechanisms of muscle fatigue in intense exercise, *J Sports Sci* 15(3):247-256, 1997.
8. Enoka RM: Mechanisms of muscle fatigue: central factors and task dependency, *J Electromyogr Kinesiol* 5(3):141-149, 1995.
9. Green HJ: Metabolic determinants of activity induced muscular fatigue. In Hargreaves M, editor: *Exercise metabolism*, pp. 211-256, Champaign, Ill, 1995, Human Kinetics.
10. Jones DA: Muscle fatigue due to changes beyond the neuromuscular junction. In Porter R, Whelan J, editors: *Human muscle fatigue: physiological mechanisms*, pp. 178-196, London, 1981, Pitman Medical.
11. McArdle WD, Katch FI, Katch VL: *Exercise physiology: energy, nutrition, and human performance*, ed 5, Philadelphia, 2001, Lippincott Williams & Wilkins.
12. Burke RE, Levine DN, Tsairis P, et al: Physiological types and histochemical profiles in motor units of the cat gastrocnemius, *J Physiol* 234(3):723-748, 1973.
13. De Luca CJ: Control properties of motor units, *J Exp Biol* 115:125-136, 1985.
14. Fitts RH, Balog EM: Effect of intracellular and extracellular ion changes on E-C coupling and skeletal muscle fatigue, *Acta Physiol Scand* 156(3):169-181, 1996.
15. Vollestad NK: Measurement of human muscle fatigue, *J Neurosci Methods* 74(2):219-227, 1997.
16. Bigland-Ritchie B: Muscle fatigue and the influence of changing neural drive, *Clin Chest Med* 5(1):21-34, 1984.
17. Guyton AC, Hall JE: *Textbook of medical physiology*, ed 10, Philadelphia, 2001, Saunders.
18. Payne AM, Delbono O: Neurogenesis of excitation-contraction uncoupling in aging skeletal muscle, *Exerc Sport Sci Rev* 32(1):36-40, 2004.
19. Warren GL, Ingalls CP, Lowe DA, et al: Excitation-contraction uncoupling: major role in contraction-induced muscle injury, *Exerc Sport Sci Rev* 29(2):82-87, 2001.
20. Guyton AC: *Textbook of medical physiology*, ed 7, Philadelphia, 1986, Saunders.
21. Clausen T: Regulation of active Na+-K+ transport in skeletal muscle, *Physiol Rev* 66(3):542-580, 1986.
22. Clausen T, Nielsen OB: The Na+,K(+)-pump and muscle contractility, *Acta Physiol Scand* 152(4):365-373, 1994.
23. Dixon IM, Hata T, Dhalla NS: Sarcolemmal Na(+)-K(+)-ATPase activity in congestive heart failure due to myocardial infarction, *Am J Physiol* 262(3 Pt 1):C664-671, 1992.
24. Allen DG, Lannergren J, Westerblad H: Muscle cell function during prolonged activity: cellular mechanisms of fatigue, *Exp Physiol* 80(4):497-527, 1995.
25. Everts ME, Clausen T: Activation of the Na-K pump by intracellular Na in rat slow- and fast-twitch muscle, *Acta Physiol Scand* 145(4):353-362, 1992.

26. Westerblad H, Lee JA, Lannergren J, et al: Cellular mechanisms of fatigue in skeletal muscle, *Am J Physiol* 261 (2 Pt 1):C195-209, 1991.

27. Moss RL, Diffee GM, Greaser ML: Contractile properties of skeletal muscle fibers in relation to myofibrillar protein isoforms, *Rev Physiol Biochem Pharmacol* 1261-1263, 1995.

28. Davies CT, White MJ: Muscle weakness following eccentric work in man, *Pflugers Arch* 392(2):168-171, 1981.

29. Moussavi RS, Carson PJ, Boska MD, et al: Nonmetabolic fatigue in exercising human muscle, *Neurology* 39(9):1222-1226, 1989.

30. Hultman E, Greenhaff PL, Ren JM, et al: Energy metabolism and fatigue during intense muscle contraction, *Biochem Soc Trans* 19(2):347-353, 1991.

31. Gaitanos GC, Williams C, Boobis LH, et al: Human muscle metabolism during intermittent maximal exercise, *J Appl Physiol* 75(2):712-719, 1993.

32. McCartney N, Spriet LL, Heigenhauser GJ, et al: Muscle power and metabolism in maximal intermittent exercise, *J Appl Physiol* 60(4):1164-1169, 1986.

33. Harris RC, Edwards RH, Hultman E, et al: The time course of phosphorylcreatine resynthesis during recovery of the quadriceps muscle in man, *Pflugers Arch* 367(2):137-142, 1976.

34. Kraemer WJ: Physiological adaptations to anaerobic and aerobic endurance training programs. In Baechle TR, Earle RW, editors: *Essentials of strength training and conditioning,* ed 2, Champaign, Ill, 2000, Human Kinetics.

35. Axen K, Axen KV: *Illustrated principles of exercise physiology.* Upper Saddle River, NJ, 2001, Prentice-Hall.

36. Daniels J: Aerobic capacity for endurance. In Foran B, editor: *High performance sports conditioning,* Champaign, Ill, 2001, Human Kinetics.

37. Baldwin J, Snow RJ, Carey MF, et al: Muscle IMP accumulation during fatiguing submaximal exercise in endurance trained and untrained men, *Am J Physiol* 277 (1 Pt 2):R295-300, 1999.

38. Korge P: Factors limiting adenosine triphosphatase function during high intensity exercise. Thermodynamic and regulatory considerations, *Sports Med* 20(4):215-225, 1995.

39. Cooke R, Franks K, Luciani GB, et al: The inhibition of rabbit skeletal muscle contraction by hydrogen ions and phosphate, *J Physiol* 395:77-97, 1988.

40. Chase PB, Kushmerick MJ: Effects of pH on contraction of rabbit fast and slow skeletal muscle fibers, *Biophys J* 53(6):935-946, 1988.

41. Freude G, Ullsperger P: Changes in Bereitschaftspotential during fatiguing and non-fatiguing hand movements, *Eur J Appl Physiol Occup Physiol* 56(1):105-108, 1987.

42. Duchateau J, Hainaut K: Behaviour of short and long latency reflexes in fatigued human muscles, *J Physiol* 471:787-799, 1993.

43. Enoka RM, Robinson GA, Kossev AR: Task and fatigue effects on low-threshold motor units in human hand muscle, *J Neurophysiol* 62(6):1344-1359, 1989.

44. Loscher WN, Cresswell AG, Thorstensson A: Central fatigue during a long-lasting submaximal contraction of the triceps surae, *Exp Brain Res* 108(2):305-314, 1996.

45. Fuglevand AJ, Zackowski KM, Huey KA, et al: Impairment of neuromuscular propagation during human fatiguing contractions at submaximal forces, *J Physiol* 460:549-572, 1993.

46. Bigland-Ritchie B, Woods JJ: Changes in muscle contractile properties and neural control during human muscular fatigue, *Muscle Nerve* 7(9):691-699, 1984.

47. Dousset E, Jammes Y: Reliability of burst superimposed technique to assess central activation failure during fatiguing contraction, *J Electromyogr Kinesiol* 13(2):103-111, 2003.

48. Merton PA: Voluntary strength and fatigue, *J Physiol* 123(3):553-564, 1954.

49. Vollestad NK, Sejersted OM, Bahr R, et al: Motor drive and metabolic responses during repeated submaximal contractions in humans, *J Appl Physiol* 64(4):1421-1427, 1988.

50. Lepers R, Hausswirth C, Maffiuletti N, et al: Evidence of neuromuscular fatigue after prolonged cycling exercise, *Med Sci Sports Exerc* 32(11):1880-1886, 2000.

51. Behm DG, St-Pierre DM: Effects of fatigue duration and muscle type on voluntary and evoked contractile properties, *J Appl Physiol* 82(5):1654-1661, 1997.

52. Bigland-Ritchie B, Kukulka CG, Lippold OC, et al: The absence of neuromuscular transmission failure in sustained maximal voluntary contractions, *J Physiol* 330:265-278, 1982.

53. Arnaud S, Zattara-Hartmann MC, Tomei C, et al: Correlation between muscle metabolism and changes in M-wave and surface electromyogram: dynamic constant load leg exercise in untrained subjects, *Muscle Nerve* 20(9):1197-1199, 1997.

54. Solomonow M, Baten C, Smit J, et al: Electromyogram power spectra frequencies associated with motor unit recruitment strategies, *J Appl Physiol* 68(3):1177-1185, 1990.

55. Millet GY, Lepers R, Maffiuletti NA, et al: Alterations of neuromuscular function after an ultramarathon, *J Appl Physiol* 92(2):486-492, 2002.

56. Debold EP, Dave H, Fitts RH: Fiber type and temperature dependence of inorganic phosphate: implications for fatigue, *Am J Physiol Cell Physiol* 287(3):C673-681, 2004.

57. Enoka RM, Stuart DG: Neurobiology of muscle fatigue, *J Appl Physiol* 72(5):1631-1648, 1992.

58. Lewis SF, Fulco CS: A new approach to studying muscle fatigue and factors affecting performance during dynamic exercise in humans, *Exerc Sport Sci Rev* 26:91-116, 1998.

6

Robert A. Donatelli

Overuse Injury and Muscle Damage

LEARNING OBJECTIVES

After studying this chapter, the reader will be able to do the following:

1. Identify the predisposing, precipitating, and perpetuating factors of muscle damage and overuse
2. Describe muscle damage secondary to metabolic overload
3. Describe muscle damage secondary to mechanical factors
4. Summarize the physiological effects of muscle damage
5. Compare the damaging effects of isometric, concentric, and eccentric exercises on the muscle
6. Identify the increased risk of muscle damage in the young athlete
7. List the classification of muscle strain
8. Describe the healing of muscle cells and fibers
9. Summarize the appropriate management of damage to muscle

Overuse use injuries result from repetitive subtraumatic forces. Breakdown of microscopic tissue occurs faster than the tissue can heal or repair itself. The results are inflammation, ligament failure, tendonitis, tendon ruptures, muscle fatigue, and muscle damage.[1,2] In 2000 approximately 60 million children between the ages of 5 and 18 years old lived in the United States.[3] Approximately 72% of middle and high school children sustained a physical activity–related injury that was treated by a physician or nurse.[3,4] Muscle injuries are the most common injury in sports. Their incidence has been reported to be as high as 55% of all injuries sustained in sports events.

In 2001 an estimated 18 million children (30% of 60 million) were treated for a sports/physical activity–related injury. Approximately 50% of those injuries (9 million) were attributed to overuse mechanisms resulting in muscle damage.[3,4]

Acute muscle strain injuries, contusions, and ruptures are a large percentage of the injuries treated by rehabilitation specialists. Muscle injuries lead to significant pain, disability, and time away from work and athletic pursuits. On the basis of the author's clinical observations, an overwhelming number of overuse injuries are related to muscle damage. The major

factors leading to damage of the muscle result from overtraining, strenuous exercises, and lack of recovery time secondary to participation in multiple sporting activities.

This chapter reviews pertinent information on the etiology of overuse and muscle damage, structural changes resulting from muscle damage, the repair of muscle, special considerations in muscle damage in children, classification of muscle strains, and the management of muscle damage.

ETIOLOGY OF OVERUSE INJURY TO MUSCLE

Factors leading to overuse injuries can be subgrouped as predisposing, precipitating, and perpetuating. The ability of the clinician to evaluate for the factors leading to overuse will determine the success of the treatment plan.

Predisposing Factors of Muscle Damage

Muscle strains occur with the highest frequency in muscles that cross two joints and in those with the highest proportion of Type II fibers.[5] In addition, eccentric exercise appears to predispose muscle to pain and damage. Eccentric exercises can cause damage to the muscle, which has been associated with delayed onset of muscle soreness (DOMS).[5] Eccentric exercises can be therapeutic or potentially damaging to the muscle and its musculotendinous junction (MTJ).[6]

Muscle is the best force attenuator in the body. Eccentric or lengthening action of muscle dampens the forces of weight bearing. At heel strike, the lower limb is slowly lowered to the ground by the action of muscle-lengthening contractions.[7] Flexion of the knee is controlled by the eccentric action of the quadriceps femoris muscle.

Muscle imbalances are commonly associated with overuse injuries. Muscle imbalances may be alterations in muscle function secondary to a dysfunction between the antagonist and agonist. The disparity may include muscle weakness, poor flexibility, and inadequate endurance for musculoskeletal performance during specific functional activities. Alterations in muscle function secondary to muscle imbalances may result in inadequate or abnormal movement patterns during activities such as running. For example, Elliot and Achland[1] used high-speed cinematography to study the effect of fatigue on the mechanical characteristics in highly skilled long-distance runners. They found that, toward the end of a race, the runners exhibited less efficient positioning of the foot at foot strike, as well as decreased stride length and stride rate. Alteration in muscle function during running may cause bones, ligaments, and tendons to be overworked, producing tissue breakdown and pathology.[8] Weakness of the hamstring muscle can cause increased strain to the anterior cruciate ligament (ACL). Hamstring muscle tightness in the presence of quadriceps femoris muscle weakness has been associated with anterior knee pain including chondromalacia patellae. In the presence of hamstring tightness, patellofemoral joint compressive forces increase during the swing-through phase of gait or recovery phase of running.[8] Quadriceps femoris muscle weakness, especially in the vastus medialis muscle, can result in lateral patellar tracking during knee flexion and extension. Because the quadriceps femoris muscle controls knee flexion during the stance phase of walking or running, weakness can result in increased shock to the ankle and knee. Weakness of the quadriceps femoris muscle places increased stress on the lower leg, resulting, with repetitive exercise, in overuse.

Imbalance among gastrocnemius-soleus muscles and weak pretibial muscles, anterior tibialis, extensor hallucis longus, and extensor digitorium longus muscles has been associated with anterior shin splints, especially during repetitive hill running.[9] During uphill running, pretibial muscles forcefully contract in the recovery phase of running to dorsiflex the ankle, allowing the foot to clear the surface of the ground. Additionally, during downhill running, at heel strike, the pretibial muscles contract eccentrically to control ankle plantar flexion and prevent foot-slap. Overactivation of these muscles can occur in the presence of tight antagonists (the gastrocnemius-soleus muscles). The result may be microtrauma and inflammation of the pretibial muscles, tendons, and bony attachments.[9]

In the shoulder rotator cuff, imbalance is often associated with overuse. The external rotators of the glenohumeral joint should be 70% of the strength of the internal rotators in overhead-throwing athletes.[10] The eccentric overload of the external rotators in the overhead-throwing athlete weakens the glenohumeral external rotators. In some cases the external rotator strength decreased to 50% of the internal rotator strength. On the basis of clinical observation, the author considers the previous ratio to be pathological and may result in damage to the glenohumeral joint or the rotator cuff muscles.

Precipitating Factors of Muscle Damage

Poorly conditioned individuals secondary to sedentary lifestyles or athletes who have experienced an injury in the past requiring a period of immobilization are predisposed to muscle imbalances. Furthermore, the injured athlete or the sedentary individual might be more susceptible to precipitating muscle damage.

Prolonged or strenuous exercise can lead to muscle overuse injuries resulting in pain and dysfunction. Fatigue may be a major precipitating factor leading to muscle damage causing pain, aches, and cramps. The term *fatigue* is typically described as a general sensation of tiredness and accompanying decrements in muscular performance. The underlying causes of fatigue include accumulation of metabolic by-products, such as lactic acid, failure of the muscle fiber's contractile mechanism, depletion of muscle glycogen, and failure of nerve impulse transmission.[11] Further discussion of muscle fatigue is discussed in depth in Chapter 5.

If the athlete pushes beyond the point of fatigue and its warning signs, further damage to the muscle and the musculotendinous junction is possible. Muscle pain, aches, and cramps may lead to ruptures. Hematoma formation, necrosis of myofibers, and inflammatory cell reaction are all precursors to tendon or muscle ruptures, or both.[12]

Demanding physical activities, either at work or sport related, require concentric and eccentric muscle contraction. The most damaging types of exercise are those requiring excessive eccentric loading, such as heavy weight training and repetitive eccentric loading activities of an overhead-throwing athlete. Maximum power can be reduced by 50% or more after damaging exercise. Muscle strength reaches its lowest value immediately after eccentric exercise and recovers slowly over 10 days.[13] In addition, the joint range of motion can be impaired immediately after exercise or as a result of muscle imbalances.[14] The combination of decreased strength and flexibility may result in significant muscle damage, such as a rupture.

Evidence-Based Clinical Application

The capacity of the muscle-tendon unit to resist stretching is directly related to the tension of the muscle: During muscle contraction twice as much force is necessary to cause a rupture than in a relaxed muscle.[12]

Perpetuating Factors of Muscle Damage

Muscle damage, especially in athletes, is often difficult to treat because the athlete usually resumes the same training or exercise regimens (precipitating factors). In addition, the same muscle deficits and imbalances continue and in many cases become worse. The perpetuating factors of muscle damage therefore are the combination of the predisposing and precipitating factors already discussed. To treat muscle damage successfully, the predisposing and precipitating factors must be eliminated or modified. For each patient the rehabilitation specialist must evaluate muscle flexibility and strength. In addition, the clinician must have a thorough understanding of the anatomical and physiological demands of the sport in which the athlete is participating. Furthermore, the clinician must determine the best type of exercise regimen to take the athlete from rehabilitation back to his or her sport.

MUSCLE DAMAGE: THE PHYSIOLOGY, EVALUATION, CLASSIFICATION AND MANAGEMENT

Muscle damage by unaccustomed or high-intensity exercise is common. Muscle strains appear to occur with the highest frequency in muscle that crosses two joints and in muscle with the highest proportion of Type II muscle fibers.[10] As previously noted, unaccustomed eccentric exercise appears to be predisposed to pain and is more likely to cause muscle damage than other types of muscular activity. Gleeson [15] demonstrated that the severity of symptoms of exercise-induced muscle damage (EIMD) is reduced by a prior bout of eccentric exercise. Because of the specificity of muscle adaptation to training or the SAID (Specific Adaptations to Imposed Demands) principle, prior concentric training increases the susceptibility of muscle to EIMD following eccentric exercise.

The clinical assessment of muscle damage is difficult. Although pain and the inability to produce a forceful contraction are the most common symptom of muscle damage, it is not a good indicator of the amount of damage. The only objective means for determining the amount of muscle damage is histological verification, which is limited even with the use of the light or electron microscope.

Two hypotheses explain muscle damage: metabolic overload and mechanical factors. Metabolic overload means the demand for ATP exceeds it production.[16-18] To support the metabolic overload theory, several observations have reported that exercise-induced muscle damage resembles ischemic muscle damage. Furthermore, creatine kinase (CK) activity in serum is frequently used as a marker for muscle damage. Although CK is used as a marker for muscle damage, its value as an adequate quantitative marker is poor. Recently, an additional metabolic marker indicating muscle damage was discovered. One study showed that downhill running induced eccentric injury as evidenced by plasma troponin-I levels.[19] The presence of proteins, such as troponin-I, might be better markers of muscle damage because of their association with the contractile apparatus of generation and regulation of tension within muscle.

Lieber and Friden[20] hypothesized that excessive strain to the sarcomeres permits extracellular or intracellular membrane disruption that may cause myofibrillar disruption. Inflammation that occurs after injury further degrades the tissue, but prevention of inflammation leads to a long-term loss in muscle function.

The second hypothesis is that mechanical factors are a cause of EIMD. Faulkner and Brooks[21] demonstrated in laboratory mice local damage to muscle fiber through overuse. The extensor digitorum longus muscle of a mouse was activated by stimulation of the peroneal nerve. The muscle was either shortened or lengthened through 20% of the fiber length. Contractions were elicited every 4 to 5 seconds over periods of 5 minutes to 30 minutes or for 5 minutes with 5 minutes of rest, repeated three times. The local damage of the muscle fiber

was determined by infiltration of phagocytes, reduced muscle spindles, and nerve and artery appearance. The ultrastructural damage of the muscle was not observable with light microscopy. Despite the relationship between the number of damaged fibers and the force deficit, the force deficit at day 3 is about 15% greater than the extent of the muscle damage observed in histological sections. The researchers concluded that the force deficit provides a better estimate of the totality of contraction-induced injury.[21] Furthermore, a greater loss of force was created after a lengthening contraction (eccentric) than a shortening contraction (concentric), and the least for isometric contractions. Although shortening and isometric contractions produced significant fatigue immediately and for several hours after the exercise protocols, there was no evidence of injury at day 3. In comparison the lengthening contraction exercise protocols demonstrated morphological changes of muscle fiber throughout the first 5 days. The changes in muscle fiber included damage to the sarcoplasmic reticulum, actin and myosin filaments, and possibly capillaries. The magnitude of the injury is a function of the duration of the lengthening contraction. Friden and Lieber[22] compared different types of muscle contractions in the limb of a rabbit. This study demonstrated similar findings to the previous study. The magnitude of force deficit was a function of the treatment method. Following 30 minutes of cyclic passive stretch the force deficit was 13%; following isometric contraction it decreased by 31%; and following eccentric contraction it decreased by 69%. Immediately after a protocol of 75 lengthening contractions the force deficit was measured at 3 and 24 hours. The initial force deficit was 35% immediately after the protocol of eccentric contractions and a maximum force deficit of 55% at day 3.

Morgan [23] demonstrated that the stretching of weak sarcomeres beyond the overlap of the myosin and actin filaments resulted in the initial injury to a protein called titin. The titin links the myosin filaments in series contributing to myofibular stability during muscle contraction.

Reduction of sarcomeres in series decreases the muscle compliance and changes the length-tension relation of muscle contraction. Concentric contractions have been recently suggested as contributing to a reduction of sarcomeres in series. Conversely, eccentric exercise contributed to an increase in sarcomeres in series, making the muscle more resistant to EIMD.[24] The secondary injury to the muscle fiber resulted from the decreased capacity of the muscles' ability to develop force.

CLINICAL IMPLICATIONS OF RESEARCH

The active tension generated by a sarcomere is a direct function of the extent of overlap between actin and myosin filaments. Low forces are produced at long and short sarcomere lengths. Higher forces are generated at intermediate lengths. Clinically, the ideal length of the muscle to generate the greatest tension is approximately 30% from the muscle's fully lengthened position.[13] Other factors influence the development of tension within the muscle including the lever arm, size of the muscle, joint angle, and fiber type.

Exercise-induced muscle injury in humans frequently occurs after unaccustomed exercise, particularly if the exercise involves a large amount of eccentric contractions. Significant myofibrillar disruption may occur secondary to a lengthening contraction that may also disrupt the titin molecule. Even an isometric contraction may produce significant myofibrillar disruption if preceded by excessive or unaccustomed eccentric exercises. Specificity of training is important to the development of fiber length and the ability to protect the muscle from excessive damage. Eston[25] showed that muscle soreness, the amount of strength loss, and increases in plasma CK activity after a downhill run were reduced when 100 maximal isokinetic eccentric exercises were performed 2 weeks earlier.

As the muscle shortening velocity increases, its force decreases. Therefore concentric exercises at high velocities are not associated with muscle damage. In contrast, during eccentric or lengthening exercises high forces are sustained and muscle damage is common. The most commonly used markers indicating muscle damage are maximal voluntary contraction force, blood protein assessment, and subjectively determined muscle soreness. Prolonged strength loss after eccentric exercise is considered to be one of the most valid and reliable indirect measures of muscle damage in humans.[24] Downhill running, which is an eccentric activity, may generate 10% to 30% force loss directly after the exercise, with recovery up to 24 hours postexercise. High force eccentric exercise can often generate up to 50% to 65% loss of force-generating capacity, lasting 1 and 2 weeks after initial damage.[24] The loss of force after excessive eccentric loading could be due to damage within the tendon attachments and the elastic elements within the muscle. Concentric exercise is typically associated with strength loss of 10% to 30% immediately after exercise, with strength returning to baseline within hours after exercise.[24]

SPECIAL CONSIDERATIONS IN CHILDREN

Overall body height and mass increases on an average from 18 kg to 55 kg in females and 18 kg to 73 kg in males between the ages of 5 and 18. Body height increases from 110 cm for males and females to 160 cm in females and 175 cm in males over the same age range.[3] The growth rate of an individual may increase the risk of injury. A muscle group may adapt quickly to rapid increases in growth. The muscle accommodates to growth spurts by either increasing size or activating a greater portion of its mass. A growth spurt may lead to muscle damage if the tendons and apophyses associated with the changing muscle group adapt slowly. The stress is then increased to the tendons and apophyses, in response to muscle forces that may exceed the strength of the tendon and apophyses.[3] For example, the thigh muscles may need to develop about 30% more force after the growth spurt to develop the same lower leg angular acceleration required during a kicking movement. If the child can produce the needed additional force and the movement is performed repetitively, muscle fatigue, tendonitis or apophyseal irritation, or both, may result.[3]

CLINICAL CLASSIFICATION OF MUSCLE STRAIN/DAMAGE

Muscle strains are classified in three categories according to severity: (1) mild (first-degree) strain: a tear of a few muscle fibers; minor swelling and discomfort with minimal or no loss of strength or function; (2) moderate (second-degree) strain: a tear of multiple muscle fibers; mild swelling and discomfort with moderate loss of strength and function; and (3) severe (third-degree) strain: a greater damage of muscle with loss of strength; extending across the whole muscle belly, with total loss of function.

Muscle strains usually result in a hematoma secondary to rupture of intramuscular blood vessels. The first type of intramuscular hematoma lacks damage to the muscle fascia, which limits the size of the hematoma. The patient experiences pain and loss of function. The second type of muscle strain results in an intramuscular hematoma when the fascia is ruptured. The patient may not experience pain as long as pressure in the area does not increase.[12]

Repair of Muscle Damage

The stages of muscle healing are all interrelated and time dependent. Necrosis/degeneration, inflammation, repair, and scar tissue formation (fibrosis) are necessary for the healing process of muscle to occur.[26] Mechanical trauma causing injury to the muscle destroys the integrity of the myofiber plasma membrane and basal lamina.[27] The injured myofibers undergo necrosis by autodigestion mediated by intrinsic enzymes called proteases.[28] Local swelling and hematoma formation occur rapidly after injury and further promote muscle degeneration. The necrotic area is invaded by small blood vessels, lymphocytes, and macrophages, which perform a wide range of functions in the inflammation process. The most important function of the cells is activation of several growth factors, such as insulin-like growth factor, epidermal growth factors, and platelet-derived growth factors. The growth factors released at the injured site regulate the satellite cells that promote myoblast proliferation and differentiation to advance muscle regeneration and repair.[29] The initial muscle degeneration and inflammation occur with the first few days after injury. Rest, elevation, and ice are important to control the inflammatory response and prevent further damage to the muscle. The regeneration process usually peaks at 2 weeks and decreases at 3 to 4 weeks after injury. The formation of scar tissue (fibrous) begins between the second and third weeks.[26]

Within each myofiber are two divisions of satellite cells dedicated to the regeneration of the muscle fiber, differentiating satellite cells (myoblasts) and stem satellite cells.[11] Immediately after the injury the satellite cells begin to differentiate into myoblasts and fuse with each other to form multinucleated myotubes. The surviving parts of the injured myofiber fuse with the multinucleated myotubes, which grow into myofibers. The sarcoplasm is filled with contractile filamentous proteins organized into myofibrils.[30] The other type of cell used in the regeneration process is the stem satellite cell, which undergoes cell division before differentiation. The stem satellite cells replenish the satellite cells used in the initial formation of myoblasts.[11]

The concentration of collagen usually increases in muscles undergoing tissue repair when necrosis is due to physical trauma. The gap between the muscle fibers is filled with a hematoma. Within the first day inflammatory cells including phagocytes, which begin disposal of the blood clot, invade the hematoma. Fibrin and fibronectin are derived from the hematoma and form a matrix that acts as a scaffold and anchorage site for the invading fibroblasts.[31,32] The invading fibroblasts give the initial strength to the scar. Fibroblasts begin to synthesize proteins, as well as proteoglycans, of the extracellular matrix. From the time of the injury until days 10 to 12, the scar is the weakest point of the injured muscle. Increased tensile strength of the scar takes place with the production of Type I collagen fiber.[33]

After regenerating myofibers fill the damaged area, they extend from the opening into the connective tissue scar. The intervening scar progressively diminishes in size, and the stumps are brought closer together. The muscle and the scar do not reach normal strength until weeks after the injury, indicating that a long time is necessary until the strength of the muscle is completely restored.[33] The muscle is reinnervated by the growth of new dendrites distal to the rupture.

Evidence-Based Clinical Application
Growing evidence suggests that tissue repair depends on the immune system. A new hypothesis is that the inflammatory response is essential for efficient muscle repair and should not be repressed.[34]

Evidence-Based Clinical Application
Delayed onset of muscle soreness (DOMS) has been shown to occur after strenuous bouts of eccentric exercise and impairs strength and motion. The introduction of aerobic exercise to alleviate DOMS was not successful, and the trend analysis suggests that the intervention slowed the normal healing process.[35]

Evidence-Based Clinical Application
Short-term immobilization for 4 days after eccentric exercise enhanced the recovery of voluntary force produced by the muscle when compared with muscles that were not immobilized.[36]

Management of Muscle Strains

Early mobilization is the method of choice in the treatment of muscle ruptures. Early mobilization induces more rapid and intensive capillary ingrowth to the injured area. In addition, early movement promotes better fiber regeneration and orientation, allowing the functional properties of muscle to return sooner to the normal level.

The importance of early mobilization should not lessen the significance of immobilization immediately after the injury. Immobilization allows newly formed granulation tissue to reach sufficient tensile strength to withstand the contractile forces of the muscle. Mobilization too soon can cause reruptures at the original injury site. Therefore immobilization protects the injured muscle while the regeneration process is initiated. On the basis of the author's clinical observation, active mobilization started within the first few days following the injury provides ideal conditions for regeneration with a more functional final outcome. (See Chapter 1 for a more detailed discussion of the effects of mobilization on healing soft tissues.)

Little agreement exists as to when an athlete can safely return to a sport following a muscle strain.[37] No testing or clinical observation is considered the gold standard. The most popular and safe approach has been that the individual can return to the sport if full range of motion, muscle strength, and functional activities can be performed at the intensity necessary to compete. However, limited scientific evidence supports this approach.[37] Factors that may contribute to the recurrence of muscle strain include the following:

- Reduced strength of the muscle due to disuse atrophy, the limitations of pain, or reflex inhibition
- Reduced flexibility of the muscle-tendon unit secondary to inhibition or scar formation, or both
- Reduced tensile strength of the scar tissue at the site of previous disruption
- Changes in movement patterns secondary to adaptive changes, such as muscle imbalances[37]

Previous injury is the one risk factor for recurrent muscle injury for which there is universal agreement. For example, if the athlete returns to play following a hamstring strain, the player is more likely to strain the quadriceps muscle group.[37] These findings suggest that changes in the biomechanics and neurological alterations of muscles and joints are important to consider during rehabilitation.

Evidence-Based Clinical Application: Muscle Training and Delayed Onset of Muscle Soreness
Aquatic plyometrics training provided the same performance as land plyometrics, but significantly reduced the perception of muscle soreness. Therefore aquatic plyometrics is a viable training option to enhance performance in athletes while reducing delayed onset of muscle soreness.[38]

A carefully structured rehabilitation program accelerates the recovery of muscle damage. The immediate treatment for muscle strain is RICE: rest, ice, compression, elevation, and antiinflammatory medications. The major goal of this treatment is to minimize bleeding from the ruptured blood vessels. The control of bleeding will prevent formation of a large hematoma, which has a direct impact on the size of the scar tissue at the end of the regeneration. A small hematoma and the limited interstitial edema accumulation at the rupture site will shorten the ischemic period in the granulation tissue and accelerate regeneration.[11]

After the primary treatment of RICE, early mobilization of the injured muscle is important to the healing process. After 3 to 5 days of the previously described treatment regimen, controlled exercises can be initiated[11]: isometric training without load and later with increasing load within the limits of pain and cautious and controlled isotonic training with minimal loads within the limits of pain. High repetition and low resistance can promote healing.

Isokinetic exercises are excellent in the early phases of muscle healing because the therapist can control the resistance by setting the speed of movement. In addition, range-of-motion limitations can be programmed into the exercise. Finally, isokinetic exercise eliminates the dangers of eccentric loading on the muscle during the early stages of healing. The therapist can program concentric exercise only.

Formation of scar (fibrous) tissue begins between the seventh and twenty-first day after injury. Stretching exercises are important during the fibrosis phase of muscle healing. Stretching the muscle increases the extensibility of the scar and improves the flexibility of the muscle. A painless stretch is important to prevent rerupture of the muscle.

Evidence-Based Clinical Application: Therapeutic Ultrasound

Ultrasound is widely recommended and used in the treatment of muscle injury. Experimental studies are not encouraging.

Therapeutic ultrasound promotes the proliferation phase of myoregeneration; however, it has no significant effect on the final outcome.[39]

SUMMARY

Muscle damage is one of the most common problems faced by the rehabilitation specialist. Muscle strain injuries are the most common type of injury seen in sports and occupational medicine. They occur frequently in certain muscles during powerful eccentric contractions. Eccentric contractions may make a muscle more prone to injury because the large forces produced by the contraction are added to the forces that are stretching the muscle. The muscles more susceptible to excessive stretching are the two-joint or biarticular muscles. In addition, muscles that are called on to slow down or control movement are more frequently injured. For example, the external rotators of the glenohumeral joint are designed to slow down the rotational movement of the humerus during the propulsive phase of overhead throwing. The eccentric overload

to the external rotator of the shoulder is damaging to the muscle and the underlying posterior glenohumeral capsule.

In order to protect the muscle from eccentric overload damage, the rehabilitation specialist must make use of the SAID principle. Specific adaptations of imposed demands means determining the muscle deficits and prescribing the specific exercise targeting the muscles that are in dysfunction. Furthermore, as previously noted, specificity of the training is important in preservation and the development of strength. To protect the muscle from eccentric overload, the training must include eccentric exercises. Once the muscle is strong it is more resistant to damage. Overuse injuries result in a breakdown in strength of muscles, tendons, ligaments, and bones. If the muscle is strong it is protective to the joint and its periarticular structures.

REFERENCES

1. Elliot B, Achland T: Biomechanical effects of fatigue on 10,000 meter running techniques, *Res Quart Ex Sports* 52:160, 1981.
2. Leadbetter WB: An introduction to sports-induced soft tissue inflammation. In Leadbetter WB, Buckwalter JA, Gordon SL, editors: *Sports-induced inflammation: clinical and basic science concepts*, pp. 3-23, Park Ridge, Ill, 1990, American Academy of Orthopaedic Surgeons.
3. Hawkins D, Metheny J: Overuse injuries in youth sports: biomechanical considerations, *Med Sci Sports Ex* 33:1701-1707, 2001.
4. Adirim T, Cheng T: Overview of injuries in the young athlete, *Sports Med* 33:75-81, 2003.
5. Douglas B, Nimmo M, Wood L: Pr*inciples of physiology: a scientific foundation of physiotherapy*, London, 1996, WB Saunders.
6. Cheung K, Hume P, Maxwell L: Delayed onset muscle soreness: treatment strategies and performance factors, *Sports Med* 33:145-164, 2003.
7. Basmajjan JV: *Muscle alive: their function revealed by electromyography*, ed 4, Baltimore, 1979, Williams & Wilkins.
8. James SL: Chondromalacia of the patella in the adolescent. In Kennedy JC, editor: *The injured adolescent knee*, pp. 214-218, Baltimore, 1979, Williams & Wilkins.
9. Subotnick SI: The shin splints syndrome of the lower extremity, *Podiatr Sports Med* 66:605-611, 1976.
10. Ellenbecker T, Mattalino AJ: Concentric isokinetic shoulder internal and external rotation strength in professional baseball pitchers, *J Orthop Sports Phys Ther* 25:323-328, 1999.
11. Wilmore JH, Costill DL: *Physiology of sports and exercise*, ed 2, Champaign, Ill, 1999, Human Kinetics.
12. Jarvinen T, Kaariainen M, Jarvinen M, et al: Muscle strain injuries, *Curr Opin Rheumatol* 12:155-161, 2000.
13. Clarkson PM, Nosake K, Braun B: Muscle function after exercise-induced muscle damage and rapid adaptation, *Med Sci Sports Ex* 24:512-520, 1992.

14. Rodenburg JB, Bar PR, De Boer RW: Relation between muscle soreness and biochemical and functional outcomes of eccentric exercise, *J Appl Physiol* 74:2976-83, 1993.

15. Gleeson NI, Eston R, Marginson V, et al: Effects of prior concentric training on eccentric exercise induced muscle damage, *Br J Sports Med* 37:119-125, 2003.

16. Armstrong RB: Mechanisms of exercise-induced delayed onset muscular soreness: a brief review, *Med Sci Sports Ex* 16:529-538, 1984.

17. Armstrong RB: Muscle damage and endurance events, *Sports Med* 3:370-381, 1986.

18. Ebbeling CB, Clarkson PM: Exercise-induced muscled damage and adaptation, *Sports Med* 7:207-234, 1989.

19. Caiozzo V, Green S: Breakout session 2: Muscle injury, *Clin Ortho Rel Res* 1:120-125, 2002.

20. Frieden J, Lieber RL: Eccentric exercise-induced injuries to contractile and cytoskeletal muscle fibre components, *Acta Physiol Scand* 171:321-326, 2001.

21. Faulkner JA, Brooks SV: Muscle damage induced by contraction: an in situ single skeletal muscle model. In Salmons S, editor: *Muscle damage*, pp. 28-40, New York, 1997, Oxford Medical Publications.

22. Frieden J, Lieber RL: Muscle damage induced by cyclic eccentric contraction: biomechanical and structural studies. In Salmons S, editor: *Muscle damage*, pp. 41-63, New York, 1997, Oxford Medical Publications.

23. Morgan DL: New insights into the behavior or muscle during active lengthening, *Biophys Sci* 57:209-221, 1990.

24. Clarkson PM, Hubal MJ: Exercise-induced muscle damage in humans, *Am J Phys Med Rehabil* 8:1-28, 2002.

25. Eston R, Finney S, Baker S, et al: Muscle tenderness and peak torque changes after downhill running following a prior bout of isokinetic eccentric exercise, *J Sports Sci* 14:291-299, 1996.

26. Huard J, Li Y, Fu FH: Muscle injuries and repair: current trends in research, *J Bone Joint Surg Am* 84:822-832, 2002.

27. Kasemkjjwattqana C, Menetrey J, Day CS, Bosch P, et al: Biological intervention in muscle healing and regeneration, *Sports Med Arthroscopy Rev* 6:95-102, 1998.

28. St. Pierre BA, Tidball JG: Differential response of macrophage subpopulations to soleus muscle reloading after rat hindlimb suspension, *J Appl Physiol* 77:290-297, 1994.

29. Honda H, Kimura H, Rostami A: Demonstration and phenotypic characterization of resident macrophages in rat skeletal muscle, *Immunology* 70-272-277, 1990.

30. Hurme T, Kalimo H: Activation of myogenic precursor cells after muscle injury, *Med Sci Sports Exercise* 24:197-205, 1992.

31. Tidball JG: Inflammatory cell response to acute muscle injury, *Med Sci Sports Exercise* 27:1022-1032, 1995.

32. Hurme T, Kalimo H, Lehto M, et al: Healing of skeletal muscle injury. An ultrastructural and immunohistochemical study, *Med Sci Sports Exercise* 23:801-810, 1991.

33. Lehto M, Duance VC, Restall D: Collagen and fibronectin in a healing skeletal muscle injury: an immunohistochemical study of the effects of physical activity on the repair of injured gastrocnemius muscle in the rat, *J Bone Joint Surg* 67B:820-828, 1985.

34. Lapointe BM, Cote CH: Repression of inflammation in exercise-induced muscle damage. Are we aiming at an enemy? *Med Sci Sports Exercise* 35:S9, 2003.

35. Millar Al, Sims JL Wright HJ, et al: The effects of aerobic exercise on DOMS measures, *Med Sci Sports Exercise* 35:S318, 2003.

36. Sayers SP, Peters BT, Knight CA, et al: Short-term immobilization after eccentric exercise. Part 1: Contractile properties, *Med Sci Sports Exercise* 35:753-761, 2003.

37. Orchard J, Best T: The management of muscle strain injuries: an early return versus the risk of recurrence, *Clin J Sport Med* 12:3-5, 2002.

38. Robinson LE, Devor ST, Merrick MA, et al: The effects of land versus aquatic plyometrics on power, torque, velocity, and muscle soreness, *Med Sci Sports Exercise* 35:S243, 2003.

39. Rantanen J, Thorsson O, Wollmer P, et al: Effects of therapeutic ultrasound on the regeneration of skeletal muscle myofibers after experimental muscle injury, *Am J Sports Med* 27:54-59, 1999.

Sharon Ann Plowman
and Denise Louise Smith

Physiological Effects of Overtraining and Detraining*

LEARNING OBJECTIVES

After studying this chapter, the reader will be able to do the following:

1. Define exercise training and identify the goal of exercise training for athletes
2. List and explain the training principles
3. Define and explain the goals of periodization
4. Describe the cycle types within each phase of periodization
5. Define and differentiate between overreaching and the overtraining syndrome (OTS)
6. Distinguish between sympathetic and parasympathetic forms of OTS
7. Discuss the major hypotheses proposed to explain the causes and mechanisms of OTS
8. Identify components important to monitor during training
9. Suggest techniques to prevent OTS
10. Identify treatment for OTS
11. Define detraining and indicate the factors that influence the magnitude and rate of loss of training adaptations
12. Describe the consequences of detraining on the metabolic system
13. Describe the consequences of detraining on the cardiorespiratory system
14. Describe the consequences of detraining on the neuromuscular system

For the athlete, training for a sport can make the difference between reaching his or her potential and failing to achieve optimal performance. This chapter discusses all aspects of exercise training principles. Specificity, progression, individualization, and maintenance are several key principles to include in the development of an exercise-training program. The athlete, in his or her enthusiasm to train hard, can overtrain. This chapter reviews the causes, mechanisms, prevention, treatment, and dangers of overtraining. Furthermore, detraining

can occur rather quickly if the athlete does not follow certain training principles to maintain the exercise adaptations. The last section of this chapter reviews the causes and consequences of detraining on various systems.

EXERCISE TRAINING

Exercise training is a consistent or chronic progression of physical activity sessions designed to improve physiological function/physical fitness for better health or sport performance. In this chapter, only sport performance is considered. To develop sport fitness, the physiological demands of the sport and specific position or event within the sport must first be analyzed. Second, each athlete must be evaluated in terms of these requirements. Finally, a specifically designed, individualized program must be devised.

Training Principles

Although much about training is unknown and new techniques always appear, there are eight well-established, fundamental guidelines that should form the basis for the development of any training program. These training principles are defined and briefly discussed as follows.

1. *Specificity.* This principle is sometimes called the SAID principle, which stands for "specific adaptations to imposed demands" (i.e., what you do is what you get). Thus the exercise program for any given athlete should work the specific musculature involved while achieving a proper balance between agonistic and antagonistic muscle groups; use the muscles in the biomechanical patterns of the sport; match the metabolic requirements; and incorporate any needed motor fitness attributes at a starting level that is appropriate. The demands of the sport will not change to accommodate the athlete. The athlete must be the one to meet the demands of the sport if success is desired.
2. *Overload.* To overload is to place a demand on the body greater than that to which it is accustomed. Three factors must be considered: frequency—the number of training

*Based on Plowman SA, Smith DL: *Exercise physiology for health, fitness, and performance,* ed 2, San Francisco, 2003, Benjamin Cummings..

sessions on a daily or weekly basis; intensity—the level of work, energy expenditure, or physiological response in relation to the maximum; and duration—the amount of time spent training per session or per day. Training volume indicates the quantity or amount of overload (frequency times duration), whereas training intensity represents the quality of overload.

3. *Rest/Recovery/Adaptation.* Adaptation is the change in physiological function that occurs in response to training. Adaptation occurs during periods of rest, when the body recovers from the acute homeostatic disruptions or residual fatigue, or both. Thus it is vitally important that exercisers receive sufficient rest between individual training sessions, after periods of increased training overload, and both before and after competition. Adaptation allows the individual to either do more work or do the same work with a smaller disruption of baseline values.

4. *Progression.* Progression is the change in overload in response to adaptation. Progression implies that the increments in training load are small, controlled, and flexible. Progression should not be thought of as a continuous unbroken increase in training overload. The best progression occurs in a series of steps, called *steploading*, in which every third or fourth change is actually a slight decrease in training load.[1,2] This stepdown allows recovery, which leads to adaptation.

5. *Retrogression/Plateau/Reversibility.* Progress is rarely linear, predictable, or consistent. When an individual's adaptation or performance levels off or gets worse, a plateau has been reached or retrogression has occurred, respectively. Too much time spent doing the same type of workout using the same equipment in the same environment can lead to a plateau. Plateaus are a normal consequence of a maintenance overload and may also occur normally, even during a well-designed and well-implemented steploading progression. Variety and rest may help a person move beyond these plateaus. However, if a plateau continues for some time or if other signs and symptoms appear, then the plateau may be an early warning signal of overtraining. Retrogression may also signal overtraining. Reversibility is the reversal of achieved physiological adaptations that occurs when training stops (detraining).

6. *Maintenance.* Maintenance refers to sustaining the achieved adaptation with the most efficient use of time and effort. At this point the individual has reached an acceptable level of fitness or training. The amount of time and effort required to maintain the individual's adaptation depends on the systems involved; it is higher, for example, in the cardiovascular system than in the neuromuscular system. In general, intensity is the key to maintenance; that is, as long as exercise intensity is maintained, frequency and duration of exercise may be decreased without losing positive adaptations.

7. *Individualization.* Individuals both require personalized exercise prescriptions based on their fitness levels and

goals and adapt differently to the same training program. The same training overload may improve physiological and performance levels in one individual, maintain physiological and performance levels in a second individual, and result in maladaptation and decrease in performance in a third. A major reason for these differences is lifestyle, particularly nutritional and sleep habits, stress levels, and substance use (e.g., tobacco or alcohol). Finally, age, sex, genetics, disease conditions, and training modality all affect individual exercise prescriptions and adaptations.

8. *Warm-up/Cool-down.* A warm-up prepares the body for activity by elevating the body temperature. Conversely, a cool-down allows for a gradual return to normal body temperature. The best type of warm-up is specific to the activity that will follow and individualized so as not to produce fatigue.

Periodization

Once a training program is designed, it should be applied in a pattern that will be most beneficial. Such a pattern is called the *training cycle* or *periodization.* Periodization is a plan for training based on a manipulation of the fitness components and training principles; the objective is to peak the athlete's performance for the competitive season or some part of it.

Figure 7-1 is an example of how periodization might be arranged for a basketball player whose season lasts approximately 4.5 months. This is intended as an example only because periodization depends on individual situations and abilities. In Figure 7-1, the time frame of 1 year—presented as 52 weeks *(outer circle)*—has been divided into four phases or cycles: the general preparatory (sometimes labeled *off-season*) phase, the specific preparatory (also known as *preseason*) phase; the competitive (or *in-season*) phase; and the transition *(active rest)* phase.[1-3] Each phase is typically divided into macrocycles that may vary in length from 2 to 6 weeks. A macrocycle is further divided into microcycles lasting 1 week.[4,5] Each type of cycle aims for an optimal mixture of work and rest. Macrocycles and microcycles have five basic goals or patterns: (1) developmental; (2) shock; (3) competitive, or maintenance; (4) tapering, or unloading; and (5) transition, or regeneration.[1]

In Figure 7-1 the first macrocycle (Figure 7-1, *A*) represents a developmental cycle for the preparatory stage and is designed to improve either general or specific fitness attributes, such as an aerobic base or sport-specific strength, progressively. Overloading is achieved by a stepwise progression from low to medium to high by gradually increasing the load for three cycles, followed by a regeneration cycle back to the level of the second load. This second load level then becomes the base for the next loading cycle. This is what is meant by steploading.

Shock cycles, illustrated in Figure 7-1, *B*, are used primarily during the preparatory phase and are designed to increase training demands suddenly. They should always be followed by a regeneration cycle that consists of a drastically reduced training load.

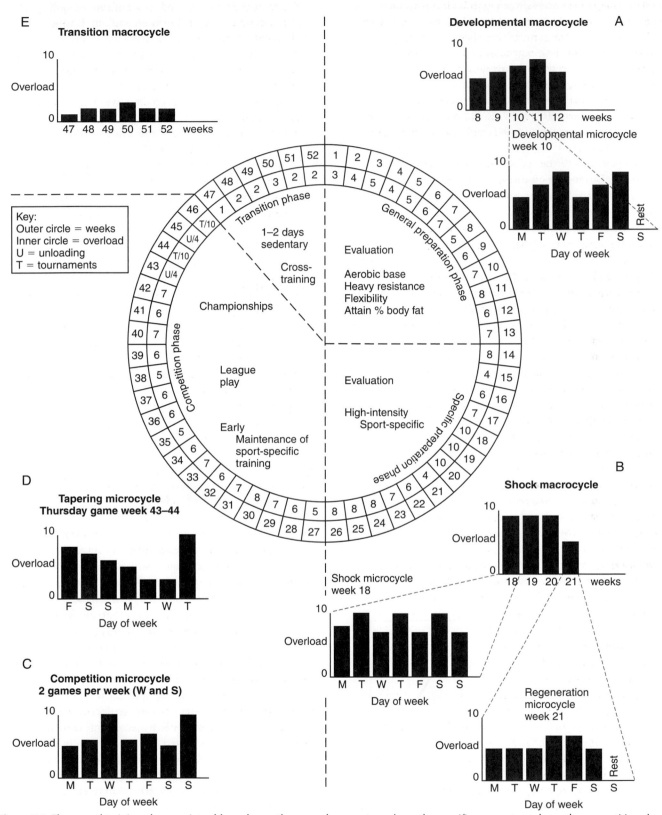

Figure 7-1 The annual training plan consists of four phases: the general preparatory phase, the specific preparatory phase, the competitive phase, and the transition phase. Overload is rated on a scale of 0 (complete rest) to 10 (maximal) on the inner circle. (From Plowman SA, Smith DL: *Exercise physiology for health, fitness, and performance*, ed 2, San Francisco, 2003, Benjamin Cummings.)

Competitive cycles (Figure 7-1, *C*) are based on maintaining physiological fitness while optimizing performance on game days. Obviously, competitive macrocycles and microcycles occur during the competitive phase.

Tapering or unloading regeneration cycles (Figure 7-1, *D*) involve systematic decreases in overload to facilitate a physiological fitness peak.[1] As noted, regeneration cycles are used both as breaks between other cycles and to form the basis of the active transition phase (Figure 7-1, *E*).[1,2,5] They are intended to remove fatigue, emphasize relaxation, and prevent overtraining.

Microcycles are further subdivided into daily workouts or lesson plans. Depending on the maturity and experience of the athlete and the level of competition, a training day may entail one, two, or three workouts.[1]

The general preparatory, or off-season, phase should be preceded by a sport-specific fitness evaluation to guide both the general and specific preparatory training programs. Another evaluation might be conducted before the season if desired, or evaluations might be conducted systematically throughout the year to determine how the individual is responding to training and to make any necessary adjustments. All evaluation testing should be done at the end of a regeneration cycle so that fatigue is not a confounding factor. The off-season is a time of general preparation when basic fitness components are emphasized to develop cardiovascular-respiratory endurance (an aerobic base), flexibility, and muscular strength and endurance. Any needed changes in body composition should be addressed during this phase.[5] An aerobic base is important for all athletes, even those whose event is primarily anaerobic. A high aerobic capacity allows the individual to work at a higher intensity before accumulating large quantities of lactic acid and becoming fatigued. A high aerobic capacity also allows the individual to recover faster, which is important both in and of itself and for allowing for a potentially greater total volume of work during interval sessions.[1]

During this general preparatory phase, overload progresses by steps in both intensity and volume (frequency times duration) with volume typically being relatively more important than intensity.[1] During the preseason phase, the athlete shifts to specific preparation for the fitness and physiological components needed to succeed in the intended sport. The training program at this time is heavy and generally occupies the 7 to 8 weeks before the first competition. About midway through the specific preparatory phase, intensity may surpass volume in importance. This will vary with the physiological demands of particular sports.[5]

Once the athlete begins the competition phase, the emphasis shifts to maintaining the sport-specific fitness that was developed during the preseason. Although both volume and intensity may be maintained, heavy workouts should immediately follow a competition instead of directly preceding one. During the late season, when the most important competitions are usually held (such as conference championships or bowl games), the athlete should do only a minimum of training or taper gradually by decreasing training volume but maintaining intensity so that he or she is rested without being detrained. For particularly important contests, both training volume and intensity might be decreased to peak for a maximal effort.[5]

The transition phase begins immediately after the last competition of the year. The athlete should take a couple of days of complete rest and then participate in active rest using noncompetitive physical activities that are not his or her primary sport. This type of activity is often called cross-training. In this transition phase, neither training volume nor intensity should exceed low levels.[5]

TRAINING ADAPTATION AND MALADAPTATION

Training and its relationship to athletic performance exist on a continuum that is best described as an inverted U (Figure 7-2).[6-8] At one end of the continuum are individuals who are undertrained and whose fitness level and performance abilities are dictated by genetics, diseases, and nonexercise lifestyle choices. Individuals whose training programs lack sufficient volume, intensity, or progression for either improvement or maintenance of fitness or performance are undertrained. The goal of optimal periodized training is the attainment of peak fitness or performance, or both. However, if the training overload is too much or improperly applied, then maladaptation is possible. The first step toward maladaptation may be overreaching (OR), a short-term decrement in performance capacity that is easily recovered from and generally lasts only a few days to 2 weeks. OR may develop into overtraining.

OR can result from either planned shock microcycles, as previously described, or, inadvertently, from too much stress and too little planned recovery.[6,7,9] If OR is planned and recovery is sufficient, positive adaptation and improved performance, sometimes called supercompensation, result (Figure 7-3, *A*). If, however, OR is left unchecked or the individual or coach interprets the decrement in performance as an indication

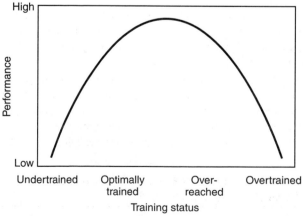

Figure 7-2 Training and performance. (From Plowman SA, Smith DL: *Exercise physiology for health, fitness, and performance*, ed 2, San Francisco, 2003, Benjamin Cummings.)

that more work must be done, OR may develop into over-training (Figure 7-3, *B*). Overtraining, more properly called the *overtraining syndrome* (OTS) (or staleness) is a state of chronic decrement in performance and ability to train, in which restoration may take several weeks, months, or even years.[7,9-11] Because the only universally apparent result of the OTS is a decrement in performance, the term *unexplained underperformance syndrome* (UPS) has been suggested.[12] Acceptance of this terminology has been slow.

The relationship between OR and OTS is often depicted as a continuum.[6] That is, as the imbalance between training and recovery increases, the complexity of the symptoms also increases and the athlete progresses from OT to OTS. However, research data to back this up do not exist.[13] Coaches and athletes often use shock microcycles to induce OR in the normal periodization of training. Therefore it is possible for scientists to follow and test athletes in such a situation. However, it is neither ethical nor reasonable to deliberately induce a state of OTS. Thus scientific data on the OTS has largely been derived retrospectively from case studies of athletes with unexplained underperformance. Data in which meaningful numbers of subjects in both resistance and endurance activities have been followed from adaptation and performance improvement through overreaching to the over-training syndrome simply do not exist.

What does exist is a long list of signs and symptoms that have been observed in athletes exhibiting unexplained per-formance decrements.[6,14] A sampling of some that may be observed by the athlete himself or herself, the coach, or athletic trainer is presented in Table 7-1.

Intentionally incomplete, this list is further complicated by the fact that two forms of the OTS probably exist: a sympa-thetic form and a parasympathetic form.[9,15-21] The sympathetic form is characterized by an increased sympathetic neural tone at rest and during exercise and down-regulation of beta (β) receptors. Restlessness and hyperexcitability dominate. For example, an elevated resting heart rate, slower heart rate recovery postexercise, decreased appetite and unintentional loss of body mass, excessive sweating, and disturbed sleep patterns are symptomatic of the sympathetic form of overtraining.[6,19] The sympathetic form of overtraining is generally considered to be an early indication of overtraining. It appears to be most closely related to high-intensity anaerobic activities.[9] The parasympathetic form of overtraining is characterized by sym-pathetic neural insufficiency, a decreased sensitivity to the pituitary and adrenal hormones, and an increase in parasympa-thetic tone at rest and during exercise. The symptoms of the parasympathetic form of overtraining are less obvious and in isolation may be difficult to distinguish from positive training adaptations.[6,19] For example, resting pulse rates may be lower, submaximal exercise heart rates and lactate responses lower, and heart rate recovery from exercise rapid; however, these responses are typically associated with early fatigue and impaired maximal work capacity markers, such as heart rate and lactate. Apathy, digestive disturbances, and altered immune and reproductive function are common. The parasympathetic form of the overtraining syndrome is the more advanced form. It appears to be most frequently associated with excessive volume training in both aerobic endurance activity and dynamic resistance exercise.[9] Individual differences in the nervous system may predispose any given individual to either up-regulation (sympathetic form) or down-regulation (parasympathetic form) of the neuroendocrine homeostasis.

The signs and symptoms of OTS are outward manifesta-tions of neuroendocrine imbalances; immune system activation or suppression, or both; or a reversal of normal physiological adaptations. They provide a starting point for research aimed at determining the physiological mechanisms behind the OTS.

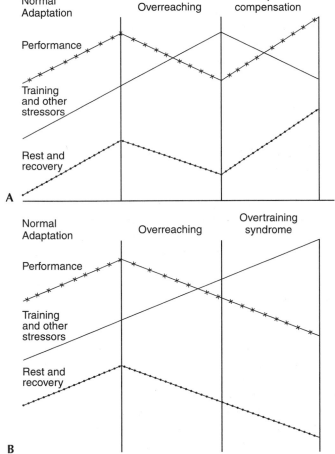

Figure 7-3 Exercise training adaptation (**A**) and maladaptation (**B**). (From Fry RW, Morton AR, Keast D: *Can J Sport Sci* 17:241-248, 1992; Kuipers H: *Med Sci Sports Exerc* 30: 1137-1139, 1998; Kreider RB, Fry AC, O-Toole ML: *Overtraining in sport*, pp. vii-ix, Champaign, Ill, 1998, Human Kinetics; Halson SL, Jeukendrup AE: *Br J Sports Med* 32: 107-110, 1998.)

Hypothesized Causes and Mechanisms of Overtraining Syndrome

The precise cause(s) and mechanism(s) of OTS are unknown. A high-volume training load performed at high intensity and applied in a monotonous manner without sufficient rest

Table 7-1	Signs and Symptoms of the Overtraining Syndrome

Type	Signs and Symptoms
Performance-related	Consistent decrement in performance
	Persistent fatigue and sluggishness that leads to several days of poor training
	Prolonged recovery from training sessions or competitive events
	Reappearance of already corrected errors
	Increased occurrence of muscular accidents/injuries
Physiological	Decreased maximal work capacities and markers
	Increased disruption of homeostasis at submaximal workloads
	Headaches or stomachaches out of proportion to life events
	Insomnia
	Persistent low-grade stiffness and soreness of the muscles and joints; feeling of "heavy" legs
	Frequent upper respiratory tract infections: sore throats, colds, or cold sores
	Constipation or diarrhea
	Loss of appetite; loss of body weight or muscle mass, or both, when no conscious attempt is being made to diet or when weight loss is undesirable
	An elevation of approximately 10% in the morning heart rate taken immediately on awakening
	Amenorrhea
Psychological/Behavioral	Feelings of depression
	General apathy, especially toward previously enjoyed activities
	Decreased self-esteem
	Emotional instability or mood changes
	Difficulty concentrating
	Loss of competitive drive or desire
	Perceived insufficient recovery

From Plowman SA, Smith DL: *Exercise physiology for health, fitness, and performance,* ed 2, San Francisco, 2003, Benjamin Cummings.

and recovery, which alters metabolic processes and leads to an accumulation of muscle trauma, appears to be the primary predisposing factor (Figure 7-4).[6,10,12,22-24] Related stressors, such as frequent competition, excessive travel, training and competing under inhospitable environmental conditions, and poor nutrition, as well as unrelated stressors, such as family, school, or work commitments, accumulate and are likely peripheral causes. In this context a stressor is defined as any activity, event, or impingement that causes stress, and stress is defined as any disruption in body homeostasis and all attempts by the body to regain homeostasis.[25] Both acute exercise and chronic training are stressors.

Attempts at explaining the physiological mechanisms by which the probable causative factors actually bring about the OTS have resulted in a number of hypotheses. It is important to remember that a hypothesis by definition is "an assumption not proved by experiment or observation. It is assumed for the sake of testing its soundness or to facilitate investigation of a class of phenomena."[26] Thus although research data may account for some observed symptoms of the OTS, they are generally insufficient to even support the use of the term theory. In short, the underlying mechanism(s) remain(s) unproven at this point.[10]

In general the hypotheses may be categorized into three major areas: biochemical/metabolic, neuroendocrine, and immunological. Figure 7-4 indicates how all of these areas may interact in producing the OTS.

Alterations of Carbohydrate, Lipid, and Protein Metabolism

Muscles obviously use fuel for the contractions that make up exercise training. Indeed, a major objective of exercise training, especially endurance training, is to increase metabolism to support the competitive events. Thus the OTS in endurance athletes may be mediated primarily through dysfunctions of carbohydrate (CHO), lipid (FAT), and/or protein (PRO) metabolism.[11,22,23,27] Glycogen depletion may become a reality if insufficient CHO ingestion follows successive training bouts. In and of itself, low glycogen can lead to the defining signs of OTS, early fatigue and poor performance.[27]

The predominant back-up fuel to CHO for exercise is, of course, FAT in the form of triglyceride-derived free fatty acids (FFAs). Although the utilization of higher amounts of FFA and the sparing of glycogen is a beneficial adaptation of training, this is typically accomplished in the presence of adequate glycogen stores. Without sufficient CHO stores and in the presence of the oxidative stress that accompanies endurance activity, alterations occur in the triglyceride/fatty acid cycle and an increase is seen in polyunsaturated fatty acids (PUFAs).

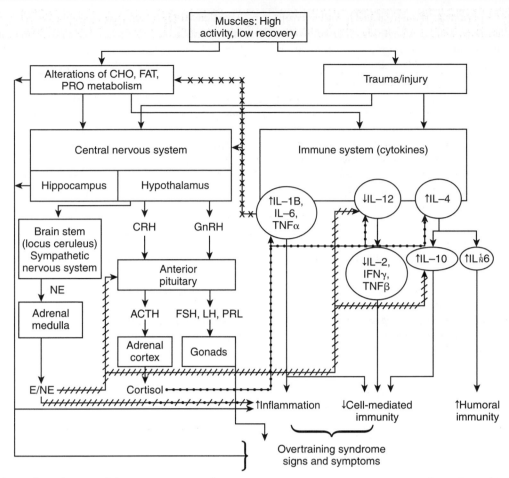

Figure 7-4 Hypothesized mechanism of the overtraining syndrome. (From Fry RW, Morton AR, Keast D: *Can J Sport Sci* 17:241-248, 1992; Kreider RB, Fry AC, O'Toole ML: *Overtraining in sports*, pp. vii-ix, Champaign, Ill, 1998, Human Kinetics; Budgett R: *Br J Sports Med* 32:107-110, 1998; Petibois C, Cazorla G, Poortmans J-R, et al: *Sports Med* 32:867-878, 2002; Petibois C, Cazorla G, Poortmans J-R, et al: *Sports Med* 33: 83-94, 2003; Smith LL: *Med Sci Sports Exerc* 32:317-331. 2000; Snyder AC: *Med Sci Sports Exerc* 30:1146-1150, 1998; Steinacker JM, Lormes W, Reissnecker S, et al: *Eur J Appl Physiol* 91:382-391, 2004; Gastmann UAL, Lehmann MJ: *Med Sci Sports Exerc* 30: 1173-1178; Robson PH: *Sports Med* 33-771-781, 2003; Chrousos GP, Gold PW: *JAMA* 267: 1244-1252, 1992; Smith LL: *Sports Med* 33:347-364, 2003; Moldoveanu AL, Shephard RJ, Shek PN: *Sports Med* 31:115-144, 2001; Keizer HA: Neuroendocrine aspects of overtraining. In Kreider RB, Fry AC, O'Toole ML, editors: *Overtraining in sports*, pp. 145-167, Champaign, Ill, 1998, Human Kinetics.)

These changes have been linked to the pathogenesis of inflammation and immunosuppression.[22,23,28] Additionally, leptin is released from adipose cells. Leptin provides feedback for satiety, may act as a metabolic hormone, and assists in the regulation of the hypothalamic-pituitary function. Movement of fatty acid from adipocytes may inhibit leptin secretion. Low plasma leptin levels activate the hypothalamus-pituitary-adrenal axis (HPAA), as well as sympathetic activity, and, as a member of the cytokine family, leptin level is closely linked to immune function.[28,29]

These alterations in CHO (insufficient) and FAT metabolism (increased FFA use) also lead to shifts in PRO metabolism. Protein comprises a substrate pool not normally used extensively as fuel. However, under conditions of high-intensity, long duration training, or competition, especially when CHO stores are inadequate, PRO, and in particular the branched

chain amino acids (BCAA) are used as fuel. Furthermore, the increase in circulating FFA, which must be transported in blood by albumin, leads to release of another amino acid (AA), tryptophan (TRY). TRY is also normally bound to albumin. In addition to competing for albumin, BCAA and TRY normally compete for the same carrier to enter the brain. The decrease in BCAAs (as they are used to supply fuel) and increase in TRY favor the entry of TRY into the brain. In the brain, TRY is converted into serotonin. Increased levels of serotonin are responsible for decreased motor excitability, decreased appetite, increased sleep, and altered neuroendocrine function, which are among the signs and symptoms often seen in OTS.[11,12,30]

Glutamine is another AA of importance; it is the most abundant AA in human muscle and plasma. Glutamine, an energy source essential to kidney function, is used by the liver during exercise for the production and release of the antioxidant glutathione and is important at the neural level in the perception of exertion, lethargy, and energy levels. Glutamine is a precursor of substances essential for immune cell replication. Specifically, macrophages cannot synthesize certain cytokines (e.g., interleukin-1 [IL-1]) if glutamine is in short supply. Cytokines are essential for communication between immune cells and other cells of the body. Muscles are the main source of glutamine. Psychological, environmental, or exercise stress, especially with insufficient rest periods between bouts, may decrease glutamine flux from muscle during recovery. As a consequence, immune function may be depressed postexercise due to the decreased availability of glutamine, and, in turn, this may be linked to the high incidence of upper respiratory tract infections (URTIs) often seen in athletes after excessive exercise, such as a marathon, or in an overreached/overtrained state.[6,12,22,23,31-33] Only cell-mediated immunity appears to be adversely affected (see Figure 7-4).

Altered neuroendocrine function is predominantly mediated through the hypothalamus. The primary neural component is called the *brainstem (locus ceruleus)–sympathetic nervous system pathway.* The primarily hormonal component, discussed earlier, is the HPAA. When an individual is presented with a stressor, the hypothalamus coordinates the response. The hypothalamus is both a neural structure and an endocrine gland. Thus it can orchestrate the body's response by stimulating both the sympathetic nervous system and endocrine glands.

The sympathetic nerve fibers originate in the brainstem and travel throughout the body to a variety of target sites. The sympathetic nerve fibers also go to and control the adrenal medulla. Norepinephrine (NE) is released by sympathetic nerve fibers, and both NE and epinephrine (E) are secreted by the adrenal medulla. The NE and E secreted by the adrenal medulla circulate in the bloodstream to the target sites, where they mimic and reinforce the actions of the sympathetic nerve fibers that innervate the same target sites. Both NE and E may also influence other endocrine glands, as indicated by the connecting line to the anterior pituitary gland in Figure 7-4.[34]

The hypothalamus directly regulates endocrine glands both neurally and hormonally through a series of releasing hormones. In the generic stress response, corticotrophin-releasing hormone (CRH) is released by the hypothalamus and stimulates the anterior pituitary to secrete adrenocorticotrophic hormone (ACTH). ACTH in turn stimulates the adrenal cortex to release cortisol, which acts on specific target sites. E, NE, and cortisol are involved in the inflammatory process directly and indirectly by stimulation of the cytokine responses.[24]

Muscle Trauma and Injury

Microtrauma or tissue injury in muscles can affect both the central nervous system (CNS) and the immune system. Activation of the CNS by cytokines provides a way of explaining many of the signs and symptoms of the OTS. Among the principal types of cytokines are interleukins (ILs), interferons (IFNs), and tumor necrosis factors (TNFs). Each IL acts on a specific group of immune cells, causing them to divide and differentiate. IFNs interfere with and hence act to limit the spread of viral infections. TNFs deal with inflammation and stimulate cytotoxicity. Certain cytokines (IL-1, IL-6, IFNγ, and TNFα) are proinflammatory and probably play a role in coordinating the response to muscle damage resulting from strenuous exercise. Other cytokines (IL-4, IL-10, and possibly IL-6 in a dual role) are antiinflammatory. The antiinflammatory cytokines determine the role of T cells. T cells divide into two distinct functional subsets: TH1, associated with cell-mediated immunity, and TH2, associated with humoral immunity. The up-regulation of TH1 cells is primarily dependent on IL-12; the up-regulation of TH2 cells is primarily dependent on IL-4. In addition, IL-4 and IL-10 coordinate to inhibit TH1 development. Thus IL-10 suppresses cell-mediated immunity and macrophage function. The response to trauma/injury is a shift to a TH2 lymphocyte response, resulting in an up-regulation of humoral immunity and down-regulation of cell-mediated immunity. The individual is thus more susceptible to URTI.[35,36] The binding of cytokines (particularly IL-6) in the hypothalamus activates the HPAA and the sympathetic nervous system, resulting in the release of E, NE, and cortisol.[28,35] These stress hormones not only bring about physical/physiological changes but are also associated with mood changes, depression, and anxiety. The activation of the hippocampus may explain loss of attention and the return of previously corrected errors.[10,24,28,35,37]

MARKERS AND MONITORING TO PREDICT OVERTRAINING SYNDROME

Research to determine the mechanisms of the OTS is important because this could lead to the identification of a marker and level or amount of change that might lead to early detection of an athlete on the brink of overtraining. Such identification or early detection could lead to intervention and ideally prevention.[12,20]

Unfortunately, despite numerous attempts to identify such a marker, the overwhelming consensus remains that there is no reliable and valid variable or index available to predict the OTS or even to distinguish among well-trained, overreached, or overtrained athletes. To make matters more difficult, there is no clear demarcation for when overload becomes overtraining load, and the margin between adaptation/supercompensation and the functional impairment of the OTS is fluid both among athletes and within individual athletes. Given these circumstances, however, there is an equally strong consensus that monitoring athletes is extremely important. The difficulty, then, is how and what to monitor.[7,14,15,38-42] Training, performance, and nutrition appear to be reasonable and practical places to begin.

Monitor Training

All athletes should be encouraged to keep a daily training log, noting the following physical aspects: body weight (with periodic evaluation of body composition); morning resting heart rate (often difficult because of compliance issues—athletes do not particularly like doing this); training goal and actual training achieved; subjective ratings of perceived exertion during the training; any muscle/tendon/joint aches/pains; and any symptoms of URTI.[43]

The athlete needs to be aware of and report any meaningful changes (a rise $\geq$ 20%) in resting heart rate, any muscle/tendon/joint soreness, or URTI symptoms that remain from the previous day before the next day's workout. These could be indications that it is necessary to cut back the volume and intensity of the workout on this day to possibly avoid longer setbacks in the future.[41]

At the end of each macrocycle the training logs need to be carefully evaluated to determine the athlete's response to the training load. The training plan for the next cycle should be based on this evaluation.[44]

Monitor Performance

The most obvious item to monitor is, of course, sport-specific performance. Not only does the outcome of the performance need attention but also the effort involved in the performance and apparent recovery from the effort. In this context performance should include training workouts. In some events specific levels of performance can be reproduced by individualized ergometric tests in the exercise physiology laboratory or training room.[14] Because athletes suffering from OTS can often start a normal training workout, race, or other event, but not complete the performance as expected, analysis should be done of splits (in relation to predetermined strategy). This also means that a two-bout exercise protocol might be best to detect differences in training status.

Meeusen et al[45] detected subtle differences in HPAA hormonal responses to two bouts of maximal exercise 4 hours apart between cyclists in a well-trained (N = 7) and in a purposely overreached state (same seven athletes), and in one diagnosed OTS motocross athlete that would have been missed had only one exercise bout been used. Unfortunately, the authors did not report heart rate or ratings of perceived exertion values that would have been more practical for application than hormonal analysis. However, performance itself was sensitive to the training status. Time to exhaustion in Bout 2 decreased only 3% from Bout 1 in the well-trained state, doubled to −6% in the overreached condition, and almost doubled again to −11% in the OTS athlete. If performance tests are used, they must be conducted after a recovery or regeneration cycle when adaptation or maladaptation can accurately be evaluated and not confused with the normal fatigue of training.[4,8] This assumes, of course, that prior baseline data have been established for each athlete.

Monitor Mood State

Subjective ratings of mood, fatigue, athletic and nonathletic stress, and muscle soreness have been suggested as the most cost-effective strategy for early detection of OTS and hence monitoring of training.[14,17,41,46] The Profile of Mood States (POMS)[47] has been most extensively studied. This is a 65-item test that provides subjective ratings of tension-anxiety, depression, anger, vigor, fatigue, confusion, and total mood. Although POMS does not diagnose the OTS, it does seem to document mood changes consistent with the condition (as increased depression and tension-anxiety and decreased vigor and total mood score) in some athletes.[41,48] The deterioration in mood states often coincides with an increase in training load and usually precedes a decrement in performance.[14] Self-analysis questionnaires involving well-being ratings relative to fatigue, stress level, muscle soreness (especially "heavy" legs), training enjoyment, health concerns, irritability, self-confidence/self-esteem, attitude toward work/study/teammates, communication with teammates and coaches, and sleep quality/disorders can prove useful. Although verbal communication is extremely important, all of these items can and should succinctly be recorded in written training logs. The subjective portions of the logs require candor and complete honesty on the part of the athlete and must be evaluated in light of training and performance. Their usefulness depends heavily on the interpretation by the coach or athletic trainer.

PREVENTION AND TREATMENT OF OVERTRAINING SYNDROME

Prevention

The key to preventing the OTS is careful periodization of training. The delicate balance between overload/progression, in which large immediate increases in overload are avoided, and sufficient rest/recovery is difficult to attain but essential for each individual.[44] Periodization allows the athlete to peak for specific competitions. Peak performance cannot be maintained indefinitely, so competitions must be prioritized and periodization phases matched to these priorities. The more the attempted peaks, the more vulnerable the athlete will be to overtraining.[44,49] Few studies have actually compared the effectiveness of periodization. However, Rhea and Alderman[50] and Steinacker[51] have published positive results for strength/power (weight lifting) and aerobic/anaerobic (rowing) programs when periodization was employed.

The main protection against OTS is the inclusion of sufficient recovery after heavy physical training. Sufficient recovery from each daily training session or competition is extremely important. To athletes and coaches indoctrinated with the philosophy of "if some is good, more is better," the concept of "less is actually more" can be difficult to accept. Possible components of daily recovery include hydration and refueling as soon as possible to deal with metabolic fatigue; light activity, stretching, and hydrotherapy (as simple as showering or as complex as pool or spa activities) to deal with neural fatigue; and unwinding with activities, such as debriefing or listening to music, to deal with psychological fatigue.[43] This should be monitored in some manner. One such system has been proposed by Kenttä and Hassmén[16] and is described in the following Evidence-Based Clinical Application box. Restful sleep of 8 to 9 hours is essential. Sufficient recovery also means within the training progression itself. This may be accomplished by the inclusion of easy days, days of active cross-training, rest days emphasizing stretching and relaxation techniques, or days of complete rest.[16] The Evidence-Based Clinical Application box also provides a technique whereby the adequacy of the variation of training may be evaluated.

Ratings of Perceived Exertion and Recovery

Researchers have begun to suggest that the adequacy of recovery from training be monitored through the use of rating scales. One system[16] proposes that recovery from training be assessed using two total quality recovery (TQR) scales. The TQR perceived (TQRper) scale is a subjective rating by the individual to the query "How do you rate your overall recovery for the previous 24 hours?" The TQR action scale (TQRact) allows the athlete to accumulate "recovery points" on the basis of his or her activities in the previous 24 hours. Up to 10 points can be awarded for nutrition and hydration; up to 4 points for sleep and rest; up to 3 points for relaxation and emotional support; and up to 3 points for stretching and active rest. Because the point values for the action items are not set in stone, but rather are determined by the athlete and his or her coach/trainer, they should be established before implementing this scale. On the basis of this system, recovery is adequate if both the TQRper and TQRact are at or above the training stress as measured by the 6-20 Borg Rating of Perceived Exertion Scale[52] for the workout preceding the recovery.

Foster[53] bases his technique on Borg's 0-10 category ratio scale (CR-10)[52] and the duration of each day's workout (multiplying the two) to obtain a training session load. Each week the mean and standard deviation of the training load is computed as an index of training variability. The monotony of the weekly training load is described by dividing the daily mean load by the standard deviation (SD). A small SD and a high quotient indicate little day-to-day variation (i.e., high monotony).

TQRper scale

6
7 very, very poor
8
9 very poor
10
11 poor
12
13 reasonable
14
15 good
16
17
18
19
20

The strain of the weekly load is determined by multiplying the daily load by 7 days per week and the monotony factor. Both consistent high training monotony and high training strain appear to be related to training maladaptation.

The following example shows how simply substituting one rest day for a long cycling ride reduces the training monotony and strain. Many elite athletes work at a training load of 4000 units per week, thus even for an elite athlete the seven day a week program would be considered excessive. This biathlete could substitute the long bike ride for the long run on alternate weeks.

Day	Training Session	Duration (min)	Perceived Exertion CR-10	Load (units)
Monday	Weight Lifting	90	4	360
Tuesday	Running (8 km)	45	3	135
Wednesday	Cycling (48 km)	120	4	480
Thursday	Weight Lifting	90	4	360
Friday	Cycling (80 km)	200	6	1200
Saturday	Track Intervals	75	7	525
Sunday	Long Run (29 km)	180	6	1080
Daily Mean Load	591			
Standard Deviation of Daily Load	396			
Monotony (daily load ÷SD)	1.49			
Weekly Load (daily load × 7)	4140			
Strain (weekly load × monotony)	6169			

Ratings of Perceived Exertion and Recovery—cont'd

Day	Training Session	Duration (min)	Perceived Exertion CR-10	Load (units)
Monday	Weight Lifting	90	4	360
Tuesday	Running (8 km)	45	3	135
Wednesday	Cycling (48 km)	120	4	480
Thursday	Rest Day	0	0	0
Friday	Weight Lifting	90	4	360
Saturday	Track Intervals	75	7	525
Sunday	Long Run (29km)	180	6	1080
Daily Mean Load	420			
Standard Deviation of Daily Load	345			
Monotony (daily load ÷SD)	1.21			
Weekly Load (daily load × 7)	2940			
Strain (weekly load × monotony)	3557			

Adequate nutrition, with the possible periodization of CHO intake to match glycogen needs as described in the following paragraphs, is also critical. One of the foremost goals is to ensure sufficient glycogen stores to support high-intensity training or competition. Maintaining blood glucose is also important in attenuating increases in stress hormones (especially cortisol), diminishing changes in immunity mediated through cytokines. Ingestion of CHO during prolonged high-intensity exercise has been shown to blunt the inflammatory response.[11,54,55]

One to two hours of high-intensity exercise or as little as 20 to 30 minutes of heavy interval training can result in glycogen depletion. Full replenishment of glycogen under optimal dietary conditions will take 20 to 24 hours. Optimal conditions include ingestion of 50 to 100 g of high glycemic CHO within 15 to 20 minutes of exercise cessation and continuing each hour for the first 4 hours of recovery at a rate of 1 to 1.2 g CHO/kg of body weight. If the next day's workout is scheduled to be moderate or heavy endurance activity, the 24-hour recovery diet should consist of 7 to 12 g CHO/kg; if moderate duration but low intensity, the 24-hour recovery diet can be 5 to 7 g CHO/kg. Extreme duration training or competition necessitates 10 to 12 g CHO/kg. From these numbers it should be obvious that "two-a-days" will not allow for full glycogen replenishment between sessions. This represents a form of metabolic underrecovery.[54]

Adequate nutrition is more than just CHO ingestion, however. The most basic consideration is that, unless the athlete is trying to lose weight during the general preparatory cycle, caloric intake must balance caloric output. Days of lower CHO intake (if CHO is periodized as suggested) will allow for increases in FAT and PRO while still maintaining caloric balance.

Both FAT and PRO ingestion are critical. Not only do low-fat diets (<20%) compromise endurance performance and lead to possible deficiencies in micronutrients, but both the quantity and quality of fats alter the immune system. Diets low in PRO (<20%) or high (>60%) both have negative effects on immune function as well. Thus diets unbalanced in FAT and PRO may be a factor in overtraining. In addition, the inclusion of PRO in the immediate postexercise nutrient intake has been shown to aid in glycogen storage.[54]

Hydration is the last critical component and should include both water and sports drinks. Thirst is not a reliable indication of the amount of fluid needed. Active individuals need at least 2350 to 2825 ml (80 to 96 oz) of fluid per day plus 400 to 600 ml (14 to 20 oz) preexercise; 200 to 400 ml (7 to 14 oz) every 15 to 20 minutes during exercise; and a volume greater than sweat lost (containing sufficient sodium to retain the fluid) postexercise.[56,57]

Treatment

If training adjustments are insufficient and OTS develops, treatment is necessary. The first step in treatment, if OTS is suspected, is a medical examination to rule out possible illnesses or injuries as the underlying cause of the decrement in performance. Once illness or injury has been ruled out, the individual must be guided through a recovery program. This must be done carefully because active—and especially competitive—individuals often resist recommendations to cut down or cease training. Rest may be a four-letter word to an athlete, but rest is the only established treatment.[58] As with recovery, rest need not mean total inactivity.

Armstrong and Van Heest[10] have pointed out that the OTS and clinical (major) depression involve similar signs and symptoms, brain structures, neurotransmitters, endocrine pathways, and immune responses and thus probably have similar causes. Given these communalities, they and others[56] have suggested treating overtrained athletes with antidepressant medications and professional psychological counseling. Research to support the use of specific antidepressants is necessary.

Just as there is no definitive marker to indicate overtraining, there is no definitive marker to indicate recovery. Resumption of training must be gradual. The best "treatment," of course, is prevention.[15,56]

DETRAINING

Decreasing training volume is an important way to treat overtraining symptoms. However, decreasing training volume or intensity often creates anxiety for athletes who fear that detraining might result. Detraining (also referred to as *deconditioning*) can be defined as a partial or complete loss of training-induced adaptations as a result of training reduction or cessation.[59] Detraining may occur due to lack of compliance with a training program, injury, illness, or a planned periodization cycle.

When discussing the extent and rate of loss of training adaptations with detraining, it is important to clarify exactly what is being discussed. As detailed earlier, exercise training or an increase in exercise stimulus results in improved physiological function that is evident in improved fitness and health benefits (see Figure 7-2). Training is evident when sedentary individuals become more active and when normally active or moderately trained individuals increase the training stimulus. It is also clear that at some point, the addition of exercise stimulus (or the combination of exercise stress and other stressors) can lead to the conditions of overreaching or overtraining in which performance is decreased despite an increase in exercise stimuli.

The consequences of detraining depend on many factors including the training status of the individual and the magnitude of the inactivity (decreased activity or cessation of activity). In overtrained individuals, it is possible that a decrease in training load (exercise stimulus) may lead to increased performance or improved physiological functioning. Maintenance refers to the condition in which a trained individual decreases training volume (but not intensity) and maintains the benefits of training. The term *detraining* is most commonly applied to the loss of physiological adaptations that occur when a highly active individual lessens his or her training (i.e., when an athlete is out of season and does not train regularly) or ceases activity (i.e., immobilization due to casting or bed rest). The term *detraining* can also be applied to the condition that occurs when a normally active individual becomes increasingly sedentary, such as happens with some job changes or during illness. Obviously, the extent of detraining in any of the aforementioned cases depends on the amount of time that detraining continues. Further complicating our understanding of detraining is the extent to which many of the detraining responses parallel normal aging. In fact, it is often not possible to distinguish between the effects of aging and detraining in an elderly population.

All available research evidence suggests that any physiological variable that is responsive to exercise training will also respond to detraining. However, the timeline for the loss of adaptation is not known for all variables or in all populations.

Furthermore, there is not uniformity within the body regarding the loss of training adaptation when a training stimulus is lessened or withdrawn. The following section will therefore discuss separately the impact of detraining on the three major systems of the body (metabolic, cardiorespiratory, and neuromuscular system).

Consequences of Detraining on the Metabolic System

Detraining is associated with several metabolic changes including shifts in fuel utilization and aerobic/anaerobic energy production. Detraining leads to increased reliance on carbohydrates as an energy substrate and a decreased reliance on lipid metabolism during exercise, as evidenced by an increase in respiratory exchange ratio (RER) values. Increased RER values during exercise after a period of detraining have been reported in recently trained individuals and highly trained athletes.[60-64] Detraining is also associated with a decline in insulin sensitivity, as evidenced by an increase in area under the insulin response curve during an oral glucose tolerance test and a decrease in GLUT-4 protein levels.[65,66] A decrease in intracellular glycogen storage has been reported in highly conditioned individuals following 4 weeks of detraining.[67,68] Several authors have also reported a decrease in oxidative enzymes in highly trained athletes following 4 to 12 weeks of detraining.[60,69]

Detraining leads to an increase in blood lactate levels during exercise at any given absolute submaximal exercise intensity, a decrease in maximal lactate values, and the occurrence of lactate thresholds at a lower percentage of $\dot{V}O_2$max. These changes have been reported in recently trained individuals and in highly trained athletes, although the magnitude of the detraining effect is greatest in the highly trained athletes.[60,62,70-72]

Consequences of Detraining on the Cardiorespiratory System

In general, detraining is associated with a decrease in maximal oxygen consumption ($\dot{V}O_2$max). Brief periods of detraining (10 to 14 days) appear not to result in a decrease in $\dot{V}O_2$max in highly trained individuals.[73,74] On the other hand, training cessation of 2 to 4 weeks results in decreases in $\dot{V}O_2$max of approximately 4% to 15%.[59,75,76] The reduction in $\dot{V}O_2$max is greater in highly trained than in recently trained individuals.[59] In 1993 Madsen[68] performed a study in which exercise training was severely reduced in highly trained athletes and reported that $\dot{V}O_2$max was maintained during the 4 weeks of detraining. These findings are likely attributable to the fact that in the Madsen study athletes severely reduced their training but did not cease to train (the athletes performed one 35-minute bout of intense training rather than their normal 6 to 10 hours a week). The effects of decreased training volume have been investigated by Hickson et al[77-79] in a series of studies designed to determine the relative influence of decreases in training frequency, duration, and intensity on $\dot{V}O_2$max (Figure 7-5). These studies suggest that $\dot{V}O_2$max can be maintained when training frequency or duration is reduced by as much as two thirds, provided that training intensity is maintained. However, when training intensity is reduced by one third, $\dot{V}O_2$max declines markedly.

As the length of detraining advances, greater losses in $\dot{V}O_2$max occur. Figure 7-6 depicts changes in $\dot{V}O_2$max over an 84-day period in a group of endurance-trained subjects.[75] These data suggest that in highly trained individuals, $\dot{V}O_2$max may decline as much as 20% with detraining but still remain above levels of sedentary individuals. Other studies report the complete reversal of $\dot{V}O_2$max to pretraining levels in individuals who are recently trained.[64]

Changes in $\dot{V}O_2$max during detraining are accompanied by reductions in maximal stroke volume and cardiac output and an increase in maximal heart rate (Figure 7-6). The decrease in stroke volume and hence cardiac output is most likely attributable to changes in blood volume. Detraining leads to decreases in blood volume of 5% to 10%, and these reductions may occur within 2 days of inactivity.[64,73] Coyle[76] investigated the effects of 2 to 4 weeks of inactivity on endurance-trained men and reported a 9% decline in blood volume and a 12% reduction in stroke volume during the detraining period. When blood volume was expanded (by infusing a dextran solution in saline) to a level equal to the trained state, both stroke volume and $\dot{V}O_2$max were increased to within 2% to 4% of the trained state.

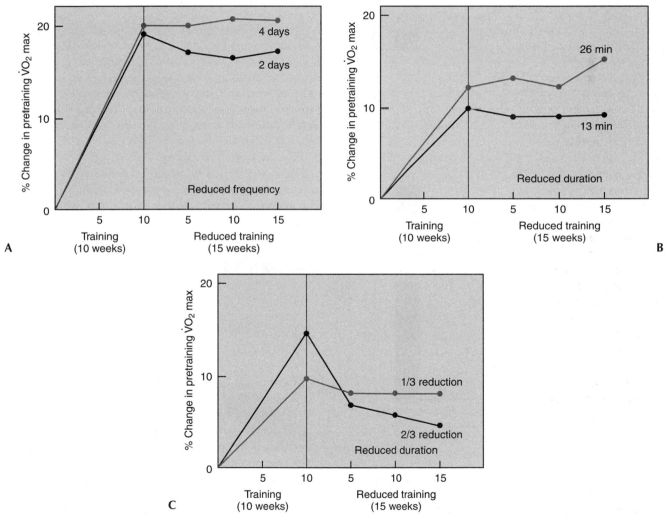

Figure 7-5 Effects of reducing exercise frequency, intensity, and duration on maintenance of $\dot{V}O_2$max. **A,** Improvements in $\dot{V}O_2$max during 10 weeks of training (bicycling and running) for 40 minutes a day, 6 days a week were maintained when training intensity and duration were maintained, but the frequency was reduced from 6 days a week to 4 or even 2 days per week. **B,** $\dot{V}O_2$max was maintained when frequency of training and intensity were maintained, but training duration was reduced to 13 minutes. $\dot{V}O_2$max continued to improve when training duration was reduced to 26 minutes. **C,** $\dot{V}O_2$max was maintained when frequency and duration were maintained and training was reduced by two thirds.(From Hickson RC, Foster C, Pollock ML, et al: *J Appl Physiol* 58:492-499, 1985; Hickson RC, Kanakis C Jr, Davis JR, et al: *J Applied Physiol* 58:225-229, 1982; Hickson RC, Rosenkoetter MA: *Med Sci Sports Exerc* 13:13-16, 1981.

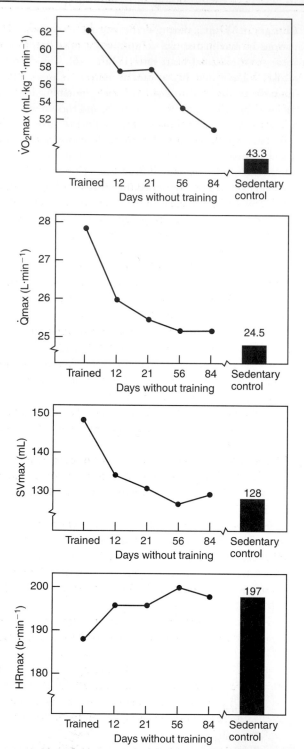

Figure 7-6 Effects of detraining on highly conditioned athletes. (From Coyle EF, Martin WH, Sinacore DR, et al: *J Applied Physiol* 57:1857-1864, 1984.)

Consequences of Detraining on the Neuromuscular System

Detraining leads to loss of neuromuscular adaptations. As with the other systems, the time course for the loss of adaptation depends on the training status of the individual and the extent to which training load is decreased. Strength-trained athletes

retain strength gains during short periods of inactivity (2 weeks) and retain significant portions of strength gains (88% to 93%) during inactivity lasting up to 12 weeks.[59,80] Thus it appears that strength gains are preserved longer than many other training adaptations.

The effect of detraining on muscle strength is not consistent in all muscle groups or for all exercises; in one study squat exercise strength decreased by only 13% following 30 to 32 weeks of detraining, whereas leg press strength decreased by 32%.[81] No differences were apparent in strength loss between genders during detraining, but evidence indicated that older individuals lose strength gains more rapidly than younger people.[82] Some evidence, in trained swimmers, indicates that muscular power (defined as a swim test) may decrease substantially during 4 weeks of inactivity even when muscular strength is maintained.[83] On the other hand, vertical jump (a field measure of muscle power) has been shown to be unchanged with 8 or 12 weeks of detraining.[84,85] Additional work remains to better identify the effect of detraining on muscular power.

Short-term detraining (2 weeks) in strength-trained athletes has resulted in a significant decrease in fast-twitch (FT) muscle fiber cross-sectional area.[86] On the other hand, short-term detraining does not appear to cause changes in muscle fiber cross-sectional area in endurance-trained athletes.[87] Longer periods of detraining (12 weeks) have been associated with a significant decrease in cross-sectional area of both FT and slow-twitch (ST) muscle fibers in strength-trained athletes[84] and in ST fiber diameter in elite rowers.[88]

Diminished neural activation (as measured by integrated electromyography) has been shown to decrease with detraining. The decrease in neural activation is associated with a decrease in fiber area and a decrease in muscle strength.[84,85,89]

REFERENCES

1. Bompa TO: *Periodization: theory and methodology of training,* Champaign, Ill, 1999, Human Kinetics.
2. Freeman WH: *Peak when it counts: periodization for American track & field,* ed 3, Mountain View, Calif, 1996, Tafnews Press.
3. Kearney JT: Training the Olympic athlete, *Sci Am* 274(6): 52-63, 1996.
4. Fry RW, Morton AR, Keast D: Periodisation and the prevention of overtraining, *Can J Sport Sci* 17:241-248, 1992.
5. Kibler WB, Chandler TJ: Sport-specific conditioning, *Am J Sport Med* 22:424-432, 1994.
6. Fry RW, Morton AR, Keast D: Overtraining in athletes: an update, *Sports Med* 12:32-65, 1991.
7. Kuipers H: Training and overtraining: an introduction, *Med Sci Sports Exerc* 30:1137-1139, 1998.
8. Rowbottom DG, Keast D, Morton AR: Monitoring and preventing of overreaching and overtraining in endurance athletes. In Kreider RB, Fry AC, O'Toole ML, editors: *Overtraining in sport,* pp. 47-66, Champaign, Ill, 1998, Human Kinetics.

9. Fry AC, Kraemer WJ: Resistance exercise overtraining and overreaching: neuroendocrine responses, *Sports Med* 23:106-129, 1997.

10. Armstrong LE, vanHeest JL: The unknown mechanism of the overtraining syndrome: clues from depression and psychoneuroimmunology, *Sports Med* 32:185-209, 2002.

11. Kreider RB, Fry AC, O'Toole ML: Overtraining in sport: terms, definitions, and prevalence. In Kreider RB, Fry AC, O'Toole ML, editors: *Overtraining in sport,* pp. vii-ix, Champaign, Ill, 1998, Human Kinetics.

12. Budgett R: Fatigue and underperformance in athletes: the overtraining syndrome, *Br J Sports Med* 32:107-110, 1998.

13. Halson SL, Jeukendrup AE: Does overtraining exist? An analysis of overreaching and overtraining research, *Sports Med* 34:967-981, 2004.

14. Urhausen A, Kindermann W: Diagnosis of overtraining: what tools do we have? *Sports Med* 32:95-102, 2002.

15. Flynn MG: Future research needs and directions. In Kreider RB, Fry AC, O'Toole ML, editors: *Overtraining in sport,* pp. 373-383, Champaign, Ill, 1998, Human Kinetics.

16. Kenttä G, Hassmén P: Overtraining and recovery: a conceptual model, *Sports Med* 26:1-16, 1998.

17. Lehmann M, Foster C, Keul J: Overtraining in endurance athletes: a brief review, *Med Sci Sports Exerc* 25:854-862, 1993.

18. Lehmann M, Foster C, Dickhuth H-H, et al: Autonomic imbalance hypothesis and overtraining syndrome, *Med Sci Sports Exerc* 30:1140-1145, 1998.

19. Lehmann M, Foster C, Netzer N, et al: Physiological responses to short- and long-term overtraining in endurance athletes. In Kreider RB, Fry AC, O'Toole ML, editors: *Overtraining in sport,* pp. 19-46, Champaign, Ill, 1998, Human Kinetics.

20. Urhausen A, Kindermann W: The endocrine system in overtraining. In Warren MP, Constantini NW, editors: *Sports endocrinology,* pp. 347-370, Totowa, NJ, 2000, Humana Press.

21. Witlert G: The effects of exercise on the hypothalamo-pituitary-adrenal axis. In Warren MP, Constantini NW, editors: *Sports endocrinology,* pp. 43-56, Totowa, NJ, 2000, Humana Press.

22. Petibois C, Cazorla G, Poortmans J-R, et al: Biochemical aspects of overtraining in endurance sports: a review, *Sports Med* 32:867-878, 2002.

23. Petibois C, Cazorla G, Poortmans J-R, et al: Biochemical aspects of overtraining in endurance sports: the metabolism alteration process syndrome, *Sports Med* 33:83-94, 2003.

24. Smith LL: Cytokine hypothesis of overtraining: a physiological adaptation to excessive stress? *Med Sci Sports Exerc* 32:317-331, 2000.

25. Selye H: *The stress of life,* New York, 1956, McGraw-Hill.

26. Thomas CL, editor: *Taber's cyclopedic medical dictionary,* ed 16, Philadelphia, 1985, FA Davis.

27. Snyder AC: Overtraining and glycogen depletion hypothesis, *Med Sci Sports Exerc* 30:1146-1150, 1998.

28. Steinacker JM, Lormes W, Reissnecker S, et al: New aspects of the hormone and cytokine response to training, *Eur J Appl Physiol* 91:382-391, 2004.

29. Saris WH: The concept of energy homeostasis for optimal health during training, *Can J Appl Physiol* 26 Suppl: S167-75, 2001.

30. Gastmann UAL, Lehmann MJ: Overtraining and the BCAA hypothesis, *Med Sci Sports Exerc* 30:1173-1178, 1998.

31. Gotovtseva EP, Surkina ID, Uchakin PN: Potential interventions to prevent immunosuppression during training. In Kreider RB, Fry AC, O'Toole ML, editors: *Overtraining in sport,* pp. 243-272, Champaign, Ill, 1998, Human Kinetics.

32. Robson PJ: Elucidating the unexplained underperformance syndrome in endurance athletes: the interleukin-6 hypothesis, *Sports Med* 33:771-781, 2003.

33. Rowbottom DG, Keast D, Morton AR: The emerging role of glutamine as an indicator of exercise stress and overtraining, *Sports Med* 21:80-97, 1996.

34. Chrousos GP, Gold PW: The concepts of stress and stress system disorders, *JAMA* 267:1244-1252, 1992.

35. Smith LL: Overtraining, excessive exercise, and altered immunity: is this a T helper-1 versus T helper-2 lymphocyte response? *Sports Med* 33:347-364, 2003.

36. Moldoveanu AL, Shephard RJ, Shek PN: The cytokine response to physical activity and training, *Sports Med* 31:115-144, 2001.

37. Keizer HA: Neuroendocrine aspects of overtraining. In Kreider RB, Fry AC, O'Toole ML, editors: *Overtraining in sport,* pp. 145-167, Champaign, Ill, 1998, Human Kinetics.

38. Achten J, Jeukendrup AE: Heart rate monitoring: applications and limitations, *Sports Med* 33:517-538, 2003.

39. Gabriel HHW, Urhausen A, Valet G, et al: Overtraining and immune system: a prospective longitudinal study in endurance athletes, *Med Sci Sports Exerc* 30:1151-1157, 1998.

40. Hartmann U, Mester J: Training and overtraining markers in selected sports events, *Med Sci Sports Exerc* 32:209-215, 2000.

41. Hooper SL, Mackinnon LT: Monitoring overtraining in athletes: recommendations, *Sports Med* 20:321-327, 1995.

42. Lac G, Maso F: Biological markers for the follow-up of athletes throughout the training season, *Pathol Biol (Paris)* 52:43-49, 2004.

43. Calder A: Recovery strategies for sports performance, *US Olympic Coach E-Magazine http://coaching.usolympicteam.com/coaching/kpub.nsf/v/3Sept03* accessed 3/11/2004.

44. Smith DJ: A framework for understanding the training process leading to elite performance, *Sports Med* 33: 1103-1126, 2003.

45. Meeusen R, Piacentini MF, Busscharert B, et al: Hormonal responses in athletes: the use of a two bout exercise protocol to detect subtle differences in (over)training status, *Eur J Appl Physiol* 91:140-146, 2004.

46. Meyers AW, Whelan JP: A systematic model for understanding psychosocial influences in overtraining. In

Kreider RB, Fry AC, O'Toole ML, editors: *Overtraining in sport,* pp. 335-369, Champaign, Ill, 1998, Human Kinetics.

47. McNair DM, Lorr M, Droppleman LF: EDITS Manual for the Profile of Mood States, pp. 1-29, San Diego, 1971, Educational and Industrial Testing Service.

48. Hawley CJ, Schoene RB: Overtraining syndrome: a guide to diagnosis, treatment, and prevention, *Phys Sportsmed* 31:25-31, 2003.

49. Bompa TO: Primer on periodization, *US Olympic Coach E- Magazine http://coaching.usolympicteam.com/coaching/kpub. nsf/v/0504b* accessed 3/11/2004.

50. Rhea MR, Alderman BL: A meta-analysis of periodized versus non-periodized strength and power training programs, *Res Q Exerc Sport* 75:413-422, 2004.

51. Steinacker JM, Lormes W, Lehman M, et al: Training of rowers before world championships, *Med Sci Sports Exerc* 30:1158-1163, 1998.

52. Borg G: Borg's perceived exertion and pain scales, Champaign, Ill, 1998, Human Kinetics.

53. Foster C: Monitoring training in athletes with reference to overtraining syndrome, *Med Sci Sports Exerc* 30: 1164-1168, 1998.

54. Coyle EF: Highs and lows of carbohydrate diets, *Gatorade Sports Sci Instit Sports Sci Exchange* 17:1-6+(Suppl), 2004.

55. Venkatraman JT, Pendergast DR: Effect of dietary intake on immune function in athletes, *Sports Med* 32:323-337, 2002.

56. American College of Sports Medicine, American Dietetic Association, Dietitians of Canada: Nutrition and athletic performance joint position statement, *Med Sci Sports Exerc* 32:2130-2145, 2000.

57. Shirreffs SM, Taylor AJ, Leipur JB, et al: Post-exercise rehydration in man: effects of volume consumed and drink sodium content, *Med Sci Sports Exerc* 28:1260-1271, 1996.

58. Pearce PZ: A practical approach to the overtraining syndrome, *Curr Sports Med Rep* 1:179-183, 2002.

59. Mujika I, Padilla S: Detraining: loss of training-induced physiological and performance adaptations. Part I, *Sports Med* 30(2):79-87, 2000.

60. Coyle EG, Martin WH III, Bloomfield SA, et al: Effects of detraining on responses to submaximal exercise, *J Applied Physiol* 59:853-859, 1985.

61. Drinkwater BL, Horvath SM: Detraining effects on young women, *Med Sci Sports* 4:91-95, 1972.

62. Graves JE, Ploutz-Snyder LL, Pollock ML: Physiological consequences of deconditioning in physically active populations. In Greenleaf JE, editor: *Deconditioning and reconditioning,* Boca Raton, Fla, 2004, CRC Press.

63. Moore RL, Thacker EM, Kelley GA, et al: Effect of training/detraining on submaximal exercise responses in humans, *J Applied Physiol* 63:1719-1724, 1987.

64. Mujika I, Padilla S: Cardiorespiratory and metabolic characteristics of detraining in humans, *Med Sci Sports Exercise* 33:413-421, 2001.

65. Arciero PJ, Smith DL, Calles-Escandon J: Effects of short-term inactivity on glucose tolerance, energy expenditure,

and blood flow in trained subjects, *J Applied Physiol* 84:1365-1373, 1998.

66. McCoy M, Proietto J, Hargreaves M: Effect of detraining on GLUT-4 protein in human skeletal muscle, *J Applied Physiol* 77:1532-1536, 1994.

67. Costill DL, Fink WJ, Hargreaves M, et al: Metabolic characteristics of skeletal muscle during detraining from competitive swimming, *Med Sci Sports Exercise* 17:339-343, 1985.

68. Madsen K, Pedersen PK, Djurhuus MS, et al: Effects of detraining on endurance capacity and metabolic changes during prolonged exhaustive exercise, *J Applied Physiol* 75:1444-1451, 1993.

69. Amigó N, Cadefau JA, Ferrer I, et al: Effect of summer intermission on skeletal muscle of adolescent soccer players, *J Sports Med Phys Fitness* 38:298-304, 1998.

70. Hardman AE, Hudson A: Brisk walking and serum lipid and lipoprotein variables in previously sedentary women—effect of 12 weeks of regular brisk walking followed by 12 weeks of detraining, *Br J Sports Med* 28:261-266, 1994.

71. Ready AE, Enyon RB, Cunningham DA: Effect of interval training and detraining on anaerobic fitness in women, *Can J Applied Sport Sci* 6:114-118, 1981.

72. Ready AE, Quinney HA: Alterations in anaerobic threshold as the result of endurance training and detraining, *Med Sci Sports Exercise* 14:292-296, 1982.

73. Cullinane EM, Sady SP, Vadeboncoeur L, et al: Cardiac size and $\dot{V}O_2$max do not decrease after short-term exercise cessation, *Med Sci Sports Exerc* 18:420-424, 1986.

74. Houston ME, Bentzen H, Larsen H: Interrelationships between skeletal muscle adaptations and performance as studied by detraining and retraining, *Acta Physiol Scand* 105:163-170, 1979.

75. Coyle EG, Martin WH, Sinacore DR, et al: Time course of loss of adaptations after stopping prolonged intense endurance training, *J Applied Physiol* 57:1857-1864, 1984.

76. Coyle EF, Hemmert MK, Coggan AR: Effects of detraining on cardiovascular responses to exercise: role of blood volume, *J Applied Physiol* 60:95-99, 1986.

77. Hickson RC, Foster C, Pollock ML, et al: Reduced training intensities and loss of aerobic power, endurance, and cardiac growth, *J Appl Physiol* 58:492-499, 1985.

78. Hickson RC, Kanakis C Jr, Davis JR, et al: Reduced training duration effects on aerobic power, endurance, and cardiac growth, *J Applied Physiol* 58:225-229, 1982.

79. Hickson RC, Rosenkoetter MA: Reduced training frequencies and maintenance of increased aerobic power, *Med Sci Sports Exerc* 13:13-16, 1981.

80. Mujika I, Padilla S: Detraining: loss of training-induced physiological and performance adaptations. Part II, *Sports Med* 30(3):145-154, 2000.

81. Staron RS, Leonardi MJ, Karapondo DL, et al: Strength and skeletal muscle adaptations in heavy-resistance-trained women after detraining and retraining, *J Applied Physiol* 70:631-640, 1991.

82. Lemmer JT, Hurlbut DE, Martel GF, et al: Age and gender responses to strength training and detraining, *Med Sci Sports Exerc* 32:1505-1512, 2000.

83. Neufer PD, Costill DL, Fielding RA, et al: Effect of reduced training on muscular strength and endurance in competitive swimmers, *Med Sci Sports Exerc* 19:486-490, 1987.

84. Häkkinen K, Alén M, Komi PV: Changes in isometric force- and relaxation-time, electromyographic and muscle fibre characteristics of human skeletal muscle during strength training and detraining, *Acta Physiol Scand* 125:573-585, 1985.

85. Häkkinen K, Komi PV, Tesch PA: Effect of combined concentric and eccentric strength training and detraining on force-time, muscle fiber and metabolic characteristics of leg extensor muscles, *Scand J Sports Sci* 3:50-58, 1981.

86. Hortobágyi T, Houmard JA, Stevenson JR, et al: The effects of detraining on power athletes, *Med Sci Sports Exerc* 25:929-935, 1993.

87. Houmard JA, Hortobágyi T, Johns RA, et al: Effect of short-term training cessation on performance measures in distance runners, *Int J Sports Med* 13:572-576, 1992.

88. Larsson L, Ansved T: Effects of long-term physical training and detraining on enzyme histochemical and functional skeletal muscle characteristics in man, *Muscle Nerve* 8:714-722, 1985.

89. Häkkinen K, Komi PV: Electromyographic changes during strength training and detraining, *Med Sci Sports Exerc* 15:455-460, 1983.

C H A P T E R

8

Michael S. Zazzali, Robert A. Donatelli, and Vijay B. Vad*

Pathophysiology of Injury to the Overhead-Throwing Athlete

LEARNING OBJECTIVES

After studying this chapter, the reader will be able to do the following:

1. Identify the phases of throwing
2. Describe the muscle activity during the phases of throwing
3. Describe the changes in soft tissues surrounding the glenohumeral joint as a result of overhead-throwing activities
4. Identify changes in the range-of-motion measurements specific to overhead-throwing athletes
5. Identify changes in the posture of the scapula specific to overhead-throwing athletes
6. Describe the different theories associated with the etiology of injury to the overhead-throwing athlete
7. Describe the appropriate management of injuries to the overhead-throwing athlete

In recent decades there has been a dramatic rise in the number of participants in overhead-throwing sports. The increase in participation has developed a concurrent increase in incidence of injury to the upper extremity. The skill of throwing a baseball with extremely high velocities and precision requires years of practice and advanced neuromuscular efficiency, not to mention natural ability to reach the upper echelons of professional competition.

The professional baseball pitcher most likely starts out early in life during Little League to begin the development of his musculoskeletal and neuromuscular systems. However, no matter how blessed the individual may be to pitch a baseball upwards of 90 miles an hour, the repetitive microtrauma that stresses the athlete's shoulder complex during the throwing motion challenges the physiological limits of the surrounding

tissues. Frequently the repetitive act of throwing a baseball has led to a variety disabilities arising from alterations in throwing mechanics secondary to fatigue, capsular shortening, or contracture versus capsular laxity; glenohumeral labral tears; muscle weakness; and imbalances around the shoulder complex, all of which can lead to tissue compromise and eventual injury.

Conte et al[1] performed a study over a 5-year period from 1995 to 1999 that determined the prevalence of upper extremity injuries in Major League Baseball. They found an injury rate of 27.8% and 22% involving the shoulder and elbow, respectively. The authors also reported in a prior study between 1989 and 1999 that 48.4% of all injuries in Major League Baseball involved pitchers.[1] The data suggest that half of all Major League Baseball injuries that necessitated removal of the athlete from the active roster and placed on the disabled list were related to pathology to the upper extremity.[1,2]

This chapter reviews the phases of throwing and details the most current concepts in the pathophysiology of the throwing shoulder compared with the past theories and practices from conservative, as well as surgical, perspectives.

The act of throwing a baseball involves a transfer of kinetic energy from the legs, through the hips, spine, shoulder, elbow, and wrist. The forces are generated through the trunk and core and expressed in the extremities. The stages of overhand throwing as it relates to pitching have been divided into the following phases: (1) windup, (2) early cocking, (3) late cocking, (4) acceleration, and (5) follow-through.

STAGES OF OVERHAND THROWING

Windup

The purpose of the windup is to organize the body beneath the arm to form a stable platform. The body must perform in sequential links to enable the hand to be in the correct position

---

*Special thanks to Jeff Cooper, MS, ATC, for his contribution to the section on phases of throwing.

in space to complete the assigned task. The scapulohumeral rhythm must place the hand in an optimal position for propulsion. The humeral head is centered in the glenoid during the first initial phase of elevation via the supraspinatus. Due to the windup phase having such individualistic styles among athletes, there is no consistent pattern of muscle activity.

Early Cocking

Early cocking is the temporal period when the dominant hand is separated from the gloved hand, and it ends when the forward foot makes contact with the mound. The scapula is fully retracted at this time and stabilized against the chest wall by the rhomboids and the serratus anterior. The humerus is brought into position of 90-degree abduction and horizontal extension, with external rotation of only approximately 50 degrees. This is accomplished with the activation of the anterior, middle, and posterior deltoid. The external rotators of the cuff are activated toward the end of early cocking, with the supraspinatus being more active than the infraspinatus and teres minor as it steers the humeral head in the glenoid. The biceps brachii and brachialis act on the forearm to develop the necessary angle of the elbow.

As the body moves forward, the humerus is supported by the anterior and medial deltoid as the posterior deltoid pulls the humerus into approximately 30 degrees of horizontal extension. At this time the static stability of the humeral head becomes dependent on the restraints of the anterior margin of the glenoid, notably the anterior band of the inferior glenohumeral ligament (IGHL) and the inferior portion of the glenoid labrum.

Late Cocking

Late cocking is the interval in the throwing motion when the lead foot makes contact with the mound, and it ends when the humerus begins internal rotation. The lead foot applies an anterior shear to slow the lower extremity and to transfer energy. The foot serves as an anchor. The forward and vertical momentum is transformed into rotational components. During this time the humerus is moved into a position more forward in relation to the trunk and begins to come into alignment with the upper body. The extreme of external rotation, an additional 125 degrees, is achieved to provide positioning for the power or acceleration phase.

The supraspinatus, infraspinatus, and teres minor are active in this phase but become quiet once external rotation is achieved. Deceleration of the externally rotating humerus is accomplished by contraction of the subscapularis. The subscapularis remains active until the completion of late cocking. The serratus anterior and the clavicular head of the pectoralis major have their greatest activity during deceleration. The biceps brachii aids in maintaining the humerus in the glenoid by producing a compressive axial load. At the end of this phase, the triceps begins activity and provides compressive axial loading to replace the force of the biceps. The capsule winds tightly in preparation for acceleration. The humeral head experiences a force of anterior translation equivalent to 40% of body weight.[3]

Acceleration

Acceleration is a ballistic action lasting less than one tenth of a second. The ball is accelerated from 4 mph to 90 mph or higher.[4] This rapid acceleration produces angular velocities that have reported as high as 9198 degrees/sec.[5] The scapula is protracted, rotated downward, and held to the chest wall by the serratus anterior. The arm continues into forward flexion and is marked by the maximal internal rotation of the humerus. The humerus travels forward in 100 degrees of abduction but adducts about 5 degrees just before release. The latissimus dorsi and pectoralis major deliver the power to the forward-moving shoulder. The subscapularis activity is at maximum levels as the humerus travels into medial rotation. The triceps develops strong action in accelerating the extension of the elbow.

The forces developed in this instant reflect the body's ability to generate power and encase itself in a protective mechanism. Pappas et al[5] reported peak accelerations approaching 6000 degrees/sec. Gainer et al[6] reported 14,000 inch lbs of rotatory torque produced at the shoulder. This torque develops 27,000 inch lbs of kinetic energy in the humerus.

Control of the ball is lost approximately midway through the acceleration phase, when the humerus is positioned slightly behind the forward-flexing trunk and at an angle of about 110 degrees of external rotation. The hand follows the ball after release and is unable to apply further force.

Follow-Through

Follow-through begins with release of the ball. Within the first tenth of a second the humerus travels across the midline of the body and undergoes a slight external rotation before finishing in internal rotation. This is an active phase for all glenohumeral muscles because the arm is decelerated. The deltoid and upper trapezius have strong activity, as does the latissimus dorsi. The infraspinatus, teres minor, supraspinatus, and subscapularis are all active while eccentric loads are produced. The biceps develops peak activity in decelerating the forearm and imposing a traction force within the glenohumeral joint.

The task of documenting the sequence of muscle activity during the act of pitching has allowed the musculature acting on the glenohumeral joint to be divided into two groups.[7] The first group of muscles consists of those that are most active during the second and third phases of throwing and early and late cocking. They are least active during the acceleration phase. The deltoid, trapezius, external rotators, supraspinatus, teres minor, and biceps brachii comprise this first group.

The second group of muscles consists of those used primarily for the fourth phase of throwing—acceleration. These muscles are necessary to protract the scapula, horizontally flex forward and internally rotate the humerus, and extend the elbow. This group consists of the subscapularis, serratus anterior, pectoralis major, latissimus dorsi, and triceps brachii. The first phase of throwing is not included in either group because of its nonspecific generalized activity.

It has been postulated that in order for the elite pitcher to reach velocities of mid to upper 90s, excessive external rotation of the glenohumeral joint must occur during the late cocking and acceleration phase of throwing. This hyperexternal rotation is often seen in elite pitchers who appear to have a set point of external rotation that they know they need to attain to throw with maximum velocities. These high-level pitchers have a proprioceptive sense of reaching their set point of hyperexternal rotation, which they call the *slot*.[8]

The amount of external rotation at the glenohumeral joint has been measured to reach upwards of 130 to 170 degrees during this phase of throwing.[8] The arm has been clocked at moving from 7000 to 9000 degrees/sec during the acceleration phase of throwing as it moves into internal rotation at the glenohumeral joint.[9] Jobe et al[10] described that one of the main reasons shoulder pain occurred during the act of throwing was an impingement-instability overlap. They postulated that repetitive throwing and this hyperexternal rotation gradually induced a serial stretching of the anterior capsuloligamentous complex. According to Jobe et al,[10] this would then lead to the anterosuperior migration of the humeral head during throwing, thus inducing subacromial impingement symptoms, and affect the athletes' throwing ability. However, these authors reported only a 50% success rate of pitchers returning to sport for 1 year following open capsulolabral reconstruction.[11]

In the past the primary rationale for the ability to reach these amounts of hyperexternal rotation was thought to be due to serial laxity of the anterior capsuloligamentous tissues.[12] This repetitive microtrauma eventually could lead to subluxation and eventually dislocation or the so-called "dead arm syndrome."

INTERNAL IMPINGEMENT

Walch et al[13] were the first to describe a condition known as *internal impingement,* which relates to intra-articular compression that occurs in all shoulders when they are in the abducted and hyperexternally rotated position. Walch described that in the position of 90 degrees of abduction and 90 degrees of external rotation position, the posterosuperior rotator cuff, mainly the supraspinatus, contacts the posterosuperior glenoid labrum and may become impinged between the labrum and the greater tuberosity (Figure 8-1). Jobe extrapolated this observation to the throwing athlete and described the propensity of internal impingement to possibly lead to injury to the rotator cuff, glenoid labrum, and osseous structures.[14] Jobe also hypothesized that internal impingement in throwers might worsen over time due to the serial stretching of the anterior capsuloligamentous structures. Jobe believed there was a hyperangulation occurring at the humeral head as opposed to hypertranslation that needed to be kept in check by the subscapularis during the act of throwing to help control this hyperexternal rotation.[14]

The thrower with internal impingement will most often complain of pain in the posterior aspect of the shoulder in the late cocking and early acceleration phases of throwing.[15] The posterior impingement sign can confirm a diagnosis of tears into the posterior labrum or rotator cuff, or both.[16,17] In this test the patient is positioned supine with the shoulder in 90 degrees of abduction and maximum external rotation (Figure 8-2). Re-creation of the patient's symptoms with the arm in this position elicits pain of a deep nature within the posterior aspect of the shoulder. Applying a posteriorly directed force (as in the relocation test) to the humeral head while in the posi-

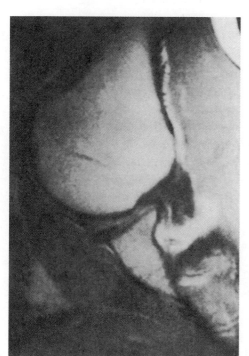

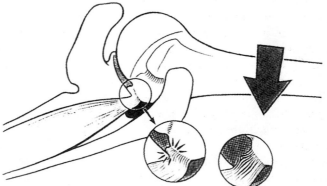

Figure 8-1 Cross section (**A**) and artist's tracing (**B**) of a cadaver shoulder frozen in forward elevation and internal rotation to mimic the impingement sign. The tuberosity and cuff are already past the acromion. The structures at risk for this mechanism are (1) greater tuberosity, (2) supraspinatus tendon, (3) superior labrum, (4) inferior glenohumeral ligament, and (5) superior glenoid bone. (From Jobe CM: *J Shoulder Elbow Surg* 11:530-536, 1995.)

tion of 90 degrees of abduction and maximum external rotation that reduces or eliminates the posterior pain may also be diagnostic.[17] The surgical approach to address the previous description of internal impingement led to anterior capsulolabral reconstruction under the hypothesis that the anterior microinstability was the underlying mechanism of the internal impingement. However, the results of this surgical intervention for throwing athletes remained unpredictable.[11,18]

Gerber and Sebesta[19] arthroscopically assessed 16 individuals who were not described as throwing athletes with moderate to severe and primarily unexplained shoulder pain provoked by anterior elevation and internal rotation and who were unresponsive to subacromial injection. None of the patients had signs of instability. The authors determined that when the subjects' arms were internally rotated and elevated below 90 degrees, impingement occurred between the deep surface of the subscapularis tendon and the anterior glenoid labrum and rim. Gerber and Sebesta's study suggests that in addition to the posterosuperior impingement of the supraspinatus tendon originally described by Walch, anterosuperior impingement of the deep surface of the subscapularis is a form of intra-articular impingement.[19] This impingement may be related to a lack of deceleration control or eccentric strength of the external rotators during the follow-through phase of throwing, which could result in an excessive amount of flexion and coupled internal rotation leading to the intra-articular subscapularis impingement.

Other authors such as Halbrecht et al[20] and Burkhart et al[8] disagreed with the premise that anterior instability would aggravate internal impingement. They felt that an anterior instability would most likely lessen the posterosuperior glenoid contact with the rotator cuff due to the fact that the unstable shoulder is subluxing anteriorly. This could be an underlying reason why anterior stabilization procedures did not appear to have predictable and promising results in the overhead-throwing athlete.

More recently, Burkhart and Morgan,[21,22] on the basis of two arthroscopic studies, clinical observation, and biomechanical data, have questioned the role of microinstability as the universal cause of throwing injuries. Burkhart et al reported on 53 baseball players, 44 of whom were pitchers, who had Type II superior labrum anterior to posterior (SLAP) lesions that were surgically repaired after failed conservative rehabilitation. Arthroscopic repair of these Type II SLAP lesions returned 87% of these athletes to a preinjury level of performance.[21] This was superior to the reported successful return of athletes after open anterior capsulolabral repairs, which ranged from 50% to 68% return to sport.[11,18] Burkhart et al do not believe that the underlying lesion is the anterior capsular laxity or microinstability but that the SLAP lesion induces a "pseudolaxity," which has led to the erroneous diagnosis of microinstability.[8]

Pitchers and throwing athletes are believed to be at risk of developing SLAP lesions due to the obligatory tightening of the posteroinferior glenohumeral capsule.[8] In studying 372 professional baseball players, Wilk and Meister[23] have reported that external rotation on average is 7 degrees greater in the throwing shoulder and internal rotation is 7 degrees greater in the nonthrowing shoulder. The average total shoulder range of motion was reported as 129.9 plus or minus 10 degrees of external rotation and 62.6 plus or minus 9 degrees of internal rotation. The authors coined the term *total motion concept* to describe total shoulder motion being equal to the summation of external and internal rotation. Thus an individual with an imbalance of external to internal rotation as such would lend to dynamic instability with overhead throwing.

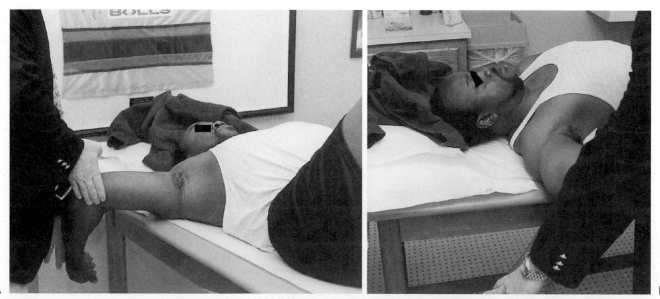

Figure 8-2 A and **B,** Test for internal impingement. The arm is placed in the plane of the scapula and in maximal external rotation of the undersurface of the rotator cuff between the humeral head and the posterosuperior glenoid, and the labrum occurs in this position. The patient will experience pain in the posterior aspect of the shoulder at the level of the glenohumeral joint if internal impingement is present. (From DeLee JC, Drez D, Miller MD: *DeLee & Drez's orthopaedic sports medicine: principles and practice*, ed 2, Philadelphia, 2002, Saunders.)

In 1991, Verna was the first to recognize the relationship between gross internal rotation deficit (GIRD) and shoulder dysfunction in the throwing athlete.[24] During a baseball season he assessed 39 professional pitchers who were determined to have 25 degrees or less of total internal rotation at spring training (GIRD, ≥35 degrees in each of these pitchers). During the course of the study and season, 60% developed shoulder problems requiring them to stop pitching. These findings of

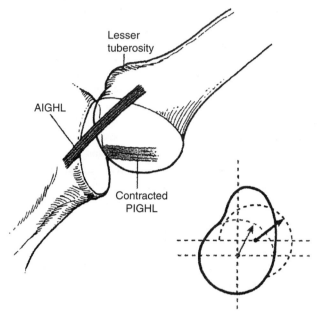

Figure 8-3 When the posterior capsule shortens (contracted posterior band), the glenohumeral contact point shifts posterosuperiorly and the allowable arc of external rotation (before greater tuberosity contacts the posterior glenoid) significantly increases *(dotted lines)*. (From Burkhart SS, Morgan C: *Orthop Clin North Am* 32:431-441, 2001.)

restricted internal rotation correlate with a tight posteroinferior capsule but can also be attributed to tightness of the external rotators and osseous adaptations of the humeral head or glenoid.[2]

Cooper manually stretched 22 Major League pitchers daily to minimize GIRD to less than 20 degrees during the 1997, 1998, and 1999 professional baseball seasons.[8] During those seasons, he reported innings lost, no intra-articular problems, and no surgical procedures in the study group. These reports help substantiate that a prophylactic-focused posteroinferior capsular stretching program is successful in minimizing GIRD and is effective in preventing secondary intra-articular problems, particularly posterior Type II SLAP lesions.[8]

According to Burkhart et al,[8] this acquired loss of internal rotation caused by the posteroinferior capsule contracture is the "essential lesion" that leads to a secondary resultant increase in external rotation. They believe this occurs via two mechanisms by which a tight posterior capsule induces hyperexternal rotation of the humerus. First, the tethering effect of the posterior capsular contracture shifts the glenohumeral contact point posterosuperiorly, allowing the greater tuberosity to clear the glenoid rim through a greater arc of external rotation before internal impingement occurs (Figure 8-3). Second, the shift in the glenohumeral contact point reduces the cam effect of the proximal humerus on the anteroinferior capsule to allow greater external rotation due to the redundancy in the capsule (Figure 8-4). They define GIRD as a loss in degrees of glenohumeral internal rotation of the throwing shoulder compared with the nonthrowing shoulder. Glenohumeral internal rotation deficits of 15 to 20 degrees have been associated with nonsymptomatic pitchers, while symptomatic pitchers have reported deficits as high as 45 degrees.[2,22]

Typically, glenohumeral internal rotation is measured with the subject supine and the shoulder elevated to 90 degrees of

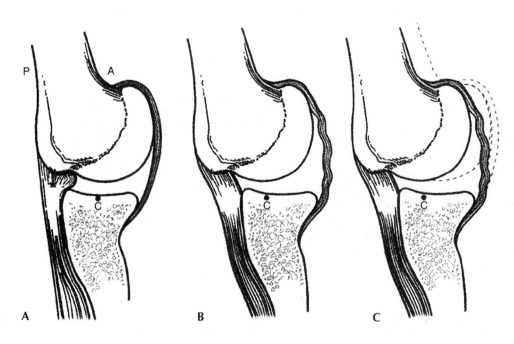

A   **B**   **C**

Figure 8-4 A, With the arm in a position of abduction and external rotation, the humeral head calcar produces a significant cam effect of the anteroinferior capsule, tensioning the capsule by virtue of the space-occupying effect. **B,** With a posterosuperior shift of the glenohumeral contact point, the space-occupying effect of the proximal humerus on the anteroinferior capsule is reduced (reduction of the cam effect). This creates a relative redundancy in the anteroinferior capsule that has probably been misinterpreted as microinstability. **C,** Superimposed neutral position *(dotted line)* shows the magnitude of the capsular redundancy that occurs as a result of the shift of the glenohumeral contact point. (From Burkhart SS, Morgan C: SLAP lesions in the overhead athlete, *Orthop Clin North Am* 32:431-441, 2001.)

abduction in the frontal plane. The examiner stabilizes the scapula by applying downward pressure on the anterior shoulder. The subject can also be assessed in the plane of the scapula, again with scapular stabilization. These measurements give the clinician an appreciation for what internal rotation is available before scapular compensation, as well as a sense of how tight the posterior capsule may be.

Tyler et al[25] proposed a method of measuring posterior capsular tightness in 22 collegiate baseball pitchers and also recorded bilateral external and internal rotation of the glenohumeral joint in 90 degrees of abduction. The alternate method involved a side-lying position in which the scapula is manually stabilized and the humerus is horizontally adducted without humeral rotation until a firm end feel is appreciated. The measurement (in centimeters) was taken from the medial epicondyle of the humerus to the surface of the examination table. When the examiners compared these linear measures with their internal rotation data, they reported that every centimeter of horizontal adduction lost corresponded with 4 degrees of internal rotation loss in the baseball pitcher.

Kibler found significant GIRD in 38 arthroscopically proven symptomatic Type II SLAP lesions in overhead athletes (average GIRD, 33 degrees, range 26 to 58 degrees).[26] Kibler also prospectively evaluated high-level tennis players and followed them for 2 years.[27] They were divided into two groups. One group performed daily posterior inferior capsular stretching to minimize GIRD, and the other (control) group did not stretch. Those who stretched had significant improvement in their internal rotation and total arm rotation compared with the control group. Furthermore, those in the stretching group had a 38% decrease in the incidence of shoulder problems compared with the control group.

BICEPS TENDON SUPERIOR LABRAL COMPLEX

Only recently has there been an appreciation for the role of the long head of the biceps tendon at the glenohumeral joint in the throwing athlete. Historically, the biceps has been thought of as having a minor role as a glenohumeral depressor. Itoi et al[28] have described the biceps as a secondary anterior stabilizer in 60 and 90 degrees of abduction. Andrews et al[12] described the biceps during the follow-through phase as an elbow stabilizer and an eccentric decelerator as the elbow extends. In 1985 Andrews et al,[12] in a study of 73 throwing athletes, observed that 60% had anterior-superior labral tears and 23% had tears in both the anterosuperior and posterosuperior regions. The majority of the athletes (73%) had a concomitant partial supraspinatus tear, and in a smaller subset of the original group 7% had partial tears of the long head of the biceps tendon.[12]

The authors hypothesized that the incidence of injury located at the superior labrum was due to the excessive eccentric-overload forces placed on the biceps tendon in an attempt to decelerate the arm during the follow-through phase of throwing. This eccentric contraction of the biceps would then cause a sudden tensile load with the potential to avulse the

biceps or labral complex.[29] Andrews also used electrical stimulation during arthroscopy that resulted in lift-off of the labrum, which he postulated as the mechanism of injury. The athletes' chief complaint was pain during the overhead throwing motion, a popping or catching sensation, as well as a sense of instability.[12]

Snyder et al[30] classified superior labral lesions after reviewing more than 700 arthroscopies. They reported that the most common mechanism of injury was a compression force to the shoulder, usually from a fall on an outstretched arm. The position of the arm was believed to be in abduction and slight forward flexion at the time of impact. Higgins et al,[29] who published a retrospective analysis of SLAP lesions, reported that despite the widespread acceptance of the classification scheme proposed by Snyder et al (1991, labral lesions), there have been no studies correlating the mechanism of injury and the injury pattern in the majority of SLAP lesions.

Rodosky et al[31] used mathematical modeling with the glenohumeral joint in the abducted and externally rotated position, simulated the throwing position and investigated the role of the long head of the biceps and its origin at the superior labrum and glenoid. They hypothesized that the biceps would help limit the hyperexternal rotation at the glenohumeral joint. They determined that the biceps gave a compressive force for the humeral head into the glenoid that in effect resisted rotation. The long head of the biceps was also found to withstand higher external rotational forces without a concomitant increase in strain at the IGHL. Their study suggests that with the increasing force at the biceps, it appears that the biceps plays a role in preventing anterior stability by augmenting torsional stability at the glenohumeral joint (Figure 8-5).

To test their theory, Rodosky et al[31] surgically induced a SLAP lesion and were able to calculate a 26% decrease in torsional rigidity and a concomitant 33% increase in strain at the IGHL. This study suggests that the biceps is a critical player in the shoulder for dynamic stability during the cocking, acceleration, and follow-through phases in throwing. This torque-attenuating capacity of the long head of the biceps helps ensure less strain along the IGHL. Thus there appears to be a clear coexistence of shoulder instability in the presence of a SLAP lesion.[32] The biceps plays a large role in the dynamic stability of the glenohumeral joint during throwing and should be a consideration in assessment and treatment in the athlete's shoulder if he or she is going to continue his or her respective sport.

Snyder et al[33] published the results of 140 superior labral injuries out of 2375 examined shoulders that were treated surgically. They discovered only 6% of all shoulder arthroscopies involved SLAP lesions, and of the 140, only in 38% was there an isolated lesion involving the superior labrum and biceps complex. They inferred that there was limited number of cases of SLAP lesions in the general population and that the mechanism of injury varied. Maffet et al,[32] after reviewing 712 surgical shoulder cases with significant superior labrum and biceps long head involvement, also suggest the etiologies and prevalence of involvement is certainly varied.

Burkhart et al[8] have observed a dynamic peel-back phenomenon arthroscopically in throwers with posterior and combined

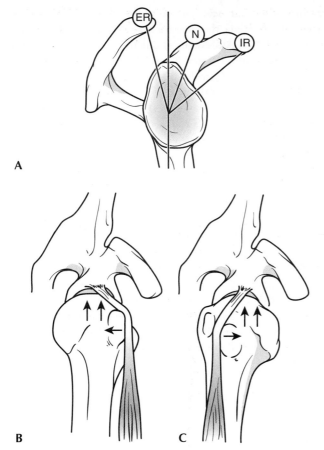

A

B   C

Figure 8-5 A diagrammatic representation of forces created with simulated contraction of the long head of the biceps brachii is shown. **A,** Rotation of the humerus changes orientation of the biceps tendon with respect to the joint. In neutral rotation *(N),* the tendon generally occupies a slightly anterior position. With internal rotation *(IR),* the tendon lies anterior to the joint. In contrast, the tendon occupies a slightly posterior position with external rotation *(ER).* **B,** With internal rotation of the humerus, the biceps seems to generate joint compressive forces *(paired arrows)* and posteriorly directed force *(arrow),* which restrain glenohumeral translation. **C,** With external rotation of the humerus, anteriorly directed force *(arrow)* seems to accompany joint compressive forces *(paired arrows).* (From Soslowsk L: *Clin Orthop* 400:55, 2002.)

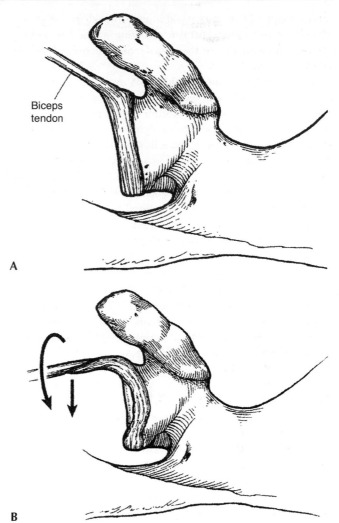

Biceps tendon

A

B

Figure 8-6 Biceps peel-back mechanism: **A,** Superior view of the biceps and labral complex of a left shoulder in a resting position. **B,** Superior view of the biceps and labral complex of a left shoulder in the abducted, externally rotated position, showing the peel-back mechanism as the biceps vector shifts posteriorly. (From Burkhart SS, Morgan C: *Orthop Clin North Am* 32:431-441, 2001.)

anteroposterior SLAP lesions. They describe the peel-back occurring when the arm is in the cocked position of abduction and external rotation and is secondary to the effect this position has on the biceps tendon. This position shifts the vector of the biceps tendon to a more posterior position in the late cocking phase of throwing and essentially produces a twist at the base of the biceps. This twist of the biceps then transmits a torsional force to the posterior superior labrum, causing it to rotate medially over the corner of the glenoid onto the posterior superior scapular neck. In addition, the biceps root shifts medially to the supraglenoid tubercle.[21]

Burkhart and Morgan[21] have observed that the biceps tendon will "peel back" over the posterior-superior corner of the labrum in patients with posterior SLAP lesions or combined anteroposterior SLAP lesions, an action that is absent in normal

shoulders. They described that, during arthroscopy, when the arm was placed in abduction and external rotation, the biceps tendon assumed a more vertical and posterior direction (Figure 8-6). The authors believe that this dynamic angle change induces a posterior shift in the biceps vector, as well as a twist at the base of the biceps, which in effect transmits a torsional force to the posterior superior labrum.

Burkhart et al believe that this peel-back phenomenon is a consistent finding in patients with posterior SLAP lesions or "thrower's SLAP," or combined anteroposterior SLAP lesions. The throwing athlete would most likely need to undergo a SLAP repair to eliminate the peel-back sign as confirmation that this torsional force had been neutralized. The stabilization of technique of choice is a suture anchor with a simple loop around the labrum. This provides enough tensile force within the suture loop to effectively resist the torsional force of the peel-back mechanism.[8] Contrary to Andrews' deceleration mechanism for biceps and labral injuries, Burkhart et al postulate an acceleration mechanism occurring in the late cocking phase of throwing due to the position of abduction and hyperexternal rotation.[8]

Using a cadaver model, Kuhn et al[34] made an experimental comparison of both acceleration versus deceleration and the effect on the biceps-superior labrum complex. They simulated the deceleration mechanism by applying a tensile force through the biceps with the arm in the follow-through position. They induced a superior labral avulsion in only 20% of the specimens with a large tensile force (340 ± 40 N). To simulate the acceleration mechanism, they loaded the biceps of the cadaver specimens in the abducted and externally rotated position to simulate late cocking and consistently produced a Type II SLAP lesion at a lesser force of 289 plus or minus 39 N, 20% less than the force used during the deceleration mechanism. The authors found that 9 of 10 specimens in the acceleration model were found to incur Type II SLAP lesions and only 2 of 10 of those in the deceleration position.[34] Thus on the basis of this experimental and clinical data, it appears that the biceps and superior labrum complex is not pulled from bone but instead peeled from bone.[8,34]

Pathophysiological Cascade

Burkhart et al[8] have proposed that the contracture of the posteroinferior capsule is the initial and ultimate etiology abnormality that initiates the pathological cascade that peaks in the late cocking phase of throwing. At the late cocking phase of throwing there is a shift in the glenohumeral contact point that causes maximum shear on the posterosuperior labrum at precisely the time when the peel-back force and the total force on the shoulder are at their maximum.

The contracted posteroinferior capsule and posterior band of the IGHL complex result in the inferior axillary pouch structures becoming imbalanced and will not provide the normal cradling or hammock effect of the humeral head as described by O'Brien et al.[35] The normal effect of the posterior band of the IGHL complex allows the shoulder to wind and unwind in abduction around a relatively fixed central glenohumeral rotation point located in the lower half of the glenoid face.[8,35] As the shoulder attempts to wind up into the cocked position, the contracted posterior band will not allow the head to fully externally rotate around the normal glenoid rotation point. Koffler et al[36] describe that the net effect is the posterior contracture acting as a check rein or tether that draws the humeral head posterosuperiorly to a new rotation point on the glenoid. In addition, the posterior band of the IGHL is now bowstrung beneath the humeral head, exerting a posterosuperiorly directed force that maintains this shift.

The posterosuperior shift of the humeral head permits abnormally excessive external rotation to occur around the new rotation point because the shift allows the anterior capsule to relax. As the thrower's shoulder excessively rotates externally around this new rotation point, a number of adverse consequences can develop according to Burkhart et al[8]: (1) Shear forces at the biceps anchor and the posterosuperior labrum

attachment increase, and both structures begin to fail at their attachment sites via the peel-back phenomenon, which produces a Type II SLAP lesion; (2) due to the acquired hyperexternal rotation from the new rotation point, a possible sequela would be augmented tensile stresses on the IGHL and, should the athlete continue to throw, the hyperexternal rotation may result in anterior capsule failure; (3) the excessive external rotation caused by the GIRD also causes increased shear and torsional forces in the articular side of the posterosuperior rotator cuff. All of these soft tissue changes are thought to be secondary to an acquired posteroinferior capsular contracture that may have been clinically silent initially.[8]

The Shoulder at Risk: The 180-Degree Rule

Pitchers and throwing athletes alike tend to acquire a tight posterior-inferior capsule due to the tensile stress on the shoulder during the deceleration phase of throwing. The development of the "dead arm syndrome" is a common sequela due to the lack of posterior-inferior capsule extensibility and concomitant lack of glenohumeral internal rotation. Burkhart and Morgan[21] reported that the healthy throwing shoulder presents with increased external rotation in abduction at the expense of internal rotation. Their term "Rotational Unity Rule" describes that if the gain of external rotation equals the loss of internal rotation, allowing a 180-degree arc of motion, problems will be avoided. However, the shoulder with a posterior inferior capsular contracture that restricts the total arc to less than 180 degrees is truly a "shoulder at risk."[21]

Asymmetry of the Scapula

All of the previously mentioned consequences are worsened by a protracted scapula that antetilts the glenoid. The antetilted scapula and thus glenoid increase the anterior tensile loads on the capsule and increase the peel-back effect posteriorly.[8] The importance of scapular symmetry should not be overlooked. No normal scapular asymmetry occurs through overhead sport; in fact, it could be the precursor to shoulder problems.[37] The fact that the rotator cuff and scapular rotators are primary players in dynamic stability of the shoulder in the act of throwing it should be one of the first assessments made. Asymmetry of the scapula, especially of the throwing shoulder, results in an inefficient length-tension of the rotator cuff and could lead to pathology.

The scapula acts as a stable platform from which forces are generated and translated from the trunk via the kinetic chain and expressed through the shoulder. Normal scapular kinematics is necessary for the upper extremity to properly throw a baseball and protect against injury. The glenoid articulation must constantly shift to coordinate proper articulation and axis of rotation with the humeral head. A protracted scapula has been shown to augment tensile strain on the anterior capsule and IGHL and possibly contribute indirectly to instability in the abducted and externally rotated position.[38]

Because the scapulothoracic joint is a physiological joint and forms the foundation for glenohumeral joint function, it is important to evaluate and objectively document the status of scapulothoracic joint position, arthrokinematics, and muscular power.[39] Kibler[40] has described the lateral scapular slide test, which is an objective method to quantify the bilateral comparison of the scapula in three positions. Kibler states that less than 1 cm of asymmetry in a bilateral comparison is within normal limits. More than 1 cm of asymmetry in two of the three test positions is correlated to impingement syndrome in the shoulder. Although Kibler's lateral slide test is an objective way to measure scapular symmetry, there are no descriptive norms in his article and it has not proven to be either reliable or valid in determining scapular asymmetry due to weakness of the scapular rotators.[41]

Davies et al[42] developed a modified lateral slide test that uses the three positions described by Kibler, as well as two additional positions. The two additional positions were added because Davies believed that patients often only complain of pain in the overhead position. The additional positions were the arms in 120 and 150 degrees of abduction. The results did not demonstrate a statistically significant change from one arm position to the next. DeVita et al[43] described a reliable method of assessing scapular position at rest using string to assess the distance from the inferior angle of the acromion to the spinous process of the third thoracic vertebrae (Figure 8-7). This method of scapular measurement was reported to have acceptable intratester and intertester reliability (ICC = 0.91 to 0.92).[43]

Johnson et al[44] demonstrated good to excellent intrarater reliability in assessing upward scapular rotation in subjects with and without shoulder pathology using two-dimensional measurements with an inclinometer with the arm at rest, in 60, 90, and 120 degrees of humeral elevation in the scapular plane. They compared their data with three-dimensional measurements obtained using a magnetic tracking device with the arm fixed and during arm movement. Anecdotally, it appears effective to assess scapular symmetry while the subject

has his or her arms resting at the side and palpating the inferior angles of the scapula to determine if they are aligned side to side. Some experts use this asymmetry as a guideline when they need to shut down their pitchers to prevent the risk of injury.[2]

Because the scapulothoracic articulation acts more as a sesamoid joint with its lack of a capsule or ligamentous support, it relies predominantly on the dynamic and stabilizing roles of the surrounding musculature. A winging of the scapula is often seen when observing scapulohumeral rhythm during elevation of the arm, especially during the eccentric phase. When the anchoring stability of the scapula is lost, the deltoid becomes less efficient, rotator cuff stabilizing strength is diminished, the humerus elevates superiorly, and the athlete develops a functional subluxation leading to suprahumeral impingement.[44,45]

McQuade et al[46] assessed the effect fatigue played on scapulohumeral rhythm when assessed under dynamic fatigued-inducing exercise. Twenty-five subjects were involved and were required to lift their arms against maximum resistance until they could no longer completely elevate overhead. Three-dimensional kinematics were assessed using an electromagnetic tracking system. Electromyographic activity was recorded for the upper trapezius, lower trapezius, serratus anterior, and the middle deltoid muscles. The results showed that from 60 to 150 degrees of elevation, the scapulohumeral rhythm decreased with fatigue and tended to result in compensatory increased motion of the scapula.

Alterations in the scapular kinematics have been demonstrated to be a key factor in subacromial impingement. When assessing the scapular kinematics, it is essential to also assess muscle strength to correlate with the observed yet subtle asymmetries seen on motion testing. Recently, Ekstrom et al[47] determined positions for manual muscle testing for the upper, middle, and lower trapezius, as well as the serratus anterior. The retractors and protractors of the scapula work together in a force couple to first properly position the arm during the throw in the fully retracted position for the late cocking phase. The rhomboids are of primary importance for stability and positioning early on in the throwing cycle. As the athlete begins the acceleration phase, the protractors need to fire to keep the scapula in line with the humeral head, yet the middle and lower trapezius need to also contract in an eccentric fashion to decelerate the scapula during the follow-through phase of motion. Any weakness in this chain of events may lead to impingement of the suprahumeral structures or excessive strain along the anterior capsule and ligamentous tissues.

Other recent studies have assessed the role the proximal humeral anatomy plays in the loss of internal rotation and gains in external rotation in the throwing athlete.[48-50] Reagan et al[49] performed a descriptive anatomical study with 54 asymptomatic college baseball players. The authors used standard assessments of dominant versus nondominant arm total range of motion and also assessed the degree of humeral retroversion radiographically. Retroversion of the humerus was defined as the acute angle, in a medial and posterior direction, between the axis of the elbow joint and the axis through the

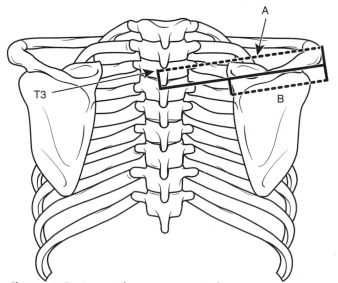

Figure 8-7 Devita scapular measurement technique.

center of the humeral head.[49] An increase in humeral retroversion allows the articulating surface of the humeral head to remain in contact with the glenoid articulating surface while the glenohumeral joint externally rotates to a higher degree before the humeral head is stabilized by the anterior capsule.[49,51]

Finally, Vad et al[52] demonstrated that overhead-throwing athletes are at risk for nerve stretch injuries, especially to the suprascapular and long thoracic nerves, similar to patients with full-thickness rotator cuff tears who are at risk for injuries to the upper trunk of the brachial plexus and axillary nerve. Therefore paying close attention, in the physical examination of overhead athletes, to excessive scapular winging or atrophy of the infraspinatus fossa is important.

Vad et al hypothesized that changes in humeral retroversion may provide an explanation for the decrease in internal rotation characteristic in overhead-throwing athletes. Theoretically, the increased retroversion may lead to restraint of the humeral head by the posterior capsule at a more limited degree of internal rotation.[49] Reagan et al[49] found total rotational motion, measured at 90 degrees of glenohumeral abduction, was 159.5 degrees for the dominant shoulder and 157.8 degrees for the nondominant shoulders. Significant mean differences found in external and internal rotation in the dominant versus nondominant extremity were 9.7 degrees and 8.2 degrees, respectively. Humeral retroversion was also found to be significantly different between the throwing and nonthrowing arm, which measured 36.6 degrees plus or minus 9.8 degrees in the dominant extremity and 26 degrees plus or minus 9.4 degrees in the nondominant extremity.

Crockett et al[50] also assessed the influence of osseous humeral adaptation and range of motion at the glenohumeral joint in professional baseball pitchers. Glenohumeral joint range of motion and laxity, along with the humeral head and glenoid version of the dominant versus nondominant shoulders, were studied in 25 professional baseball pitchers and 25 nonthrowing subjects. Each subject underwent a computed tomography scan to determine bilateral humeral head and glenoid versions. A comparison of the dominant shoulders of the two groups indicated that both external rotation at 90 degrees and humeral head retroversion were significantly greater in the throwing group. The throwing group also demonstrated a significant increase in dominant shoulder versus nondominant shoulder in humeral head retroversion, glenoid retroversion, external rotation at 90 degrees, and external rotation in the scapular plane. Internal rotation was decreased in the dominant shoulder.[50]

SUMMARY

The authors of this chapter have identified that the pathology of the throwing shoulder has a large variety of etiological factors. Clinically, it is important for the clinician to evaluate the total range of motion, with an emphasis on identifying internal rotation deficits. The etiology of microtrauma to the shoulder in the overhead-throwing athlete is associated with

tightness and contracture of the posterior band of the inferior glenohumeral capsule. As noted earlier, the dysfunction of the posterior band of the inferior glenohumeral capsule changes the biomechanics of the shoulder joint. In addition, asymmetry of the scapula alerts the position of the glenohumeral posture, which in turn changes the length tension of the rotator cuff muscles.

The authors have observed clinically that the successful treatment of the overhead-throwing athlete must include a detailed evaluation to determine the soft tissue deficits. Once the deficits have been determined, specific stretching and mobilization techniques are critical in restoring normal range-of-motion and shoulder mechanics. In order to maintain the range of motion, the athlete needs to strengthen the glenohumeral and scapula thoracic rotators and continue with a maintenance program of stretching exercises.

REFERENCES

1. Conte S, Requa R, Garrick J: Disability days in major league baseball, *Am J Sports Med* 29:413, 2001.
2. Cooper J Donley P, Morgan C: Throwing injuries. In Donatelli R, editor: *Physical therapy of the shoulder*, ed 4, pp. 29-55, St Louis, 2004, Churchill Livingstone.
3. Altchek D, Hobbs W: Evaluation and management of shoulder instability in the elite overhead thrower, *Orthop Clin North Am* 32:423-430, 2001.
4. Dillman CJ, Fleisig G, Andrews JR: Biomechanics of pitching with emphasis upon shoulder kinematics, *J Orthop Sports Phys Ther* 18:402, 1993.
5. Pappas AM, Zawacki R, Sullivan TJ: Biomechanics of baseball pitching: a preliminary report, *Am J Sports Med* 14:216, 1985.
6. Gainor BJ, Piotrowski G, Puhl J, et al: The throw: biomechanics and acute injury, *Am J Sports Med* 8:114, 1980.
7. Gowan ID, Jobe F, Tibone JE, et al: A comparative electromyographic analysis of the shoulder during pitching, *Am J Sports Med* 15:586, 1987.
8. Burkhart S, Morgan CD, Kibler B: The disabled throwing shoulder: spectrum of pathology part I: pathoanatomy and biomechanics, *Arthroscopy* 19:404-420, 2003.
9. Fleisig GS Dillman C, Andrews JR: Biomechanics of the shoulder during throwing. In Andrews JR WK, editor: *The athlete's shoulder*, pp. 360-365, New York, 1994, Churchill Livingstone.
10. Jobe FW Tibone J, Jobe CM, et al: The shoulder in sports. In Rockwood CA and Matsen F, editor: *The shoulder*, pp. 963-967, Philadelphia, 1990, Saunders.
11. Jobe F, Giangarra C, Kvitne Rea: Anterior capsulobral reconstruction of the shoulder in athletes in overhand sports, *Am J Sports Med* 19:428, 1991.
12. Andrews JR, Carson WJ Jr., McCleod WD: Glenoid labrum tears related to the long head of the biceps, *Am J Sports Med* 13:337-341, 1985.
13. Walch G, Boileau J, Noel E, et al: Impingement of the deep surface of the supraspinatus tendon on the posterior

superior glenoid rim: an arthroscopic study, *J Shoulder Elbow Surg* 1:238-243, 1992.

14. Jobe CM : Superior glenoid impingement, *Clin Orthop Rel Res* 330:98-107, 1996.

15. Meister K: Injuries to the shoulder in the throwing athlete, *Am J Sports Med* 28:265-275, 2000.

16. Gross ML, Brenner S, Esformes I, et al: Anterior shoulder instability in weightlifters, *Am J Sports Med* 21:599-603, 1993.

17. Meister K, Batts J, Gilmore M: The posterior impingement sign: evaluation of internal impingement in the overhead athlete, *Orthop Trans* 1998.

18. Rubenstein DL, Jobe F, Glousman RE, et al: Anterior capsulolabral reconstruction of the shoulder in athletes, *J Shoulder Elbow Surg* 1:229-237, 1992.

19. Gerber C, Sebesta A: Impingement of the deep surface of the subscapularis tendon and the reflection pulley on the anterosuperior glenoid rim: a preliminary report, *J Shoulder Elbow Surg* 9:483-490, 2000.

20. Halbrecht JL, Tirman P, Atkin D: Internal impingement of the shoulder: comparison of findings between the throwing and nonthrowing shoulders of college baseball players, *Arthroscopy* 15:253-258, 1999.

21. Burkhart SS, Morgan C: SLAP lesions in the overhead athlete, *Orthop Clin North Am* 32:431-441, 2001.

22. Morgan CD, Burkhart S, Palmeri M, et al: Type II SLAP lesions: three subtypes and their relationship to superior instability and rotator cuff tears, *Arthroscopy* 14:553-565, 1998.

23. Wilk K, Meister K, Andrews JR: Current concepts in the rehabilitation of the throwing athlete, *Am J Sports Med* 30:136-151, 2002.

24. Verna C: Shoulder flexibility to reduce impingement, *Presented at the 3rd Annual PBATS (Professional Baseball Athletic Trainer Society) Meeting*, Mesa, Ariz, 1991.

25. Tyler FT, Roy T, Nichlas SJ, et al: Reliability and validity of a new method of measuring posterior shoulder tightness, *J Orthop Sports Phys Ther* 29:262, 1999.

26. Kibler W: SLAP lesions and their relationship to glenohumeral internal rotation deficit. Submitted for publication, 2002.

27. Kibler W: The relationship of the glenohumeral internal rotation deficit to shoulder and elbow injuries in tennis players: a prospective evaluation of posterior capsular stretching, *Presented at the Annual Closed Meeting of the American Shoulder and Elbow Surgeons*, New York, 1998.

28. Itoi E Kuechle D, Newman SR: Stabilizing function of the biceps in stable and unstable shoulders, *J Bone Joint Surg* 75B:546, 1993.

29. Higgins L, Warner J: Superior labral lesions: anatomy, pathology, and treatment, *Clin Orthop Rel Res* 390:73-82, 2001.

30. Snyder S, Karzel R, Del Pizzo W, et al: SLAP lesions of the shoulder, *Arthroscopy* 6:274-279, 1990.

31. Rodosky MW, Harner C, Fu FH: The role of the long head of the biceps muscle and superior glenoid labrum in anterior stability of the shoulder, *Am J Sports Med* 22:121, 1994.

32. Maffett MW, Gartsman G, Moseley B: Superior labrum-biceps tendon complex lesions of the shoulder, *Am J Sports Med* 23:93, 1995.

33. Snyder S, Banas M, Karzel R: An analysis of 140 injuries to the superior glenoid labrum, *J Shoulder Elbow Surg* 4:243-248, 1995.

34. Kuhn JED Lindholm S, Huston LJ, et al: Failure of the biceps-superior labral complex in the throwing athlete: a cadaveric biomechanical investigation comparing the late cocking and early deceleration, The Arthroscopy Association of North America Specialty Day, AAOS Annual Meeting, Anaheim, Calif, 1999.

35. O'Brien S, Neves M, Arnoczky SP et al: The anatomy and histology of the inferior glenohumeral ligament complex of the shoulder, *Am J Sports Med* 18:449-456, 1990.

36. Koffler KM, Bader D, Eager M, et al: The effect of posterior capsule tightness on glenohumeral translation in the late cocking phase of pitching. A cadaveric study. The 21st Annual Meeting of the Arthroscopic Association of North America, Washington, DC, 2002.

37. Warner JP Micheli LJ, Arslanian L, et al: Patterns of laxity, flexibility, and strength in normal shoulders and shoulders with instability and impingement, *Am J Sports Med* 18:366, 1990.

38. Weiser WM, Lee T, McMaster WC, et al: Effects of simulated scapular protraction on anterior glenohumeral instability, *Am J Sports Med* 27:801, 1999.

39. Davies G, Dickoff-Hoffman S: Neuromuscular testing and rehabilitation of the shoulder complex, *J Orthp Sports Phys Ther* 18:448-459, 1993.

40. Kibler W: Role of the scapula in the overhead throwing motion, *Contemp Orthop* 22:525-533, 1991.

41. Gibson M, Goebel G, Jordan T, et al: A reliability study of measurement techniques to determine static scapular position, *J Orthop Sports Phys Ther* 21:100-106, 1995.

42. Davies GJ, Jones B: Isokinetic testing of scapulo-thoracic protraction/retraction and correlation to a modified lateral slide test. Unpublished research at the University of Wisconsin-LaCrosse, Wis, 1992-1993.

43. DeVita J, Walker M, Skibinski B: Relationship between performance of selected scapular muscles and scapular abduction in standing subjects, *Phys Ther* 70:470-476, 1990.

44. Johnson M, McClure P, Karduna A: A new method to assess scapular upward rotation in subjects with shoulder pathology, *J Orthop Sports Phys Ther* 31:81-89, 2001.

45. Glousman R, Jobe F, Tibone J, et al: Dynamic electromyographic analysis of the throwing shoulder with glenohumeral instability, *J Bone Joint Surg* 70A:220-226, 1988.

46. McQuade K, Dawson J, Smidt G: Scapulothoracic muscle fatigue associated with alterations in scapulohumeral rhythm kinematics during maximum resistive shoulder elevation, *J Orthop Sports Phys Ther* 28:74-80, 1998.

47. Eckstrom R, Donatelli R, Soderberg G: Selective exercises for the scapular rotators with electromyography, *J Orthop Sports Phys Ther* 33(5): 247-258, 2003.

48. Osbahr D, Cannon D, Speer K: Retroversion of the humerus in the throwing shoulder of college baseball pitchers, *Am J Sports Med* 30:347-353, 2002.

49. Reagan KM, Meister K, Horodyski M: Humeral retroversion and its relationship to glenohumeral rotation in the shoulder of college baseball players, *Am J Sports Med* 30:354-360, 2002.

50. Crockett H, Gross L, Wilk K et al: Osseous adaptation and range of motion at the glenohumeral joint in professional baseball pitchers, *Am J Sports Med* 30:20-26, 2002.

51. Jobe CM, Iannotti J: Limits imposed on glenohumeral motion by joint geometry, *J Shoulder Elbow Surg* 4:281-285, 1995.

52. Vad V, Southern D, Warren R, et al: Prevalence of peripheral neurologic injuries in full thickness rotator cuff tears, *J Shoulder Elbow Surg* 12:333-336, 2003.

9

Robert A. Donatelli

The Anatomy and Pathophysiology of the CORE

LEARNING OBJECTIVES

After studying this chapter, the reader will be able to do the following:

1. Define the hip and trunk CORE
2. Evaluate the CORE muscles and structure
3. Delineate the difference between local and global muscles on the back
4. Identify the muscles of the abdominal area that are considered stabilizing
5. Identify the spinal muscles that stiffen the spine
6. Evaluate the CORE dysfunction
7. Instruct patients in exercises designed to strength hip and trunk muscles
8. Identify the correlation between muscle weakness in the hip and lower extremity injuries

INTRODUCTION AND DEFINITION

This chapter defines the CORE, identifies the anatomical structures within the CORE, and discusses the pathophysiology of muscle imbalances. The evaluation of the CORE and strength training concepts are discussed in Chapter 12.

For the purposes of this chapter the CORE is defined as a clinical manifestation in which a delicate balance of movement and stability occurs simultaneously. The author of this chapter describes the upper quadrant CORE to include the glenohumeral joint and the scapulothoracic joint and the lower quadrant CORE to include the hip and trunk. This chapter discusses the function and special considerations of the muscles of the CORE. In addition, muscle imbalances and dysfunction of the CORE are discussed.

Speed is allegedly an innate talent and cannot be changed with training. However, muscle imbalances, joint restrictions, and pain may prevent the athlete from achieving his or her maximum innate abilities. The job of the sports-specific rehabilitation specialist is to identify deficits within the CORE and design a rehabilitation program to promote an increase in strength, power, and endurance specific to the muscles and joints that are in a state of dysfunction. Specificity of the rehabilitation program can help the athlete overcome musculoskeletal system deficits and achieve maximum potentials of his or her talents. A combination of power, strength, and endurance is critical for the muscles of the CORE to allow the athlete to perform at his or her maximum capabilities.

The lower quadrant CORE is identified by the muscles, ligaments, and fascia that produce a synchronous motion and stability of the trunk, hip, and lower extremities. The initiation of movement in the lower limb is a result of activation of certain muscles that hold onto bone, referred to as *stabilizers,* and other muscles that move bone, referred to as *mobilizers.* The muscle action within the CORE depends on a balanced activity of the stabilizers and mobilizers. If the stabilizers do not hold onto the bone, the mobilizing muscles will function at a disadvantage. The lack of harmony between the stabilizers and the mobilizers can result in muscle imbalances and injury.

Thirty-five muscles attach directly to the sacrum or innominate, or both. This chapter is not intended to describe the detailed anatomy of each of these muscles but rather to highlight the muscle groups and their specific application to movement and stabilization. In addition, the chapter presents evidence of how the muscle groups within the trunk and hip CORE are important to the athletes' performance and prevention of injuries. The CORE trunk muscles include the abdominals, thoracolumbar, lumbar, and lateral thoracolumbar muscles. The CORE hip muscles include the hip flexors, extensors, adductors, abductors, and internal and external rotators.

CORE MUSCLES OF THE TRUNK AND HIP

The CORE muscles of the trunk include the thoracolumbar muscles (longissimus thoracic pars thoracis, and the iliocostalis lumborum pars thoracis), the lumbar muscles (lumbar multifidus, iliocostalis lumborum pars lumborum, longissimus thoracic pars lumborum, intertransversarii, interspinalis and rotatores), the lateral thoracolumbar muscle, the quadratus lumborum, and the abdominal muscles (the transverses abdominis, rectus abdominis, internal and external oblique abdominals). Although the thoracodorsal fascia is not a contractile tissue, it does enhance CORE trunk stability as a result of the contraction of several trunk muscles attached to it.

The CORE hip muscles include psoas, iliacus, gluteus maximus, gluteus medius (anterior and posterior fibers), rectus femoris, and the hamstring muscle group. The external and internal rotators of the hip include a large group of muscles. These muscles are important to the hip and trunk for movement and stability. Lack of strength and power of the muscles noted as follows can contribute to injury of the lower extremity or reduced performance, or both.

External Rotators

The external rotators are the piriformis, superior/inferior gemellus, obturator internus and externus, quadratus femoris, gluteus maximus two thirds attached to tensor fasciae latae, iliopsoas, sartorius, and biceps femoris.

Internal Rotators

The internal rotators are the medial hamstrings, anterior portion of the gluteus medius, tensor fascia, iliotibial band, gluteus minimus, pectineus, and gracilis.

FUNCTIONAL ANATOMY OF THE MUSCLES OF THE TRUNK AND HIP

This section discusses the specific function of individual muscle groups within the CORE and their importance to performance in the athlete. Muscle is the body's best force attenuator. Eccentric control of rapid movement is critical for performance enhancement and prevention of injury. In addition, muscles create forces that play a role in the production of movement and in stabilizing of joints for safety and performance.

The physiological cross-sectional area (PCSA) of muscle determines the force-producing potential, while the line of pull and moment arm determine the effect of the force on movement and stabilization.[1] The small muscle of the thoracic and lumbar spine includes the intertransversarii, interspinales, and rotatores. These muscles have small cross-sectional areas and

> ### Evidence-Based Clinical Application
> The intertransversarii, interspinales, and rotatores are considered length transducers and therefore sense the positioning of each spinal motion. These structures are likely affected during active and passive end-range rotational movements, such as a baseball swing, a golf swing, passive stretch, or an end-range lumbar rotational mobilization technique.

work through a small moment arm.[1] Their total contribution to rotational axial twisting and bending torque is minimal. Bogduk[2] and McGill[1] hypothesized that these small muscles may not predominate as mechanical stabilizers but instead have a proprioceptive role. The rotatores and intertransversarii muscles are highly rich in muscle spindles, 4.5 to 7.3 times more than the multifidus.[3] Muscle spindles are the proprioceptors of muscle. These receptors are stimulated by stretch.

The major extensors of the thoracolumbar spine are the longissimus, iliocostalis, and multifidus groups. According to Bogduk[4] and McGill and Norman,[5] the longissimus and iliocostalis are divided into lumbar and thoracic portions, longissimus thoracis pars lumborum and pars thoracic, and iliocostalis lumborum pars lumborum and pars thoracis (Figure 9-1, A). The pars thoracis component of these two muscles attaches to the ribs and vertebral components and has

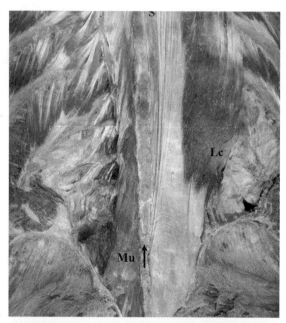

A

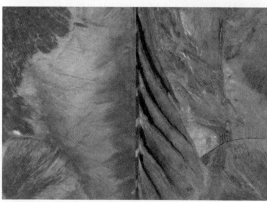

B

Figure 9-1 A, Longissimus and Iliocostalis muscles. **B,** Multifidus muscle. (**A** From Willard FH: The muscular, ligamentous and neural structure of the low back and its relation to back pain. In Vleeming A, Mooney V, Dorman T, et al, editors: *Movement, stability and low back pain,* Edinburgh, 1997, Churchill Livingstone. **B** From Lee D: *The pelvic girdle: an approach to the examination and treatment of the lumbopelvic-hip region,* ed 3, Edinburgh, 2004, Churchill Livingstone. Courtesy Gracovetsky personal library.)

relatively short contractile fibers with long tendons that run parallel to the spine attaching to the sacrum and iliac crest. These muscles have the greatest extensor moment with a minimum of compression to the spine.[1] The lumbar components of these muscle groups have a line of pull that is not parallel to the spine but rather have a posterior and caudal direction that causes them to generate posterior shear and an extensor moment to the spine.[1] The multifidus muscles have a low density of muscle spindles and are involved in producing extensor torque with small amounts of twisting and side-bending torque.[1] The lumbar multifidus muscles span two to three spinal segments. Therefore their forces affect only local areas of the spine. The multifidus is a good example of a muscle that stiffens the spine, acting as a stabilizer (Figure 9-1, *B*) (Table 9-1).

> ### Evidence-Based Clinical Application
> Biering-Sorensen[6] showed that in young, healthy subjects the back extensors demonstrate the greatest endurance of all three muscles groups within the trunk CORE. In addition, decreased torso extensor endurance predicts those who are at greatest risk of developing back problems. Increased endurance of the back extensors is critical for the athlete for stability, prevention of injury, and improved performance.

The abdominals are an important part of the trunk CORE muscles. The three layers of the abdominal wall muscles (external oblique, internal oblique, and transverse abdominis) perform several functions. All three are involved in flexion because of their attachment to the linea semilunaris, which changes the line of pull of the oblique muscle forces to the rectus sheath, increasing the flexor moment arm (Figure 9-2).[7] The oblique abdominal muscles are mobilizers, involved with torso rotational forces and lateral bending.[7] Because the oblique abdominal muscles' role is to produce trunk rotational forces, they have been identified as an important CORE muscle in the baseball and golf swing. The rectus abdominis appears to be the strongest trunk flexor and is the most active during sit-ups and curl-ups.[8] The rectus is divided by fascial tissue. This has been referred to as the "beaded" effect (see Figure 9-2). Porterfield and DeRosa[9] have determined that the beaded rectus performs an additional role of lateral transmission of forces from the oblique muscles forming a continuous hoop around the abdomen, thus increasing stability to the spine.

The transverse abdominis has been the focus of many researchers. The muscle has been identified as an important stabilizer of the trunk because of its attachment into the anterior abdominal fascia and the posterior attachment to the lumbodorsal fascia (Figure 9-3). The resulting corset-like containment, described earlier, provides stiffness that assists with spinal stability. Richardson et al.[10] have demonstrated early activation of the transverse abdominis before arm and leg movements, thus signifying that the trunk must be stable

before movement. In addition, a cocontraction of the transverse abdominis and the paraspinal muscles is assisted when the trunk is perturbed and a mass is added to the upper limb.[11]

> ### Evidence-Based Clinical Application
> Training the athlete to cocontract the transverse abdominis and the paraspinal muscles can be achieved while standing on an unstable surface and catching a medicine ball off a rebounder. This activity provides perturbing forces to the trunk while adding a mass to the upper limb.

The last muscle of the trunk CORE is the all-important quadratus lumborum (QL). The QL acts as a strong stabilizer by its attachment to each lumbar vertebra and the pelvis and rib cage. The functional aspects of the QL are unique. Specifically, the fibers of the QL have a large lateral moment arm via the attachments to the transverse processes, and thus the QL could support lateral shear instability, which may result from excessive compressive forces to the spine.[1]

McGill[12] determined that the QL hardly changes length during any spine motion, suggesting that when it contracts it is practically always isometric. The QL seems to be active during several different movement patterns, such as flexion-dominant, extensor dominant, and lateral bending tasks. The QL is an important stabilizing muscle for the lumbar spine in a wide variety of movements.[1]

> ### Evidence-Based Clinical Application
> The quadratus lumborum (QL) is an important stabilizer to the lumbar spine in many movement patterns important to improving the athlete's performance and prevention of injuries to the low back. Exercises designed to enhance the strength and endurance of the QL play an important role in the CORE program for the athlete. Isometric exercises would simulate the function of the muscle.

GLOBAL AND LOCAL MUSCLE SYSTEMS

As noted previously, the muscles described earlier can be classified as stabilizers or mobilizers. Richardson et al[10] has the best definition and description of trunk or lumbopelvic stability. The author of this chapter is in agreement that a stabilizing muscle acts as a dynamic process of controlling static position when appropriate to the functional movements. The dynamic process of stability allows the trunk to move with control in dynamic activities exemplified by athletes. Movement of the spine from flexion to extension should be a controlled sequence of intervertebral rotation and translation movements.[2] Bergmark[13] described the local stabilizing system as a group of muscles that have their origin or insertion on the lumbar

Table 9-1	CORE Muscle Tables	

Trunk CORE Structures by Group	Stabilizing Action	Mobilizing Action
Thoracolumbar Muscles		
Longissimus thoracis		X
Iliocostalis lumborum		X
Lumbar Muscles		
Lumbar multifidus*	X	
Iliocostalis lumborum	X	
Longissiums thoracic	X	
Intertransversarii	Proprioception	
Interspinales	Proprioception	
Rotatores	Proprioception	
Lateral Thoracolumbar Muscle		
Quadratus lumborum	X	
Abdominal muscles		
Transversus abdominis*	X	
Rectus abdominis		X
Internal obliques (posterior fibers)	Posterior fibers	X
External obliques	X	X
Thoracolumbar fascia	Stabilizes via muscle attachment	
Myofascial Slings (transfer load UE ↔ LE)	**Muscles and Fascia**	
Posterior oblique sling	Lat dorsi	
	Glut max	
	Thoracodorsal fascia	
Anterior oblique sling	External oblique	
	Anterior abdominal fascia	
	Contralateral internal oblique	
	Hip adductors	
Longitudinal sling	Peronii	
	Biceps femoris	
	Sacrotuberous ligament	
	Deep lamina of thoracodorsal fascia	
	Erector spinae	
Lateral sling	Gluteus med/min	
	Tensor fascia latea	
	Lateral stabilizers of thoracopelvis region	

Hip CORE Structure by Group	Stabilizing Action	Mobilizing Action
Psoas (posterior fibers)	Posterior fibers	X
Iliacus		X
Gluteus maximus		X
Gluteus medius *posterior fibers and anterior fibers*	X	
Rectus femoris		X
Hamstrings		X
External hip rotators	Piriformis, gemeli, oburator	X
Piriformis, gemeli, obturator interior/exterior, quadratus femoris, gluteus maximus *(aspect attached to TFL),* iliacus, sartorius, biceps femoris	interior/exterior	
Internal hip rotatores	TFL	X
Med hamstrings, gluteus medius *(anterior fibers),* TFL, ITB, gluteus minimus, pectineus, gracilis	ITB	
	Gluteus medius (anterior fibers)	

Table 9-1	CORE Muscle Tables—cont'd		
Upper Quadrant CORE by Group		Stabilizing Action	Mobilizing Action
Scapulohumeral			
Supraspinatus		X	
Infraspinatus		X	
Teres major			X
Teres minor		X	
Subscapularis		X	
Long head of biceps		X	
Deltoids			X
Thoracohumeral			
Pectoralis major			X
Latissimus dorsi		X	X
Scapulothoracic			
Upper trap			X
Middle trap			X
Lower trap			X
Rhomboids		X	
Levator scap		X	
Serratus anterior			X
Pectoralis minor		X	

ITB, Iliotibia band; *TFL*, tensor fascia latea.
*Lumbar multifidus and transversus abdominis are local trunk stabilizers.

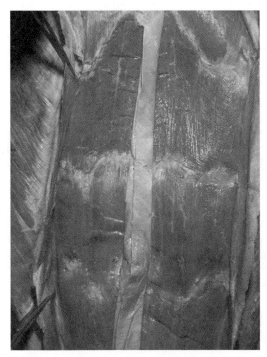

Figure 9-2 Linea semilunaris, which changes the line of pull of the oblique muscle forces to the rectus sheath, increasing the flexor moment arm. (From DeRosa C: Functional anatomy of the lumbar spine and sacroiliac joint. In Proceedings from the 4th Montreal Proceedings of the Interdisciplinary World Congress on Low Back and Pelvic Pain, Montreal, 2001.)

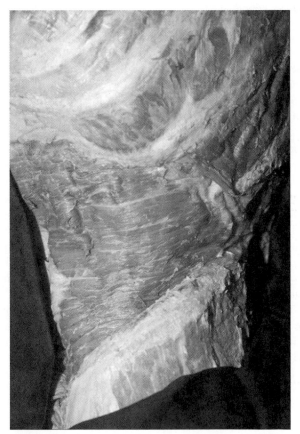

Figure 9-3 Transverse abdominis. (From DeRosa C: Functional anatomy of the lumbar spine and sacroiliac joint. In Proceedings from the 4th Montreal Proceedings of the Interdisciplinary World Congress on Low Back and Pelvic Pain, Montreal, 2001.)

vertebrae. These muscles are capable of controlling the stiffness of the spinal segments and postures of the lumbar spine. The lumbar multifidus with the segmental attachments is a prime example of a local muscle responsible for stiffening the lumbar segments. The posterior fibers of the obliquus internus abdominis and the transverse abdominis, which attach to the thoracolumbar fascia, form part of the local system. The medial fibers of the quadratus lumborum, iliocostalis lumborum pars lumborum, and the longissimus thoracis pars lumborum are also included in the local system (see Table 9-1).

The global muscle system includes the large, superficial muscles of the trunk that do not have direct attachment to the vertebrae. These muscles are the torque generators for spinal motion and act like guy ropes to control spinal orientation, balance the external loads to the trunk, and transfer load from the thorax to the pelvis.[10,13] The global muscles include the obliquus internus and externus abdominis, rectus abdominis, lateral fibers of the quadratus lumborum, longissimus thoracic pars thoracis, and iliocostalis lumborum pars thoracis (see Table 9-1).[13]

THE HIP CORE MUSCLES

Hip CORE muscle strengthening is an important part of the athlete's CORE program of exercises. The gluteus maximus and medius have always been considered strong stabilizers to the lumbar spine and pelvis. The gluteus maximus has a strong attachment to the thoracolumbar fascia proximally, and 80% of the gluteus maximus attaches into the iliotibial band distally. The gluteus maximus acts as a mobilizer. The gluteus maximus is an extensor and lateral rotator of the hip. In addition, the upper one half of the muscle abducts the hip, and the lower one half adducts the hip.[14] Decreased strength of the gluteus maximus in addition to decreased performance of the other posterior muscles of the hip, such as the gluteus medius posterior fibers, gluteus minimus, and the external rotators, compromise the control of the femur in the acetabulum. The anterior fibers of the gluteus medius abduct, medially rotate, and assist in flexion of the hip. In the clinical experience of the author of this chapter the anterior fibers of the gluteus medius are often found to be stronger than the posterior fibers of the gluteus medius in patients with lower extremity dysfunction. When testing the posterior fibers of the gluteus medius, the examiner must hold the leg in abduction and extension.

The piriformis muscle is a two-joint muscle extending over the sacral iliac joint and the hip joint. The piriformis extends, abducts, and externally rotates the hip. The obturator, internus and externus, and superior and inferior gemelli muscles are all lateral rotators. In the clinical experience of the author of this chapter, these lateral rotators frequently become weak. Nadler et al[15] indicated that alterations in side-to-side muscle strength might occur secondary to altered weight bearing, anthropometrics, lateral dominance, or gender. In this study athletes with previous lower extremity injury or low back pain were found to have differences in hip strength of the hip extensors and abductors, as compared with athletes without injury. Leetun et al[16] demonstrated that athletes who did not sustain an injury were significantly stronger in hip abduction and external rotation. Furthermore, analysis revealed that hip abduction and external rotator strength was the only useful predictor of injury status. A recent study by Tsai et al[17] demonstrated that the hip muscles play an important role in balancing the forces transferred between the lower body and upper extremities during the golf swing. Stronger hip muscles may provide better trunk stability. This study measured isometric hip abductor and adductor strength in golfers. A significantly stronger left hip abductor was found in the better golfers.

The semimembranosus and semitendinosus rotate the hip medially and flex and rotate the knee medially. The gracilis and pectineus muscles adduct the hip and internally rotate and flex the knee. The biceps femoris rotates the hip laterally and flexes and rotates the knee laterally. In the clinical experience of the author of this chapter, hamstring strains result from weakness of the CORE hip abductors, extensors, and rotators and CORE trunk muscles.

The psoas muscle function has been determined to be a primary hip flexor, along with the secondary hip flexor, the rectus femoris. The myoelectric evidence suggests that the psoas muscle activation is minimally linked to the spine demands.[8] The psoas counteracts the hip flexor torque created by the iliacus muscle. If the iliacus functioned alone, an anterior pelvic tilt force would force the spine into extension. The psoas provides stiffness between the spine and the pelvis and can be thought of as a stabilizer to the spine in the presence of a significant hip flexor torque.[1] The iliacus and psoas muscles produce compressive and anterior shearing forces to the spine.[13] Bogduk[18] points out that the psoas muscle is divided into anterior and posterior fibers. The posterior fibers arriving from the transverse processes of the lumbar vertebrae provide a compressive force to the spine, which is stabilizing. The anterior fibers make a larger contribution to hip flexion.

Evidence-Based Clinical Application

The iliopsoas participates strongly during sit-up exercises performed with the hips and knees flexed or extended.

The psoas muscle is activated during push-up exercises.

Maximum activity of the psoas occurs with resistance to hip flexion.[8]

FUNCTION OF THE TRUNK AND HIP MUSCLES

In the athlete the hip and trunk provide the stability and mobility needed to perform their sport. The greater the synchronization between the exact timing of the trunk muscles to stabilize movement and the hip muscles to create movement, the better the athlete performs with reduced risks of injury.

Trunk muscles transfer the forces to the hip and lower extremity. The trunk muscles are by design better stabilizers. Stiffness or stability of the lumbopelvic region is important for load transfer. The muscles of the trunk, pelvis, and lower limb, through a synchronized effort, provide a safe load transfer. The transfer of load protects the joints from the excessive forces of weight bearing, such as compressive and torsion forces. They provide a stabile spine and pelvis for the hip and lower leg to move against.

Performance in an athlete depends heavily on rotational movements of the trunk and hips. The initiation of powerful rotational movement, such as a baseball swing, golf swing, and tennis serve, occurs within the trunk and hips. Shaffer et al[19] demonstrated peak activity of the vastus medialis, hamstrings, gluteal muscles, erector spinae, and abdominal obliquus during a baseball swing. Watkins et al[20] indicated that the transfer of torque in an overhead-throwing athlete was achieved by the activation of the gluteus maximus, lumbar spine paraspinalis, and abdominal oblique muscles.

Watkins et al[20] emphasized the importance of hip and trunk muscles, the gluteus medius, the gluteus maximus, and lumbar spine erectors in stabilizing and controlling the loading response for maximum power and accuracy in golf swing. Tasi et al[17] demonstrated that significantly stronger left hip abduction strength was correlated with the more elite golfers and that hip strength in general was correlated to improved performance. Shaffer et al[1] established peak activity of the vastus medialis, hamstrings, gluteal muscles, erector spinae, and abdominal obliquus during a baseball swing. Watkins et al[21] confirmed the dynamic transfer of torque from the trunk to the lower extremity in professional baseball pitchers.

Several studies have demonstrated the capacity of the lumbar spine muscles to increase the spinal segmental stiffness.[22-25] Kaigle et al[22] demonstrated that combined activation of the muscles surrounding the spine including the multifidus, lumbar portions of the erector spinae, quadratus lumborum, and psoas stabilized the segmental movement in an injured segment. Goel et al[23] studied the effects of the action of the interspinalis, intertransversarii, the lumbar multifidus, and the quadratus lumborum. Activation of these muscles imparted stability to the ligamentous system, and the load bearing of the zygapophyseal joints increased. Panjabi et al[24] concluded that the intersegmental nature of the deep multifidus gave a significant advantage to the stability of the lumbar segment. Wilke et al[25] indicated that the multifidus was responsible for restricting the lumbar spinal range of motion in all directions except rotation.

In summary, the trunk and hip CORE muscles work together to attain a stable base around which movement occurs. A combined effect of the abdominals, back extensor muscles, and the lateral quadratus lumborum muscles provide the stability within the trunk to allow the hip muscles to develop explosive power. Isometric, concentric, and eccentric muscle contractions of the CORE muscles provide the movement and stability, through cocontraction of the agonist and antagonist muscles. The evaluation and CORE exercises are discussed in length in Chapters 12 and 13.

THE CONNECTION BETWEEN THE TRUNK AND HIP CORE TO THE UPPER QUADRANT CORE

For the purposes of this chapter, the muscles of the upper quadrant CORE include the rotators of the glenohumeral joint and scapula. On the basis of the author's clinical experience, the importance of rotation range of motion of the glenohumeral joint and the strength of the scapula and glenohumeral rotator muscles in the overhead-throwing athlete are critical in preventing injuries and improving performance. Monte et al[26] strengthened only the glenohumeral rotators in skilled tennis players and were able to demonstrate a significant increase in the velocity of the tennis serve. Wooden et al[27] demonstrated in teenage baseball pitchers a significant increase in ball velocity after strengthening the glenohumeral rotators.

Although more emphasis has been placed on the lower CORE for prevention and improvement in the ability to swing a golf club or a baseball bat, several studies have demonstrated an important role of the upper quadrant CORE.[28-30] Jobe et al[28] studied the muscle activity, in professional golfers, of the rotator cuff, deltoid, pectoralis major, and the latissimus dorsi muscles during a golf swing. The study used electromyographic analysis and high-speed photography to determine the muscle activity during the phases of the golf swing. The study demonstrated that the subscapularis muscle was the most active of all the rotator cuff muscles throughout the swing. The supraspinatus, infraspinatus, and all portions of the deltoid muscle had low levels of activity throughout the swing. The most active mobilizers of the upper limbs during the golf swing were the pectoralis major and latissimus dorsi (Figure 9-4). The previously mentioned muscle groups seemed to provide power bilaterally to the golf swing. In another study, using electromyographic analysis of the shoulder muscles during a golf swing demonstrated similar results.[29] The infraspinatus and supraspinatus muscles were active predominantly at the extremes of shoulder range of motion, and the deltoid muscles were again relatively noncontributory. Once again, the subscapularis, pectoralis major, and latissimus dorsi muscles were the propulsive muscles of the swing and maintained activity during acceleration and the forward swing. Finally, Kato et al[30] described the role of the scapular muscles in the golf swing. The study determined that the golf swing and uncoiling action require that the scapular muscles work in synchrony to maximize swing arc and club head speed. The anterior serratus muscle activity was the most active through all phases of the swing, which could indicate that fatigue could be an etiology of shoulder problems in high-demand golfers. Kato et al's study also indicated the stabilizing effect of the rhomboid and levator scapulae muscles during the majority of the swing.

Vleeming et al[31] and Snijders et al[32] described a connection of muscle systems that stabilize the pelvis between the thorax and legs. Four slings of muscle systems exist: (1) The posterior oblique sling contains the connection between the latissimus dorsi and the gluteus maximus through the thoracodorsal

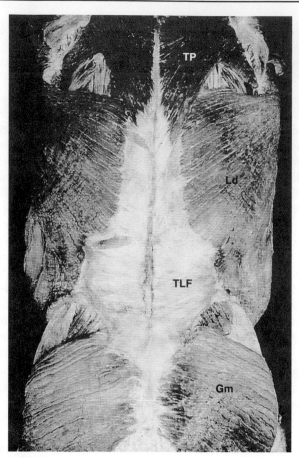

Figure 9-4 The latissimus dorsi is an important muscle to the posterior oblique sling, connecting the upper quadrant CORE to the lower quadrant CORE by its connection to the thoracolumbar fascia. (From Willard FH: The muscular, ligamentous and neural structure of the low back and its relation to back pain. In Vleeming A, Mooney V, Dorman T, et al, editors: *Movement, stability and low back pain*, Edinburgh, 1997, Churchill Livingstone.)

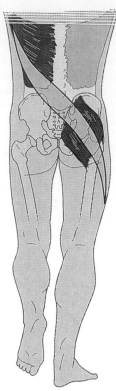

Figure 9-5 Posterior oblique sling contains the connection between the latissimus dorsi and the gluteus maximus through the thoracodorsal fascia. (Redrawn from Vleeming A, Pool-Goudzwaard AL, Stoeckart R, et al: The posterior layer of the thoracolumbar fascia: its function in load transfer from spine to legs, *Spine* 20:753, 1995.)

fascia (Figure 9-5); (2) the anterior oblique sling contains connections among the external oblique, the anterior abdominal fascia, and the contralateral internal oblique abdominals and the adductors of the thigh; (3) the longitudinal sling connects the peronei, the biceps femoris, the sacrotuberous ligament, the deep lamina of the thoracodorsal fascia, and the erector spinae; and (4) the lateral sling contains the gluteus medius/minimus and tensor fascia latea and the lateral stabilizers for the thoracopelvis region. These integrated muscle systems produce slings of forces that assist in transfer of load.

As previously noted, the posterior sling is the connection between the upper quadrant CORE and the lower quadrant CORE. Transfer of torque from the upper quadrant to the lower quadrant is important to the athlete. As noted earlier, the serratus and trapezius muscle groups are largely responsible for dynamic stability of the scapula as it moves through the shoulder range of motion. One could argue that the function and strength of the latissimus depends on the position of the humeral head on the glenoid. After evaluating numerous athletes, a clinical observation of this author demonstrates that scapula asymmetry alters the central position of the humerus on the glenoid and leads to muscle weakness of the glenohumeral rotators. Because the latissimus muscle is an internal rotator and depressor of the humeral head, posture of the scapula may be important to the mechanical advantage of the latissimus muscle in order to perform mobility and stabilizing roles within the shoulder and the trunk.

CORE DYSFUNCTION

The lower kinetic chain is a linkage system, which includes a series of joints, such as the ankle, knees, hips, and trunk, making possible the transmission of forces into the trunk and hips during running, jumping, kicking, and throwing. Dysfunction of any one of the joints within the lower kinetic chain linkage system may result in dysfunction elsewhere within the chain. Kinetic chain injuries may result from muscle imbalances, joint restrictions, and inadequate rehabilitation of previous injuries. Beckman and Buchanan[33] noted a significant delay in latency of the gluteus medius muscle in patients with chronic ankle instability as compared with normal controls. Devita et al[34] demonstrated alteration in firing of the proximal hip musculature in patients with anterior cruciate insufficiency. Jaramillo et al[35] found significant strength deficits of the ipsilateral gluteus medius in patients who had knee surgery. Yamamoto demonstrated an increased injury rate in individuals with weaker hamstrings and a decreased hamstring-to-quadriceps ratio.[36]

Nadler et al[37] demonstrated that only in female athletes the left hip abductors were weaker. This study indicated that female athletes had a more significant probability of requiring treatment for low back pain, secondary to the hip abductor weakness. The hip musculature plays a significant role in transferring forces from the lower extremity to the spine during upright activities and theoretically may influence the development of low back pain. Poor endurance and delayed firing of the hip extensors (gluteus maximus) and abductors (gluteus medius) have been noted in individuals with lower extremity instability and low back pain.[37-39] Hip extensors play a major role in stabilizing the pelvis during trunk rotation or when the center of gravity is grossly shifted.[37]

As previously noted, Leetun et al[16] demonstrated that CORE stability played an important role in injury prevention during sporting activities. Athletes who experienced an injury over the course of the season generally demonstrated lower CORE stability measures than those who did not. The results of the study indicated that in an athletic population, isometric hip strength measures, particularly in abduction and external rotation, are more accurate predictors of back and lower extremity injury than trunk endurance measures.[16]

Management of overuse injuries within the upper and lower limbs must include an assessment of CORE deficits, followed by the appropriate treatment. According to the clinical experience of the author of this chapter, patellofemoral pain, hamstring strains, lateral hip pain, chronic ankle sprains, and in some cases low back pain in the athlete result from lower-quadrant CORE muscle deficits. Mascal et al[40] reported that strengthening the hip, pelvis, and trunk musculature resulted in a significant reduction in patellofemoral pain and improved lower-extremity kinematics and the patients' ability to return to their original levels of function. The hip abductors, extensors, and internal/external rotators were the key muscles strengthened. Ireland et al[41] measured hip abduction and external rotation strength in 15 female subjects with patellofemoral pain. The subjects demonstrated 26% less hip abduction strength and 36% less hip external rotation strength than similar age-matched controls. Lastly, Sherry and Best[42] compared two rehabilitation programs in the treatment of acute hamstring strains. This study demonstrated that progressive agility and trunk stabilization exercises are more effective than a program emphasizing isolated hamstring stretching and strengthening in promoting return to sports and preventing a recurrence of the hamstring injury.

The literature is void of a relationship between overuse injuries of the upper quadrant CORE and muscle strength deficits. However, based on this author's clinical experience, assessment of muscle strength of the glenohumeral and scapula rotators is essential in the treatment of shoulder problems in the athlete.

SUMMARY

This chapter has identified the muscles of the upper and lower quadrant CORE (see Table 9-1). The upper quadrant CORE muscles include the rotators of the glenohumeral joint and scapula. The lower quadrant CORE comprises the muscles in the trunk and hip. In both cases the CORE is an area in which mobility and stability occur simultaneously. Electromyographic analysis and strengthening programs involving the muscles of the upper and lower quadrant CORE demonstrate that athletic performance is based on the mobilizing and stabilizing effect these muscles have on the shoulder, trunk, and hip.

Dysfunction of the upper and lower quadrant CORE can result in shoulder, elbow, low back, and lower limb pain and injuries. The author of this chapter has discovered through clinical observation that muscle imbalances within the CORE can be a major etiology of poor athletic performance, which can lead to injury. Strengthening of the upper and lower quadrant CORE muscles is oftentimes the major treatment approach for many overuse injuries identified in the athlete.

REFERENCES

1. McGill S: *Low back disorders: evidence-based prevention and rehabilitation,* Champaign, Ill, 2002, Human Kinetics.
2. Bogduk N: *Clinical anatomy of the lumbar spine and sacrum,* ed 3, Edinburgh, 1997, Churchill Livingstone.
3. Nitz AJ, Peck D: Comparison of muscle spindle concentrations in large and small human epaxial muscles acting in parallel combinations, *Am Surg* 52:273-277, 1986.
4. Bogduk N: A reappraisal of the anatomy of the human erector spinae, *J Anat* 131(3):525, 1980.
5. McGill SM, Norman RW: Effects of an anatomically detailed erector spinae model on L4/L5 disc compression and shear, *J Biomechanics* 20(6):591, 1987.
6. Biering-Sorensen F: Physical measurements as risk indicators for low-back trouble over a one-year period, *Spine* 9:106-119, 1984.
7. McGill SM: A myoelectrically based dynamic 3-D model to predict loads on lumbar spine tissues during lateral bending, *J Biomechanics* 25(4):395-399, 1992.
8. Juker D, McGill SM, Kropf P: Quantitative intramuscular myoelectric activity of lumbar portions of psoas and the abdominal wall during cycling, *J Applied Biomechanics* 14(4):428-438, 1998.
9. Porterfield JA, DeRosa C: *Mechanical low back pain: perspectives in functional anatomy,* Philadelphia, 1998, Saunders.
10. Richardson C, Hodges P, Hides J: *Therapeutic exercise for lumbopelvic stabilization. A motor control approach for the treatment and prevention of low back pain,* Philadelphia, 2004, Elsevier.
11. Hodges PW: Changes in motor planning of feedforward postural responses of the trunk muscle in low back pain, *Exp Brain Res* 141:261-266, 2001.

12. McGill SM: The kinetic potential of the lumbar trunk musculature about three orthogonal orthopaedic axes in extreme postures, *Spine* 16(7):809-815, 1991.

13. Bergmark A: Stability of the lumbar spine. A study in mechanical engineering, *Acta Orthopaedica Scand* 230: 20-24, 1989.

14. Sahrmann S: *Diagnosis and treatment of movement impairment syndromes,* St Louis, 2002, Mosby.

15. Nadler S, Malanga G, Deprince M, et al: The relationship between lower extremity injuries, low back pain, and hip muscle strength in male and female collegiate athletes, *Clin J Sport Med* 10(2):89-97, 2000.

16. Leetun D, Ireland ML, Willson JD, et al: Core stability measures as risk factors for lower extremity injury in athletes, *Med Sci Sports Ex* 36(6):926-934, 2004.

17. Tasi YS, Sell TC, Myers JB, et al: The relationship between hip muscle strength and golf performance, *Med Sci Sports Ex* 36(5):2-9, 2004

18. Bogduk N, Pearcy M, Hadfield G: Anatomy and biomechanics of the psoas major, *Clin Biomechanics* 7:109-119, 1992.

19. Saffer B, Jobe F, Perry J, et al: Baseball batting. An electromyographic study, *Clin Orthop* 292:285-293, 1993.

20. Watkins, Uppal J, Perry M, et al: Dynamic electromyographics analysis of trunk musculature in professional golfers, *Am J Sports Med* 24:535-538, 1996.

21. Watkins RG: Dynamic EMG analysis of torque transfer in professional baseball pitchers, *Spine* 14(4):404-408, 1989.

22. Kaigle AM, Holm SH, Hansson TH: Experimental instability in the lumbar spine, *Radiology* 55:145-149, 1995.

23. Goel VK, Gilbertson L: A combined finite element and optimization of lumbar spine mechanics with and without muscles, *Spine* 18:1531-1541, 1993.

24. Panjabi M, Abumi K, Duranceau J, et al: Spinal stability and intersegmental muscle forces. A biomechanical model, *Spine* 14:194-200, 1989.

25. Wilke HJ, Wolf S, Claes LE, et al: Stability increase of the lumbar spine with different muscles groups. A biomechanical in vitro study, *Spine* 20:192-198, 1995.

26. Monte MA, Cohen DB, Campbell KR, et al: Isokinetic concentric versus eccentric training of shoulder rotators with functional evaluation of performance enhancement in elite tennis players, *Am J Sports Med* 22(4) 513-517, 1994.

27. Wooden M, Greenfield B, Johanson M, et al: Effects of strength training in throwing velocity and shoulder muscle performance in teenage baseball pitchers, *J Ortho Sports Phys Ther* 15(5):223-227, 1992.

28. Jobe FW, Moynes DR, Antonelli DJ: Rotator cuff function during golf swing, *Am J Sports Med* 14(5):388-392, 1986.

29. Pink M, Jobe FW, Perry J: Electromyographic analysis of the shoulder during a golf swing, *Am J Sports Med* 18(2):137-140, 1990.

30. Kao JT, Pink M, Jobe FW, et al: Electromyographic analysis of the scapular muscles during a golf swing, *Am J Sports Med* 23:19-23, 1995.

31. Vleeming A, Pool-Goudzwaard AL, Stoeckart R, et al: The posterior layer of the thoracolumbar fascia: its function in load transfer from spine to legs, *Spine* 20:753-762, 1995.

32. Snijders CJ, Vleeming A, Stoeckart R: Transfer of lumbosacral load in iliac bones and legs. 1: Biomechanics of self-bracing of the sacroiliac joints and its significance for treatment and exercise, *Clin Biomechanics* 8:285-292, 1993.

33. Beckman SM, Buchanan TS: Ankle inversion injury and hypermobility: effect on hip and ankle electromyography onset latency, *Arch Phys Ked Rehabil* 76:1138-1143, 1995.

34. Devita P, Hunter PB, Skelly WA: Effects of functional knee brace in biomechanics of running, *Med Sci Sports Exer* 24:797-806, 1992.

35. Jaramillo J, Worrell TW, Ingersoll CD: Hip isometric strength following knee surgery, *J Orthop Sport Phys Ther* 20:160-165, 1994.

36. Yammamoto T: Relationship between hamstring strains and leg muscle strength. A follow up study of collegiate track and field athletes, *J Sport Med Phys Fitness* 33:194-199, 1993.

37. Nadler SF, Malanga GA, Fienberg JH, et al: Functional performance deficits in athletes with previous lower extremity injury, *Clin Sport Med* 12(2):73-78, 2002.

38. Kankaanpaa M, Taimela D, Laaksonen O, et al: Back and hip extensor fatigability in chronic low back pain patients, and controls, *Arch Phys Med Rehabil* 79:412-417, 1998.

39. Leinonen V, Kankaapaa O, Airaksinen O, et al: Back and hip extensor activities during trunk flexion/extension: effects of low back pain and rehabilitation, *Arch Phys Med Rehabil* 81:32-37, 2000.

40. Mascal C, Landel R, Powers C: Management of patellofemoral pain targeting hip, pelvis, and trunk muscles function: 2 case reports, *J Ortho Sports Phys Ther* 33(11):647-660, 2003.

41. Ireland ML, Wilson JD, Ballantyne BT, et al: Hip strength in females with and without patellofemoral pain, *J Ortho Sports Phys Ther* 33(11):671-676, 2003.

42. Sherry MA, Best TM: A comparison of 2 rehabilitation programs in the treatment of acute hamstring strains, *J Ortho Sports Phys Ther* 34(3):116-125, 2004.

From the CORE to the Floor—Interrelationships*

LEARNING OBJECTIVES

After studying this chapter, the reader will be able to do the following:

1. Identify interdependency, linkage, and function between proximal and distal joints in the lower extremity
2. Describe abnormal mechanics from the foot up the kinetic chain
3. Describe abnormal mechanics from the core down the kinetic chain
4. List structural malalignments of the lower extremity and their influence on lower extremity pathomechanics
5. Identify features of gait and functional assessment
6. Describe functional exercise concepts that maximize core-to-the-foot interdependency
7. Summarize the science of foot orthotic invention in sport.
8. Describe foot orthotic strategies in the treatment of abnormal foot mechanics and common pain patterns

During sport activity, the lower extremity moves in a myriad of motion planes with linkage to the body's core. Speed variations, changes in directions, upper extremity requirements, and opposing player disturbances all challenge the athlete's postural stability. Restoration of dysfunction in the athlete must be viewed from a total kinetic chain, sport-specific, and core-to-the-floor perspective. Recovery from injury depends on reestablishing mobility and neuromuscular control, often with underlying factors of less than optimal structural alignment. In the spontaneous environment of sport, the body's core provides muscular stability as the foot and ankle serve as the interface to the grass, court, or track surface. The foot and ankle provide shock absorption, contact balance, and spontaneous propulsion in all motion planes. The body's core is interdependent with the foot and ankle because it benefits from mobility and stability characteristics from which it can absorb and generate

*The author extends acknowledgment to Diane Voelker, Hamot Medical Center, for her typing and process expertise and to Robert Madia for his photography skills.

forces required during running and jumping in sport.[1] Often in sport rehabilitation, a joint- or muscle-specific treatment approach is taken. Practitioners can miss total kinetic chain interdependencies and lead the athlete through suboptimal rehabilitation. A joint- or muscle-specific treatment focus may place added overuse stress to the area that is painful. A total kinetic chain approach, however, with attention given from above and below the injured area, assists mechanoreceptor stimulation and imparts functional mobility and stability feed to the injured site.

Sources from above and below the injured site are often the primary origins of dysfunction. Consider the knee positioned halfway between the body's center of gravity at $\frac{1}{2}$ inch anterior to the sacral segment and the foot–ground interface. Muscle control influences driven from the trunk down that affect knee and patellar stability are discussed in this chapter. The foot's role in the mechanics of concomitant tibial rotation influences to the lower extremity is reviewed. This chapter describes the interrelationships of normal and abnormal core, knee, and lower leg mechanics. Treatment strategies focus on a total kinetic chain functional exercise approach and foot orthotic intervention.

INTERRELATIONSHIPS OF THE CORE, KNEE, ANKLE, AND FOOT

As the athlete moves, responds, accelerates, and decelerates, dependency exists between the stability and power offered by the body's core and the mobility and kinesthetic directives to the kinetic chain provided by the foot and ankle (Figure 10-1).[2] Kibler[3] describes the significant role the trunk and scapula play in the tennis athlete. His premise for upper extremity overuse pathophysiology is that altered proximal function places increased burden on the distal joint. Kibler[3] describes the kinetic chain linkage in the tennis stroke that allows ground reaction forces and large leg and trunk muscles to generate forces that are summated and passed distally with contributions from each successive link: legs, trunk, shoulder, elbow, and wrist.

Evidence-Based Clinical Application: Core Trunk Influence to the Upper Extremity

Kibler[3] writes that during the tennis stroke 51% of the total kinetic energy and 54% of the total force are developed in the leg-hip-trunk linkage. The large forces developed in the proximal links are funneled through the shoulder to the hand and racquet by soft tissue constraint systems of the shoulder. The shoulder relies on its position as a link in the kinetic chain and depends on the generation and transfer of forces from the lower extremity and core to the hand.

Evidence-Based Clinical Application: Proximal Segment Weaknesses That Result in Distal Segment Pathology

A strong core aids muscle stabilization, balance, coordination, and kinesthesia. Nicholas and Marino[4] reported on the thigh strength of 134 athletes with residual chronic pain patterns after their injury was thought to have been healed. The authors report that their foot and ankle–injured athletes demonstrated significant weakness of the hip abductors and adductors when compared with the uninvolved side through isokinetic testing.

Similarly, jumping and jump landing require summated acceleration and deceleration forces between the foot and the core. Nicholas and Marino[4] describe this kinetic chain linkage enabling stronger muscles to support weaker movements. They propose that weakness of one segment can disrupt the entire kinetic chain and eventually promote weakness that can migrate throughout the chain. They examined the relationship between proximal thigh strength in athletes with lower extremity pain patterns and related deficiencies to ankle pain.

Similarly, Beckman and Buchanan[5] studied the interrelationship between hip muscle recruitment and ankle instability.

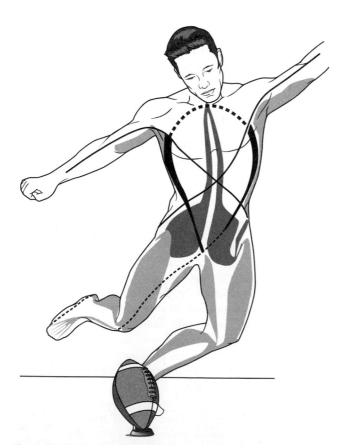

Figure 10-1 From the trunk to the foot, interdependencies exist as the kinetic chain acts and reacts in sport.

They describe a neuromuscular response of lowered hip muscle activation thresholds of the gluteus medius in response to a protective steady state ability to respond to ankle inversion.

Bullock-Saxton et al[6] found alterations in electromyographic activity of proximal core muscles in subjects who had sustained a significant ankle sprain. Gribble et al,[7] when studying the effect of chronic ankle instability on postural control, proposed that disruptions to a joint may lead to altered neural activity and compensatory muscle recruitment at neighboring joints and corresponding movement patterns. The authors state "the injured athlete may be able to complete a gross motor task, but the method of completion may be altered and less than optimal and/or efficient creating the potential threat of reinjury."[7]

Postural stability is defined as the ability to control the body's center of mass within specific boundaries (stability limits).[8] It depends on mobility, stability, and kinesthesia from the core to the floor. Consider jump landing with poor core stability resulting in less than optimal control of postural orientation on landing. Body sway and postural instability require the foot to act as a balance adapter and adjuster. If end range of motion is required, the foot may load beyond its physiological limits and become injured. Hewett et al[9] write that an athlete is at risk for injury if the lower extremity is not properly aligned or if the foot is in an unusual position on landing from a jump. The avoidance of excessive valgus or varus forces at the knee on jump landing minimizes the risk of knee injury.[10] A total kinetic chain, core-to-the-floor thinking process enables the practitioner to think beyond the area of localized pain to the multifaceted potential causes of mechanical breakdown. When considering patellofemoral joint pain, an understanding of kinetic chain influences is imperative. Post et al[11] describe patellofemoral pathogenesis in dynamic foot-to-the hip function terms: "bony malalignment, joint geometry, soft tissue restraint, neuromuscular control and functional demands combine to produce symptoms as a result of abnormally directed loads that exceed the physiologic threshold of the tissues" (Figure 10-2).[11]

Weakness of hip abductors, extensors, and external rotators is related to the body's ability to control frontal and transverse plane motion at the knee (Figure 10-3).[12] Targeting core hip muscles through strength facilitation has been shown to alleviate patellofemoral pain and change knee mechanics.[12,13]

Evidence-Based Clinical Application: Targeting Hip, Pelvis, and Trunk Muscle Function in the Treatment of Patellofemoral Pain

Mascal et al[12] reports on two patellofemoral joint patients with weakness of hip abductors, extensors, and external rotators as demonstrated by hand-held dynometry testing. A 14-week period of training included a progression from non–weight-bearing exercise, weight-bearing exercise, to functional training. Posttesting demonstrated a greater than 50% increase in gluteus medius force production in a greater than 90% gluteus maximus force production in these cases with objective kinematic improvement in step-down tasks, as well as a significant reduction in visual analog scale pain rating.

Fulkerson[14] correlates hip weakness to anterior cruciate ligament injury and patellofemoral pain patterns. He particularly identifies hip external rotators as key stabilizers to dampen the functional internal rotation of the hip during landing mechanics. McConnell[15] describes exercise strategies in the treatment of patellofemoral pain with a focus on the gluteus medius as being critical to normal mechanics of the patellofemoral joint. Gluteus medius posterior fiber training aims to decrease excessive closed chain hip internal rotation and its resultant knee valgus vector force.

Ireland et al[16] found hip weakness related to patellofemoral joint pain. When comparing patellofemoral pain subjects with normals, a 26% decrease in hip abduction strength and a 36% decrease in external rotation strength were found in the group with patellofemoral joint dysfunction. Leetun et al[17] also found a relationship in pain patterns related to hip abduction and hip external rotation weakness. Forty-one injuries were studied in 140 athletes, and core stability measures were found as primary risk factors for injury in basketball and cross-country college athletes.

Concomitant with hip muscle stability, the abdominals provide a critical role in core stabilization for kinetic chain activity. Abdominal, paraspinal, and pelvic muscles integrate upper and lower extremity motions. Core trunk muscles act as synergistic stabilizers[4,18,19] as they act as a hub where trunk and ground reactions converge and are modulated.[20] Hodges and Richardson[21] found that the transverse abdominis is the first muscle that is active during movement of the lower limb following contralateral weight shifting. They provide evidence that the central nervous system initiates contraction of abdominal muscles in a feed-forward manner in advance of lower limb motion, hence the interdependency and linkage between the trunk and lower limb in the control of postural stability.

ABNORMAL MECHANICS OF THE LOWER EXTREMITY LINKAGE SYSTEM

The lower extremity is designed as a locomotor unit providing shock absorption, stability, propulsion, and energy conserva-

tion during sport activity.[22] The accumulative amount of force generation and dissipation that the kinetic chain responds to is enormous. During running and jumping sports, the lower kinetic chain moves in various forms of airborne-to-landing impacts thousands of times each training and competition session.[23] Running 5 km requires an estimated 2500 foot fall with landing forces described as high as 8 times body weight.[1] Jump landing forces are reported to be as high as 20 times body weight.[24] Simple stairway descent requires shock absorption of as much as 3.7 times body weight.[4] Abnormal loading and landing mechanics, when performed repetitively, can place microstress and strain throughout the lower extremity. Inflexibility, hypermobility, neuromuscular weakness, altered kinesthesia, and structural malalignment contribute individually or in combination to abnormal running and jumping mechanics.

Foot and Ankle Influences to the Kinetic Chain (Bottom Up)

Mobility and structure of the foot and ankle greatly influence proximal segments of the lower extremity during shock absorption and propulsion requirements.[25] The foot and ankle act as the first unloaders to ground reaction forces protecting

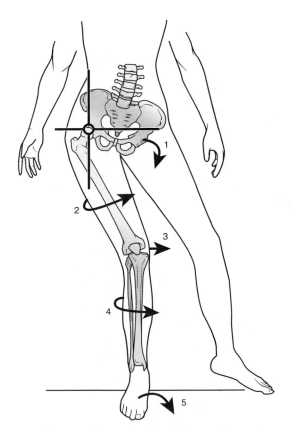

Figure 10-2 Schematic showing kinetic chain reaction to abnormal functional alignment potentially related to weakness or structural malalignment, or both: *1,* contralateral pelvic crest drop, *2,* excessive femoral internal rotation, *3,* knee adduction/valgus, *4,* excessive tibial internal rotation, *5,* excessive foot pronation.

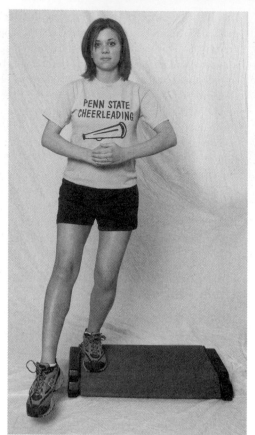
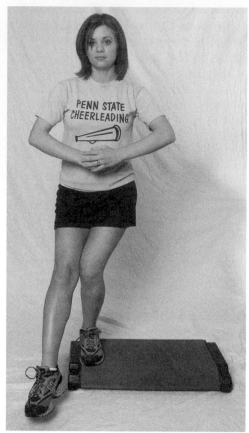

Figure 10-3 A, Anterior balance reach test demonstrating neutral knee postural stability. **B,** Weakness at posterior proximal hip and quadriceps produces femoral adduction and internal rotation with resultant knee valgus stress.

the entire kinetic chain from shock impact. Subtalar and midtarsal mobility enable triplanar pronation and supination, providing the kinetic chain with shock absorption and torque conversion of the femoral and tibial rotation at the foot–ground interface.[26] The foot is uniquely designed with 26 bones and more than 30 articulations, each with 6 degrees of freedom of movement to serve as the body's interface with the ground.[25] During jump landing the foot acts to decrease the downward velocity of the center of mass, thereby attenuating impact force.[2] The foot responds to ground reaction forces when jump landing from a plantarflexed position and absorbs landing forces by dorsiflexing at the ankle and pronating at the foot. Bobbert describes the angular velocity of foot dorsiflexion during jump landing as ranging from 578 degrees per second to 1025 degrees per second with varying heights of 20 cm and 60 cm, respectively.[27] Valiant and Cavanagh[28] reported that basketball players who land flat-footed versus the typical toe heel pattern had increased vertical impact forces and peak landing pressures on landing.

Dananberg and Guiliano[30] write that the rocker effect of ankle dorsiflexion, calcaneus bone curvature, and hallux extension while walking and running serve to absorb landing forces and propel the body forward in the sagittal plane (Figure 10-4). Motion restrictions with sagittal plane ankle dorsiflexion or hallux extension, or both, will alter gait mechanics, shock absorption, and propulsion. Restoration of restricted foot and

---

Evidence-Based Clinical Application: Sensory Influences of the Foot on the Lower Kinetic Chain

Sensory deprivation of the feet has been shown to significantly alter lower extremity kinetic chain response and postural reflexes. O'Connell[29] reported on the postural reflex response of four subjects ejected from a swing under the conditions of controlled jumps, blindfolded jumps, and anesthetized feet (20 minutes with feet suspended in ice water). During the controlled drops each subject landed and achieved an effortless erect posture. When visually deprived (subject blindfolded), three of the subjects responded with greater knee flexion than during the controlled ejections. However, with subjects blindfolded and feet chilled in ice water, no subject was able to regain erect posture as their postural reflex and postural stability was completely impaired. The necessity for feedback from sensory organs of the feet to coordinate a positive supporting reaction of the kinetic chain was demonstrated.

ankle motion in the athlete relates to improved shock absorption and propulsion throughout the kinetic chain. Functional retraining through dynamic mobilization and weight-bearing exercise purportedly stimulates a neuromuscular response.[31-33] Mulligan[33] writes that when motion is gained in weight

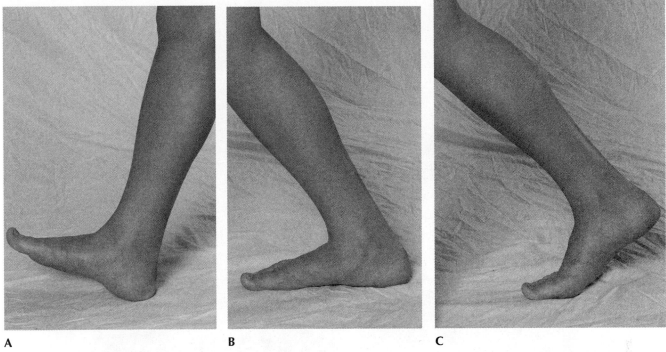

Figure 10-4 Rocker effect in the sagittal plane. **A,** Calcaneus bone curvature. **B,** Ankle dorsiflexion. **C,** Hallux extension.

bearing, it is better retained in function than non–weight-bearing techniques (Figures 10-5 through 10-10). Kaufman et al[34] describe insufficient ankle dorsiflexion as a primary risk factor for injury among 449 Navy Seal candidates. They relate the 149 injuries to a prescreening assessment profile of flexibility and foot mechanics when following the Navy Seal candidates over 25 weeks of intensive training. Ankle dorsiflexion restriction, abnormal pronation, and supination foot mechanics, as well as hypermobility of ankle inversion, were all found to be risk factors for this Navy Seal group (Figures 10-11 through 10-12).

Evidence-Based Clinical Application: Static Stretching versus Dynamic Functional Stretching

Improving gastrosoleus flexibility is particularly difficult due to the shortening influence of the muscle tendon unit during sleeping hours when the foot is in end range of plantar flexion. Youdas et al[35] reported on the effects of a 6-week program of static calf musculature stretching with 101 adults. A 6-week once-per-day static stretching regimen for up to 2 minutes was not sufficient to increase active dorsiflexion range of motion in this group.

Functional gastrosoleus stretching exercises include dynamic movement and neuromuscular training into the direction of desired motion. Ryerson and Levit[31] describe movement reeducation training to stimulate firing patterns of the foot and ankle with weight shift and foot posturing strategies for neuromuscular reeducation.

Closed kinetic chain pronation defined as calcaneal eversion, talar adduction, and talar plantar flexion links to tibial rotation and knee flexion and thereby directly influences the knee and patellofemoral joints.[26] Hreljac et al[36] write that foot pronation during stance provides dissipation of stress protecting the lower extremity by attenuating high-impact forces. When comparing injury-free runners with runners with a history of lower extremity pain patterns, they found that the injury-free group pronated more rapidly during the stance phase of running. They postulated that this may have assured foot stability before push off. Excessive, inadequate, or mistimed pronation and supination relate to deficiency in the lower extremities' ability to absorb shock, provide ground reaction stability, and propel the lower extremity forward. The repetitive nature of abnormal foot mechanics can cascade into a myriad of lower extremity injury patterns including iliotibial band syndrome, patellofemoral dysfunction, stress fracture, ankle instability, posterior tibialis tendon dysfunction, shin splints, Achilles' tendonitis, and plantar fasciitis.[37-47] Williams and McClay[48] studied injury history patterns and lower extremity mechanics in a group of 20 runners classified as high-arched pes cavus feet and 20 runners with low-arched planus feet (Figure 10-13). Low-arched runners had significantly more medial, soft tissue, and knee injuries, while high-arched pes cavus foot types sustained more lateral, bony, and foot injuries. The authors describe that the injury patterns correlated planus foot types with greater rearfoot motion and higher velocities stressing more medial and soft tissue structures. Conversely, high-arched cavus foot types run with stiffer gait patterns and higher vertical load rates, sustaining more shock-related problems, such as stress fractures.

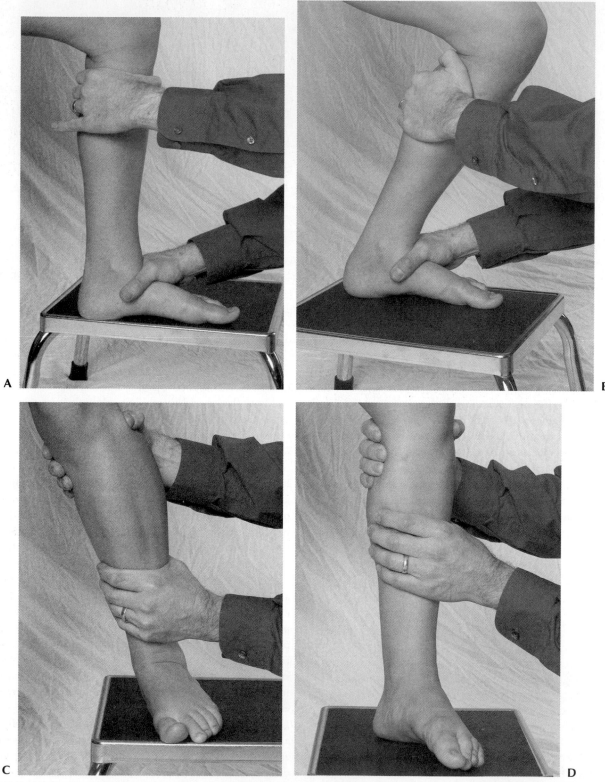

Figure 10-5 Mobilization with motion. **A** and **B**, Ankle dorsiflexion. **C** and **D**, Subtalar pronation and supination linked with tibial rotation and knee flexion-extension.

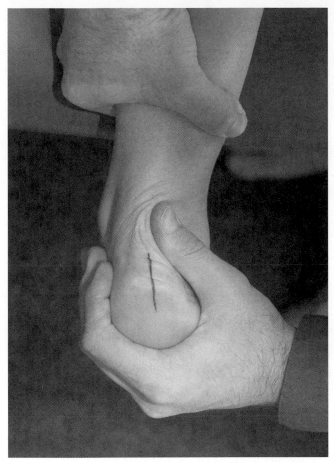

Figure 10-6 Open chain calcaneal eversion mobilization to increase pronation motion.

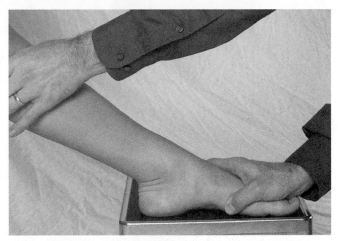

Figure 10-7 Top-down–influenced ankle plantar flexion stretching in semi–weight bearing.

The cavovarus-type foot strikes the ground in an inverted position, and rearfoot eversion motion is typically limited, diminishing the shock-absorbing capacity of the subtalar joint. This excessively supinating foot type commonly presents with a plantarflexed first metatarsal. Laterally directed overload can occur with resultant ankle instability, Jones fracture of the fifth metatarsal, metatarsalgia, peroneal tendon pathologies, and sesamoiditis.[43] Linkage to excessive external rotation of the tibia may result in varus strain at the knee joint and iliotibial band friction syndrome.[53]

Core Influences to the Kinetic Chain (Top Down)

Proximal core weakness at the trunk, pelvis, and hip has significant ramifications for the athlete's ability for shock absorption and postural stability. The gluteus medius, upper gluteus maximus, and posterior tensor fascia lata stabilize the pelvis in the frontal plane during rapid transfer of the body weight onto the loading leg when running (Figure 10-14).[22] These muscles provide an active lateral stabilization of the pelvis over the hip. Muscle stabilization is required because the base of the body vector shifts to the supporting foot while controlling the center of gravity. Weight transfer while running produces a large medial torque at the hip that causes the unsupported side of the pelvis to drop, hence the stabilization requirement of hip muscles firing at approximately 35% of maximal muscle tension even with simple walking. Internal rotation of the limb in the transverse plane also must be controlled during the loading response. The lower extremity is neurophysiologically wired for concomitant knee flexion, tibial and femoral internal rotation, and foot pronation when loading from airborne to landing postures. Muscular stability provides boundary to this knee flexion, hip internal rotation, and hip adduction pattern. Excessive internal rotation and adduction of the femur lead to potentially injurious transverse and frontal plane motions. Hip internal rotation is decelerated by the external rotational effects of the gluteus maximus muscle action.

During running, maximum pronation occurs at approximately 45% of the total stance time when measured by rearfoot calcaneal eversion angle.[49] Similarly, maximum knee flexion occurs also at approximately 45% of stance, followed by kinetic chain propulsion with knee extension. Subtalar joint pronation is linked to tibial internal rotation and knee flexion.[11] The complementary relationship between knee flexion and pronation provides kinetic chain loading and shock absorption. Knee extension and concomitant lower leg external rotation and supination provides propulsion stability. Buchbinder et al[50] theorized that excessive pronation causes prolonged lower extremity internal rotation in late stance phase when it would normally undergo external rotation. Disruption of this normal timing relationship may result in tissue overload and injury patterns throughout the lower kinetic chain.[1] The relationship of excessive pronation to patellofemoral mechanics is well accepted.[51] McClay and Manal[52] describe the increased valgus position of the tibial femoral joint related to excessive foot pronation. Powers et al[13] report on an alignment profile of excessive foot pronation; excessive heel angle; and an associated increased, laterally directed resultant quadriceps and patellar tendon forces in the frontal plane. They describe the lateral resultant force production with increased contact forces and contact pressures on the lateral aspect of the patellofemoral joint.

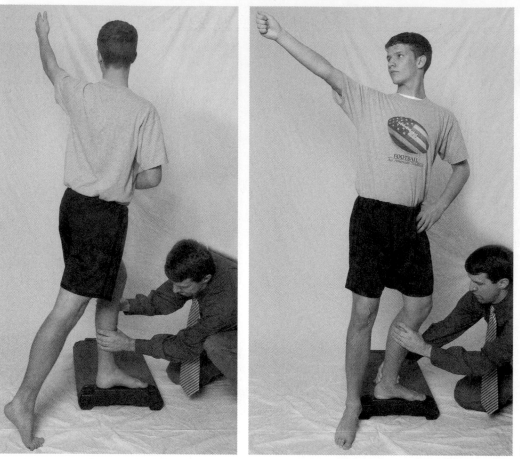

Figure 10-8 **A,** Therapist-assisted mobility training linking supination with tibial external rotation. **B,** Pronation and tibial internal rotation–linked mobility training.

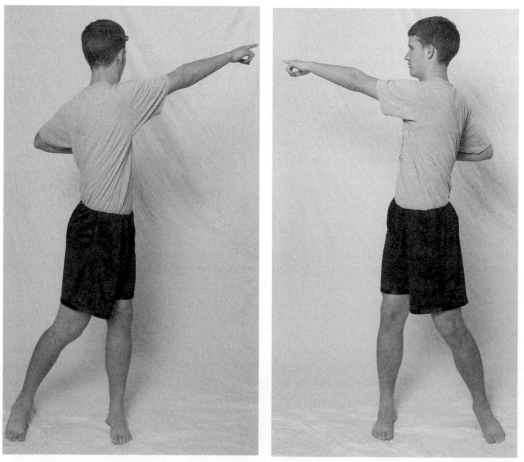

Figure 10-9 Functional pronation and supination mobility exercise linked to total leg rotation.

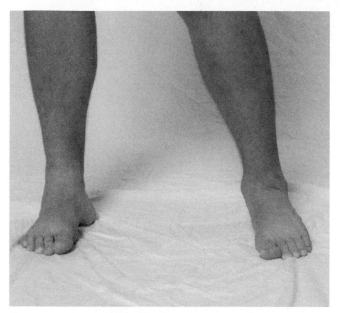

Figure 10-10 Supination with external rotation right leg. Pronation with internal rotation left leg.

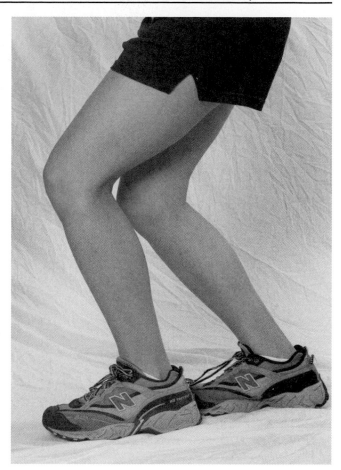

Figure 10-11 Static ankle dorsiflexion stretch.

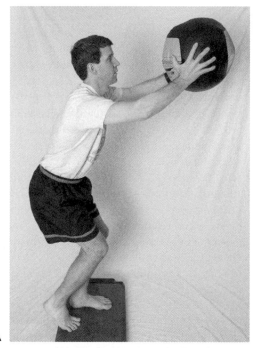

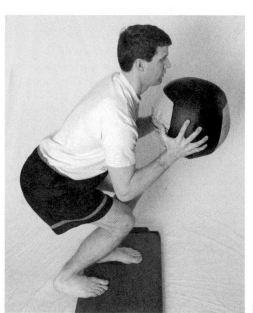

A   B

Figure 10-12 A, Dynamic ankle dorsiflexion squat stretch with functional stimulation from upper extremities, hip, and knee. **B,** Note ankle dorsiflexion end-range stretch.

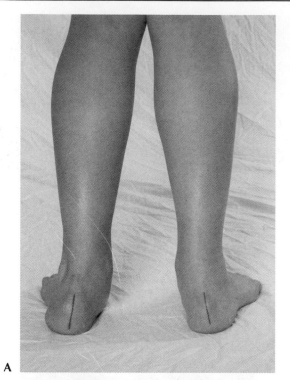

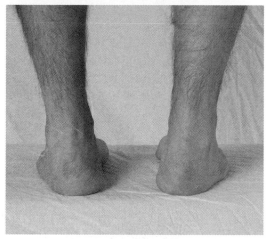

A

B

Figure 10-13 A, Pes planus feet tend to have greater medially directed lower extremity stress. **B,** Pes cavus feet tend to have greater laterally directed lower extremity stress.

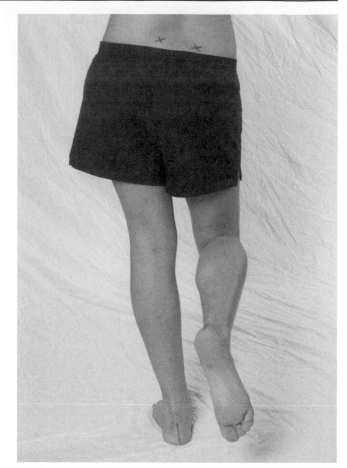

Figure 10-14 Inability of the gluteus medius, upper gluteus maximus, and posterior tensor fascia lata to stabilize the pelvis over the hip.

Powers et al[13] describe altered lower extremity kinematics of the femur and tibia in the transverse and frontal planes and its effects on patellofemoral joint mechanics. They describe bottom up and top down influences to the patellofemoral joint and its movement mechanics. Excessive frontal plane valgus and transverse plane tibial and/or femoral rotation increase the Q-angle as the patella displaces medially relative to anterior superior iliac spine. In contrast, misbalance and altered mechanics could result in excessive knee varus load placed in the frontal plane. Excessive knee varus or valgus loading necessitates a kinetic chain response to control the center of gravity in space. Therefore excessive ankle, knee, or hip muscle activation may be required, creating a potentially overstressed joint

environment. Geraci[54] describes a relationship between muscle weakness patterns of the hip and lower extremity injury patterns. Muscle imbalance patterns are described in which the gluteus medius, maximus, and abdominals can have neural reflexive inhibition resulting in functional weakness. In contrast, the antagonist hip adductors, hip flexors, and erector spinae are related to tendencies for shortening and tightening restrictions. Janda[55] describes neuromuscular imbalances in which pain and dysfunction in a motion segment can initiate weakness in phasic muscles and tightness in postural muscles. Sale[56] describes a concept of neural adaptation in which focused strength facilitation exercises may cause changes within the neuromuscular system that enable an individual to better coordinate the activation of muscle groups, thereby affecting a greater net force even in the absence within the muscles themselves. Facilitation techniques involve stretching the antagonist of the inhibited weak gluteus medius and gluteus maximus (Figure 10-15). Geraci[54] describes a neurological release to the inhibition through functional retraining. The recruitment of mechanoreceptor input through functional closed kinetic chain exercise patterns includes patterns of postural muscle flexibility and phasic muscle dynamic strength recruitment (Figure 10-16).

STRUCTURAL MALALIGNMENT OF THE HIP, KNEE, AND TIBIA

Faulty mechanics during running, jump propulsion, and landing may be predisposed by skeletal malalignment. Post et al[11] write that normal bony alignment allows weight transfer to be balanced in a manner tolerated by the core and lower extremities. Conversely, malalignment can cause the transfer of body weight to be unbalanced and asymmetric and potentially cause overload somewhere along the kinetic chain.[11] Lower extremity malalignment, compensations, and potential pain patterns occur from the pelvis down and from the foot up in the kinetic chain. Skeletal malalignment includes static deformities present in individual bone segments (i.e., tibial torsion), as well as joint deformities (i.e., genu valgus).[57]

The most common types of malalignment are axial and rotational. Axial alignment refers to the longitudinal relationships of the limb segments.[58] Axial alignment is described in reference to the angle made by the segments in relation to a straight line. Deviation toward the midline would relate to the term *valgus*. Deviation away from the midline is termed *varus*. Rotational alignment refers to the twisting of the limb around its longitudinal axis.[58] Joint deformities, such as genu valgus, may increase in magnitude when assessed from a static non–weight-bearing position in contrast to more functional positions, such as unilateral limb weight bearing due to ground reaction forces coupled with foot pronation.[57]

Normal characteristics at the hip include an inwardly rotated relationship between the femoral neck relative to the femoral condyles of the femur in the transverse plane called *femoral anteversion.* Normal femoral anteversion ranges from 13 to 18 degrees in adults.[11,57,59,60] Measurement of hip anteversion can be performed in the prone position by recording the angle of the lower leg from the vertical when the greater trochanter is placed in its most lateral and prominent position.[11,57,61,62] Excessive femoral anteversion influences the knee joint medially, giving rise to a cascade of biomechanical stresses and compensations (Figure 10-17).[11] An inwardly rotated knee creates excessive laterally directed shear forces resulting in increased stress in the medial patellofemoral ligaments and increased lateral patellofemoral compressive forces.[11] The trochlea is pushed medially and forward against the patella, creating resultant excessive posterolateral pull on the patella. Lee et al[63] describe that excess of femoral internal rotation of 30 degrees increases contact pressures on the lateral facets of the retropatellar surface. Riegger-Krugh and Keysor[64] report possible femoral anteversion compensations in the kinetic chain as including excessive tibial external torsion, excessive pelvic external rotation, and excessive ipsilateral lumbar spine rotation. Predisposition for altered mechanics as described by Powers et al[13] is set up by excessive femoral anteversion. Clinically, the requirement for strong muscular stability from the hip and pelvis to limit knee stress is amplified.

Femoral retroversion is defined as excessive external rotation of the femoral neck relative to the femoral condyles in the transverse plane. Excessive external rotation of the femur

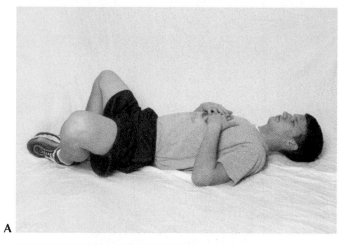

A

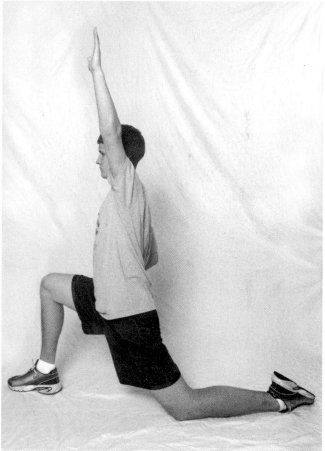

B

Figure 10-15 A, Stretching the hip adductors assists a neurological release to inhibited gluteus medius muscle. **B,** Stretching the hip flexor assists a neurological release to inhibited gluteus maximus muscle.

magnifies retropatellar articular surface stress along the medial facet.[65] Compensations include excessive tibial internal rotation and pelvic internal rotation with contralateral lumbar spine rotation.[64] Physical examination of excessive femoral anteversion and retroversion demonstrates distinctive range of motion differences. An excessively anteverted hip will demonstrate an excess of hip internal rotation and limitation of external rotation.[66,67] Conversely, a retroverted hip will demonstrate

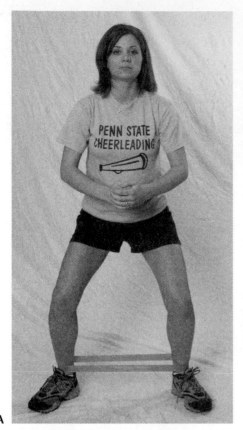

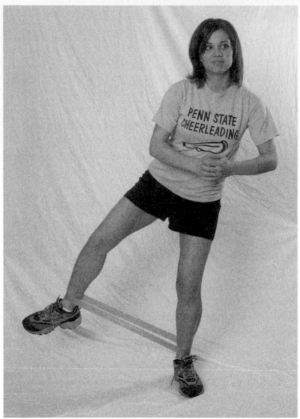

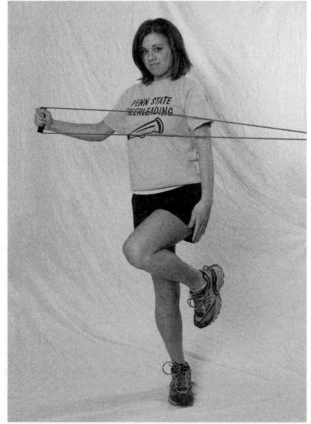

Figure 10-16 A, Resistive band walking recruits core hip and pelvis muscles. **B,** After multiple multiplanar steps, several active hip abduction repetitions produce fatigue in both weight-bearing and non–weight-bearing legs. **C,** Tubing exercise with top-down–driven rotational resistance strengthens the hip external rotators in the closed chain.

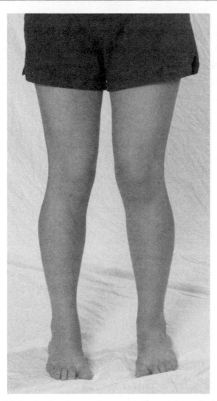

Figure 10-17 Excessive femoral anteversion with squinting patella.

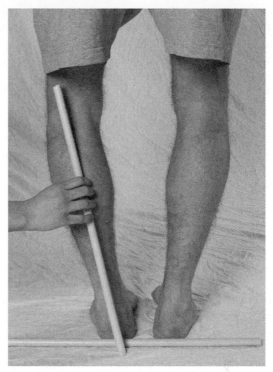

Figure 10-18 Excessive tibial varum in double-limb stance. Distal one third of the tibia is angled medially in the frontal plane.

excessive hip external rotation and limitation of hip internal rotation.

Genu valgus is defined as the angle formed at the knee between the femur and tibia in which the knee angulates toward the midline with the tibia angulating away from the midline.[58] Frontal plane knee valgus posturing in weight bearing is considered normal at approximately 6 degrees.[57,68] Excessive knee valgus correlates with excessive pronation as gravity influences the lower limb toward the midline in weight bearing.[64] Radiographically and clinically, this can be measured by the angle bisecting the midline position of the distal femur with the midline position of the proximal tibia.[57] Excessive valgus results in disproportionate compressive forces laterally and distractive tensile forces medially. Conversely, knee varus posturing produces compressive forces medially and increased tensile forces laterally.[57] Genu varum is defined as the angle formed by the femur at the knee directing away from the midline and the tibia angling back toward the midline.[58] This contact stress asymmetry leads to structural failure, such as arthrosis and chondromalacia.[11]

Excessive tibial varum is a common congenital osseous deformity in which the distal one third of the leg is angled medially in the frontal plane (Figure 10-18).[40,69] The varum angle occurs within the shaft of the tibia as opposed to the angulation occurring at the joint in the genu varum deformity condition. Measurements of tibial varum are described in three positions: double-limb stance with subtalar joint in the resting position, double-limb stance with the subtalar joint in neutral, and single-limb stance with the subtalar joint in the resting position.[70] Lohmann recorded tibial vara measurement in

uninjured subjects and found the single-limb stance measurement to be the largest at 6.35 degrees and double-limb stance with the subtalar joint in neutral to be the smallest at 4.62 degrees relative to these three test positions. Tomaro[40] found a significant difference in the amount of tibial varum between the involved and uninvolved extremities in 20 patients with various lower extremity overuse injuries. He found an increased tibial varum measurement on the side of overuse symptoms with measurements at 5.3 degrees compared with 4 degrees on the uninvolved extremity. Increased tibial varum is related to compensatory excessive subtalar joint pronation because this malalignment tends to elevate the medial foot from the

Evidence-Based Clinical Application: Leg Length Inequality

Brady et al[71] advised the following after studying 58 articles related to limb length inequality, classification criteria, etiological factors, assessment, and intervention:
1. Palpation of bony landmarks with block correction is preferable over tape measurement.
2. Excessive foot pronation relates to functional shortening of a long limb.
3. Radiological assessment provides the most accurate and reliable measure.
4. Clinicians should use caution in intervening with a lift device with a clinically measured limb difference of 5 mm or less.
5. Lift therapy should be implemented gradually in small increments.

support surface, requiring increased pronation to achieve foot flat. Ross and Schuster[41] describe a concept of total varus imbalance that includes the summation of tibial varum, rearfoot varus, and forefoot varus measurements. Tibial varum was measured in stance, while rearfoot and forefoot varus were measured non–weight bearing. A preseason screening examination of 63 runners was then correlated to the summation of varum measurements. A low injury rate was described with individuals of less than 8 degrees of total varus, and a high injury rate was found in runners with more than 18 degrees of total varum summation.

Tibial torsion is a static bony measurement of the distal tibia relative to the proximal tibia. Mean values in adults are reported to range between 20 and 30 degrees of external tibial torsion. Excessive external tibial torsion will present with an excessively toed-out foot placement when weight bearing.[57] A 5-degree toe-out alignment is considered to be normal in the adult population.[72] Running over an excessively toed-out foot posture will require excessive and prolonged pronation, particularly at the midfoot. External tibial torsion has been associated with a variety of patellofemoral dysfunctions including compression syndrome and instability.[73,74] Lee et al[65] reported that fixing the tibia in 15 degrees of external tibial rotation beyond neutral resulted in significant increases in both peak and average patellofemoral joint contact pressures. Increased pressure was localized to the lateral patellar articular facets. Fixing the tibia in excessive internal rotation had minimal effect on pressures or contact areas.[65]

STRUCTURAL MALALIGNMENT OF THE FOOT

McClay[75] writes that describing foot function by both static measures and dynamic measures has both identifiable strengths and shortcomings. Intrinsic foot malalignment relates to both excessive pronation and supination functional mechanics. Static foot deformities related to excessive foot pronation include rearfoot varus and forefoot varus measured in non–weight-bearing postures. Forefoot varus is defined as inversion of the forefoot on the rearfoot with the subtalar joint in neutral position (Figure 10-19).[76,77] Functionally, a forefoot varus deformity requires compensatory subtalar joint motion to enable sufficient weight bearing to the medial aspect of the foot.[57] Forefoot varus of greater than 7 degrees has been implicated as a factor in contributing to postural instability.[78] Gray[79] describes that a compensated forefoot varus deformity is the foot type that is most likely to produce proximal dysfunction as excessive subtalar joint pronation links with internal rotation influence up the kinetic chain. Garbalosa et al[76] examined a normal population of 240 feet and found 86.67% had a forefoot varus alignment. The mean forefoot varus in this group was 7.8 degrees.[76] Astrom et al[80] identified 6 degrees as the mean varus alignment in a study of normals. Glasoe et al[81] classified foot types in a group of 60 normals as being forefoot valgus, forefoot neutral (defined as 0 to 10 degrees of varus) or forefoot varus (defined as ≥ 11 degrees of varus). The authors

chose this varus classification because 11 degrees is one standard deviation larger than the 6-degree mean varus alignment measured by Astrom and Arvidson when they introduced the jig-goniometer as a reliable measure.[80]

Rearfoot varus is an intrinsic frontal plane deformity in which the calcaneus is inverted relative to the tibia when measured from a non–weight-bearing subtalar neutral position.[42] A rearfoot varus malalignment functionally inverts the foot relative to the ground, requiring subtalar compensation (dependent on calcaneal eversion mobility). Garbalosa reported a mean of 2.5 degrees of calcaneal varus in the normal population of 240 feet. Powers reported greater rearfoot varus mean values in a group of 30 female subjects.[42] A mean value of 8.9 degrees of rearfoot varus was found with a group of 15 patellofemoral pain patients and a mean value of 6.8 degrees of rearfoot varus was found with 15 controls.

Forefoot valgus is defined as an everted position of the frontal plane of the forefoot relative to the rearfoot with the subtalar joint held in neutral non–weight-bearing position (Figure 10-20).[26,57] The forefoot valgus deviation exists when the head and neck of the talus exceeds the necessary valgus torsion at 35 to 40 degrees relative to the trochlear of the talus.[82] All five metatarsal heads are everted relative to the calcaneal bisection.[83] Garbalosa found that forefoot valgus was present in 8.75% of the 240 feet that were studied. The mean value of forefoot valgus in this foot type was 4.7 degrees. The midtarsal joint is supinated with the forefoot valgus deformity, enabling the lateral aspect of the foot to be brought in contact with the ground.[57]

A plantarflexed first ray structural deformity is defined as the first metatarsal being dropped and plantarflexed relative to metatarsal bones two through five.[84] The neutral position of first ray occurs when the first metatarsal head lies in the same transverse plane as the second through fourth metatarsal heads when they are maximally dorsiflexed.[77] A plantarflexed first ray produces an everted forefoot when the forefoot alignment includes the first through fifth metatarsal heads.[83] If congenital, this structural malalignment describes a pes cavus foot.[77]

A plantarflexed first ray is described as the most common form of an everted forefoot and is generally acquired as a compensation from excessive tibial varum with concomitant restricted calcaneal eversion.[85] The first ray plantarflexes to enable the medial aspect of the foot to make contact with the ground. A plantarflexed first ray and a forefoot valgus alignment are conditions that cause the forefoot to be everted relative to the rearfoot.[81] Both result in excessive supination during the stance phase of running. A rigid or hypomobile plantarflexed first ray will necessitate excessive weight bearing to the first metatarsal head and sesamoids, creating callus formation and potential painful overloading.

DYNAMIC ASSESSMENT OF THE CORE AND FOOT MECHANICS

Dynamic assessment of the athlete during functional movement provides critical information of potential weakness,

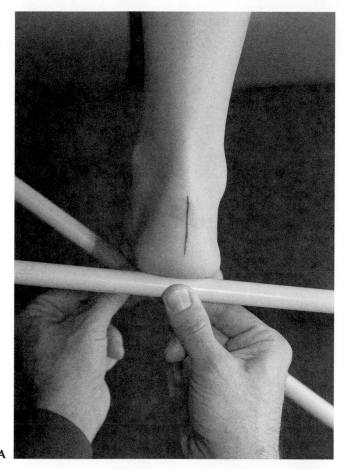

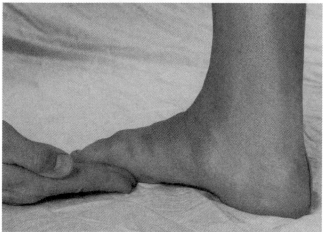

Figure 10-19 A, Forefoot varus deformity. Inversion of the forefoot on the rearfoot with the subtalar joint in neutral position. **B,** Forefoot varus deformity in the closed chain. Inversion of the forefoot relative to the rearfoot. Bringing the ground up to the foot eliminates the need for compensatory excessive subtalar pronation.

motion restrictions, and abnormal joint stress contributing to pathomechanics. Although varying in complexity, walking, running, jumping, and hopping all share common functional patterns. Sport requires hundreds of acceleration, deceleration, and multiplanar changes of direction. Perry[22] defines the locomotor unit in the lower kinetic chain as the two lower limbs and pelvis providing 11 articulations. The lumbosacral spine,

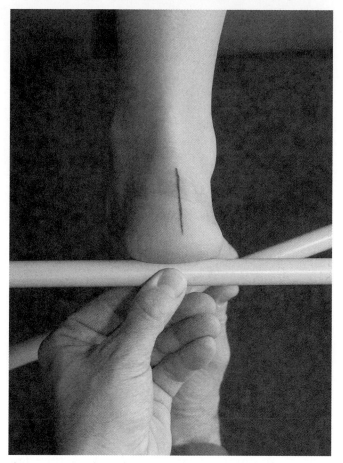

Figure 10-20 Forefoot valgus deformity. Eversion of the forefoot on the rearfoot with the subtalar joint in neutral position.

hip, knee, ankle, subtalar, mid tarsal, and metatarsophalangeal (MTP) joints form this locomotor unit. When walking and running, the magnitude and timing of motions in each lower limb is controlled by 57 muscles acting in selective fashion.[22] Jumping and hopping involve a highly orchestrated sequence with neuromuscular control requirements of both two-joint and one-joint muscles. The core and lower extremities provide four distinctive functions: propulsion, stance stability, shock absorption, and energy conservation. Deficiency in any of these four functions can relate to soft tissue overload and injury.

Gait Analysis

Gait analysis can be as simple as observational screening to note abnormalities detectable by the naked eye. Systematic gait analysis incorporating a top-down and bottom-up visual orientation is optimal when investigating subtle deviations. A top-down orientation provides data on symmetry, quantity, and quality of arm swing; pelvic rotation; pelvic tilt; and lateral trunk shift. Next, knee and lower leg motions are observed. The bottom-up orientation provides assessment of ankle, subtalar, midfoot, and hallux motion symmetry, quantity, and quality. The observer studies this top-down and bottom-up gait assessment with focus of potential exaggerated motion or insufficient ability of the locomotor unit to provide propulsion, stance stability, shock absorption, and energy conservation. Core postural muscle instability is suspected when excessive pelvis crest drop and pelvic rotation are observed. Further testing of gluteal muscle function in open and closed kinetic chain positions would be warranted. Excessive hip adduction with knee valgus producing an increased dynamic quadricep angle is a significant observation. Knee varus trust defined as a lateral knee shift may be indicative of lateral knee complex instability or osteoarthritis of the medial knee compartment. Early heel rise during propulsion is a common compensation for hallux limitus, sesamoiditis, or ankle equinus. Dananberg and Guiliano[30] describe a relationship between hallux limitus and spine pain related to deficient hallux extension in late stance phase when walking. A contralateral increased lateral shift is described as the lower extremity adapting to the loss of hallux extension with the concomitant decrease in hip extension at midstance. Spine pain patterns are related to the hallux limitus, and Dannenberg and Guiliano[30] describe a 36% improvement with custom foot orthotics described to neutralize the deleterious effects of hallux extension loss.

Excessive foot pronation is visualized by three potential observations: excessive calcaneal eversion, medial midfoot collapse, and excessive toe out. Abnormal foot supination is visualized by calcaneal inversion, excessive medial midfoot arch height, and disproportionate weight bearing on the lateral foot. Large callus formation may develop under the first and fifth metatarsal heads. Excessive toe-out posturing in stance phase may represent compensation for hallux limitus, ankle equinus, excessive tibial external torsion, or excessive foot pronation. Toe-out walking patterns place increased medially directed elongation stresses and laterally directed compressive stresses along the soft tissues of the ankle joint. Excessive toe-in posturing in stance phase represents most commonly metatarsus adductus or excessive tibial internal torsion. Gait assessment of running includes all of those previously described with attention given to initial foot strike. First foot contact may be observed at the calcaneus, midfoot, forefoot, or toes. Early-stance phase heel strike enables ankle joint dorsiflexion and foot pronation to provide weight-bearing loading and shock absorption. Forefoot and toe strike as the initial foot contact is the norm in running sports' requirement for speed and change of direction. Prolonged straight-ahead running with forefoot and toe strike as the initial contact relates to decreased shock absorption capability.

Clinical single-camera videotaping during observational gait analysis provides a significant tool both for assessment and patient instruction. Video captures 60 images per second compared with the naked eye, which can capture only 4 to 6 images per second.[22] Immediate playback provides pause frame and advance abilities enhancing clinical study and patient feedback. Instrumented gait analysis systems include motion analysis, dynamic electromyography, and force plate measurement. Motion analysis systems are designed to define the magnitude and timing of individual joint action. Dynamic electromyography provides muscle function data defining timing and contraction intensity. Force plate systems measure weight-bearing loading characteristics.

Functional Movement Analysis

Analysis of functional movement patterns focuses on kinetic chain stability, mobility, postural control, and symmetry in a varying progression of specific task-related motion patterns.[86] Functional movement analysis includes observation of the initiation phase in which the body starts or initiates movement.[87] A movement is initiated when the body moves to position itself for the task or changes its position relative to its base of support. The second stage in the functional movement sequence is called *transition.* The transition point is defined as the time in the movement sequence when there is a change in the active muscle groups, the direction of motion, or the body's relationship to its base of support.[87] Functional exercise training helps to reestablish patterns of coordinated extremity movement sequencing multiple body segments with symmetry, efficiency, and postural stability.[88,89]

Evidence-Based Clinical Application
The use of video for functional analysis and training is an effective means of motor learning and reeducation. Video can be used for direct training purposes, home exercise program documents, and for communication purposes to physicians, parents, and coaches. Onate et al[90] reported on augmented feedback using video in the training of reduction of jump landing forces. Subjects given video feedback regarding jump landing reduced ground reaction forces significantly greater compared with controls.

Gray[91] describes a strategy in functional measurement involving a battery of tests called *a total body functional profile.* This series includes balance, balance reach, excursion, lunge, squat, jump, and hop tests in multiplanar positions. Sports-specific movement patterns are simulated in a progression from simple to complex and conscious to subconscious. The STAR excursion balance test is a dynamic stability test in which the athlete balances unilaterally while reaching with the contralateral leg in eight different planes of motion.[91-93] Olmsted et al[94] found significant asymmetry in the STAR excursion balance test when studying 20 subjects with chronic ankle instability matched with uninjured subjects (70.6 cm vs. 82.8 cm). Gribble et al[7] also reported the use of the STAR excursion measurement tool studying the effects of fatigue and ankle instability on postural control. Ankle instability and fatigue disrupted balance reach values when comparing ankle instability subjects with controls.

Faulty jump landing mechanics have been implicated as a primary cause of knee injury, especially with females.[9,10,95,96] Hewett et al[9] studied 181 middle school and high school soccer and basketball players. Dynamic control of the knee joint was measured kinematically by assessing jump land response, medial knee motion, and lower extremity valgus angles. Hewett et al found that female athletes landed with greater total medial rotation of the knees in greater maximum lower extremity valgus than did male athletes. Huston et al[95] found significant gender differences in knee flexion angles on jump landing from 20- and 30-inch heights. Women landed at a mean flexion angle of 7 degrees compared with 16 degrees for men. Landing with a straighter, more extended knee is related to poor loading and shocking absorption mechanics in the sagittal plane, potentially leading to increased transverse plane stresses at the knee. Multiple studies have demonstrated the value of teaching proper mechanics through functional neuromuscular exercise training.[97-99]

EXERCISE CONCEPTS FROM THE CORE TO THE FLOOR

Closed chain exercise integrates combined weight-bearing and shear forces that are mediated by eccentric muscle activity.[100] Functional exercise training incorporates an interdependent series of skeletal reaction that involves stabilizers, synergists, neutralizers, and antagonists all working in harmony to accelerate, decelerate, and stabilize the body in three body planes.[101] Functional strength is the ability of the neuromuscular system to act and react with dynamic concentric, eccentric, and isometric stabilization in response to gravity, momentum, and ground reaction forces.[102] Whether the athlete is running, jumping, throwing, pulling, pushing, or lifting, movement involves lifting one leg onto the other. Functional sport training incorporates this pattern. This assists a proprioceptively enriched training pattern that incorporates the complex interdependencies that the locomotor system performs in sport activity.

Evidence-Based Clinical Application: Neuromuscular Control of the Hip and Pelvis

Muscle strength testing of the hip is described in both open-chain and functional closed-chain positions.[103,104] Functional neuromuscular training requires weight-bearing motor control stimulation.[31] Paterno et al[89] report on hip, pelvis, trunk, strengthening, and balance training in a group of 41 female high school athletes. Functional hip, pelvis, and trunk training was done in closed-chain posturing over a 6-week period with pre– and post–single-limb postural stability testing. Significant improvement was made in postural stability as measured by the Biodex stability system following the training regimen.

Pelvic stability is critical to whole body linking. During sport activity and functional training, the closer the body's center of gravity is to its base of support, the more stable it is.[105] A low strong center allows the athlete to change body position with agility in sport action and reaction, as well as for the avoidance of contact if necessary. Legs generate power through a stable pelvis and torso and thereby enable a well-coordinated transfer of stability to the upper extremities. There

can be a fourfold increase in power when generating a push motion when using the legs and total body versus the upper extremities alone.[106]

Multiplanar lunges provide dynamic stabilization functional muscle recruitment patterns (Figures 10-21 and 10-22). For example, during hamstring activity while running and sprinting, the foot strikes the ground with the hamstring immediately eccentrically decelerating tibial internal rotation, femoral internal rotation, and hip flexion. The hamstring works synergistically with the gluteus maximus and piriformis, providing stability to the knee.[102] The lunge exercise recruits these muscles in a neuromuscular functional pattern feed for the kinetic chain.

Multiplanar balance reach training requires significant gluteus medius muscle control because pelvic deviation must be stabilized as the non–weight-bearing lower extremity moves through a variety of functional patterns. Consider the muscle group classically described as the groin including the hip adductors and hip flexors. The posterior medial and lateral rotation balance reach exercise creates muscle coupling inclusive of the gluteus medius, gluteus maximus, piriformis, abdominals, and erector spinae, in harmony with the anterior muscle groups including the hip flexors and hip adductors (Figure 10-23).[91]

Bilateral and unilateral squat exercise provides isolation of gluteus, quadricep, and hamstring muscles in varying degrees depending on depth and plane of motion (Figure 10-24). Squat exercise requires strong stabilization of the pelvis through eccentric action of the biarticular hamstring muscles with cocontraction of the quadriceps, abdominals, and spine muscles to control an erect position of the trunk.[107] Focused quadricep isolation occurs with vertical posturing during squatting exercise versus greater gluteus muscle isolation during a more horizontally directed trunk and torso.

FOOT ORTHOTIC STRATEGIES IN SPORT

Shoe modifications and foot orthoses are widely prescribed with the primary goal of altering patterns of movement and lower extremity joint alignment.[108] Foot orthoses are intended to provide a mechanical advantage for feet that are negatively influenced by malalignment (excessive pronation/supination), intrinsic joint restrictions (hallux limitus), and feet affected by a localized microtrauma (sesamoiditis/plantar fasciitis). Foot orthotics are categorized as being either biomechanical or accommodative. Biomechanical orthotics are fabricated to provide motion control. Accommodative foot orthotics are designed to dampen the painful effects of stress and shear to localized areas of foot pain. Foot orthotics may provide a blend of both biomechanical and accommodative features.

Historically, evidence supporting the use of foot orthotics is found with studies showing subjective symptom relief but controversial mechanical validity.

Multiple kinetic variables are reported to increase an athlete's risk for overuse injuries including excessive or inadequate pronation, high eversion velocity, excessive tibial

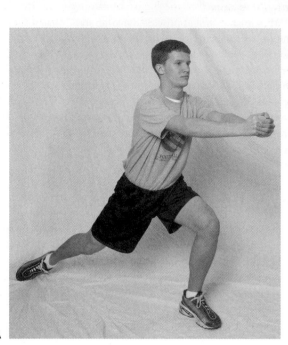
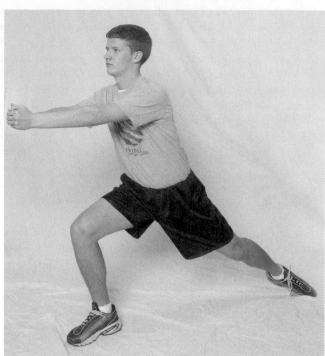

Figure 10-21 A, Left leg anterior lateral lunge. **B,** Right leg anterior lateral lunge.

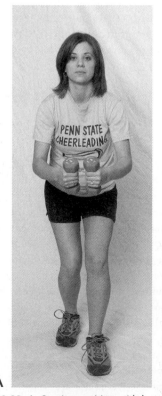
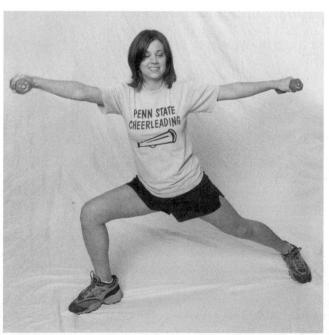

Figure 10-22 A, Starting position with hand weights. **B,** Multiplanar arm exercises add to stability requirement during lunge.

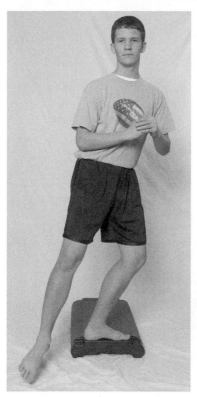

Figure 10-23 Posterior lateral balance reach off a 4-inch step recruits groin muscle activity in a functional pattern.

Evidence-Based Clinical Application: Kinematic Influence of Foot Orthotics for the Lower Extremity

1.6 degrees of decreased internal tibial rotation with pronation controlling orthotic use[109]

2.2 degrees' reduction in maximal calcaneal angle with pronation controlling orthotic use[110]

15% reduction in calcaneal eversion velocity with foot orthotic use[111]

---

internal rotation, excessive loading and impact rate of vertical ground reaction force, and excessive knee abduction and external rotation moments.[36,109-112] The foundational goal in foot orthotic intervention is that performance should improve with an optimal orthotic.[108] A functional profile of walking, running, balance reach, squatting, lunging, as well as jump and hop performance skills should all improve in terms of floor-to-the-core stability for a foot orthotic to be deemed valuable. Certainly, the athlete's subjective comfort and pain reduction response should coexist with functional advantage for a foot orthotic device to be implemented.

Foot Orthosis Design

A common type of custom sport foot orthotic is a device termed *a total contact orthosis.* This is a custom-fabricated foot insert made from a model of the patient's foot, thereby achieving total contact with the plantar surface of the foot.[113] As previously described, a biomechanical foot orthosis is designed to influence foot motion or dampen the velocity of pronation, or both. Biomechanical orthoses are designed to alter the position or mechanics of the foot, or both, in an attempt to establish foot function near a subtalar neutral position.[114] Foot orthoses may be fabricated by posting wedge material at the forefoot or rearfoot to bring the ground up to the foot and support a foot deformity, such as forefoot varus or forefoot valgus.[1] Extrinsic posting involves wedging material added to the outer shell of the orthotic device. Intrinsic posting involves influencing foot alignment on the basis of the cast molding of the foot by creating a twist within the orthotic shell and thereby supporting a varus or valgus forefoot deformity.

Foot Orthotic Strategies for the Excessively Pronating Foot

The primary goal in foot orthotic control in the overpronating foot is to provide boundary and a speed-dampening effect to excessive subtalar and midtarsal motion. Strategies can include a deep heel cup in an attempt to limit calcaneal eversion, total contact support along the medial longitudinal arch, and medial forefoot and rearfoot posting to lessen compensatory motion.[110,111,115-117] Johanson et al[115] report on three different posting strategies in treating compensated forefoot varus feet, rearfoot posting alone, forefoot posting alone, and combined forefoot and rearfoot posting. A 2.3-degree reduction in maximal calf to calcaneus angle was found with combined rearfoot and forefoot posted orthotics compared with controls using running shoe inserts alone. No difference was found in pronation control when comparing forefoot and rearfoot combined posting with rearfoot posting alone. The least effective posting strategy was found for forefoot posting alone. Donatelli et al[117] reported on 53 subjects in a retrospective study of qualitative pain relief with the use of biomechanical pronation controlling foot orthotics. They reported the average forefoot varus deformity at 8.4 degrees in the open chain and the

---

Evidence-Based Clinical Application: Strength-Training Effects on Pronation Kinematics and Running

Nineteen muscles are attached to the foot. Intrinsic foot muscle stability has been reported to limit pronation when running. Feltner et al[118] chose 18 runners out of 71 volunteers whose videotape running captured the greatest amount of pronation. Runners were split into a nonisokinetic group performing a variety of closed chain exercises, such as balance boards, resistive tubing exercise, step-ups, hop and jump exercises, and functional running drills. An isokinetic training group performed concentric and eccentric repetitions at 20, 90, and 180 degrees per second. Each group trained three times per week for a period of 8 weeks. Maximal calcaneal eversion measurements of pronation were decreased by 2.2 degrees in the isokinetic trained group, whereas the closed chain exercise group did not demonstrate kinematic pronation changes.

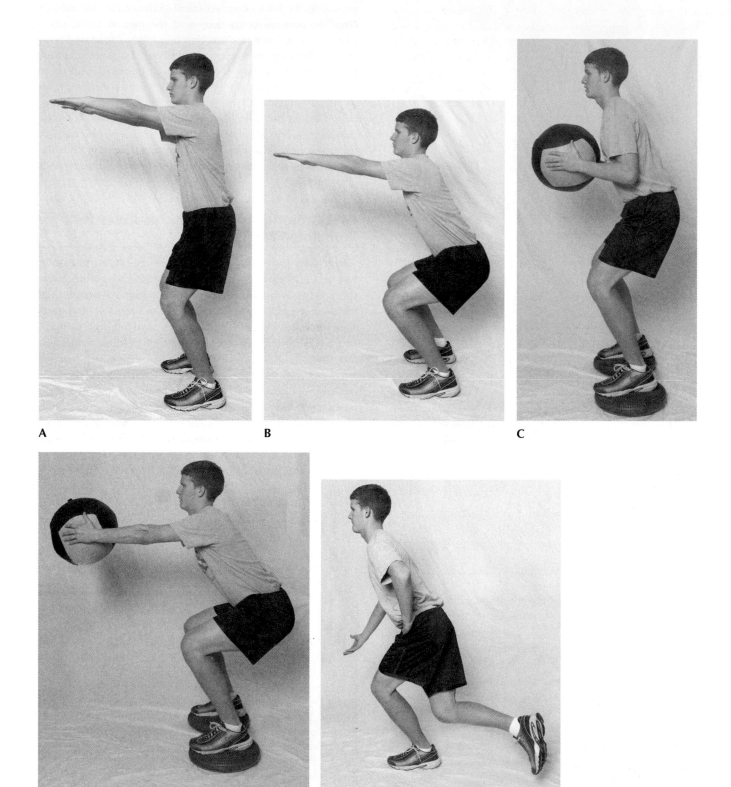

Figure 10-24 A, Level surface double-leg squat. **B,** Observe hamstring recruitment. **C** and **D,** Double-leg squat on uneven surface with medicine ball for greater stabilization requirement. **E,** Single-leg squat enhances quadriceps recruitment.

average rearfoot everted position in standing at 7.8 degrees. The average forefoot varus post used was 5.2 degrees, and the average rearfoot varus post used was 4.5 degrees. Ninety-six percent of the patients reported pain relief with the use of the prescribed orthotic. Sixty-one percent of the patients' forefoot varus deformities were supported by posting, and 57% of the rearfoot deformities were supported by posting in this subject group.

Foot Orthotic Strategies for the Excessively Supinating Foot

A forefoot valgus deformity is treated with lateral posting (Figure 10-25). Theoretically, the lateral posting brings the ground up to the forefoot, lessening thereby compensatory subtalar joint supination. Tolerance to lateral rearfoot posting depends on adequate passive motion into calcaneal eversion. Laterally posting the rearfoot in a maximum of 4 degrees is recommended, if the calcaneus can passively move into 4 degrees of eversion.[114] An orthotic designed to influence the

cavus foot type moves the foot toward subtalar neutral and away from its function in end range of supination. Manoli and Graham describe a device termed the *cavus foot orthosis* (CFO).[43] The CFO is made of ethylvinylacetate and has an elevated heel, intrinsic lateral heel wedge, lessened longitudinal arch height, a first metatarsal head cutout, and a lateral forefoot wedge.

Foot Orthotic Strategies for Turf Toe

An estimated 40% of body weight is born by the toes at the propulsion stage of push off during the gait cycle.[119] The greatest amount of loading hinges through the first MTP joint.[120] The Clanton classification of turf toe injury defines three levels of trauma to the first metatarsal capsuloligamentous complex including compression injury of the articular surface.[121] The etiology of turf toe can be either a traumatic event or repetitive overuse in the hyperextension plane.[122] The forceful hyperextension mechanism of injury to the first MTP joint is often related to unyielding characteristics of synthetic turf or a firm court surface. Poor forefoot stability within sport footwear also relates to inadequate protection of extension forces born in sport (Figure 10-26). Preexisting extension range of motion limitations to the first MTP also can play a role in the onset of turn-toe injury. The primary foot orthotic strategy is to limit the first MTP joint extension within a pain-free range (Figure 10-27).[123] Orthotic strategies include a total contact orthosis with a Morton's extension fabricated from a nonyielding material for rigidity at the first MTP joint. Strategies also include the use of a steel shank or carbon fiber plate designed to stiffen the last of the shoe (Figure 10-28).

Foot Orthotic Strategies for Sesamoiditis

Sesamoid bone injury involves either a fracture or repetitive stress–type injury.[124,125] Sesamoid injury can be extremely painful and difficult for the athlete because sport involves continuous extended toe push-off positioning. The goal for orthotic intervention is to accommodate and relieve painful

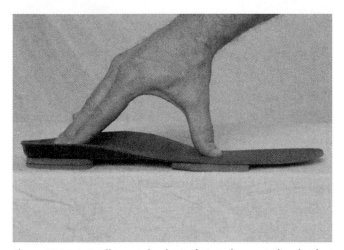

Figure 10-25 Laterally posted orthotic designed to neutralize forefoot valgus and influence the foot toward pronation.

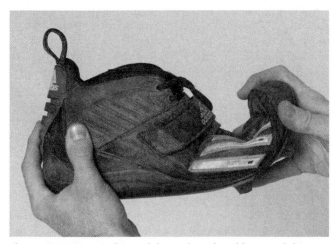

Figure 10-26 Poor toe box stability making the athlete at risk for great toe injury.

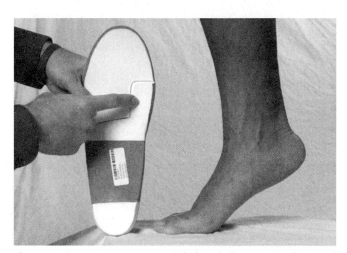

Figure 10-27 Morton's extension with firm shell material to limit and protect hallux extension at push off.

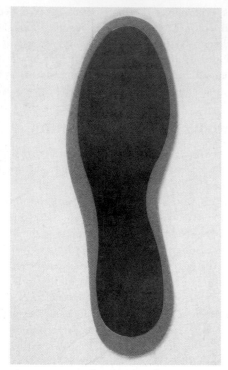

Figure 10-28 Turf toe insert with steel shank.

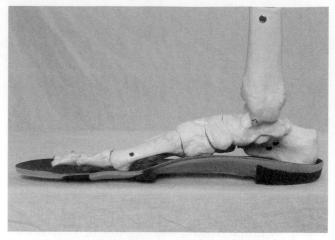

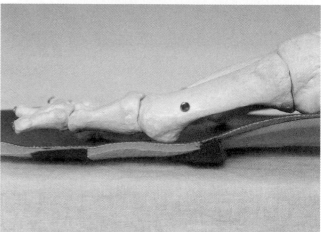

Figure 10-29 Kinetic wedge device designed to provide mechanical advantage to hallux limitus at push off (Langer Biomechanics Group Inc.).

weight-bearing pressure beneath the first metatarsal head region. This can be accomplished by an accommodative design, such as a first ray cutout or custom padding to unload and distribute weight bearing along the boundary of the sesamoids (Figures 10-29 through 10-31).[126] Weight-bearing accommodation coupled with forefoot orthotic and shoe toe box firmness to dampen hallux extension both provide stress relief.

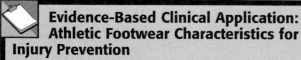

Evidence-Based Clinical Application: Athletic Footwear Characteristics for Injury Prevention

Athletes should shop for shoes after a training session when their feet are their largest.

Toe box length should be 1 fingerbreadth from the end of the toe box to the end of the longest toe.

Firm outsole for toe protection during push off and propulsion

Firm heel counter for subtalar joint motion control and plantar heel fat pad containment

Varying lacing strategies can accommodate for bony prominences and adjusting shoe support[127]

Foot Orthotic Strategies for Plantar Heel Pain

Plantar fasciitis is the most common cause of plantar heel pain and is reported to constitute approximately 15% of all foot-related problems.[45,128-130] Biomechanically, the plantar heel is stressed in the athlete both on heel weight-bearing loading, as well as at propulsion push off as the windlass effect creates tension of the plantar aponeurosis.[131-135] Shoe characteristics of

heel outsole cushioning and heel counter stability for fat pad containment are advised for the protection of the plantar heel in sport.[127] Wilk et al[136] describe the significant role a faulty shoe plays in a triathlete with plantar fasciitis as he reports on defective footwear as a contributing factor to injury. Shoe modifications consisting of a steel shank and anterior rocker bottom are reported as strategies to lessen plantar fascia loading.[137] Mizel et al[138] treated 71 feet with plantar fasciitis symptoms of greater than 6 months with a shoe steel shank modification and reported a 67% success in either complete resolution or improvement in this patient group. Lynch et al[130] found that taping and foot orthoses proved to be the most effective intervention in a randomized, prospective study involving 103 plantar fasciitis patients assigned to one of three treatment categories: antiinflammatory, accommodative modalities, and taping or foot orthoses.

Pfeffer et al[139] report on the five different treatment strategies for 236 patients with plantar heel pain from 15 different orthopedic facilities. The authors concluded that when used in conjunction with a stretching program, a prefabricated insert gave greater resolution in symptoms than a custom polypropylene foot orthosis.[139] This study met with significant controversy, however, regarding the potentially inadequate design

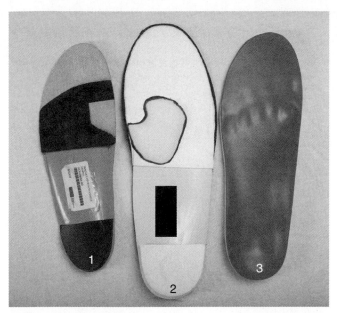

Figure 10-30 *1,* Kinetic wedge device from Langer Biomechanics Group Inc., *2,* Hapad Inc. first ray cutout relief pad, *3,* AMFIT accommodative relief device.

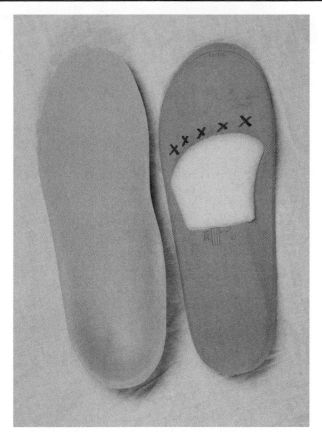

Figure 10-31 Metatarsal bar device from Hapad Inc.

and features of the polypropylene orthotic.[140,141] The literature supports orthotic design characteristics of a deep heel cup for fat pad containment, cushioning plantar heel material, longitudinal medial arch support, and customized posting based on individual foot alignment characteristics (Figure 10-32).[45] Kogler et al[142] reported on the effect of heel elevation on strain within the plantar aponeurosis. They found that elevations of the heel did not significantly alter strain in the plantar aponeurosis. Kogler et al also reported on in vivo method for evaluating the effectiveness of the longitudinal arch support mechanism of a foot orthosis. They described a dampening effect on plantar aponeurosis tension with the longitudinal arch support of a custom foot orthotic.

Foot orthotic design specific to plantar fasciitis was described by Seligman et al[143] as including a 4-degree sorbothane medial heel wedge with a customized insertion of a low-density Plastazote material heel pad. This soft molded orthotic with a cork arch fill was found to provide significant pain relief in a pilot study of 10 patients using verbal and Likert type scales. Gross et al[45] report a 66% reduction in pain ratings and 75% reduction in disability ratings with orthotic treatment in a group of 15 patients who averaged more than 21 months of plantar fasciitis pain. The custom semirigid foot orthotic consisted of four shock-absorbing layers including a thermal cork material used for longitudinal arch containment and custom posting. Gross et al describe a time requirement of 1 hour and 45 minutes for patient evaluation and orthotic fabrication.

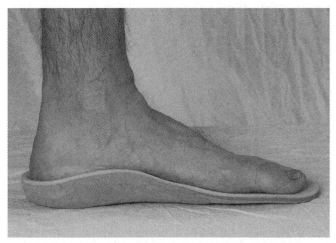

Figure 10-32 Orthotic features include deep heel cup, longitudinal arch support, and heel cushioning for plantar heel pain relief.

NEW RESEARCH TRENDS

Case Study

Subject

A 120-lb, 15-year-old, three-sport athlete was referred for physical therapy consultation by her orthopaedic surgeon at the conclusion of her spring high school track and field season. She reported an 8-week history of bilateral medial lower leg pain both during and after running. Pain patterns interfered with her high school track and field performance, and concern was voiced about her upcoming cross-country and soccer seasons, only 2 months away. Her goal for the upcoming sports season was to participate in both soccer and cross-country running simultaneously.

Physical Examination

Diffuse palpation tenderness along the medial crest of the tibias was noted bilaterally. No swelling was observed. Tibia radiographs were normal.

Top-down Assessment

Bilateral hip and pelvis muscle deficiency was observed symmetrically. Unilateral mini squat demonstrated pelvic crest drop on the non–weight-bearing leg and excessive femoral internal rotation and adduction with the weight-bearing lower extremity. The entire weight-bearing limb demonstrated excessive internal rotation as excessive foot pronation influenced the knee into excessive valgus posturing. Star excursion balance reach testing also revealed postural instability as an increased functional Q angle at the knee reflected the excessive femoral adduction and internal rotation coupled with excessive pronation of the foot.

Bottom-up Assessment

Tightness of the gastrosoleus was impressive. Ankle dorsiflexion measurement was completed by measuring its angle with a goniometer while passively dorsiflexing the non–weight-bearing ankle from subtalar neutral position with 0 degrees of extension at the knee. Ankle dorsiflexion range of motion was distinctly tight at 0 degrees bilaterally. Subtalar, midtarsal, first MTP joints all had normal mobility. Static lower extremity alignment was observed from both weight-bearing and non–weight-bearing vantage points. In the closed kinetic chain, excessive foot pronation was observed, demonstrated by calcaneal valgus, navicular drop, and forefoot abduction (toe out). Non–weight-bearing static foot assessment was done with the patient in prone position. With the subtalar joint positioned from a neutral alignment, forefoot varus and mild rearfoot varus malalignments were identified. Walking and running gait assessment was performed next. Excessive foot pronation was apparent as expected on the basis of static alignment. Excessive calcaneal eversion and medial midfoot drop was recognized during walking visual assessment. With the increased speed of running, excessive calcaneal eversion and median midfoot drop accentuated and toe-out posturing of the forefoot was observed. Additionally, excessive medially directed forces were observed at the knee at midstance as excessive femoral adduction and internal rotation coupled with prolonged internal rotation at the tibia and pronation of the foot.

The athlete's footwear was evaluated and found to be adequate. Motion control features for both running and soccer shoes were discussed for future purchases.

Functional Goals

1. Improve shock absorption mechanics to negate overuse stress to the lower extremities.
2. Increase ankle dorsiflexion to 15 degrees.
3. Increase stability of the proximal core with a focus on hip and pelvic muscle strengthening.
4. Restore postural stability as demonstrated by mini squat and Star excursion balance reach with knee over midfoot alignment and foot functioning near subtalar neutral, not at end range of pronation.
5. Enable foot pronation control with custom foot orthotics.
6. Provide cross-training alternatives for 6 weeks during the injury recovery stage.
7. Advance to sport conditioning to prepare for fall sport participation.
8. Participate in pain-free soccer and cross-country running during the fall season.

Treatment

Slipper foot casts were made for custom foot orthotics. Slipper casting was performed from a prone position with the sequence tagged site (STS) slipper sock material. The slipper sock material is a knitted, polyester, slipper-shaped sock impregnated with extra fast-setting, slippery, polyurethane resin (STS Company, 655 Redwood Highway, Suite 203, Mill Valley, California 94941). The STS casting method required $2\frac{1}{2}$ minutes of casting time per foot. The slipper casts were shipped with the product selection order form to Podiatry Arts Lab (Podiatry Arts Lab, 1805 Riverway Drive, Pekin, IL 61554) via second day air-mail. The System 3.0 orthotic (semiflexible procarbolene product) was ordered. This total contact orthotic featured pronation controlling extrinsic medial rearfoot and intrinsic forefoot posts.

Exercise Training

Three 40-minute exercise training sessions were performed with one-on-one teaching, demonstration, and performance feedback. The exercise program progressed from simple to more complex on the basis of quality success and from conscious to subconscious for kinesthesia facilitation. The program consisted of the following:

Closed Kinetic Chain

1. Hamstring and gastrosoleus and flexibility exercise with the use of the ProStretch Motion Enhancement System (Prism Technologies, 7492 Reindeer Trail, San Antonio, TX 78238).
2. Single leg squats.
3. Double leg squats.
4. Multiplanar lunges. Exercises 2 through 4 provided dynamic flexibility lengthening for the tight gastrosoleus and functional postural stability strength-

ening. Lunges included upper extremity exercise with 2-lb hand weights for shoulder abduction during side lunges and shoulder flexion during forward and backward lunges.

5. Multiplanar resistive band walking. Focus was placed on hip external rotation, extension, and abduction facilitation.

6. Balance reach exercise in frontal, sagittal, and horizontal planes.

7. Bosu training (Bosu Balance Trainer, DW Fitness, LLC, PO Box 452, Chatham, NJ 07928). Bosu training included 360-degree walking, balance squats, and balance stepovers.

Open Kinetic Chain Training

8. Exercise ball training with a 65-cm ball. Abdominal sit-up crunches and prone quadruped alternate arm and leg extensions, isolating scapular, paraspinal, and gluteus maximus training.

9. Hip abduction/adduction with Cybex Eagle equipment.

10. Resisted ankle dorsiflexion with resistance pad on dorsum of feet bilaterally while patient positioned sitting on Nautilus hamstring machine.

11. Cross-training aerobic work (elliptical trainer, Stairmaster, and recumbent cycling).

Progression Toward Independent Training

After three one-on-one sessions, the patient joined a fitness center adjacent to our office. The functional closed kinetic chain training exercises were performed on a cushioned aerobics-type surface in front of a 20′ × 10′–height mirror providing feedback for quality alignment during all exercises.

She worked on the exercise program three times per week independently over a period of 6 weeks. A walk/jog progression was initiated after becoming pain free 4 weeks into her program. Cross-country running training started 6 weeks after the physical therapy program began.

Results

The patient successfully completed both soccer and cross-country seasons (participated in both of these sports simultaneously pain free). Ankle dorsiflexion was increased from 0 to 10 degrees bilaterally. A significant improvement was noted in postural stability with the mini-squat and balance-reach exercise techniques. She could maintain neutral knee alignment and neutral foot posturing during these functional tests with increased mini-squat and balance-reach excursions. The athlete returned for a 1-year follow-up and reported success throughout her sports year without pain patterns until her foot orthotics began to show signs of excessive wear. One new pair of foot orthotics was fabricated, and the previous pair was refurbished, allowing one specific pair to be worn in her soccer cleats and one pair to be designated for her running shoes.

The focus during this case was given to teaching the athlete her responsibility to optimize her body's ability to absorb ground reaction landing forces required in the high volume of running during soccer and cross-country participation. She demonstrated compliance to core hip and pelvis stability training, as well as foot ankle gastrosoleus flexibility enhancement. She found the foot orthotics to be a successful adjunct in treatment of and future prevention of her lower leg pain patterns.

SUMMARY

Understanding pathomechanics of the lower extremity requires an appreciation of the linkage and interrelationships of the kinetic chain. From the bottom up, alignment and mobility of the foot and ankle influence proximal segments of the knee, hip, and pelvis. Foot mobility provides shock attenuation, balance response, and propulsion capabilities. Malalignment predisposes excessive pronation and supination mechanics linking to a myriad of multiplanar stresses throughout the kinetic chain. From the top down, the body's trunk and pelvis provide proximal stabilization and postural stability from which the lower extremity can efficiently move in sport. Joint restriction patterns, malalignment of the hip and knee, and neuromuscular weakness at the proximal chain are all factors that need to be influenced for injury recovery and prevention.

Functional exercise training assists a total kinetic chain response requiring kinesthesia and postural stability related to dynamic sport-specific movement. Sequencing from simple to complex and conscious to subconscious enables the athlete to gain confidence in graduation from rehabilitation to sport training and competition.

Shoe and foot orthotic intervention can provide protection to a myriad of foot-specific pain patterns and influence overuse syndromes related to excessive pronation and supination. Foot orthotic strategies include biomechanical and accommodative features specific to the diagnosis, alignment, and dynamic functional qualities of the foot.

REFERENCES

1. Holt KG, Hamill J: Running injuries and treatment: a dynamic approach. In Sammarco GJ, editor: *Rehabilitation of the foot and ankle*, pp. 241-258, St Louis, 1995, Mosby.

2. Hamill J, Holt K, Derrick T: Biomechanics of the foot and ankle. In Sammarco GJ, editor: Rehabilitation of the Foot and Ankle, p. 25, St Louis, 1995, Mosby.

3. Kibler WB: Biomechanical analysis of the shoulder during tennis activities, *Clin Sports Med* 14:79-85, 1995.

4. Nicholas JA, Marino M: The relationship of injuries of the leg, foot, and ankle to proximal thigh strength in athletes, *Foot Ankle* 7:218-228, 1987.

5. Beckman SM, Buchanan TS: Ankle inversion injury and hypermobility: effect on hip and ankle muscle elec-

tromyography onset latency, *Arch Phys Med Rehabil* 76:1138-1143, 1995.

6. Bullock-Saxton JE, Janda V, Bullock MI: The influence of ankle sprain injury on muscle activation during hip extension, *Int J Sports Med* 5:330-334, 1994.

7. Gribble PA, Hertel J, Denegar CR, et al: The effects of fatigue and chronic ankle instability on dynamic postural control, *J Athl Train* 39:321-329, 2004.

8. Shumway-Cook A, Woollacott MH: *Motor control: theory and practical applications,* Baltimore, 1995, Williams & Wilkins.

9. Hewett TE, Myer GD, Ford KR: Decrease in neuromuscular control about the knee with maturation in female athletes, *J Bone Joint Surg* 86A:1601-1608, 2004.

10. Hewett TE, Lindenfeld TN, Riccobene JV, et al: The effect of neuromuscular training on the incidence of knee injury in female athletes. A prospective study, *Am J Sports Med* 27:699-706, 1999.

11. Post WR, Teitge R, Amis A: Patellofemoral malalignment: looking beyond the viewbox, *Clin Sports Med* 21:521-546, 2002.

12. Mascal CL, Landel R, Powers C: Management of patellofemoral pain targeting hip, pelvis, and trunk muscle function: 2 case reports, *J Orthop Sports Phys Ther* 33:647-660, 2003.

13. Powers CM, Ward SR, Fredericson M, et al: Patellofemoral kinematics during weight-bearing and non-weight-bearing knee extension in persons with lateral subluxation of the patella: a preliminary study, *J Orthop Sports Phys Ther* 33:677-685, 2003.

14. Fulkerson JP: Diagnosis and treatment of patients with patellofemoral pain, *Am J Sports Med* 30:447-456, 2002.

15. McConnell J: The physical therapist's approach to patellofemoral disorders, *Clin Sports Med* 21:363-387, 2002.

16. Ireland ML, Willson JD, Ballantyne BT, et al: Hip strength in females with and without patellofemoral pain, *J Orthop Sports Phys Ther* 33:671-676, 2003.

17. Leetun DT, Ireland ML, Willson JD, et al: Core stability measures as risk factors for lower extremity injury in athletes, *Med Sci Sports Exerc* 36:926-934, 2004.

18. Knott M, Voss DE: *Proprioceptive neuromuscular facilitation: patterns and techniques,* New York, 1968, Hoeber.

19. Schmeir AA: Research work on a more precise method of determining muscle strength and poliomyelitis patients, *J Bone Joint Surg* 27:317-326, 1945.

20. Gambetta V: *From the core. The Gambetta Method,* Sarasota, FL,1998, Gambetta Sports Training System.

21. Hodges PW, Richardson CA: Contraction of the abdominal muscles associated with movement of the lower limb, *Phys Ther* 77:132-144, 1997.

22. Perry J: *Gait analysis: normal and pathological function,* Thorofare, NJ, 1992, Slack.

23. Cavanagh PR: The biomechanics of lower extremity action in distance running, *Foot Ankle* 7:197-217, 1987.

24. Skelly WA, Devita PL: Compressive and shear forces on the tibia and knee during landing. Proceedings of 6th Biannual Conference of the Canadian Society for Biomechanics, Quebec, August 1990, pp. 59-60.

25. Davis IS: How do we accurately measure foot motion? *J Orthop Sports Phys Ther* 34:502-503, 2004.

26. Donatelli RA: Normal anatomy and biomechanics. In Donatelli RA, editor: *The biomechanics of the foot and ankle,* Philadelphia, 1990, FA Davis Company.

27. Bobbert MF, Huijing PA, van Ingen Schenau GJ: Drop jumping. II. The influence of dropping height on the biomechanics of drop jumping, *Med Sci Sports Exerc* 19:339-346, 1987.

28. Valiant GA, Cavanagh PR: A study of landing from a jump: implications for the design of a basketball shoe. In Winter DA, Norman RW, Wells RP, et al, editors: *Biomechanics IX-B,* pp. 117-122, Champaign, Ill, 1985, Human Kinetics.

29. O'Connell AL: Effect of sensory deprivation on postural reflexes, *Electromyography* 11:519-527, 1971.

30. Dananberg HJ, Guiliano M: Chronic low-back pain and its response to custom-made foot orthoses, *J Am Podiatr Med Assoc* 89:109-117, 1999.

31. Ryerson S, Levit K: Walking. In Ryerson S, Levit K, editors: Functional movement reeducation, pp. 433-477, New York, 1997, Churchill Livingstone.

32. Albert M: Physiologic and clinical principles of eccentrics. In Albert M, editor: *Eccentric muscle training in sports and orthopaedics,* pp. 11-23, New York, 1991, Churchill Livingstone.

33. Mulligan BR: The extremities. Mobilisations with Movements (MWMS). In Mulligan BR, editor: *Manual therapy, "Nags," "Snags," "MWMS," etc.,* ed 4, pp. 87-119, Wellington, New Zealand, 1999, Plane View Services Ltd.

34. Kaufman KR, Brodine SK, Shaffer RA, et al: The effect of foot structure and range of motion on musculoskeletal overuse injuries, *Am J Sports Med* 27:585-593, 1999.

35. Youdas JW, Krause DA, Egan KS, et al: The effect of static stretching of the calf muscle-tendon unit on active ankle dorsiflexion range of motion, *J Orthop Sports Phys Ther* 33:408-417, 2003.

36. Hreljac A, Marshall RN, Hume PA: Evaluation of lower extremity overuse injury potential in runners, *Med Sci Sports Exerc* 32:1635-1641, 2000.

37. James SL, Bates BT, Osternig LR: Injuries to runners, *Am J Sports Med* 6:40-50, 1978.

38. Clement DB, Taunton JE, Smart GW, et al: A survey of overuse running injuries, *Phys Sports Med* 9:47-58, 1981.

39. Viitasalo JT, Kvist M: Some biomechanical aspects of the foot and ankle in athletes with and without shin splints, *Am J Sports Med* 11:125-130, 1983.

40. Tomaro J: Measurement of tibiofibular varum in subjects with unilateral overuse symptoms, *J Orthop Sports Phys Ther* 21:86-89, 1995.

41. Ross CF, Schuster RO: A preliminary report on predicting injuries in distance runners, *J Am Podiatry Assoc* 73:275-277, 1983.

42. Powers CM, Maffucci R, Hampton S: Rearfoot posture in subjects with patellofemoral pain, *J Orthop Sports Phys Ther* 22:155-160, 1995.

43. Manoli A II, Graham B: Cavus foot diagnosis determines treatment, *Biomechanics* VIII:55-69, 2001.

44. Solis G, Hennessy MS, Saxby TS: Pes cavus: a review, *Foot Ankle Surg* 6:145-153, 2000.

45. Gross MT, Byers JM, Krafft JL, et al: The impact of custom semirigid foot orthotics on pain and disability for individuals with plantar fasciitis, *J Orthop Sports Phys Ther* 32:149-157, 2002.

46. Gross ML, Davlin LB, Evanski PM: Effectiveness of orthotic shoe inserts in the long-distance runner, *Am J Sports Med* 19:409-412, 1991.

47. Gross MT, Foxworth JL: The role of foot orthoses as an intervention for patellofemoral pain, *J Orthop Sports Phys Ther* 33:661-670, 2003.

48. Williams DS, McClay IS: Lower extremity mechanics and injury patterns in runners with pes cavus and pes planus. Proceedings of the Foot Classification Conference: Keynote Address, *J Orthop Sports Phys Ther* 34:156, 2001.

49. Hamill J, Bates BT, Holt KG: Timing of lower extremity joint actions during treadmill running, *Med Sci Sports Exerc* 24:807-813, 1992.

50. Buchbinder MR, Napora NJ, Biggs EW: The relationship of abnormal pronation to chondromalacia of the patella in distance runners, *J Am Podiatry Assoc* 69:159-162, 1979.

51. Tiberio D: The effect of excessive subtalar joint pronation on patellofemoral mechanics: a theoretical model, *J Orthop Sports Phys Ther* 9:160-165, 1987.

52. McClay I, Manal K: A comparison of three-dimensional lower extremity kinematics during running between excessive pronators and normals, *Clin Biomech* 13:195-203, 1998.

53. Renne JW: The iliotibial band friction syndrome, *J Bone Joint Surg* 57A:1110-1111, 1975.

54. Geraci MC Jr: Rehabilitation of the hip, pelvis, and thigh. In Kibler WB, Herring A, Press JM, et al, editors: *Functional rehabilitation of sports and musculoskeletal injuries,* pp. 216-243, Gaithersburg, Md, 1998, Aspen Publishers.

55. Janda V: Muscle weakness and inhibition (pseudoparesis) in back pain syndromes. In Grieve GP, editor: *Modern manual therapy of the vertebral column,* pp. 197-201, New York, 1986, Churchill Livingstone.

56. Sale D: Neural adaptation in strength and power training. In Jones NL, McCartney N, McComas AJ, editors: *Human muscle power,* Champaign, Ill, 1986, Human Kinetics Publishers.

57. Gross MT: Lower quarter screening for skeletal malalignment—suggestions for orthotics and shoewear, *J Orthop Sports Phys Ther* 21:389-405, 1995.

58. Reider B: Terms and techniques. In Reider B, editor: *The orthopaedic physical examination,* pp. 2-18, Philadelphia, 1999, Saunders.

59. Yoshioka Y, Cooke TD: Femoral anteversion: assessment based on function axes, *J Orthop Res* 5:86-91, 1987.

60. Braten M, Terjesen T, Rossvoll I: Femoral anteversion in normal adults. Ultrasound measurements in 50 men and 50 women, *Acta Orthop Scand* 63:29-32, 1992.

61. Magee DJ: Hip. In Magee DJ, editor: *Orthopedic physical assessment,* ed 2, Philadelphia, 1992, Saunders.

62. Ruwe PA, Gage JR, Ozonoff MB, et al: Clinical determination of femoral anteversion. A comparison with established techniques, *J Bone Joint Surg* 74A:820-830, 1992.

63. Lee TQ, Anzel SH, Bennett KA, et al: The influence of fixed rotational deformities of the femur on the patellofemoral contact pressures in human cadaver knees, *Clin Orthop* (302):69-74, May 1994.

64. Riegger-Krugh C, Keysor JJ: Skeletal malalignments of the lower quarter: correlated and compensatory motions and postures, *J Orthop Sports Phys Ther* 23:164-170, 1996.

65. Lee TQ, Yang BY, Sandusky MD, et al: The effects of tibial rotation on the patellofemoral joint: assessment of the changes in *in situ* strain in the peripatellar retinaculum and the patellofemoral contact pressures and areas, *J Rehabil Res Dev* 38:463-469, 2001.

66. Bleck EE: Developmental orthopaedics. III: Toddlers, *Dev Med Child Neurol* 24:533-555, 1982.

67. Greenfield B: Evaluation of overuse syndromes. In Donatelli RA, editor: *The biomechanics of the foot and ankle,* pp. 3-31, Philadelphia, 1990, FA Davis.

68. Oswald MH, Jakob RP, Schneider E, et al: Radiological analysis of normal axial alignment of femur and tibia in view of total knee arthroplasty, *J Arthroplasty* 8:419-426, 1993.

69. Tiberio D: Pathomechanics of structural foot deformities, *Phys Ther* 68:1840-1849, 1988.

70. Lohmann KN, Rayhel HE, Schneiderwind WP, et al: Static measurement of tibia vara. Reliability and effect of lower extremity position, *Phys Ther* 67:196-202, 1987.

71. Brady RJ, Dean JB, Skinner TM, et al: Limb length inequality: clinical implications for assessment and intervention, *J Orthop Sports Phys Ther* 33(5):221-234, 2003.

72. Holden JP: Foot angles during walking and running. In Winter DA, Norman RW, Wells RP, et al, editors: *Biomechanics IX-A,* pp. 451-457, Champaign, Ill, 1985, Human Kinetics.

73. Larson RL, Cabaud HE, Slocum DB, et al: The patellar compression syndrome: surgical treatment by lateral retinacular release, *Clin Orthop* (134):158-167, 1978.

74. Fox TA: Dysplasia of the quadriceps mechanism: hypoplasia of the vastus medialis muscle as related to the hypermobile patella syndrome, *Surg Clin North Am* 55:199-226, 1975.

75. McClay I: Proceedings of the foot classification conference, *J Orthop Sports Phys Ther* 31:153-160, 2001.

76. Garbalosa JC, McClure MH, Catlin PA, et al: The frontal plane relationship of the forefoot to the rearfoot in an asymptomatic population, *J Orthop Sports Phys Ther* 20:200-206, 1994.

77. Root ML: *Normal and abnormal function of the foot,* Los Angeles, 1977, Clinical Biomechanics Corporation.

78. Cobb SC, Tis LL, Johnson BF, et al: The effect of forefoot varus on postural stability, *J Orthop Sports Phys Ther* 34:79-85, 2004.

79. Gray GC: *When the foot hits the ground everything changes,* seminar course book, Toledo, Ohio, Rehabilitation Network, 1985.

80. Astrom M, Arvidson T: Alignment and joint motion in the normal foot, *J Orthop Sports Phys Ther* 22:216-222, 1995.

81. Glasoe WM, Allen MK, Ludewig PM: Comparison of first ray dorsal mobility among different forefoot alignments, *J Orthop Sports Phys Ther* 30:612-623, 2000.

82. Subotnick SI: Biomechanics of the subtalar and midtarsal joint, *J Am Podiatr Assoc* 65:756-764, 1975.

83. Hunt GC, Brocato RS: Gait and foot pathomechanics. In Hunt GC, editor: *Clinics in physical therapy: physical therapy of the foot and ankle,* ed 2, vol. 15, New York, 1988, Churchill Livingstone. pp. 39-57,

84. Fromherz WA: Examination. In Hunt GC, editor: *Clinics in physical therapy: physical therapy of the foot and ankle,* ed 2, vol 15, New York, 1988, Churchill Livingstone. pp. 59-90.

85. Magee DJ: Lower leg, ankle, and foot. In Magee DJ, editor: *Orthopedic physical assessment,* ed 2, pp. 448-515, Philadelphia, 1992, Saunders.

86. Geraci MC, Brown W: *Functional evaluation and treatment of the athlete: where function meets science,* seminar course book, Buffalo Spine and Sports Medicine Institute, Williamsville, New York, 2004.

87. Ryerson S, Levit K: Functional movement: a practical model for treatment. In Ryerson S, Levit K, editors: *Functional movement reeducation,* pp. 1-13, New York, 1997, Churchill Livingstone.

88. Cerulli G, Benoit DL, Caraffa A, et al: Proprioceptive training and prevention of anterior cruciate ligament injuries in soccer, *J Orthop Sports Phys Ther* 31:655-661, 2001.

89. Paterno MV, Myer GD, Ford KR, et al: Neuromuscular training improves single-limb stability in young female athletes, *J Orthop Sports Phys Ther* 34:305-316, 2004.

90. Onate JA, Guskiewicz KM, Sullivan RJ: Augmented feedback reduces jump landing forces, *J Orthop Sports Phys Ther* 31:511-517, 2001.

91. Gray GW: *Total body functional profile,* Adrian, Mich, 2001, Wynn Marketing.

92. Kinzey SJ, Armstrong CW: The reliability of the star-excursion test in assessing dynamic balance, *J Orthop Sports Phys Ther* 27:356-360, 1998.

93. Hertel J, Miller JS, Denegar CR: Intratester and intertester reliability during the Star Excursion Balance Tests, *J Sport Rehabil* 9:104-116, 2000.

94. Olmsted LC, Carcia CR, Hertel J, et al: Efficacy of the Star excursion balance tests in detecting reach deficits in subjects with chronic ankle instability, *J Athl Train* 37:501-506, 2002.

95. Huston LJ, Vibert B, Ashton-Miller JA, et al: Gender differences in knee angle when landing from a drop-jump, *Am J Knee Surg* 14:215-220, 2001.

96. Hewett TE, Stroupe AL, Nance TA, et al: Plyometric training in female athletes. Decreased impact forces and increased hamstring torques, *Am J Sports Med* 24:765-773, 1996.

97. Prapavessis H, McNair PJ: Effects of instruction in jumping technique and experience jumping on ground reaction forces, *J Orthop Sports Phys Ther* 29:352-356, 1999.

98. Williams GN, Chmielewski T, Rudolph K, et al: Dynamic knee stability: current theory and implications for clinicians and scientists, *J Orthop Sports Phys Ther* 31:546-566, 2001.

99. Caraffa A, Cerulli G, Projetti M, et al: Prevention of anterior cruciate ligament injuries in soccer. A prospective controlled study of proprioceptive training, *Knee Surg Sports Traumatol Arthrosc* 4:19-21, 1996.

100. Albert M. Introduction. In Albert M, editor: *Eccentric muscle training in sports and orthopaedics,* pp. 1-9, New York, 1991, Churchill Livingstone.

101. Gambetta V, Clark M: Hard core training, *Training Conditioning* 9:34-40, 1999.

102. Gambetta V, Clark M: A formula for function. *Training Conditioning* 7:24-29, 1998.

103. Kendall FP, Provance PG, McCreary EK: *Muscles: testing and function with posture and pain,* ed 4, Baltimore, 1993, Williams & Wilkins.

104. Sahrmann S: Diagnosis and treatment of movement impairment syndromes, St Louis, 2001, Mosby.

105. Schafer RC: *Clinical biomechanics: musculoskeletal actions and reactions,* Baltimore, 1983, Williams & Wilkins.

106. Plotke RJ: *The power of the center,* Physical Therapy Forum, January 1994.

107. Albert M, Lathrop J: Free weight training. In Albert M, editor: *Eccentric muscle training in sports and orthopaedics,* pp. 133-151, New York, 1991, Churchill Livingstone.

108. Nawoczenski DA, Janisse DJ: Foot orthoses and rehabilitation—what's new, *Clin Sports Med* 23:157-167, 2004.

109. Stacoff A, Reinschmidt C, Nigg BM, et al: Effects of foot orthoses on skeletal motion during running, *Clin Biomech* 15:54-64, 2000.

110. Genova JM, Gross MT: Effect of foot orthotics on calcaneal eversion during standing and treadmill walking for subjects with abnormal pronation, *J Orthop Sports Phys Ther* 30:664-675, 2000.

111. Smith LS, Clarke TE, Hamill CL, et al: The effects of soft and semi-rigid orthoses upon rearfoot movement in running, *J Am Podiatr Med Assoc* 76:227-233, 1986.

112. McClay I: The evolution of the study of the mechanics of running. Relationship to injury, *J Am Podiatr Med Assoc* 90:133-148, 2000.

113. Janisse DJ: Pedorthotics in the rehabilitation of the foot and ankle. In Sammarco GJ, editor: *Rehabilitation of the foot and ankle,* pp. 351-364, St Louis, 1995, Mosby.

114. Donatelli R, Brasel J, Brotzman SB: Foot orthoses. In Brotzman SB, editor: *Clinical orthopaedic rehabilitation,* pp. 343-370, St Louis, 1996, Mosby.

115. Johanson MA, Donatelli R, Wooden MJ, et al: Effects of three different posting methods on controlling abnormal subtalar pronation, *Phys Ther* 74:149-161, 1994.

116. Nawoczenski DA, Ludewig PM: The effect of forefoot and arch posting orthotic designs on first metatarsophalangeal joint kinematics during gait, *J Orthop Sports Phys Ther* 34:317-327, 2004.

117. Donatelli R, Hurlbert C, Conaway D, et al: Biomechanical foot orthotics: a retrospective study, *J Orthop Sports Phys Ther* 10:205-212, 1988.

118. Feltner ME, MacRae HS, MacRae PG, et al: Strength training effects on rearfoot motion in running, *Med Sci Sports Exerc* 26:1021-1027, 1994.

119. Stokes IA, Hutton WC, Stott JR: Forces acting on the metatarsals during normal walking, *J Anat* 129:579-590, 1979.

120. Mann RA, Hagy JL: The function of the toes in walking, jogging and running, *Clin Orthop* (142):24-29, 1979.

121. Claton TO, Brotzman SB, Graves SG: In Griffin LY, editor: *Orthopaedic knowledge update: sports medicine,* Rosemont, Ill, 1994, American Academy of Orthopaedic Surgeons.

122. Cailliet R: *Foot and ankle pain,* ed 2, Philadelphia, 1968, FA Davis.

123. Herrmann TJ: The foot and ankle in football. In Sammarco GJ, editor: *Rehabilitation of the foot and ankle,* pp. 259-268, St Louis, 1995, Mosby.

124. Grace DL: Sesamoid problems, *Foot Ankle Clin* 5:609-627, 2000.

125. Vanore JV, Christensen JC, Kravitz SR, et al: Clinical Practice Guideline First Metatarsal Joint Disorders Panel of the American College of Foot and Ankle Surgeons. Diagnosis and treatment of first metatarsophalangeal joint disorders. Section 4: Sesamoid disorders, *J Foot Ankle Surg* 42:143-147, 2003.

126. Wilder RP, Sethi S: Overuse injuries: tendinopathies, stress fractures, compartment syndrome, and shin splints, *Clin Sports Med* 23:55-81, 2004.

127. Frey C: The shoe in sports. In Baxter DE, editors: *The foot and ankle in sport,* pp. 353-367, St Louis, 1995, Mosby.

128. Barrett SJ, O'Malley R: Plantar fasciitis and other causes of heel pain, *Am Fam Physician* 59:2200-2206, 1999.

129. Gibbon WW, Long G: Ultrasound of the plantar aponeurosis (fascia), *Skeletal Radiol* 28:21-26, 1999.

130. Lynch DM, Goforth WP, Martin JE, et al: Conservative treatment of plantar fasciitis. A prospective study, *J Am Podiatr Med Assoc* 88:375-380, 1998.

131. Cornwall MW, McPoil TG: Plantar fasciitis: etiology and treatment, *J Orthop Sports Phys Ther* 29:756-760, 1999.

132. Hicks JH: The mechanics of the foot. II. The plantar aponeurosis and the arch, *J Anat* 88:25-30, 1954.

133. Perry J: Anatomy and biomechanics of the hindfoot, *Clin Orthop* (177):9-15, 1983.

134. Mann RA: Surgical implications of biomechanics of the foot and ankle, *Clin Orthop* (146):111-118, 1980.

135. Fuller EA: The windlass mechanism of the foot. A mechanical model to explain pathology, *J Am Podiatr Med Assoc* 90:35-46, 2000.

136. Wilk BR, Fisher KL, Gutierrez W: Defective running shoes as a contributing factor in plantar fasciitis in a triathlete, *J Orthop Sports Phys Ther* 30:21-31, 2000.

137. Ng A: Treatment of plantar fasciitis with night splint and shoe modifications consisting of a steel shank and anterior rocker bottom, *Foot Ankle Int* 18(7):458, 1997.

138. Mizel MS, Marymont JV, Trepman E: Treatment of plantar fasciitis with a night splint and shoe modification consisting of a steel shank and anterior rocker bottom, *Foot Ankle Int* 17:732-735, 1996.

139. Pfeffer G, Bacchetti P, Deland J, et al: Comparison of custom and prefabricated orthoses in the initial treatment of proximal plantar fasciitis, *Foot Ankle Int* 20:214-221, 1999.

140. Heel pain study colloquy, *Biomechanics* 4:15, 1997.

141. Pfeffer GB: Heel pain study colloquy, *Biomechanics* 4:16, 1997

142. Kogler GF, Solomonidis SE, Paul JP: In vitro method for quantifying the effectiveness of the longitudinal arch support mechanism of a foot orthosis, *Clin Biomech* 10:245-252, 1995.

143. Seligman DA, Dawson DR: Customized heel pads and soft orthotics to treat heel pain and plantar fasciitis, *Arch Phys Med Rehabil* 84:1564-1567, 2003.

CHAPTER

11

Todd S. Ellenbecker

Evaluation of Glenohumeral, Acromioclavicular, and Scapulothoracic Joints in the Overhead-Throwing Athlete

LEARNING OBJECTIVES

After studying this chapter, the reader will be able to do the following:

1. Identify the key clinical tests used for evaluation of the rotator cuff, labrum, and scapula
2. Characterize scapular pathology on the basis of the Kibler Classification Scheme
3. Break down and evaluate throwing mechanics and understand the consequences of foot placement and stride characteristics in the lower extremity and their effect on upper extremity function
4. Perform and interpret manual and instrumented muscular strength tests

The return of function to the patient with a proximal upper extremity injury requires a comprehensive evaluation of the upper extremity kinetic chain, as well as a specific, evidence-based rehabilitation program. Additionally, an evaluation of the patient's sport biomechanics is an essential part of this comprehensive program to prevent reinjury and optimize performance. The purposes of this chapter are to outline several key concepts in proximal upper extremity anatomy and biomechanics and present evaluation methods and key treatment concepts to enable the transition from thorough clinical rehabilitation to functional activity.

One of the key concepts in upper extremity rehabilitation is the scapular plane concept. The scapular plane has ramifications in treatment, evaluation, and even in functional activity in sports. According to Saha,[1] the scapular plane is defined as being 30 degrees anterior to the coronal or frontal plane of the body. Placement of the glenohumeral joint in the scapular plane optimizes the osseous congruity between the humeral

head and the glenoid and is widely recommended as an optimal position for both the performance of various evaluation techniques, as well as during many rehabilitation exercises.[1,2] With the glenohumeral joint placed in the scapular plane, bony impingement of the greater tuberosity against the acromion does not occur due to the alignment of the tuberosity and acromion in this orientation.[1]

Another important general concept of relevance for this chapter is that of muscular force couples. One of the most important biomechanical principles in shoulder function is the deltoid rotator cuff force couple.[3] This phenomenon, known as a "force couple," can be defined as two opposing muscular forces working together to enable a particular motion to occur, with these muscular forces being synergists, or agonist/antagonist pairs.[3] The deltoid muscle provides force primarily in a superior direction when contracting unopposed during arm elevation.[4] The muscle tendon units of the rotator cuff must provide both a compressive force, as well as an inferiorly or caudally directed force to minimize superior migration and minimize contact or impingement of the rotator cuff tendons against the overlying acromion.[3] Failure of the rotator cuff to maintain humeral congruency leads to glenohumeral joint instability, rotator cuff tendon pathology, and labral injury.[5] Imbalances in the deltoid rotator cuff force couple, which primarily occur during inappropriate and unbalanced strength training, as well as through repetitive overhead sport activities, can lead to development of the deltoid without concomitant increases in the rotator cuff strength and increase the superior migration of the humeral head provided by the deltoid, leading to rotator cuff impingement.

Additionally, the serratus anterior and trapezius force couple is the primary muscular stabilization and prime mover of upward rotation of the scapular during arm elevation. Bagg

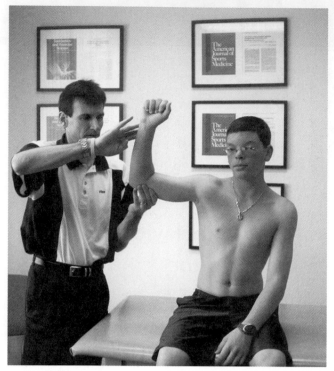

Figure 11-1 Position of testing for the infraspinatus with the glenohumeral joint in 90 degrees of coronal plane abduction and 90 degrees of external rotation.

and Forest[6] have shown how the upper trapezius and serratus anterior function during the initial (0 to 80 degrees of) arm elevation, providing upward scapular rotation and stabilization. Due to a change in the lever arm of the lower trapezius that occurs during the lateral shift of the scapulothoracic instantaneous center of rotation with arm elevation, the lower trapezius and serratus anterior function as the primary scapular stabilizer in phases II and III (80 to 140 degrees) of elevation.[6] Knowledge of the important muscular force couples in the human shoulder and scapulothoracic region is imperative and can lead to proper evaluation and ultimately treatment via strengthening and monitoring proper strength balance of these important muscular pairings.

MUSCULAR AND RANGE OF MOTION TESTING IN THE SHOULDER IN THE OVERHEAD ATHLETE

The most clinically relevant method used to assess strength of the shoulder girdle is manual muscle testing (MMT). Since its initial development in the early 1900s during the study of muscle function in patients with poliomyelitis, MMT has become a standard practice during the physical evaluation of patients with both neurological and orthopaedic injuries.[7,8] Although several limitations exist in the use of MMT in the athletic shoulder, the application of this important technique has high clinical relevance, especially in the absence of more sophisticated methodology, such as hand-held dynamometers or isokinetic testing.[9]

Key Positions Used for Manual Muscle Testing of the Rotator Cuff

Kelly et al[10] used electromyography (EMG) to determine the optimal position for testing the muscles of the rotator cuff in human subjects. Four criteria were used to establish which position was optimal for each rotator cuff muscle. These were: maximal activation of the muscle, minimal contribution from shoulder synergists, minimal provocation of pain, and good test-retest reliability. Kelley et al[10] found the optimal muscle testing position for the supraspinatus to be at 90 degrees of elevation, with the patient in a seated position. The scapular plane position was used (in this research this represented 45 degrees of horizontal adduction from the coronal plane) with external rotation of the humerus such that the forearm was placed in neutral and the thumb was pointing upward toward the ceiling. This position was termed the *Full Can Testing position*. Another frequently used test position to assess the strength of the supraspinatus muscle-tendon unit is termed the *Empty Can Test*. This test position has been advocated by Jobe[11] and has been found to have high levels of supraspinatus muscular activation using indwelling EMG.[12]

Kelly et al[10] reported the optimal position to test for infraspinatus strength is with the patient in a seated position, with 0 degrees of glenohumeral joint elevation and in 45 degrees of internal rotation from neutral. An alternative position for testing the infraspinatus has been recommended by Jenp et al.[13] They recommend testing the infraspinatus in 90 degrees of elevation in the sagittal plane, with the arm in half maximal external rotation. The author of this chapter highly recommends the use of the 90-degree abducted position for testing the infraspinatus in a functionally specific position and 90 degrees of external rotation as pictured (Figure 11-1). To test the teres minor muscle, use of the Patte test to best isolate the teres minor has been recommended by both Walch et al[14] and Leroux et al.[15] The position of the glenohumeral joint for the Patte test[16] to isolate the teres minor has been reported as 90 degrees of glenohumeral joint abduction in the scapular plane and 90 degrees of external rotation.

Finally, Kelley et al[10] reported the optimal position for subscapularis muscular activation to be in the Gerber lift-off position.[17] This position involves placing the dorsal aspect of the hand in lumbar lordosis and pressing posteriorly away from the back.

Relationship between Manual Muscle Testing and Isokinetic Testing

Ellenbecker[18] compared isokinetic testing of the shoulder internal and external rotators to MMT in 54 subjects exhibiting manually assessed, symmetrical, normal-grade (5/5) strength. Isokinetic testing found 13% to 15% bilateral differences in external rotation and 15% to 28% bilateral differences in internal rotation. Of particular significance was the large variability in the size of this mean difference between extremities, despite bilaterally symmetrical MMT. The use of MMT is an integral part of a musculoskeletal evaluation. MMT provides a time efficient, gross screening of muscular strength of multiple muscles using a static, isometric muscular contraction, particularly in situations of neuromuscular disease or in patients with large muscular strength deficits. The limitations of MMT appear to be most evident when only minor impairment of strength is present, as well as in the identification of subtle isolated strength deficits. Differentiation of agonist/antagonist muscular strength balance is also complicated using manual techniques, as opposed to using isokinetic instrumentation.[18]

Use of Isokinetic Testing for the Shoulder Complex

The initial position used for isokinetic testing of the shoulder typically involves the modified base position. The modified base position is obtained by tilting the dynamometer approximately 30 degrees from the horizontal base position.[19] The patient's glenohumeral joint is placed in 30 degrees abduction and 30 degrees forward flexion into the plane of the scapula or scaption, and with a 30-degree diagonal tilt of the dynamometer head from the transverse plane. This position has also been termed the *(30/30/30) internal/external rotation position* by Davies.[19] The modified base position places the shoulder in the scapular plane 30 degrees anterior to the coronal plane.[1] The scapular plane is characterized by enhanced bony congruity and a neutral glenohumeral position, which results in a midrange position for the anterior capsular ligaments and enhances the length tension relationship of the scapulohumeral musculature.[1] This position does not place the suprahumeral structures in an impingement situation and is well tolerated by patient populations.[19]

Isokinetic testing using the modified base position requires consistent application of the patient to the dynamometer. Studies have demonstrated significant differences in internal and external rotation strength, with varying degrees of abduction, flexion, and horizontal abduction/adduction of the glenohumeral joint.[20-22] The modified base position uses a standing patient position on many dynamometer systems, which can lead to compromises in both glenohumeral joint isolation and test-retest reliability. Despite these limitations, valuable data can be obtained early in the rehabilitative process using this neutral, modified base position, which is a safe, comfortable position for most patients with most pathologies and post-surgical considerations.[9,19] Knops et al[23] conducted a test-retest reliability study of the modified neutral position for internal/external rotation of the glenohumeral joint. This position of testing produced high test-retest reliability, with intraclass correlation coefficients ranging from 91 to 96.

The most functionally specific isokinetic testing position for the assessment of internal and external rotation strength is performed with 90 degrees of glenohumeral joint abduction (Figure 11-2). Specific advantages of this test position are greater stabilization in either a seated or supine test position on most dynamometers, as well as placement of the shoulder in

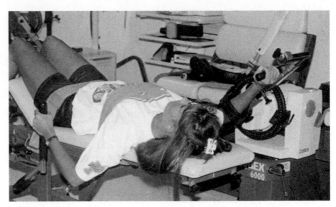

Figure 11-2 Position used for isokinetic testing with 90 degrees of abduction in the coronal plane on the Cybex 6000 isokinetic dynamometer. (From Ellenbecker TS: *Clinical examination of the shoulder*, Philadelphia, 2004, Elsevier-Saunders.)

an abduction angle corresponding to the overhead-throwing position used in many sport activities.[24] Utilization of the 90-degree abducted position of isokinetic strength assessment will more specifically address muscular function required for overhead activities.[25] Descriptive data profiles for throwing athletes,[26,27] as well as for elite junior tennis players,[28] are listed in Tables 11-1 through 11-3. These data provide objective information regarding the normal torque to body weight ratios, as well as external/internal rotation ratios used in the interpretation of instrumented upper extremity strength testing. Muscular imbalances due to the repetitive and forceful internal rotation during the acceleration of the throwing motion, tennis serve, and forehand can lead to unilateral muscular imbalances on the dominant arm between the external and internal rotators and jeopardize optimal muscular stabilization.[26-28] Use of instrumented testing is an important part of a comprehensive evaluation of the throwing athlete.[9]

Isokinetic dynamometers have also been extensively used in the measurement of muscular fatigue.[29,30] Isokinetic muscular fatigue tests typically consist of measuring the number of repetitions of maximum effort that are required to reach a 50% reduction in torque, work, or power from the beginning to the end of a certain time period or number of contractions. Relative fatigue ratios consist of comparing the work in the last half of a preset number of muscular contractions with the work performed in the first half.[19,30]

Relative fatigue ratios have been studied in elite tennis players and have produced clinically applicable information. Ellenbecker and Roetert[29] measured the relative fatigue response in the internal and external rotators of 72 elite junior tennis players, using 20 maximal effort concentric testing repetitions at 300 degrees per second in the supine position, with 90 degrees of glenohumeral joint abduction. They found the external rotators to fatigue to a level of 69%, while the internal rotators only fatigued to a level of 83%. This is significant, due to the substantial contribution the external rotators play in humeral deceleration during overhead throwing and serving activities,[24] as well as dynamic stabilization of the humeral head in the glenoid.[25] Because the external rotators appear to

| Table 11-1 | Isokinetic Data from the Biodex Isokinetic Dynamometer from Professional Baseball Pitchers for Shoulder Internal/External Rotation |

Isokinetic Peak Torque–to–Body Weight Ratios from 150 Professional Baseball Pitchers*

Speed	Internal Rotation		External Rotation	
	Dominant Arm	Nondominant Arm	Dominant Arm	Nondominant Arm
180 degrees/sec	27%	17%	18%	19%
300 degrees/sec	25%	24%	15%	15%

Unilateral External Rotation/Internal Rotation Ratios in Professional Baseball Pitchers

Speed	Dominant Arm	Nondominant Arm
180 degrees/sec		
Torque	65	64
300 degrees/sec		
Torque	61	70

Data from Wilk KE, Andrews JR, Arrigo CA, et al: *Am J Sports Med* 21:61-66, 1993.
*Data were obtained on a Biodex Isokinetic Dynamometer.

| Table 11-2 | Isokinetic Data from the Cybex Isokinetic Dynamometer from Professional Baseball Pitchers for Shoulder Internal/External Rotation |

Isokinetic Peak Torque–to–Body Weight and Work–to–Body Weight Ratios from 147 Professional Baseball Pitchers*

Speed	Internal Rotation		External Rotation	
	Dominant Arm	Nondominant Arm	Dominant Arm	Nondominant Arm
210 degrees/sec				
Torque	21%	19%	13%	14%
Work	41%	38%	25%	25%
300 degrees/sec				
Torque	20%	18%	13%	13%
Work	37%	33%	23%	23%

Unilateral External Rotation/Internal Rotation Ratios in Professional Baseball Pitchers

Speed	Dominant Arm	Nondominant Arm
210 degrees/sec		
Torque	64	74
Work	61	66
300 degrees/sec		
Torque	65	72
Work	62	70

Data from Ellenbecker TS, Mattalino AJ: *J Orthop Sports Phys Ther* 25:323-328, 1997.
*Data were obtained on a Cybex 350 Isokinetic Dynamometer.

| Table 11-3 | Isokinetic Data from the Cybex 6000 Isokinetic Dynamometer for Shoulder Internal/External Rotation |

Isokinetic Peak Torque–to–Body Weight Ratios and Single Repetition Work–to–Body Weight Ratios in Elite Junior Tennis Players*

Arm	Dominant Arm		Nondominant	
	Peak Torque (%)	Work (%)	Peak Torque (%)	Work (%)
ER				
Male, 210 degrees/sec	12	20	11	19
Male, 300 degrees/sec	10	18	10	17
Female, 210 degrees/sec	8	14	8	15
Female, 300 degrees/sec	8	11	7	12
IR				
Male, 210 degrees/sec	17	32	14	27
Male, 300 degrees/sec	15	28	13	23
Female, 210 degrees/sec	12	23	11	19
Female, 300 degrees/sec	11	15	10	13

Isokinetic ER/IR Ratios in Elite Junior Tennis Players[†]

ER/IR ratio	Dominant Arm		Nondominant	
	Peak Torque (%)	Work (%)	Peak Torque (%)	Work (%)
Male, 210 degrees/sec	69	64	81	81
Male, 300 degrees/sec	69	65	82	83
Female, 210 degrees/sec	69	63	81	82
Female, 300 degrees/sec	67	61	81	77

From Ellenbecker TS, Roetert EP: *J Sci Med Sport* 6(1):63-70, 2003.

Note: A Cybex 6000 series Isokinetic Dynamometer and 90 degrees of glenohumeral joint abduction were used.

ER, External rotation; *IR,* internal rotation.

*Data are expressed in foot-pounds per unit of body weight for ER and IR.

[†]Data are expressed as ER/IR ratios representing the relative muscular balance between the external and internal rotators.

fatigue more quickly and to a greater extent than the internal rotators, this further supports the current concepts of preventative conditioning and balancing of the shoulder external rotators in unilaterally dominant upper extremity athletes.

Range of Motion Testing

Discussing range-of-motion testing in depth is beyond the scope of this chapter; however, the measurement of one of the most important movement patterns (humeral rotation) will be covered, along with the concept of total rotation range of motion (ROM). A thorough objective documentation of the cardinal movements of the glenohumeral joint is recommended, and the reader is referred to two texts[31,32] for a more complete discussion.

Technique for Measurement of Humeral Rotation

Several important principles should be discussed to optimize the measurement of humeral rotation in the overhead-throwing athlete. One of these is the contribution of the scapulothoracic joint to glenohumeral motion, which has been widely documented.[3,33] This is one of the variables that can

lead to extensive variation of rotational measurement in the human shoulder. In a study by Ellenbecker et al,[34] active rotational ROM measures were taken bilaterally in 399 elite junior tennis players using two differing measurement techniques and a universal goniometer. Two hundred fifty-two subjects were simply measured in the supine position for internal and external rotation with 90 degrees of glenohumeral joint abduction using no attempt to stabilize the scapula. One hundred forty-seven elite junior tennis players were measured for internal and external rotation active ROM in 90 degrees of glenohumeral joint abduction using scapular stabilization. This stabilization was provided by a posteriorly directed force applied by the examiner's hand placed over the anterior aspect of the shoulder, over the anterior acromion and coracoid process (Figure 11-3). Results of the two groups showed significantly less internal rotation ROM when using the measurement technique with scapular stabilization (18% to 28% reduction in ROM). Changes in external rotation ROM were smaller between groups, with 2% to 6% reductions in active ROM measured.

One common finding confirmed in this research is the finding of significantly less (≈10 to 15 degrees) dominant arm glenohumeral joint internal rotation in elite junior tennis

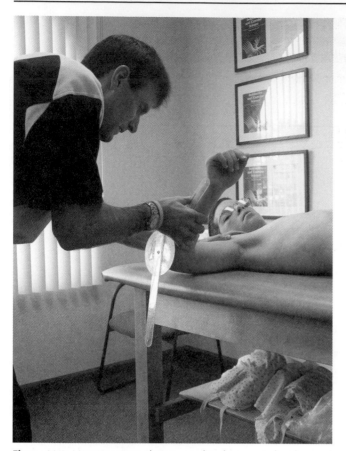

Figure 11-3 Measurement technique used to document glenohumeral joint internal rotation with 90 degrees of glenohumeral abduction in the coronal plane. The examiner's hand is on the anterior aspect of the coracoid and acromion to stabilize the scapula, thus minimizing the presence of scapular upward rotation and protraction during measurement.

players.[35,36] The significance in this present research, however, lies in the fact that this difference between extremities in internal rotation ROM was only identified in the condition where the scapula was stabilized. Failure to stabilize the scapula did not produce glenohumeral joint internal rotation ROM measurements that identified a deficit. Only measuring this population with scapular stabilization identified the characteristic ROM limitation in internal rotation. This study clearly demonstrates the importance of using consistent measurement techniques when documenting ROM of glenohumeral joint rotation. On the basis of these study results, the author of this chapter highly recommends the use of scapular stabilization during the measurement of humeral rotation to obtain more isolated and representative values of shoulder rotation.

Total Rotation Range of Motion Concept

One final concept to be discussed in this section on ROM measurement is the total rotation ROM concept. This concept simply combines the glenohumeral joint internal and external rotation ROM measure by summing the two numbers to have a numerical representation of the total rotation ROM available

at the glenohumeral joint. Recent research by Kibler et al[37] and Roetert et al[38] has identified decreases in the total rotation ROM arc in the dominant extremity of elite tennis players correlated with increasing age and number of competitive years of play. Most recently, Ellenbecker et al[39] measured bilateral total rotation ROM in professional baseball pitchers and elite junior tennis players. The findings of this study showed the professional baseball pitchers to have greater dominant arm external rotation and significantly less dominant arm internal rotation, when compared with the contralateral nondominant side. The total rotation ROM, however, was not significantly different between extremities in the professional baseball pitchers (145 degrees dominant arm, 146 degrees nondominant arm). This research shows that, despite bilateral differences in the actual internal or external rotation ROM, or both, in the glenohumeral joints of baseball pitchers, the total arc of rotational motion should remain the same.

In contrast, Ellenbecker et al[39] tested 117 elite male junior tennis players. In the elite junior tennis players, significantly less internal rotation ROM was found on the dominant arm (45 degrees vs. 56 degrees), as well as significantly less total rotation ROM on the dominant arm (149 degrees vs. 158 degrees). The total rotation ROM did differ between extremities (Table 11-4). Approximately 10 degrees less total rotation ROM can be expected in the dominant arm of the uninjured elite junior tennis player, as compared with the nondominant extremity.

Utilization of normative data from population specific research, such as this study, can assist clinicians in interpreting normal ROM patterns and identify when sport-specific adaptations or clinically significant maladaptations are present. The data in this table contain the descriptive data from the professional baseball pitchers and elite junior tennis players.[39] Further research on additional subject populations is necessary to further outline the total rotation ROM concept.

Clinical application of the total rotation ROM concept is best demonstrated by a case presentation of a unilaterally dominant upper extremity athlete. If, during the initial evaluation of a high-level baseball pitcher, the clinician finds a range of motion pattern of 120 degrees of external rotation and only 30 degrees of internal rotation, some uncertainty may exist as to whether that represents a ROM deficit in internal rotation that requires rehabilitative intervention via muscle tendon unit stretching and possibly via the use of specific glenohumeral joint mobilization. However, if measurement of that patient's nondominant extremity rotation reveals 90 degrees of external rotation and 60 degrees of internal rotation, the current recommendation based on the total rotation ROM concept would be to avoid extensive mobilization and passive stretching of the dominant extremity because the total rotation ROM in both extremities is 150 degrees (120 external rotation [ER] + 30 internal rotation [IR] = 150 dominant arm/90 ER and 60 IR = 150 total rotation nondominant arm). In elite-level tennis players, the total active rotation ROM can be expected to be up to 10 degrees less on the dominant arm before a clinical treatment to address internal rotation ROM restriction would be recommended or implemented.

Table 11-4	Bilateral Comparison of Isolated and Total Rotation Range of Motion from Professional Baseball Pitchers and Elite Junior Tennis Players	
Subjects	Dominant Arm	Nondominant Arm
Baseball Pitchers		
ER	103.2 ± 9.1 (1.34)	94.5 ± 8.1 (1.19)
IR	42.4 ± 15.8 (2.33)	52.4 ± 16.4 (2.42)
Total rotation	145.7 ± 18.0 (2.66)	146.9 ± 17.5 (2.59)
Elite Junior Tennis Players		
ER	103.7 ± 10.9 (1.02)	101.8 ± 10.8 (1.01)
IR	45.4 ± 13.6 (1.28)	56.3 ± 11.5 (1.08)
Total rotation	149.1 ± 18.4 (1.73)	158.2 ± 15.9 (1.50)

From Ellenbecker TS, Roetert EP, Bailie DS, et al: *Med Sci Sports Exerc* 34(12):2052-2056, 2002.
All measurements are expressed in degrees. Standard error of the mean in parentheses.
ER, External rotation; *IR*, internal rotation.

This total rotation ROM concept can be used as illustrated to guide the clinician during rehabilitation, specifically in the area of application of stretching and mobilization, to best determine what glenohumeral joint requires additional mobility and which extremity should not have additional mobility, due to the obvious harm induced by increases in capsular mobility and increases in humeral head translation during aggressive upper extremity exertion.

Burkhart et al[5] describe this loss of internal rotation ROM as GIRD, or glenohumeral *i*nternal *r*otation *d*eficit. Because a loss of internal rotation in the dominant shoulder is common in the glenohumeral joint of the elite thrower, Burkhart et al[5] have further described what they term as an *acceptable level* of GIRD as less than 20 degrees of limitation of internal rotation compared with the nonthrowing shoulder, or less than 10% loss of total rotation ROM compared with the contralateral shoulder. Burkhart et al[5] further state that approximately 90% of all throwers with symptomatic GIRD (>25 degrees of internal rotation loss compared with the contralateral non-throwing shoulder) respond favorably to a compliant posterior-inferior capsular stretching program and reduce GIRD to the acceptable levels. Use of the "sleeper stretch" has been advocated by these authors[5] and consists of the athlete sidelying on the dominant shoulder in varied positions of glenohumeral joint abduction while internally rotating the glenohumeral joint, using body weight to stabilize the lateral border of the scapula. Further research using controlled experimental designs is necessary to better understand the effectiveness of stretching for the throwing shoulder.

The loss of internal rotation ROM is significant for several reasons. The relationship between internal rotation ROM loss (tightness in the posterior capsule of the shoulder) and increased anterior humeral head translation has been scientifically identified.[40,41] The increase in anterior humeral shear force reported by Harryman et al[42] was manifested by a horizontal adduction cross-body maneuver, similar to that incurred

during the follow-through of the throwing motion or tennis serve. Tightness of the posterior capsule has also been linked to increased superior migration of the humeral head during shoulder elevation.[43]

Recent research by Koffler et al[44] studied the effects of posterior capsular tightness in a functional position of 90 degrees of abduction and 90 degrees or more of external rotation in cadaveric specimens. They found, with imbrication of either the inferior aspect of the posterior capsule or imbrication of the entire posterior capsule, that humeral head kinematics were changed or altered. In the presence of posterior capsular tightness, the humeral head will shift in an anterior superior direction, as compared with a normal shoulder with normal capsular relationships. With more extensive amounts of posterior capsular tightness, the humeral head was found to shift postero-superiorly. These effects of altered posterior capsular tensions experimentally representing in vivo posterior glenohumeral joint capsular tightness highlight the clinical importance of using a reliable and effective measurement methodology to assess internal rotation ROM during examination of the shoulder. Additionally, Burkhart et al[5] have clinically demonstrated the concept of posterior superior humeral head shear in the abducted externally rotated position with tightness of the posterior band of the inferior glenohumeral ligament.

SPECIAL TESTS FOR EVALUATING THE SHOULDER OF THE OVERHEAD-THROWING ATHLETE

Again, it is beyond the scope of this chapter to completely outline the specifics of the special tests used during the comprehensive evaluation of the shoulder in the overhead-throwing athlete. However, an overview of the most important tests used will be undertaken. During the evaluation process it is imperative to determine the underlying mobility status of the athlete's shoulder. However subtle, the presence of instability and the ability of the clinician to identify this presence are of critical importance.

Instability Tests

Several authors believe that the most important tests to identify shoulder joint instability are humeral head translation tests.[45,46] These tests attempt to document the amount of movement of the humeral head relative to the glenoid through the use of carefully applied directional stresses to the proximal humerus. Harryman et al[47] measured the amount of humeral head translation in vivo in healthy, uninjured subjects using a three-dimensional spatial tracking system. They found a mean of 7.8 mm of anterior translation and 7.9 mm of posterior translation using an anterior and posterior drawer test. Translation of the human shoulder in an inferior direction was evaluated using a multidirectional instability (MDI) sulcus test. During the in vivo testing of inferior humeral head translation, an average of 10 mm of inferior displacement was measured. The results from this detailed laboratory-based research study indicate that approximately a 1:1 ratio of anterior-to-posterior humeral head translation can be expected in normal shoulders with manual humeral head translation tests. No definitive interpretation of bilateral symmetry in humeral head translation is available from this research.

One key test used to evaluate the stability of the athlete's shoulder is the MDI sulcus test. This test is the primary test to identify the patient with MDI of the glenohumeral joint. Excessive translation in the inferior direction during this test most often indicates a forthcoming pattern of excessive translation in either the anterior or posterior direction or both the anterior and posterior directions. This test, when performed in the neutral adducted position, directly assesses the integrity of the superior glenohumeral ligament and the coracohumeral ligament.[48] These ligaments are the primary stabilizing structures against inferior humeral head translation in the adducted glenohumeral position.[49] To perform this test it is recommended that the patient be examined in the seated position with the arms in neutral adduction, resting gently in the patient's lap. The examiner grasps the distal aspect of the humerus using a firm but unassuming grip with one hand, while several brief, relatively rapid downward pulls are exerted to the humerus in an inferior (vertical) direction (Figure 11-4). A visible "sulcus sign" (tethering of the skin between the lateral acromion and humerus from the increase in inferior translation of the humeral head and widening subacromial space) is usually present in patients with MDI.[50]

Gerber and Ganz[51] and McFarland et al[45] believe that testing for anterior and posterior shoulder laxity is best performed with the patient in the supine position due to greater inherent relaxation of the patient. This test allows the patient's extremity to be tested in multiple positions of glenohumeral joint abduction, thus selectively stressing specific portions of the glenohumeral joint anterior capsule and capsular ligaments. Figure 11-5 shows the preferred technique to assess and grade the translation of the humeral head in both anterior and

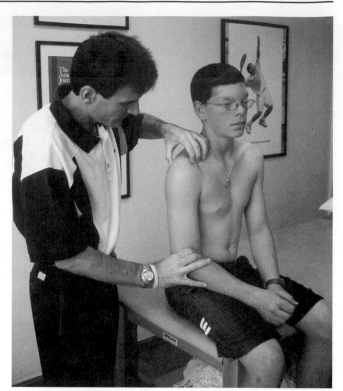

Figure 11-4 Multidirectional instability sulcus test position and hand placements.

posterior directions. Importantly, the direction of translation must be along the line of the glenohumeral joint with an anteromedial and posterolateral direction being used due to the 30-degree version of the glenoid.[7] Grading this test is performed using the classification of Altchek[52] with grade I translation representing humeral translation within the glenoid, and grade II indicating translation of the humeral head up over the glenoid rim with spontaneous return on removal of the stress. The presence of grade 2 translation in either an anterior or posterior direction without symptoms does *not* indicate instability but instead represents merely laxity of the glenohumeral joint. Unilateral increases in glenohumeral translation in the presence of shoulder pain and disability can ultimately lead to the diagnosis of glenohumeral joint instability.[7,53]

The last and possibly most important test for the overhead-throwing athlete to be discussed in this section is the subluxation/relocation test. Originally described by Jobe,[11] the subluxation/relocation test is designed to identify subtle anterior instability of the glenohumeral joint. Dr Peter Fowler has also been given credit for the development and application of this test.[54] Fowler described the diagnostic quandary of microinstability (subtle anterior instability) versus rotator cuff injury or both in swimmers and advocated the use of this important test to assist in the diagnosis. The subluxation/relocation test is performed with the patient's shoulder held and stabilized in the patient's maximal, end range of external rotation at 90 degrees of abduction. The examiner then provides a mild anterior subluxation force (Figure 11-6, *A*). The patient is then asked if this subluxation reproduces his or her symptoms.

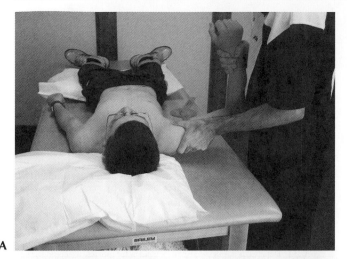

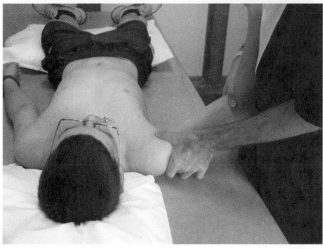

Figure 11-5 A, Test for anterior humeral head translation using the scapular plane and anteromedial direction of translation. **B,** Posterior humeral head translation test using the posterolateral direction of translation.

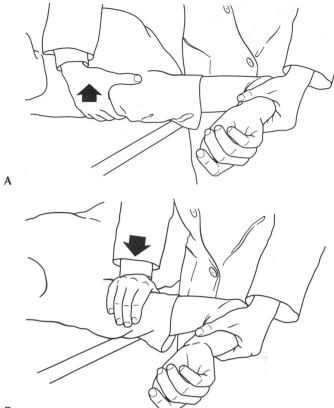

Figure 11-6 Subluxation relocation test. **A,** Subluxation applied at end-range external rotation and 90 degrees of coronal plane abduction. **B,** Demonstrates the relocation portion of the test maintaining end-range external rotation and abduction position. (Adapted from Jobe FW, Bradley JP: *Clin Sports Med* 8(3):427,1989.)

Reproduction of patient symptoms of either anterior or posterior shoulder pain with subluxation leads the examiner to then reposition his or her hand on the anterior aspect of the patient's shoulder and perform a posterior-lateral directed force using a soft, cupped hand to minimize anterior shoulder pain from the hand/shoulder (examiner/patient) interface (Figure 11-6, *B*).

Failure to reproduce the patient's symptoms with end-range external rotation and 90 degrees of abduction leads the examiner to reattempt the subluxation maneuver with 110 and 120 degrees of abduction. This modification has been proposed by Hamner et al[55] to increase the potential for contact between the undersurface of the supraspinatus tendon and the posterior superior glenoid. In each position of abduction (90, 110, and 120 degrees of abduction), the same sequence of initial subluxation and subsequent relocation is performed as previously described.

Reproduction of anterior or posterior shoulder pain with the subluxation portion of this test, with subsequent diminution or disappearance of anterior or posterior shoulder pain with the relocation maneuver, constitutes a positive test. Production

of apprehension with any position of abduction during the anteriorly directed subluxation force phase of testing would indicate occult anterior instability. The primary ramifications of a positive test would indicate subtle anterior instability and secondary glenohumeral joint impingement (anterior pain) or posterior or internal impingement in the presence of posterior pain with this maneuver. A posterior type II superior labrum anterior to posterior (SLAP) lesion has also been implicated in patients with a positive subluxation relocation test.[56]

Differentiating between Primary and Secondary Impingement

Application of the traditional impingement tests of Neer (forced forward flexion)[57] and Hawkins[58] (internal rotation at 90 degrees of abduction in the scapular plane), as well as the cross arm adduction impingement[7] tests, can be used to determine whether the patient's symptoms can be reproduced by compression of the rotator cuff against the overlying acromion. The presence of a positive reproduction of pain with these tests, coupled with general joint hypomobility (grade 1 humeral head translation tests) physiological range of motion loss

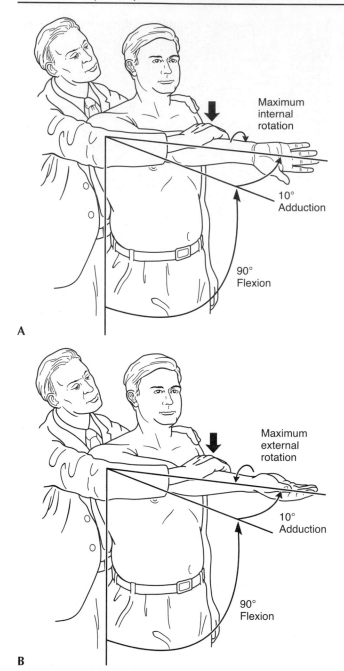

Figure 11-7 OBrien's or active compression test for superior labral injury and acromioclavicular joint dysfunction. **A,** Initial position used for testing. **B,** Second position for force application and testing. (Adapted from O'Brien SJ, Pagnani MJ, Fealy J, et al: *Am J Sports Med* 26(5):611, 1998.)

and muscular weakness, are paramount signs of primary impingement.[7,57]

In evaluation of the overhead-throwing athlete's shoulder, the clinician must be aware that positive impingement symptoms alone do not always indicate the primary cause of the athlete's apparent rotator cuff dysfunction. Instead, when positive impingement signs are coupled with unilateral or occasionally bilateral glenohumeral joint increases in humeral head translation (grade II anterior/posterior) or a positive MDI

sulcus sign and/or positive subluxation/relocation sign, these apparent impingement symptoms are indeed secondary to the underlying instability in the athlete's shoulder. Although this may at first appear to be solely a semantic issue or exercise in nomenclature, it instead gives the clinician the ability to identify and subsequently treat each type of impingement (primary or secondary) differently and with a greater degree of success.[11,59] Care must be taken to integrate the findings of the impingement tests with the instability tests discussed in this chapter to most clearly arrive at a correct understanding of the true cause of the impingement so that an effective treatment program can be developed.[60]

Special Tests to Evaluate the Glenoid Labrum and Acromioclavicular Joint

Evaluation of the glenoid labrum in the throwing athlete is important due to the incidence of labral injury, especially detachment of the superior part of the labrum from the glenoid near the bicep anchor (SLAP lesion).[5] Pain located deep within the shoulder, especially during arm cocking[56] or during follow-through when high distraction forces as much as 1090 Newtons have been reported in the human shoulder,[61] may lead the clinician to suspect subtle underlying instability of the glenohumeral joint and superior labral injury. Cheng and Karzel[62] have shown increases of up to 120% in the inferior glenohumeral ligament complex with laboratory simulation of a superior labral injury in cadaveric specimens.

Although many tests have been advocated for labral testing including the Clunk test,[63] Crank test,[64] and Anterior Slide Test,[65] it is beyond the scope of this chapter to review these in their entirety. One test showing favorable psychometric variables with clinical inquiry is the O'Brien test.[66] This test can be performed on the patient while seated or standing and begins with the patient's shoulder in 90 degrees of shoulder flexion, 10 degrees of horizontal adduction, and full internal rotation (Figure 11-7, *A*). The clinician then produces a downward pressure similar to that performed during manual muscle testing using two fingers of pressure on the ulnar styloid process. The patient is then asked whether this produces pain and, specifically, where this pain is produced. If the patient reports pain deep in the anterior aspect of the shoulder or on top of the shoulder over the acromioclavicular (AC) joint, the examiner then proceeds to the second part of the test, in which a similar humeral position of 90 degrees shoulder flexion, 10 degrees horizontal adduction, and full-external-rotation (palm-up) position is used with a manual muscle test–type downward pressure applied to the distal aspect of the extremity (Figure 11-7, *B*). For the O'Brien test to be considered positive for a superior labral tear, the deep anterior pain that was present with the internal rotation position of testing must be abated or absent during the external rotation or palm-up position of testing.[66] Although the initial psychometric variables (specificity of 98.5% and sensitivity of 100% for SLAP lesions) reported in O'Brien's study[66] have not been replicated in other studies,[67,68] the O'Brien test remains a popular and reasonably effective test that can be used without creating apprehension and guarding inherent in other labral tests that complicate the initial evaluation of the overhead-throwing athlete for labral injury.

Additional application of the O'Brien or active compression test is warranted for the AC joint. Reproduction of pain directly over the AC joint with the internal rotation test position with abatement of the superiorly directed pain with the external-rotation (palm-up) position indicates AC joint involvement. Additionally, the cross arm impingement test has been used to identify AC joint pathology when force horizontal adduction recreates pain directly over the AC joint.[69] Coupling these AC joint tests with a history of laterally based trauma or contact to the shoulder, along with visible dyscongruity of the AC joint, leads to the diagnosis of AC joint involvement.

Utilization of the special tests discussed in this brief overview allows the clinician to test the static and dynamic stabilizers of the glenohumeral joint to obtain an accurate diagnosis that will enable a comprehensive plan of care for both rehabilitation and preventative conditioning programs. One additional area that needs further and more specific discussion, however, is the role of postural evaluation of the scapulothoracic joint for the overhead-throwing athlete.

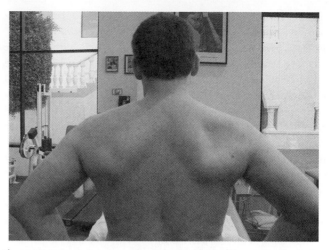

Figure 11-8 Posterior view of a patient with significant atrophy in the infraspinous fossa photographed in the "hands-on-hips" position, indicating probable involvement of the suprascapular nerve. (From Ellenbecker TS: *Clinical examination of the shoulder*, Philadelphia, 2004, Elsevier Saunders.)

Role of Posture in the Evaluation of the Scapulothoracic Joint

The evaluation of posture for the overhead-throwing athlete begins with shoulder heights evaluated in the standing position, as well as use of the hands-on-hips position to evaluate the prominence of the scapula against the thoracic wall. Typically, the dominant shoulder is significantly lower than the nondominant shoulder in neutral, nonstressed standing postures, particularly in unilaterally dominant athletes like baseball and tennis players. Although the exact reason for this phenomenon is unclear, theories include increased mass in the dominant arm, leading the dominant shoulder to be lower secondary to the increased weight of the arm, as well as elongation of the periscapular musculature on the dominant or preferred side secondary to eccentric loading.

Another typical finding often observed during the postural evaluation is the finding of "tennis shoulder," a term used by Priest and Nagel[70] in their research. As they explained, "It is said that oarsman of ancient galleys developed a corporeal deformity when rowing only on one side of the ship, and that a favor the slave master could bestow upon an oarsman was to alternate him from one side of the ship to the other, allowing maintenance of symmetrical physique." Priest and Nagel describe tennis shoulder as a developmental characteristic in the dominant arm of tennis players, in which the dominant shoulder droops inferiorly with an apparent scoliosis. The position of the shoulder girdle and scapula is one of depression, protraction, and often downward rotation. Tennis shoulder exists in unilaterally dominant athletes, such as tennis players, baseball players, volleyball players, and individuals who ergonomically use one extremity without heavy or repeated exertion of the contralateral extremity.[70-72]

In the standing position the clinician can observe the patient for symmetrical muscle development and, more specifically, focal areas of muscle atrophy. One of the positions that is recommended, in addition to observing the patient with the arms at the sides in a comfortable standing posture, is the hands-on-hips position, which simply places the patient's shoulders in approximately 45 to 50 degrees of abduction with slight internal rotation. The hands are placed on the iliac crests of the hips such that the thumbs are pointed posteriorly. Placement of the hands on the hips allows the patient to relax the arms and often enables the clinician to observe focal pockets of atrophy along the scapular border, as well as more commonly over the infraspinous fossa of the scapula. Thorough visual inspection using this position can often identify excessive scalloping over the infraspinous fossa present in patients with rotator cuff dysfunction, as well as in patients with severe atrophy who may have suprascapular nerve involvement. Impingement of the suprascapular nerve can occur at the suprascapular notch and spinoglenoid notch and from paralabral cyst formation commonly found in patients with superior labral lesions.[73] Figure 11-8 shows the isolated atrophy present in the infraspinous fossa of an overhead athlete who presented with anterior shoulder pain. Further diagnostic testing of the patient with extreme wasting of the infraspinatus muscle is warranted to rule out suprascapular nerve involvement.

CLASSIFICATION OF SCAPULAR DYSFUNCTION IN THE OVERHEAD ATHLETE

The most widely described and overused term pertaining to scapular pathology is *scapular winging*, which describes gross disassociation of the scapula from the thoracic wall.[74] Scapular winging is typically obvious to a trained observer when simply viewing a patient from the posterior and lateral orientation and becomes even more pronounced with active or resistive movements to the upper extremities. True scapular winging occurs secondary to involvement of the long thoracic nerve.[74] Isolated paralysis of the serratus anterior muscle with resultant "winged scapula" was first described by Velpeau in 1837.[74] The cause of winged scapula is peripheral in origin and is ultimately derived from involvement of the fifth, sixth, and seventh spinal cord segments.[74] Isolated serratus anterior muscle weakness due to nerve palsy will create a prominent superior medial border of the scapula and depressed acromion, while isolated trapezius muscle weakness due to nerve palsy will create a protracted inferior border of the scapula and elevated acromion.[72]

Although it is possible that some patients with shoulder pathology may present with true scapular winging, most patients with shoulder pathology present with less obvious and less severe forms of scapular dysfunction.

Kibler Scapular Dysfunction Classification

Kibler[72,75] has developed a more specific scapular classification system for clinical use that allows clinicians to categorize scapular dysfunction on the basis of common clinical findings obtained via visual observation of both static posture– and dynamic goal–directed upper extremity movements. Kibler has identified three specific scapular dysfunctions or patterns, termed *inferior* or *type I, medial* or *type II,* and *superior* or *type III.* The dysfunctions are named for the area of the scapula that is visually prominent during clinical evaluation. In the Kibler classification system, normal symmetrical scapular motion is characterized by symmetrical, scapular, upward rotation such that the inferior angles translate laterally away from the

midline and the scapular medial border remains flush against the thoracic wall with the reverse occurring during arm lowering.[75]

Inferior or Inferior Angle Dysfunction Type I

In this classification of scapular dysfunction the primary external visual feature is the prominence of the inferior angle of the scapula (Figure 11-9). This pattern of dysfunction involves anterior tilting of the scapula in the sagittal plane, which produces the prominent inferior angle of the scapula. No other abnormality is typically present with this dysfunction pattern; however, the prominence of the inferior angle of the scapula does increase oftentimes in the hands-on-hips position, as well as during active goal-directed movements of the upper extremities. According to Kibler,[75] inferior angle dysfunction or prominence is most commonly found in patients with rotator cuff dysfunction. The anterior tilting of the scapula places the acromion in a position closer to the rotator cuff and humeral head, compromising the subacromial space.

Medial or Medial Border Dysfunction Type II

In this classification of scapular dysfunction, the primary external visual feature is the prominence of the entire medial border of the scapula (Figure 11-10). This pattern or dysfunction involves internal rotation of the scapula in the transverse plane. The internal rotation of the scapula produces a prominent medial border of the scapula. Similar to the inferior or inferior angle dysfunction, the medial or medial border dysfunction often increases in the hands-on-hips position, as well as during active goal-directed movements of the upper extremity. According to Kibler[75] and Saha,[1] the medial border scapular dysfunction most often occurs in patients with instability or rotator cuff dysfunction secondary to glenohumeral joint instability.

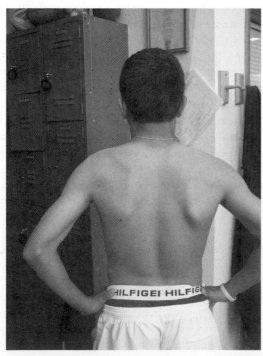

Figure 11-9 Patient with Kibler type I (inferior) scapular dysfunction. The inferior angle of the scapula is prominent.

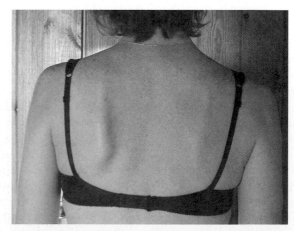

Figure 11-10 Patient with Kibler type II (medial) scapular dysfunction. The entire medial border of the scapula is prominent. (From Ellenbecker TS: *Clinical examination of the shoulder*, Philadelphia, 2004, Elsevier Saunders.)

Superior Dysfunction Type III

This type of scapular dysfunction is characterized by excessive and early elevation of the scapula during arm elevation (Figure 11-11). This has been referred to as a shoulder shrug or "hiking" of the shoulder girdle by clinicians and is most often present with rotator cuff dysfunction and deltoid–rotator cuff force couple imbalances.[3] This superior movement of the scapula is thought to occur as a compensatory movement pattern to aid with arm elevation.

Evaluation Sequence for Kibler Scapular Dysfunction

The specific sequence recommended for scapular evaluation includes both static and dynamic aspects. Both are critical for obtaining the clinical cues that allow the clinician to determine the often subtle, scapular dysfunction present in patients with shoulder pathology.

Static

Evaluation of the patient, as mentioned earlier, occurs in the standing position with arms held comfortably against the sides of the body. The clinician should note the outline of the scapula and compare the scapulae bilaterally. Although many variations exist in standing posture, the clinician should be particularly discriminating when there are bilateral differences in scapular posture and, most notably, when greater prominence of the scapula is present on the involved side. Bilateral symmetry, with respect to scapular position and scapular prominence in

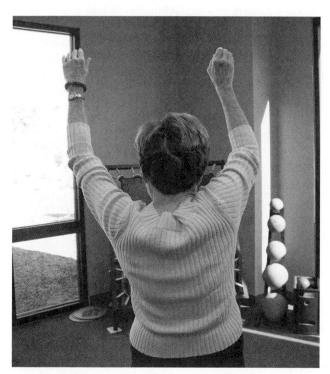

Figure 11-11 Patient with Kibler type III (superior) scapular dysfunction. Superior elevation of the scapula exists on the involved side.

the patient with unilateral shoulder dysfunction, is not necessarily an indicator of scapular dysfunction.

After examination of the patient with the arms in complete adduction at the sides of the body, the patient is then examined in the hands-on-hips position. The Kibler Lateral Slide Test can be used to objectively document scapular position in the resting position (arms at side), hands-on-hips position, and at 90 degrees of coronal plane abduction with full internal rotation.[72] Measurement is performed with a tape measure from the inferior angle of the scapula to the corresponding vertebral spinous process in the transverse plane. A bilateral difference of greater than 1.5 cm in any or all of the three positions is considered positive for scapular dysfunction.[72]

Dynamic

Following the static examination, the patient is asked to bilaterally elevate the shoulders using a self-selected plane of elevation. The clinician should be directly behind the patient to best observe the movement of the scapula during concentric elevation and especially during eccentric lowering. Excessive superior movement of the scapula during concentric arm elevation, as well as inferior angle and medial border prominence during the eccentric phase, is commonly encountered in patients with scapular dysfunction. Repeated bouts of arm elevation to confirm initial observations, as well as to determine the presence and location of symptoms (location in/on the shoulder and the ROM where symptoms occur), are recommended. Additionally, the effect of repeated movements is also of critical importance to assess the effects of fatigue on scapular stabilization.

Burkart et al[76] have also identified a characteristic scapular dysfunction in elite-level throwing athletes. They have termed this the *SICK scapula* (*scapular malposition, inferior medial border prominence, coracoid pain and malposition, and dyskinesis of scapular movement*). Alterations in both static and dynamic scapular function are inherent in the SICK scapula. The hallmark feature of the SICK scapula is the asymmetric malposition of the scapula in the dominant throwing shoulder, which usually appears on examination as if one shoulder is lower than the other. In addition to the lower dominant scapula, Burkart et al[76] point out the presence of the increase in lateral displacement or protraction compared with the nondominant shoulder. In a sample of 64 throwing athletes with arthroscopically confirmed superior labral pathology, Burkhart et al[76] reported 94% of these throwing athletes to have the characteristics of the SICK scapula on clinical examination. This scapular dysfunction commonly associated with the symptomatic throwing athlete highlights the need for longitudinal scapular evaluation and specific exercise programs designed to improve scapular stabilization.

Evaluation of Throwing Biomechanics

The component parts of a clinical shoulder evaluation have been presented in the earlier portions of this chapter. Although these are clinically useful and important parts of a thorough evaluation of the overhead athlete with shoulder pain, failure by the clinician to obtain information regarding the athlete's throwing or overhead sport biomechanics severely jeopardizes the evaluation process. Although it is not feasible for many clinicians to use sophisticated three-dimensional equipment to perform this evaluation, a thorough and most often completely effective analysis can be performed with the use of appropriately timed or staged digital still photographs or digital video obtained using commonly available video or digital camcorders.[7,77] For the purposes of this chapter, the throwing mechanics are discussed in the traditional stages for ease of analysis, with typical abnormal or injury-producing pathomechanics discussed for each stage.

For the purposes of evaluation, the throwing motion has been divided into four primary phases[78]: wind-up, cocking, acceleration, and follow-through (Figure 11-12). The wind-up phase begins with the initial motion of the pitcher and ends when the ball leaves the glove.[77,78] Little muscular activation is required in the throwing shoulder during this phase; therefore few injuries or episodes of pain provocation are typically described during this phase.

One essential aspect to analyze during the end of the wind-up phase, however, is the presence of proper balance.[77] The lead leg (left leg in a right-handed throwing athlete) is lifted and rotated around the plant leg (right leg in a right-handed throwing athlete). This rotation must be achieved in a balanced fashion and should be evaluated in reference to the shoulder because an unstable base during this phase of throwing may have drastic consequences as the player moves into external rotation and begins the sequential segmental rotation during acceleration later in the throwing motion. A digital photo or video pause near the end of the wind-up phase with the pitcher in the balance position is one of the first checkpoints recommended.

The cocking phase is often divided into two phases.[77,78] The early cocking phase begins as the ball leaves the glove and continues until the lead foot contacts the ground. During the early cocking phase the arm is brought backward away from the body, coupled with a forward drive of the lead leg. As the lead leg is extended forward, it strikes the mound. This is termed *foot contact.* At front foot or lead foot contact another critical marker or evaluation point takes place. At the time the foot strikes the mound, the throwing elbow should be flexed 90 degrees and the throwing shoulder should be externally rotated to at least the neutral position.[77] Failure of the athlete to achieve this arm position at foot contact can lead to a "lagging" behind of the arm as the hips rotate forward in preparation for ball release. This places the arm in a "catch-up" type situation as the rest of the body is too far ahead of the arm at this point in the movement pattern. A static photo or video pause at this position allows the clinician to evaluate and provide critical feedback.

Additional information critically important to the glenohumeral joint is the stride characteristics of the lower extremity during the foot contact portion of the throwing motion. Fleisig et al[79] outlined the stride characteristics during baseball pitching. They reported stride length (distance from ankle to ankle) to range between 70% and 80% of the athlete's height. Fleisig et al[79] also report that at foot contact the angle of the lead foot should be closed (angled inward) between 5 and 25 degrees rather than pointing straight ahead toward home plate. An open stance or stride angle would increase the opening or early rotation of the pelvis and may lead to hyperangulation and arm lag, increasing stress on the medial elbow and shoulder. Excessively closed stride angles would block rotation of the pelvis and decrease the contribution from the lower extremity segments.

Additionally, the lead foot should land directly in front of the rear foot or in a position with a few centimeters' closed stance (lead foot a few centimeters to the right of the rear foot in a right-handed thrower). Again, if the lead foot lands in a position too closed, pelvic rotation will be impeded, forcing the pitcher to throw across his body, which minimizes the contribution from the lower extremity.[79] Consequently, landing in a "too open" position leads to early pelvic rotation and dissipation of the ground reaction forces and lower extremity contri-

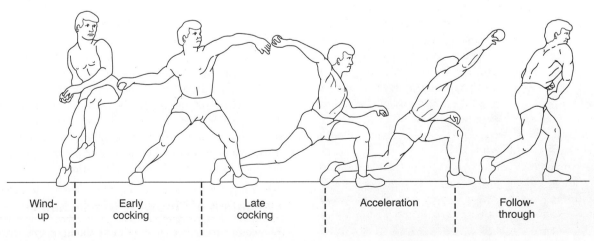

| Wind-up | Early cocking | Late cocking | Acceleration | Follow-through |

Figure 11-12 Four stages of the throwing motion. (From Glousman RE, Barron J, Jobe FW, et al: *Am J Sports Med* 20(3):312, 1992.)

bution and leads to arm fatigue and throwing with "too much arm."[79] Careful documentation of foot position using video or digital photography can again give valuable insight into possible mechanisms of arm injury stemming from lower extremity pathomechanics.

Late cocking occurs following foot contact and continues until maximal external rotation of the throwing shoulder occurs.[78] By the end of the cocking phase, the shoulder can obtain a nearly horizontal position of 180 degrees of external rotation. This amount of external rotation, however, is combined with scapulothoracic and trunk articulation and gives the appearance of the artificially high external rotation value at the shoulder joint.[77]

At the time of maximal external rotation in the throwing arm, it is important to note that the scapulothoracic joint must be in a retracted position.[5,72] The scapula actually translates 15 to 18 cm during the throwing motion.[72] Failure to retract the scapula leads to an increase in the ante-tilting of the glenoid due to a protracted scapular position and can exacerbate the instability continuum and create anterior instability and suboptimal performance, leading to injury.[5,72] Recent research has demonstrated that in late cocking, the abduction and external rotation position places the posterior band of the inferior glenohumeral ligament in a "bowstrung" position under the humeral head such that tightness in this structure can lead to a postero-superior shift in the humeral head, which can lead to rotator cuff and labral pathology.[5] Improper scapular positioning coupled with increases in horizontal abduction during late cocking and the transition into the acceleration phase has been termed *hyperangulation* and leads to aggravation of undersurface rotator cuff impingement and labral injury derangement (Figure 11- 13).

The acceleration phase begins after maximal external rotation and ends with ball release. During the delivery phase, the arm initially starts in −30 degrees of horizontal abduction (30 degrees behind the coronal plane).[80] As acceleration of the arm continues, the glenohumeral joint is moved forward to a position of +10 degrees of horizontal adduction (10 degrees of horizontal adduction anterior to the coronal plane).[80] During acceleration, the arm moves from a position of 175 to 180 degrees of composite external rotation to a position of nearly vertical (105 degrees of external rotation) at release. This is another point that the video can be paused or a digital image generated for analysis. When viewed from the side, the forearm will be nearly in a vertical position, yet the arm will appear to be 10 to 15 degrees behind the trunk because the trunk is flexed forward at ball release. This internal rotation movement following maximal external rotation will be difficult to capture on video and with digital images because it occurs at more than 7000 degrees per second.[77,80]

Another important variable to monitor during arm cocking and acceleration is the abduction angle of the glenohumeral joint. Research has consistently shown that the abduction angle for the throwing motion ranges between 90 and 110 degrees.[80,81] Importantly, this angle is relative to the trunk with varying amounts of trunk lateral flexion changing the actual release position, while keeping the abduction angle

remarkably consistent across individuals and major pitching styles.[61,77,80,81] Elevation of the glenohumeral abduction angle to greater than 110 degrees can subject the rotator cuff to impingement stresses from the overlying acromion. Careful monitoring of this abduction angle during the throwing motion is recommended, again using still digital images or video.

Follow-through is the stage following ball release and contains high levels of eccentric muscular activity in the posterior rotator cuff and scapular region.[79] Additional movements of the entire body to help dissipate the energy of the arm are necessary. Critical monitoring during this stage of the throwing motion is also recommended to ensure that an abrupt upright posture is not assumed by the pitcher and that a continuation of the forward momentum is gradually dissipated by wrapping the arm across the body with trunk rotation. Additionally, the rear leg should come forward to assist in this process, leaving the pitcher again in a balanced finish position.

Failure at any one of these stages in the throwing motion can have profound implications on the throwing shoulder. As mentioned throughout this section, use of digital still photography from multiple sides of the throwing athlete, as well as the use of video, can enhance the evaluation process and clearly improve biofeedback and education with the injured athlete, parent, and coach. Removal of the shirt when applicable in males and use of a sports bra or sleeveless shirt will enhance the ability to estimate arm-trunk relationships. Even

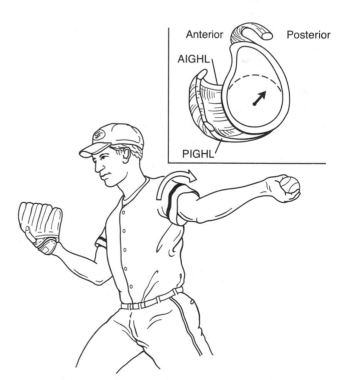

Figure 11-13 In the late cocking phase, there is twisting of the capsule, shifting the PIGHL under the head of the humerus such that tightness in this structure can lead to a posterior-superior shift in the humeral head. (From Burkhart SS, Morgan CD, Kibler WB: *Arthroscopy* 19(4): 416, 2003.) *AIGHL,* Anterior inferior glenohumeral ligament; *PIGHL,* posterior inferior glenohumeral ligament.

with careful clinical monitoring at this level, more extensive biomechanical analysis may be necessary to more clearly identify deviations from normal movement patterning. Referral to a biomechanist who has access to three-dimensional motion analysis programs and noted experience in analyzing the complex kinetic chain sequences inherent in highly skilled throwing athletes is indicated in many cases.

SUMMARY

The information in this chapter provides the clinician with information important for inclusion in the comprehensive evaluation of the overhead athlete. The specific concepts regarding glenohumeral joint total rotation ROM, muscular force couple testing, musculoskeletal manual evaluation methods for glenohumeral joint instability and impingement, and labral and AC joint testing are all required elements that enable the clinical evaluation by the therapist to result in objectively based treatment and rehabilitation strategies. Finally, the classification system for scapular dysfunction and phase-based throwing biomechanics evaluation are additional components of the clinical examination that are required to most appropriately treat the overhead-throwing athlete and allow for the transition from rehabilitation to functional activity.

REFERENCES

1. Saha AK: Mechanism of shoulder movements and a plea for the recognition of "zero position" of glenohumeral joint, *Clin Orthop* 173:3-10, 1983.
2. Ellenbecker TS: Rehabilitation of shoulder and elbow injuries in tennis players, *Clin Sports Med* 14(1):87-110, 1995.
3. Inman VT, Saunders JB, Abbott LC: Observations on the function of the shoulder joint, *J Bone Joint Surgery* 26(1): 1-30, 1944.
4. Weiner DS, MacNab I: Superior migration of the humeral head, *J Bone Joint Surg Br* 52:524-527, 1970.
5. Burkhart SS, Morgan CD, Kibler WB: The disabled throwing shoulder: Spectrum of pathology Part I: pathoanatomy and biomechanics, *Arthroscopy* 19(4):404-420, 2003.
6. Bagg SD, Forrest WJ: A biomechanical analysis of scapular rotation during arm abduction in the scapular plane, *Arch Phys Med Rehabil* 238-245, 1988.
7. Ellenbecker TS: *Clinical examination of the shoulder*, Philadelphia, 2004, Saunders.
8. Daniels L, Worthingham C: *Muscle testing: techniques of manual examination,* ed 4, Philadelphia, 1980, Saunders.
9. Ellenbecker TS, Davies GJ: The application of isokinetics in testing and rehabilitation of the shoulder complex, *J Athletic Training* 35(3):338-350, 2000.
10. Kelly BT, Kadrmas WH, Speer KP: The manual muscle examination for rotator cuff strength. An electromyographic investigation, *Am J Sports Med* 24:581-588, 1996.
11. Jobe FW, Bradley JP: The diagnosis and nonoperative treatment of shoulder injuries in athletes, *Clin Sports Med* 8:419-437, 1989.
12. Malanga GA, Jenp YN, Growney ES, et al: EMG analysis of shoulder positioning in testing and strengthening the supraspinatus, *Med Sci Sports Exercise* 28:661-664, 1996.
13. Jenp YN, Malanga BA, Gowney ES, et al: Activation of the rotator cuff in generating isometric shoulder rotation torque, *Am J Sports Med* 24:477-485, 1996.
14. Walch F, Boulahia A, Calderone S, et al: The 'dropping' and 'hornblower's' signs in evaluation of rotator cuff tears, *J Bone Joint Surgery Br* 80-B:(4):624-628, 1998.
15. Leroux JL, Thomas E, Bonnel F, et al: Diagnostic value of clinical tests for shoulder impingement syndrome, *Rev Rhum* 62(6):423-428, 1995.
16. Patte D, Goutallier D, Monpierre H, et al: Over-extension lesions, *Rev Chir Orthop* 74:314-318, 1988.
17. Gerber C, Krushell RJ: Isolated rupture of the tendon of the subscapularis muscle: clinical features in 16 cases, *J Bone Joint Surgery Br* 73:389-394, 1991.
18. Ellenbecker TS: Muscular strength relationship between normal grade manual muscle testing and isokinetic measurement of the shoulder internal and external rotators, *Isokinetics Exercise Sci* 6:51-56, 1996.
19. Davies GJ: *A compendium of isokinetics in clinical usage and rehabilitation techniques,* ed 4, Onalaska, Wis, 1992, S & S Publishing.
20. Hageman PA, Mason DK, Rydlund KW, et al: Effects of position and speed on eccentric and concentric isokinetic testing of the shoulder rotators, *J Orthop Sports Phys Ther* 11:64-69, 1989.
21. Soderberg GJ, Blaschak MJ: Shoulder internal and external rotation peak torque production through a velocity spectrum in differing positions, *J Orthop Sports Phys Ther* 8:518-524, 1987.
22. Walmsley RP, Szybbo C: A comparative study of the torque generated by the shoulder internal and external rotator muscles in different positions and at varying speeds, *J Orthop Sports Phys Ther* 9:217-222, 1987.
23. Knops JE, Meiners TK, Davies GJ, et al: *Isokinetic test retest reliability of the modified neutral shoulder test position.* Unpublished masters thesis, University of LaCrosse, Wis.
24. Elliott B, Marsh T, Blanksby B: A three dimensional cinematographic analysis of the tennis serve, *Int J Sport Biomechanics* 2:260-271, 1986.
25. Basset RW, Browne AO, Morrey BF, et al: Glenohumeral muscle force and moment mechanics in a position of shoulder instability, *J Biomechanics* 23:405-415, 1994.
26. Wilk KE, Andrews JR, Arrigo CA, et al: The strength characteristics of internal and external rotator muscles in professional baseball pitchers, *Am J Sports Med* 21:61-66, 1993.
27. Ellenbecker TS, Mattalino AJ: Concentric isokinetic shoulder internal and external rotation strength in professional baseball pitchers, *J Orthop Sports Phys Ther* 25:323-328, 1999.

28. Ellenbecker TS, Roetert EP: Age specific isokinetic glenohumeral internal and external rotation strength in elite junior tennis players, *J Sci Med Sport* 6(1):63-70, 2003.

29. Ellenbecker TS, Roetert EP: Testing isokinetic muscular fatigue of shoulder internal and external rotation in elite junior tennis players, *J Orthop Sports Phys Ther* 1999; 29:275-281.

30. Kannus P, Cook L, Alosa D: Absolute and relative endurance parameters in isokinetic tests of muscular performance, *J Sport Rehabil* 1992;1:2-12.

31. Berryman-Reese N, Bandy WD: Joint range of motion and muscle length testing, Philadelphia, 2002, Saunders.

32. Norkin CC, White DJ: *Measurement of joint motion: a guide to goniometry,* ed 2, Philadelphia, 1995, FA Davis.

33. Mallon WJ, Herring CL, Sallay PI, et al: Use of vertebral levels to measure presumed internal rotation at the shoulder: a radiographic analysis, *J Shoulder Elbow Surg* 5:299-306, 1996.

34. Ellenbecker TS, Roetert EP, Piorkowski PA: Shoulder internal and external rotation range of motion of elite junior tennis players: a comparison of two protocols, *J Orthop Sports Phys Ther* 17(1):65, 1993 (Abstract).

35. Ellenbecker TS: Shoulder internal and external rotation strength and range of motion in highly skilled tennis players, *Isok Exerc Sci* 2:1-8, 1992.

36. Ellenbecker TS, Roetert EP, Piorkowski PA, et al: Glenohumeral joint internal and external rotation range of motion in elite junior tennis players, *J Orthop Sports Phys Ther* 24(6):336-341, 1996.

37. Kibler WB, Chandler TJ, Livingston BP, et al: Shoulder range of motion in elite tennis players, *Am J Sports Med* 24(3):279-285, 1996.

38. Roetert EP, Ellenbecker TS, Brown SW: Shoulder internal and external rotation range of motion in nationally ranked junior tennis players: a longitudinal analysis, *J Strength Cond Res* 14(2):140-143, 2000.

39. Ellenbecker TS, Roetert EP, Bailie DS, et al: Glenohumeral joint total rotation range of motion in elite tennis players and baseball pitchers, *Med Sci Sports Exerc* 34(12): 2052-2056, 2002.

40. Tyler TF, Roy T, Nicholas SJ, et al: Reliability and validity of a new method of measuring posterior shoulder tightness, *J Orthop Sports Phys Ther* 29(5):262-274, 1999.

41. Gerber C, Werner CML, Macy JC, et al: Effect of selective capsulorraphy on the passive range of motion of the glenohumeral joint, *J Bone Joint Surg* 85-A(1):48-55, 2003.

42. Harryman DT, Sidles JA, Clark MJ, et al: Translation of the humeral head on the glenoid with passive glenohumeral motion, *J Bone Joint Surg* 72A:1334-1343, 1990.

43. Matsen FA III, Artnz CT: Subacromial impingement. In Rockwood CA Jr, Matsen FA III, editors: *The shoulder,* Philadelphia, 1990, Saunders.

44. Koffler KM, Bader D, Eager M, et al: The effect of posterior capsular tightness on glenohumeral translation in the late-cocking phase of pitching: a cadaveric study. Abstract

(SS-15) presented at Arthroscopy Association of North America Annual Meeting, Washington, DC, 2001.

45. McFarland EG, Torpey BM, Carl LA: Evaluation of shoulder laxity, *Sports Med* 22:264-272, 1996.

46. Gerber C, Ganz R: Clinical assessment of instability of the shoulder with special reference to anterior and posterior drawer tests, *J Bone Joint Surg* 66B(4):551-556, 1984.

47. Harryman DT, Sidles JA, Harris SL, et al: Laxity of the normal glenohumeral joint: in-vivo assessment, *J Shoulder Elbow Surg* 1:66-76, 1992.

48. Pagnani MJ, Warren RF: Stabilizers of the glenohumeral joint, *J Shoulder Elbow Surg* 3:73-90, 1994.

49. O'Brien SJ, Beves MC, Arnoczky SJ, et al: The anatomy and histology of the inferior glenohumeral ligament complex of the shoulder, *Am J Sports Med* 18:449-456, 1990.

50. Hawkins RJ, Mohtadi NGH: Clinical evaluation of shoulder instability, *Clin J Sports Med* 1:59-64, 1991.

51. Gerber C, Ganz R: Clinical assessment of instability of the shoulder with special reference to anterior and posterior drawer tests, *J Bone Joint Surg Br* 66(4):551-556, 1984.

52. Altchek DW, Dines DW: The surgical treatment of anterior instability: selective capsular repair. *Op Tech Sports Med* 1:285-292, 1993.

53. Hawkins RJ, Schulte JP, Janda DH, et al: Translation of the glenohumeral joint with the patient under anesthesia, *J Shoulder Elbow Surg* 5:286-292, 1996.

54. Speer KP, Hannafin JA, Altchek DW, et al: An evaluation of the shoulder relocation test, *Am J Sports Med* 22(2): 177-183, 1994.

55. Hamner DL, Pink MM, Jobe FW: A modification of the relocation test: arthroscopic findings associated with a positive test, *J Shoulder Elbow Surg* 9:263-267, 2000.

56. Morgan CD, Burkhart SS, Palmeri M, et al: Type II SLAP lesions: three subtypes and their relationships to superior instability and rotator cuff tears, *Arthroscopy* 14:553-565, 1998.

57. Neer CS: Anterior acromioplasty for the chronic impingement syndrome in the shoulder, *J Bone Joint Surg Am* 54:41-50, 1972.

58. Hawkins RJ, Kennedy JC: Impingement syndrome in athletes, *Am J Sports Med* 8:151-158, 1980.

59. Greenfield BH, Donatelli RA, Thein-Brody L: Impingement syndrome and impingement related instability. In Donatelli RA, editor: *Physical therapy of the shoulder,* ed 4, Philadelphia, 2004, Churchill Livingstone.

60. Morrison DS, Frogameni AD, Woodworth P: Non-operative treatment of subacromial impingement syndrome, *J Bone Joint Surg Am* 79:732-737, 1997.

61. Fleisig GS, Andrews JR, Dillman CJ, et al: Kinetics of baseball pitching with implications about injury mechanisms, *Am J Sports Med* 23:233, 1995.

62. Cheng JC, Karzel RP: Superior labrum anterior posterior lesions of the shoulder: operative techniques of management, *Op Tech Sports Med* 5(4):249-256, 1997.

63. Andrews JR, Gillogly S: Physical examination of the shoulder in throwing athletes. In Zarins B, Andrews JR,

Carson WG, editors: *Injuries to the throwing arm,* Philadelphia, 1985, Saunders.

64. Liu SH, Henry MH, Nuccion S, et al: Diagnosis of glenoid labrum tears. A comparison between magnetic resonance imaging and clinical examinations, *Am J Sports Med* 24(2):149-154, 1996.

65. Kibler WB: Specificity and sensitivity of the anterior slide test in throwing athletes with superior glenoid labral tears, *Arthroscopy* 11(3):296-300, 1995.

66. O'Brien SJ, Pagnani MJ, Fealy S, et al: The active compression test: a new and effective test for diagnosing labral tears and acromioclavicular joint abnormality, *Am J Sports Med* 26(5):610-613, 1998.

67. Stetson WB, Templin K: The crank test, the O'Brien test, and routine magnetic resonance imaging scans in the diagnosis of labral tears, *Am J Sports Med* 30(6):806-809, 2002.

68. McFarland EG, Kim TK, Savino RM: Clinical assessment of three common tests for superior labral anterior-posterior lesions, *Am J Sports Med* 30(6):810-815, 2002.

69. Davies GJ, DeCarlo MS: *Examination of the shoulder complex: current concepts in rehabilitation of the shoulder,* LaCrosse, Wis, 1995, Sports Phys Ther Assoc Home Study Course.

70. Priest JD, Nagel DA: Tennis shoulder, *Am J Sports Med* 4(1):28-42, 1976.

71. Kibler WB: Role of the scapula in the overhead throwing motion, *Contemp Orthop* 22(5):525-532, 1991.

72. Kibler WB: The role of the scapula in athletic shoulder function, *Am J Sports Med* 26(2):325-337, 1998.

73. Piatt BE, Hawkins RJ, Fritz RC, et al: Clinical evaluation and treatment of spinoglenoid notch ganglion cysts, *J Shoulder Elbow Surg* 11:600-604, 2002.

74. Zeier FG: The treatment of winged scapula, *Clin Orthop Rel Res* 91:128-133, 1973.

75. Kibler WB, Uhl TL, Maddux JWQ, et al: Qualitative clinical evaluation of scapular dysfunction: a reliability study, *J Shoulder Elbow Surg* 11:550-556, 2002.

76. Burkhart SS, Morgan CD, Kibler WB: The disabled throwing shoulder: spectrum of pathology Part III: the SICK scapula, scapula dyskinesis, the kinetic chain and rehabilitation, *Arthroscopy* 19(6): 641-661, 2003.

77. Fleisig GS, Dillman CJ, Andrews JR: Proper mechanics for baseball pitching, *Clin Sports Med* 1:151-170, 1989.

78. Glousman R, Jobe FW, Tibone JE, et al: Dynamic electromyographic analysis of the throwing shoulder with glenohumeral joint instability, *J Bone Joint Surg* 70-A: 220-226, 1988.

79. Fleisig GS, Jameson EG, Dillman CJ, et al: Biomechanics of overhead sports. In Garrett WE, Kirkendall DT, editors: *Exercise and sport science,* Philadelphia, 2000, Lippincott Williams & Wilkins.

80. Dillman CJ, Fleisig GS, Werner SL, et al: *Biomechanics of the shoulder in sports: throwing activities. Post graduate studies in sports physical therapy.* Berryville, Va, 1991, Forum Medicum.

81. Atwater AE: Biomechanics of overarm throwing movements and of throwing injuries, *Exerc Sport Sci Rev* 7: 43-85, 1979.

Evaluation of the Trunk and Hip CORE

LEARNING OBJECTIVES

After studying this chapter, the reader will be able to do the following:

1. Discuss the inherent difficulties in evaluating athletic patients
2. Describe the components of the trunk and hip CORE evaluation
3. Understand the different levels of evidence supporting the CORE evaluation tests and measures
4. Summarize the cluster of underlying CORE impairments commonly found with athletes

Evaluation of the athlete presents unique challenges to the rehabilitation professional. Even in an injured state, athletes can often outperform many uninjured subjects in standard tests and measures. Thus the examination tools must be sensitive enough to measure higher levels of performance. On the other hand, research demonstrates that the recurrent nature of athletic injuries is often secondary to previously unidentified relative weaknesses or residual impairments from previous injuries.[1-3] Therefore the sports therapist must use tests and measures specific enough to identify the underlying impairments that preclude an athlete to injury or reinjury.

This chapter describes select methods to evaluate the performance of the trunk and hip CORE structures identified in Chapter 11. The goal of this chapter is to describe evaluation methods geared toward identifying the CORE impairments that predispose athletes to injury or reinjury. Whenever possible the authors have attempted to provide valid and reliable tests. However, many evaluation tools still lack evidence as to their efficacy. In these cases the authors attempted to discuss the theories behind assessment techniques to allow the reader to judge their worth as clinical tools.

Providing a comprehensive evaluation of the trunk and hip is not the goal of this chapter. The authors refer the reader to numerous excellent references, such as Magee's *Orthopedic Physical Assessment*, ed 3, McGill's *Low Back Disorders: Evidence-Based Prevention and Rehabilitation*, Lee's *The Pelvic Girdle*, ed 3, and the American Physical Therapy Association's (APTA's) *Guide to Physical Therapy Practice*.[4-7]

HISTORY

A thorough history is a crucial first component of any evaluation. The authors assume that the reader will perform a comprehensive systems screening to rule out conditions not appropriate for therapy as described by the APTA's *Guide to Physical Therapy Practice*.[6]

With trauma, the interview should obtain the mechanism of injury. A description of training habits or lack thereof is often helpful for evaluating chronic injuries. Changes in training programs, environment, event, or position often precede injury. Does the athlete allow enough recovery time between bouts of exercise to adapt to training? Likewise, poor- or ill-fitting equipment can also contribute to injury. As with all patients, a description of current symptoms, location, severity, and provoking factors will be helpful in evaluating athletes.[4]

Clinical Application
The history also provides the therapist his or her first opportunity to identify functional limitations in the area of participation in sports. Undoubtedly the patient or his or her supporters will ask the therapist for a time frame on return to sports. Athletes' expectations are often unrealistic as they revolve around specific sporting events or psychological pressures. The wise therapist will structure goals on the basis of physiology versus an athlete's, coach's, or parent's desire. Educating the athlete and family in this area is an advisable way to avoid confusion and frustration for all involved.

OBSERVATION

Along with history, a thorough observation of biomechanics is crucial to any physical therapy examination. This chapter focuses on observations commonly seen in athletes who have impairments of the trunk and hip CORE. The relationship of core impairments to abnormal lower extremity biomechanics was previously described in Chapter 9. Observation of the lower extremity during CORE evaluation will guide the therapist in his or her selection of CORE tests and measures.

Sagittal Plane

Abnormalities observed in lumbo-pelvic posture are a hallmark of impairment in trunk and hip motion, strength, and stabilization. Patients with normal alignment of the pelvis in the sagittal plane will demonstrate the anterior superior iliac spine at 15 degrees lower than the posterior sacroiliac spine (Figure 12-1, A).[7] Comparisons of the superior iliac spines should use this normal as reference for determining anterior or posterior pelvic tilt.

An anterior tilted pelvis suggests poor recruitment of abdominal stabilizers (Figure 12-1, B). It may also suggest weak hamstrings, weak gluteales, and relative shortening of the rectus femoris. Increased lumbar lordosis will usually accompany anterior tilted pelvis. A posterior tilted pelvis suggests possible relative shortening of the hamstrings (Figure 12-1, C).[8-11]

Impairments in the trunk and hip CORE may also cause irregularities distally in the closed kinetic chain. Athletes with an anteriorly tilted pelvis will often display hyperextended knees or genu recurvatum.[8,9]

Transverse and Frontal Planes

Observation of the iliac crest will provide a rough estimate of the alignment of the pelvis in the frontal plane. Comparisons should first be made in normal stance (Figure 12-2, A). Comparisons with feet together (Figure 12-2, B) and feet apart (Figure 12-2, C) provide a quick method to screen for functional leg-length differences.[7] The presence of obvious lateral trunk shifting should also be noted and warrants further testing to rule out lumbar disk pathology.[4,12]

Weakness in hip abductors can manifest as genu valgus or "knock knees" (Figure 12-3). Likewise, weakness of the hip external rotators can lead to excessive femoral internal rotation in stance and with gait.[8,9,13-16]

The *single-legged squat* is an excellent screening test for this same pattern of excessive genu valgus or hip internal rotation, or both, during lower extremity closed kinetic chain motion (Figure 12-4). Zeller et al,[17] using surface electromyography (EMG) and video motion analysis, demonstrated that female college athletes exhibited greater genu valgus than male subjects with single leg squatting. Although their study does not demonstrate the validity or reliability of unassisted observation of single leg squatting as a clinical test, it does suggest it is a useful screening tool to identify athletes who require detailed motion and strength testing of the hip.[17]

Similarly, Noyes et al[18] used computer-assisted digital video analysis to study lower extremity motion in the frontal plane during a *drop-jump screening test* (Figure 12-5). Subjects were fitted with markers of hip, knee, and ankle joint centers and then videotaped while performing a depth jump from a 12-inch–high box, immediately followed by a maximal vertical jump. They found this method to have excellent test-retest and within-test reliability in measuring relative hip, knee, and ankle motion in the frontal plane. Again, not everyone has access to video analysis systems, but their work suggests that observation of drop-jump for excessive genu valgus will guide the clinician to further test hip strength.[18]

Gait

Athletes with relative shortening of the hip flexors and accompanying weakness of hip extensors will exhibit decreased hip extension at terminal stance phase or "toe off." Athletes who lack hip extension may also exhibit related limitation in great toe extension. Often these athletes will show decreased wear under the great toe aspect of their shoe sole and relative increased wear under the more lateral toes. These athletes may also demonstrate increased hip flexion at initial contact or "heel strike" in an effort to make up for the shorter stride length caused by limited hip extension. In patients with knee instability this will contribute to hyperextension or "giving way" of the knee.[13]

Athletes with marked weakness of the hip abductors will exhibit the classic Trendelenburg gait pattern. Hallmarks of the Trendelenburg gait pattern are depression of the swing phase pelvis (as the stance phase hip abductors cannot resist the pull of gravity on the unsupported side of the body).[4,8,13] Athletes often find ways to compensate for a relative weakness, such as with a compensated Trendelenburg gait pattern. With this pattern the athlete exhibits increased deviation of the body in the frontal plane toward the stance leg. This causes a decrease in the moment arm of gravitational forces pulling on the unsupported half of the body and a relative decreased load on the stance phase hip abductors (Table 12-1).[8,13]

TRUNK SCREENING

The following tests and measures are included in the CORE evaluation as a means to screen for conditions, such as lumbar disk herniation or sacroiliac dysfunction, that warrant more thorough evaluation.

Trunk Motion

Trunk flexion, extension, and side bending can be measured with goniometry, tape measure along the spinous processes, inclinometry, or visual estimation of motion. Disagreement regarding the intratester and intertester reliability of all methods currently used to measure trunk motion exists in the literature.[19] Still, an attempt should be made to quantify trunk motion during evaluation. McKenzie also endorses performing knees to chest and prone prop or the sphinx position to further assess trunk flexion and extension, respectively (Figure 12-6).[12,20]

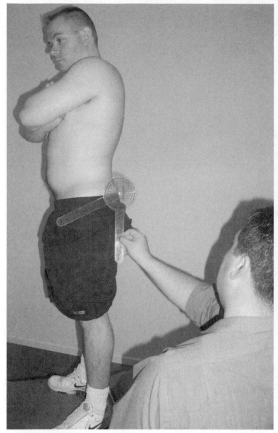

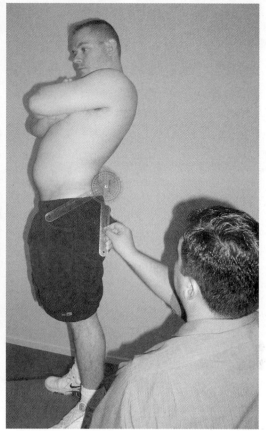

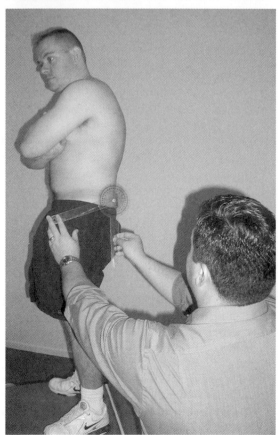

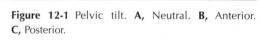

Figure 12-1 Pelvic tilt. **A,** Neutral. **B,** Anterior. **C,** Posterior.

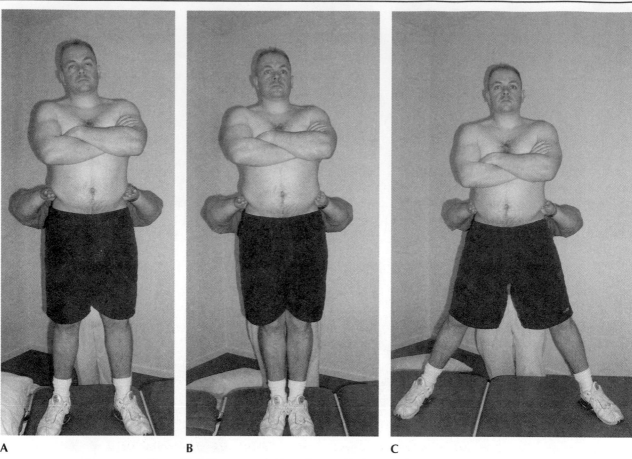

Figure 12-2 Iliac crests. **A,** Normal stance. **B,** Feet together. **C,** Feet apart.

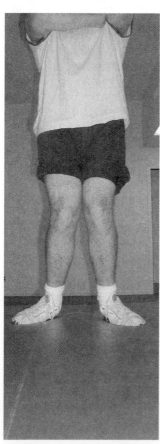

Figure 12-3 Genu valgus.

Peripheralization/Centralization Phenomenon

The therapist should note the presence of peripheralization (lower extremity symptoms moving distally) or centralization (moving proximally) with any of trunk motions described earlier (Table 12-2). The presence of either or both phenomena is commonly associated with lumbar disk derangement.[4,12,20-22]

Slump Test

Butler[21] hypothesized that pathologies of the nervous system restrict the normal motion of neural tissues. These researchers advocate the slump test to detect this "adverse neural tension" via the combined movements of the trunk and lower extremity. The patient sits in full gross trunk flexion (chin to chest, slouched, bent-forward posture). The patient then slowly extends the knee and notes any reproduction of symptoms. The patient then dorsiflexes the ankle and again notes reproduction or worsening of symptoms. Many patients, even if they are healthy, will experience pain with these tests as they stress neurological tissues. The slump test is considered positive only if it reproduces the patient's complaint of symptoms.[4,21,22]

Confirmation of positive testing is to see if reproduction of symptoms can be increased or decreased by manipulating the "sensitizing" aspects of the test. For example, reproduction of posterior lower extremity pain and "numbness" with slump testing would be considered a positive test. Elimination of

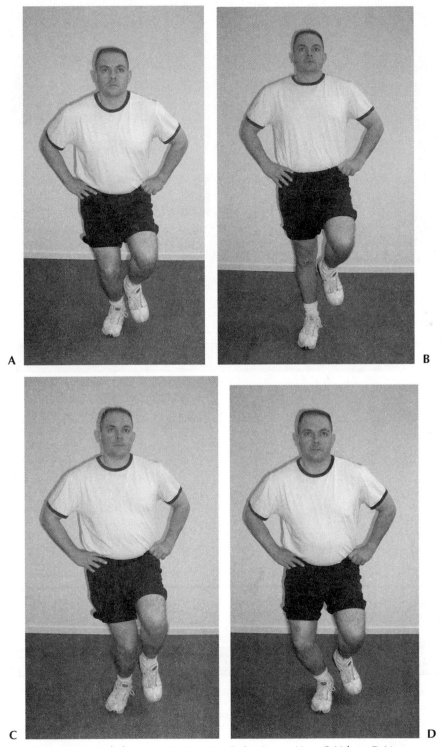

Figure 12-4 Single-leg squat. **A,** Negative. **B,** Starting position. **C,** Valgus. **D,** Varus.

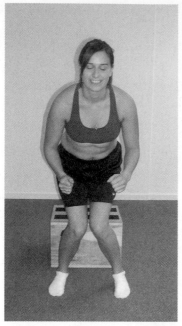

Figure 12-5 Positive drop-jump screen.

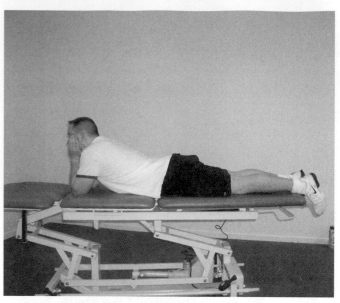

Figure 12-6 McKenzie prone prop or sphinx.

Table 12-1	Sample of Observation Section of CORE Evaluation Sheet

Observation

	Date	Date	Date	Date
Anterior Pelvic Tilt				
Posterior Pelvic Tilt				
Iliac Crest Asymmetry				
Feet together				
Feet apart				
Genu Recurvatum				
Genu Valgus				
Single-Leg Squat				
Drop-Jump Screening				
Gait				

Table 12-2	Sample of Trunk Motion Section of CORE Evaluation Sheet

Trunk Motion (note motion, peripheralization, or centralization)

	Date	Date	Date	Date
Flexion				
Extension				
R Side Bending				
L Side Bending				
Knees to chest				
Prone Prop				

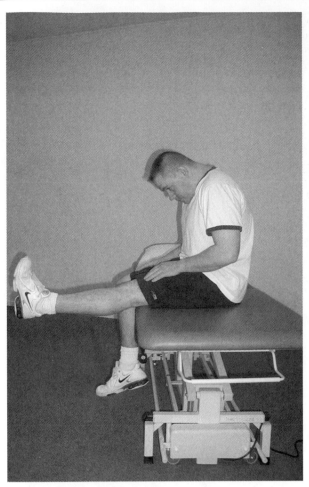

Figure 12-7 Slump test.

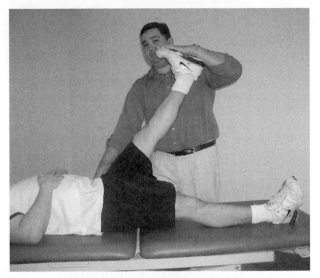

Figure 12-8 Straight leg raise.

these symptoms with plantarflexing the ankle (desensitizing the neural tissues) would further confirm a positive slump test (Figure 12-7).[21]

Straight Leg Raise Testing

Passive straight leg raise testing is the most commonly used test for lumbar discopathy and nerve root irritation. The patient lies supine while the therapist passively raises the patient's leg. Reproduction of low back pain with radiating pain to the posterior thigh noted before 60 degrees of elevation is associated with disk protrusion. Back pain with motion past 70 degrees is typically associated with the sacroiliac or lumbar spine joints because this range of motion causes negligible further nerve root deformation.[4,20-23]

Another useful special test is the *opposite straight leg raise* or well-leg raising test (Figure 12-8). The test procedure is the same as described earlier, but a positive test is reproduction of symptoms with raising the unaffected leg. The opposite straight leg raise has low sensitivity but high specificity for lumbar disk herniation. Thus positive testing does not rule in a significant intervertebral disk protrusion, but negative testing is useful in ruling out disk protrusion.[4,20,22,23]

Prone Instability Test

This test for segmental spinal instability relies on the stabilizing action of the iliocostalis lumborum pars thoracis described in Chapter 11. To perform the test, the patient is positioned in prone position on a plinth, with hips at the edge of the plinth and feet touching the floor. The therapist then applies a posterior to anterior pressure through the lumbar spinous process to be tested. The same procedure is repeated with the patient lifting his or her feet off the floor to activate the iliocostalis and thus stabilize the segment. The test is considered positive with reproduction of pain with the first position, which is reduced or eliminated with feet off the floor. Unlike the posterior shear test, the prone instability test has been shown to have good reliability (Figure 12-9).[4,24]

Facet Scour

Also known as the *lumbar quadrant test,* this test can be used as a screening tool for lumbar facet joint pathology and radiculopathy. The patient sits with arms folded across his or her chest. The therapist guides the patient into combined lumbar extension and rotation, increasing compression and shear in the facet joints. Reproduction of localized low back pain suggests possible facet joint pathology, but evidence as to the accuracy of this test is lacking.[4,23] Reproduction of radiating lower extremity pain is typically associated with narrowing of the lumbar neural foramen.

Sacroiliac Joint Tests

The following sacroiliac pain provocation tests have been found to have good to excellent interrater reliability. The authors have listed multiple tests because confirmation of three or more positive provocation tests greatly improves the likelihood index with diagnosis. All of the following tests are considered positive if they reproduce the patient's pain.[20]

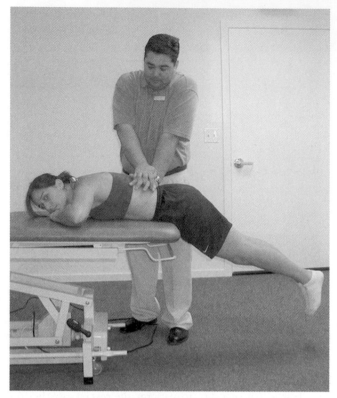

Figure 12-9 Prone instability test.

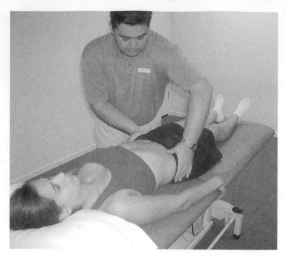

Figure 12-10 Sacroiliac joint distraction.

Distraction Test

With the patient in supine position the therapist applies an anterior to posterior force to both anterior superior iliac spines (Figure 12-10).

Thigh Thrust

The patient is positioned in supine lying with one hip flexed to 90 degrees and slightly adducted. The therapist hand stabilizes the sacrum by cupping in from underneath. Using the other arm and the body, the therapist applies pressure to axially load the femur into the table, thus producing the posterior shear force on the sacroiliac joint (Figure 12-11).

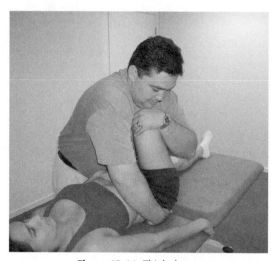

Figure 12-11 Thigh thrust.

Gaenslen's Test

The patient lies supine with one leg hanging over the edge of the table. The therapist flexes the other hip and knee toward the patient's chest. The therapist then applies firm pressure to move the legs apart and torsion the sacroiliac joint (Figure 12-12).

> ### Clinical Application
> Performing this test immediately following the Thomas test, described as follows, is easy because they begin in nearly the same position.

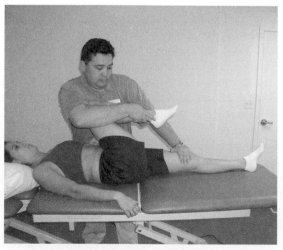

Figure 12-12 Gaenslen's test.

Compression

In sidelying, the patient flexes his or her hips and knees to 90 degrees. The examiner applies force down through the top iliac crest to compress the sacroiliac joints (Figure 12-13).

Sacral Thrust

With the patient in prone lying the therapist applies a posterior to anterior glide to the center of the sacrum to produce shearing of both sacroiliac joints (Figure 12-14).

TESTS OF SACROLIAC JOINT DYSFUNCTION

Estimations of sacroiliac joint alignment or symmetry via visual estimation, palpation, inclinometry, and the assistance of

calipers have all been found unreliable.[24] Likewise, studies of tests commonly used to determine sacroiliac "joint dysfunction" or "positional diagnosis" show them to be unreliable (Table 12-3).[25,26]

HIP TESTING

Hip Motion

Unlike trunk motion, goniometry of the lower extremity joints has been shown to be reliable to within 5 degrees of motion (Table 12-4).[19] A thorough description of all hip goniometry is provided by Norkin and White.[19]

Stabilization of the pelvis to prevent compensation is key to obtaining accurate measurement of true hip motion. Likewise, observation of compensations often provides as much informa-

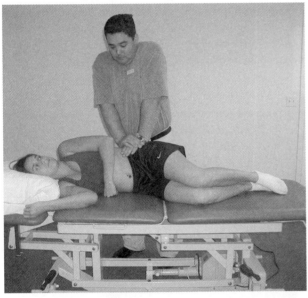

Figure 12-13 Sacroiliac joint compression.

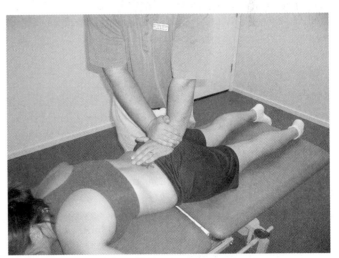

Figure 12-14 Sacral thrust.

Table 12-3	Sample of Trunk Special Tests Section of CORE Evaluation Sheet

Trunk Special Tests

	Date	Date	Date	Date
Slump Test				
SLR				
Prone Instability				
Facet Scour				
SIJ				
Distraction				
Thigh Thrust				
Gaenslen's Compression				
Sacral Thrust				

SIJ, Sacriliac joint; *SLR,* straight leg raise.

tion as the actual goniometry. The authors also recommend testing of hip rotation in both the sitting and prone positions to assess the impact of hip extension on hip rotation.

In their combined clinical practice the authors most commonly observe impairments in hip extension and rotation. The following tests are useful in identifying the hip structures that may be limiting hip motion.

Thomas Test

The authors have found that hip extension in athletes is most commonly limited by adaptive shortening of the rectus femoris. The Thomas test can be used to determine the impact of rectus femoris tightness on hip and knee position.[4,8,9,11,19]

The patient lies supine with his or her hips nearly off the edge of the plinth. The patient is cued to hold the contralateral knee into his or her chest to prevent lumbar hyperextension and anterior pelvic tilt compensations. With a negative test the down thigh will stay on the plinth while the knee remains flexed. With a positive test the down thigh will rise from the plinth and may be accompanied by knee extension. The therapist can record the hip and knee position with goniometry to further quantify the Thomas test (Figure 12-15). The therapist should also watch for hip abduction of the down leg or "J-sign," which suggests iliotibial band tightness.[4,11]

Ober's Test

This test assesses tissue extensibility in the iliotibial band and tensor fascia latae. The patient is positioned in sidelying with the test side up. The down leg is positioned in hip and knee flexion to stabilize the patient. The therapist extends and abducts the hip while stabilizing the pelvis to prevent a "rolling back" compensation. The Ober test was originally described with the test leg in knee flexion, but on the basis of recent anatomical studies that show knee extension further tensions the iliotibial band, the authors recommend using knee

Table 12-4	The American Academy of Orthopedic Surgeons' Established Mean Normal Values for Hip Motion

AAOS Hip Range of Motion Normal Values

Flexion	120 degrees
Extension	30 degrees
Abduction	45 degrees
Adduction	30 degrees
Medial Rotation	45 degrees
Lateral Rotation	45 degrees

extension (Figure 12-16). The therapist then slowly allows the up leg to fall with gravity. With a positive test the up leg will remain abducted even after support has been removed.[4]

Craig's Test

Craig's test is a clinical measure of femoral antero/retroversion or the degree to which the femoral neck angulates forward or backward in the transverse plane in relation to the plane of the femoral condyles (Figure 12-17).

Clinical Application

A good way for clinicians to remember this is to point their index fingers straight ahead to represent the femur and then move their thumbs up and down as when striking the space bar on a keyboard. Movement of the thumb upward is likened to femoral anteroversion, and downwards to retroversion.

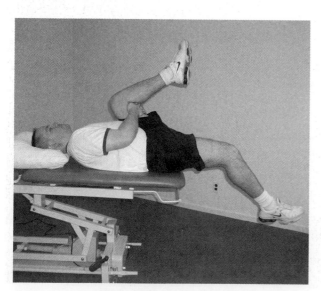

Figure 12-15 Thomas test.

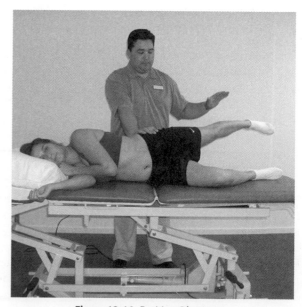

Figure 12-16 Positive Ober's test.

| Table 12-5 | Sample of Hip Motion Section of CORE Evaluation Sheet | | | | | | | |

Hip Motion

	Date		Date		Date		Date	
	R	L	R	L	R	L	R	L
Flexion								
Extension								
Abduction								
Adduction								
Sitting IR/ER								
Prone IR/ER								
Thomas Test								
Ober's Test								
Craig's Test								

ER, External rotation; *IR,* internal rotation.

To perform the test the patient lies prone with the knee flexed to 90 degrees. The therapist palpates the greater trochanter of the hip while passively rotating the hip via the lower leg, stopping when the trochanter is parallel to the floor. The angle of the lower leg in relation to vertical will provide a clinical estimate of femoral anteroversion/retroversion. When the lower leg points laterally (internal hip rotation), the patient has anteroversion. The normal amount of femoral anteroversion in the adult is 8 to 15 degrees. When the lower leg points medially (hip external rotation), the patient has retroversion (Table 12-5).[4]

HIP AND TRUNK CORE STABILIZATION TESTS

Local Stabilization Tests

As described in Chapter 11, there has been extensive recent research into the role of the local stabilizers transversus abdominis, lumbar multifidus, and pelvic floor in preventing and rehabilitating low back pain, sacroiliac pain, and groin pain. Delays in muscle activation of these muscles are thought to allow excessive motion between bony segments of the CORE, leading to increased shear forces and inefficient use of mobilizer muscles. The majority of the research used fine-wire EMG alone or in combination with diagnostic or real-time ultrasound (RTUS) to identify abnormal muscle activation patterns in patients with low back and sacroiliac pain.[27-30] However, there is a relative lack of evidence supporting many commonly used clinical assessments of local stability not dependent on technology.

Richardson et al[27] propose a three-tiered system consisting of simple screening tests, clinical measures, and diagnostic measures to assess neuromuscular control of the local stabilization system.

Screening Tests

Richardson et al[27] describe a "clinical assessment" of the abdominal drawing in action without spinal or pelvic motion based on observation and palpation. Although this is a commonly used evaluation method, even primary researchers

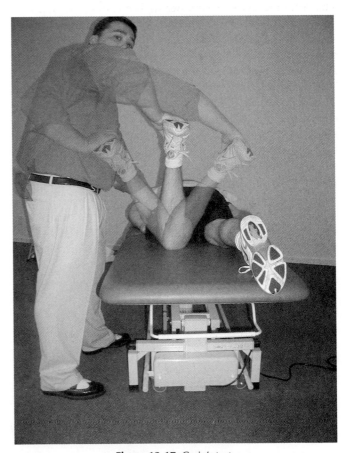

Figure 12-17 Craig's test.

acknowledge further research is necessary to validate these screening tests as evaluation tools.

Clinical Application

The authors also note anecdotally that they and all other therapists they have encountered who have used the RTUS technology in the clinic have reported they did not feel their "clinical assessment" skills compared favorably with RTUS. Hopefully this technology will be affordable to all clinicians in the near future.

Clinical Measures of Local Stability

Abdominal Drawing-in Test

This test is similar to the screening test described earlier with the addition of the use of pressure biofeedback and positioning the patient in prone. Richardson et al[27] recommend instructing the patient in the motor skill to be tested by cueing the patient to "draw in the abdominal wall" and educating the patient in the corset-like anatomy of the transversus abdominis. It may also be necessary to begin by instructing the patient in the kneeling-on-all-fours position before actual testing.

For testing the patient is positioned in prone lying with arms at sides. A pressure biofeedback unit is positioned beneath the paitent's abdomen with the navel in the center of the bladder and the distal edge of the bladder aligned with the anterior iliac spines. The bladder is inflated to 70 mm Hg in the conditions described earlier. The patient is cued to "breathe in and out and then, without breathing in, slowly draw in the abdomen so that it lifts up off the pad, keeping the spinal position steady." The therapist monitors the patient for any compensation from other muscles, which would cause movement of the pelvis.

According to Richardson et al,[27] a correct isolated transversus abdominis contraction will reduce pressure in the biofeedback unit by 6 to 10 mm Hg as the drawing-in action of the transversus abdominis moves the abdominal wall away from the pressure bladder. A drop in pressure less than 6 mm or an increase in pressure indicates a "poor" transversus abdominis contraction. If correct recruitment of the transversus abdominis is observed, then muscular endurance is assessed with 10-second isometric holds for up to 10 repetitions.

Hodges et al[31] examined the relationship between laboratory study of local stabilizers and clinical testing used to assess local stabilization patterns. They reported "good agreement" between subjects with a poor ability to decrease pressure with the drawing-in test and those with delayed transversus abdominis activation in the laboratory. However, to the authors' knowledge Hodges et al did not statistically demonstrate this relationship.[31]

Segmental Palpation of Lumbar Multifidus

Richardson et al[27] also advocate palpation to detect wasting and activation of the lumbar multifidus. For palpation the patient is positioned in prone as for the drawing-in test. First the clinician palpates the lumbar multifidus in a relaxed state, comparing bilaterally for atrophy spanning a defined two-vertebra segment.

Multifidus Atrophy

Hides et al[32] studied the agreement between RTUS and palpation in assessing "the most affected level" of lumbar multifidus atrophy and abnormal activation in patients with acute and subacute low back pain. In their study blinded examiners were asked to determine the "most affected vertebral level of lumbar multifidus using palpation." The examiners agreed with RTUS in 24 of 26 cases. Palpation may not be useful in assessment of patients with chronic low back pain because generalized atrophy or infiltration of fatty tissue, or both, into the lumbar multifidus can confound findings.[32]

Multifidus Activation

Next the multifidus is palpated during contraction. Cues for correct muscle action are the same as for the "drawing-in test" with the addition of the command "gently swell out your muscles under my fingers without moving your spine or pelvis. Hold the contraction while breathing normally." The examiner notes differences in timing and level of muscle contraction bilaterally.

Hides et al[33] report evidence supporting abnormal muscle activation in patients following spontaneous resolution of acute low back pain. However, to the authors' knowledge, no evidence exists supporting palpation as a reliable test of lumbar multifidus activation compared with the RTUS method used in laboratory study.[33]

Active Straight Leg Raise Test

Another clinical test of the local lumbopelvic stabilizers available to all clinicians is the active straight leg raise (ASLR) test. The subject lies supine with his or her arms at the sides. The subject then actively raises one leg 12 inches from the plinth and notes any reproduction of posterior back or pelvic pain. The test is performed again with the therapist simulating the action of the transversus abdominis by pushing inward from the lateral border of the pelvis or using a pelvic support belt to compress the pelvis in the frontal plane.[34-36]

A positive test is reproduction of lumbopelvic pain with the first trial and reduction or elimination of symptoms with simulation of the TrA action. A positive test suggests that a patient will respond well to local stabilization exercise. The ASLR has also been correlated with the Quebec Back Pain Disability Score in patients with posterior pelvic pain after pregnancy.[34,35] Cowan et al[36] also demonstrated delayed onset of the transversus abdominis in Australian Rules Football players with long-standing groin pain while performing the ASLR. This test holds promise as a nontechnological clinical assessment of local stabilization, but further research is required to determine reliability (Figure 12-18).

Table 12-6	Global Stabilization Test Norms		
	Male	Female	Combined M & F
Bridging with Extended Knee	Not Established	Not Established	Not Established
Bird Dog Position	Not Established	Not Established	Not Established
Right Side Bridge	95 sec	75 sec	83 sec
Left Side Bridge	99 sec	78 sec	86 sec
Abdominal Bracing	136 sec	134 sec	134 sec
Back Extensor Endurance	160 sec	185 sec	173 sec

Diagnostic Measures

The third tier of local stabilization suggested by Richardson et al is the use of fine-wire EMG, diagnostic ultrasound, and RTUS to quantify the timing of transversus and multifidus muscle action.[27] These are reliable and valid means of assessing muscle activation patterns.[37,38] However, the invasive nature of fine-wire EMG and the currently high cost of RTUS prevent many clinicians from employing these assessment tools. As practice acts evolve and this technology becomes more affordable, the authors hope to see more widespread use of these methods of local stabilizer assessment. As discussed earlier, the clinical assessment tools of local stabilizers currently lack evidence.

GLOBAL STABILIZATION

Global stabilization refers to the actions of muscles that cross more than one joint to prevent excessive motion in the trunk and hip CORE. The research into local stabilization already discussed suggests that excessive activation patterns or activation of global muscles before the local stabilizers is linked to low back, sacroiliac, and groin pain.[27-34,36] However, in the presence of normal local stabilization, global stabilization is necessary for all athletic motions. Many studies show that global stabilizers are active throughout sports motions.[7,39-42] The following tests are designed to test the muscle activation and endurance of these global CORE stabilizers in standardized positions.

Bridging Test with Knee Extended

Closed kinetic chain bridging tests the muscular endurance of all stabilizers of the trunk and hip CORE. The patient begins in supine hook lying position and then recruits the transversus abdominis and multifidus with a cue of "drawing in." The patient then uses the gluteus maximus and hamstrings to extend the hips and raise the trunk and hips from the plinth. During this motion the quadratus lumborum is active to maintain stability in the frontal plane. The gluteus medius is also active, stabilizing the hip in the frontal plane and combining with the other hip rotators to stabilize the hip in the transverse plane. To increase the test challenge, the patient lifts one leg.

Endurance is measured in consecutive seconds the patient can maintain this position.[7]

Bird Dog Test

This test is based on research showing that reciprocal upper extremity and lower extremity motion correlates to activation of the lumbar multifidus and iliocostalis pars thoracis.[7,27,32,33] The patient is positioned kneeling on all fours. The patient then actively raises one arm and the opposite leg until level with the trunk. As no established norms exist for this test, endurance is measured in consecutive seconds the patient can maintain this position.

Side Bridge Test

This test was shown to produce significant EMG activity in all of the trunk and hip stabilizers, especially an isometric bilateral muscle action by the quadratus lumborum. Established normal values for this test make it attractive for use in quantifying goals.[7] Normal values are displayed in Table 12-6.

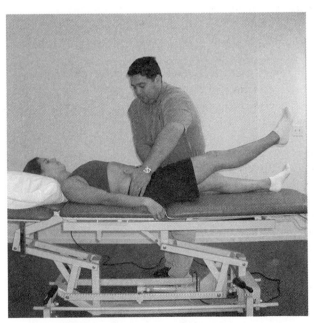

Figure 12-18 Active straight leg raise test.

Table 12-7	**Sample of Trunk Stabilization Section of CORE Evaluation Sheet**						

Trunk Stabilization

	Date		Date		Date		Date	
TrA Drawing in Multifidus Palpation	R	L	R	L	R	L	R	L

Active SLR
Leg Loading Test
Bird dog
Side bridge
   Normal: R SB: M/F =83s, M= 95s, F=75s L SB: 86s M/F, M= 99s, F=78s
Abdominal Bracing
   Normal is M/F = 134 seconds, M = 136 seconds, F = 134 seconds
Back Extensor Test
   Normal is M/F = 173 seconds, M = 160 seconds, F = 185 seconds

M/F, Male/female; *R SB,* right side bridge; *L SB,* left side bridge; *SLR,* straight leg raise; *TrA,* transversus abdominis.

The patient begins lying on his or her side with the upper body propped up on an elbow and the top leg crossed over the bottom with both feet touching the plinth. Timing begins when the patient raises his or her body off the plinth and is supported only by the feet and down forearm.[7]

Abdominal Bracing

Abdominal bracing tests the endurance of the rectus abdominis to hold the trunk in a flexed position (Figure 12-19). The patient is positioned with a 60-degree wedge placed behind the trunk as in a sit-up. The wedge is removed, and patient holds the position for as long as possible.[7] This test also has normal values displayed in Table 12-6.

Back Extensor Endurance Test

Biering-Sorensen showed that poor endurance in the lumbar extensors is associated with increased risk of low back problems.[39] Unlike manual muscle testing, this test measures the endurance of the lumbar erector spinae in their capacity to stabilize the spine in neutral curve (Figure 12-20). The patient begins in prone lying on the plinth. The patient then moves forward until the pelvis is at the edge of the plinth but still supported. The therapist must apply considerable pressure to stabilize the patient's pelvis and lower extremities on the plinth. The patient is timed for as long as the trunk can be maintained parallel to the floor (Table 12-7).[39] Normal values are displayed in Table 12-6.

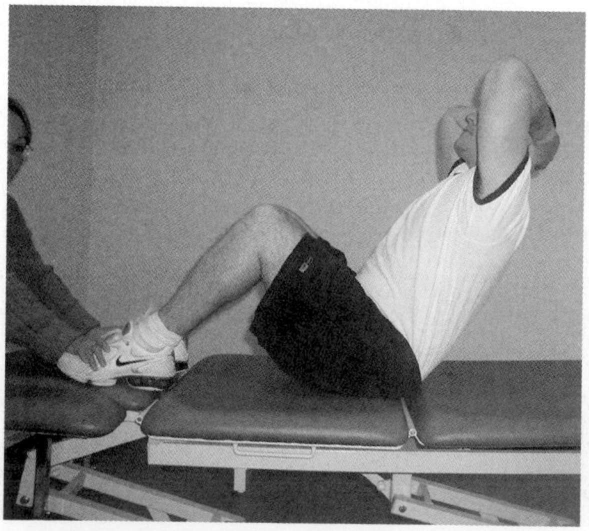

Figure 12-19 Abdominal bracing for endurance.

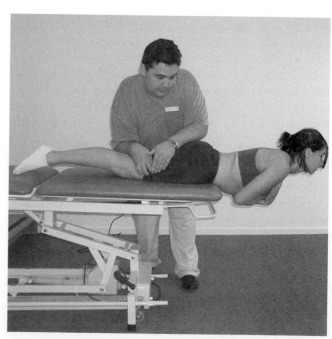

Figure 12-20 Back extensor for endurance.

Table 12-8	Manual Muscle Test Procedures
Motion Tested	**Test Procedure**
Hip Abduction	Patient lying on side with underside knee flexed. Test hip is abducted to midrange, slightly extended, and slightly externally rotated.
	Many patients will rotate the pelvis backward to compensate for a weak posterior gluteus medius with the tensor fascia latae
Hip Adduction	Patient is positioned in side lying with the leg to be tested in the down position. The therapist supports with top leg while resisting hip adduction on the medial distal femur of the down leg.
Hip Extension	Patient positioned prone with the knee flexed to 90 degrees. The hip is extended by lifting the thigh from the plinth. Downward pressure is applied by the therapist against the distal posterior thigh while stabilizing the pelvis with the other hand.
Hip Flexion	Patient seated on the edge of the plinth with knees flexed to 90 degrees. Patient flexes the hip to midrange. Therapist applies resistance against distal anterior thigh while stabilizing the trunk with one hand on the anterior shoulder.
Hip Internal Rotation	Patient is seated on the edge of the plinth with knees flexed to 90 degrees. Examiner medially rotates the femur by moving the lower leg laterally to midrange. Therapist applies pressure in a medial direction against the lateral lower leg while stabilizing the hip and pelvis with a hand on the thigh.
Hip External Rotation	Patient is positioned as with internal rotation. Therapist moves the test leg into midrange of external hip rotation by moving the lower leg medially. Resistance is now applied laterally against the medial distal lower leg.

MOBILIZER TESTS

Many of the muscles of the trunk and hip CORE function as mobilizers, muscles that produce force to cause movement across a joint. Strength is defined as the maximal amount of force produced by a muscle action; in other words, strength is a measure of muscle performance as a mobilizer. Clinicians can employ a variety of methods for measuring strength.

Isometric Manual Muscle Testing

Manual muscle tests have been a staple of physical therapy since the epidemic of polio necessitated a rapid and reliable method of assessing strength without equipment. Table 12-8 describes commonly accepted test positions used to assess trunk and hip mobilzers.[8,39]

If performed correctly using standardized testing positions with the 0 to 5 grading scale, manual muscle testing has been shown to be a reliable measure of isometric muscle strength.[8,43-45] Table 12-9 describes the 0 to 5 grading system for manual muscle testing.

However, this grading system is often not sensitive enough to detect relative weakness seen in strong athletes (i.e., some injured athletes will still demonstrate 5/5 strength with muscle testing). Conversely, this means any athlete not testing at 5/5 with manual muscle testing has an obvious strength impairment that should be addressed. Hand-held dynamometers have been shown to be a reliable and more sensitive measure of isometric strength testing and can be employed with the established test positions for manual muscle testing.[44-46]

Drop Leg Test

Clinical Application

On the basis of the clinical experience of the authors of this chapter, the hip abduction manual muscle test is often not sensitive enough to detect weakness in the posterior fibers of the gluteus medius even when performed as described earlier. Instead, they recommend taking the hip passively to the end-of-range abduction and extension and then asking the patient to hold the leg there. At end range, weak posterior fibers of the gluteus medius will cause the leg to drop 6 to 12 inches once the therapist's stabilization of the limb is removed (Figure 12-21).

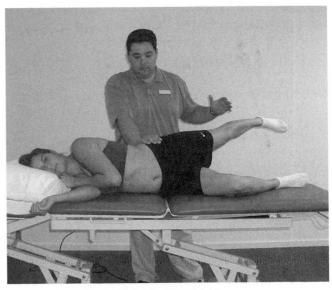

Figure 12-21 Positive drop leg test.

Table 12-9	0-5 Grading System for Manual Muscle Testing	
Grade	Value	Criteria
5	Normal	Complete range of motion against gravity with maximal resistance
4	Good	Complete range of motion against gravity with moderate resistance
3	Fair	Complete range of motion against gravity
2	Poor	Complete range of motion with gravity eliminated position
1	Trace	Evidence of slight contraction but no observable joint motion
0	Zero	No contraction palpated

Table 12-10	Hip Abductor-to-Adductor Isokinetic Muscle Force Ratios	
Male	Female	Combined Male and Female
1:2.09	1:2.46	1:2.46

Table 12-11	Ratios for Calculation of One Repetition Maximum
Number of Repetitions Lifted	Conversion Factor (Multiply Weight Lifted by This Factor to Calculate One Repetition Maximum)
1	1.00
2	1.03
3	1.06
4	1.09
5	1.13
6	1.16
7	1.20
8	1.24
9	1.29
10	1.33

Isokinetic Testing

Isokinetic testing enjoyed great favor in the 1980s and early 1990s as a means of testing strength. However, it has recently come into disfavor because of alleged limitations as a "functional test" and high operating costs. Isokinetic testing is indeed limited to testing strength at a constant joint speed, which critics are quick to point out does not occur with natural sports motions.

However, the authors take issue with other researchers' definition of "functional testing." Mont et al[47] showed that increases in isolated rotator cuff strength, as measured by isokinetic testing, increased tennis serve velocity by 10%. Most players and fans would agree that a faster serve improves performance in the sport of tennis, a functional activity as defined by the Nagi model of disability. This begs the question, "How is a reliable measure of rotator cuff strength not a functional test?" Despite its limitations, isokinetic testing remains a reliable method of strength testing and inferring agonist/antagonist imbalance.

Donatelli et al[48] found established normal hip abductor–to-adductor ratios for adults, which are displayed in Table 12-10.

Isotonic Repetition Maximums

One Repetition Maximum

Single repetition maximum lifts are still considered the gold standard for measuring muscular strength.[49-51,53] If one asks most football players what their bench press maxiumum is, they will answer without hesitation. This is because most strength training programs use one repetition maximum (rep max) to measure strength. This is also why most strengthening programs specify performing sets at a percentage of their one rep max.

However, many rehabilitation professionals fail to use one rep max to assess strength because they fear further injuring the athlete with a maximal production of force. Safety with testing is understandable, but not at the cost of preventing

accurate assessment of strength and thus inaccurate development of strength training. Identification and quantification of weakness is a necessary part of addressing it with strength training.

8 to 12 Repetition Maximum

An alternative solution is to use the 8 to 12 rep max recommended for novice trainers by the American College of Sports Medicine.[51,52] The athlete simply performs the desired motion against isotonic resistance, such as cable resistance, hydraulic machines, or free weights. Resistance is increased until the athlete is unable to maintain correct form or fails to achieve the desired number of repetitions. This method will still establish a baseline criterion reference while avoiding true maximal force production.

Calculated One Repetition Maximum

Another alternative is to calculate one rep max via the formula studied by Brzycki.[53] Table 12-11 reflects the conversion factors for calculating one rep max. For example, if a patient can safely perform 8 repetitions at 5 lb, then multiplying the 5 lb by a conversion factor of 1.24 provides a calculated one rep max of 6.2 lb. The advantage of calculating a one rep max is that it will provide the therapist with the most widely accepted measure of strength without the risks associated with one rep max testing.

Table 12-12	Sample of Hip Mobilizer Section of CORE Evaluation Sheet

Hip Mobilizer Testing
Leg Drop Test–(Abduction & Extension)

	Date		Date		Date		Date		Date		Date	
	R	L	R	L	R	L	R	L	R	L	R	L
Unable to hold												
Unable to resist												

MMT

	Date		Date		Date		Date		Date		Date	
	R	L	R	L	R	L	R	L	R	L	R	L
Abduction												
Adduction												
Extension												
Flexion												
IR Sitting												
ER Sitting												

ER, External rotation; *IR,* internal rotation; *MMT,* manual muscle test.

Although one rep max calculators are readily available online at websites, clinicians should be careful to look for citation referring to the work of Brzycki.[53] One website endorsed by many rehabilitation and fitness professionals is *http://www.exrx.net/Calculators/OneRepMax.html.*

Clinical Application

The following recommendations are universal for establishing repetition maximums, regardless of what number repetition maximum is to be performed. The athlete should begin with a 5 to 10 rep warm-up using approximately 50% of an estimated repetition max. Next, the athlete should perform trials of 70%, 90%, and then 100% of estimated rep max. Rest periods of 2 to 3 minutes should be allowed between each trial to prevent muscular fatigue. The athlete should continue trials with higher weight at whatever specified number of reps the therapist chose until he or she fails. The last successfully completed trial with correct form is the athlete's repletion max (Table 12-12).[49,50]

POWER

Power is defined as the amount of work (force × distance) produced in a given period of time.[49-52] In the realm of sports this typically means moving the body or an object over a distance in a period of seconds or milliseconds. For example, a baseball pitcher has power if he or she can use the entire body to produce enough force to move the ball the distance from the mound to home plate in a fraction of a second. A sprinter is extremely powerful if he or she can move his or her body weight over a distance of 100 yards in the 9- to 10-second range. Thus clinical measures of power can be excellent functional or sports-specific tests. Several clinical tests of lower extremity power are described as follows.

T-Test

The T-test has been shown to be a highly reliable measure of power, agility, and speed.[54] The athlete sprints around a "T"-shaped course measuring 10 meters long by 10 meters wide on the gym floor.

Shuttle Run

All that is required to perform the shuttle run test is two lines taped 6.7 m (22 ft) apart on the floor (Figure 12-22). The athlete must run the total length of the course three times (start at one line A, run to touch the other line B, return to touch line A, and finally run to line B). Nadler et al[1] studied previously injured and uninjured National College Athletic Association Division I freshman athletes with this test. Their data for uninjured freshman athletes are displayed in Table 12-13.

Cycle Ergometer Testing

An old standard of exercise physiologists, the cycle ergometer test of lower extremity power, is reliable and has established norms for peak power, as well as power output–to–body weight ratios. This test is most appropriate when testing cyclists but is also helpful when assessing power in postsurgical patients not yet ready for plyometric activity.

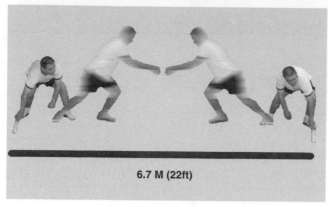

6.7 M (22ft)

Figure 12-22 Shuttle run.

Table 12-13	Shuttle Run Times for Uninjured National College Athletic Association Freshman Athletes

Males	5.7 seconds
Females	6.4 seconds

The athlete sits atop a cycle ergometer equipped with pedal straps and a power monitor (power can be calculated by revolutions per minute and resistance on older models). The athlete pedals as fast as possible for 10 or 30 seconds. Table 12-14 displays the percentile ranking for cycle ergometer peak power and power output-to-body weight ratio.[55]

Countermovement Vertical Jump Testing

Rehabilitation professionals, exercise physiologists, and coaches have all used maximal vertical jumping as a measure of lower extremity power. All that is required is a clear landing area and vertical wall. The athlete marks the highest point of reach with feet flat on the floor. The athlete performs his or her maximum vertical jump. He or she can gather the lower extremities and use upper extremity pumping motion, but no steps are allowed. The therapist calculates the vertical jump from the highest point reached during jump-minus-baseline reach. Automated systems, such as the Vertec and Just Jump, automatically calculate the vertical jump for the clinician and ease standardization of measurement.

Studies into normal values for vertical jump in athletes vary widely, most likely because of variance in methodology. Patterson and Peterson[57] established vertical jump normal for college students who were 21 to 24 years old. Their normal values are listed in Table 12-15.

Medicine Ball Throws

Stockbrugger and Haennel demonstrated the *backward overhead medicine ball toss* to be a reliable measure of total body power.[58]

Table 12-14	Percentile Ranking for Cycle Ergometer Power and Power-to–Body Weight Ratio

Percentile Rank	Power in Watts		W/kgBW	
	Male	Female	Male	Female
95	676.6	483	8.63	7.52
90	661.8	469.9	8.24	7.31
85	630.5	437	8.09	7.08
80	617.9	419.4	8.01	6.95
75	604.3	413.5	7.96	6.93
70	600.0	409.7	7.91	6.77
65	591.7	402.2	7.70	6.65
60	576.8	391.4	7.59	6.59
55	574.5	386	7.46	6.51
50	564.6	381.1	7.44	6.39
45	552.8	376.9	7.26	6.2
40	547.6	366.9	7.14	6.15
35	534.6	360.5	7.08	6.13
30	529.7	353.2	7	6.03
25	520.6	346.8	6.79	5.94
20	496.1	336.5	6.59	5.71
15	484.6	320.3	6.39	5.56
10	470.9	306.1	5.98	5.25
5	453.2	286.5	5.56	5.07
Mean	562.7	380.8	7.28	6.35
Minimum	441.3	235.4	4.63	4.53
Maximum	711	528.6	9.07	8.11
SD	66.5	56.4	0.88	0.73

SD, Standard deviation.

Table 12-15	Average Values for Jump Height, Body Mass Index, and Power

Gender	Ages	N	Jump (inches)	Power (W)*
Women	21-30	224	14.1	834
	21-25	182	14.1	833
	26-30	42	14	837
Men	21-30	500	22.1	1332
	21-25	312	22.2	1309
	26-30	188	21.9	1370

*Power calculated via Lewis Power Equation: Power = $2.21 \times$ wt (kg) $\times \sqrt{\text{jump (m)}}$

To perform this test the clinician will need a large area, such as a baseball outfield, in which the athlete throws the medicine ball safely. The athlete stands with his or her back to the scratch line and throws the ball backward, overhead as far as possible using the entire body to generate force. Horizontal distance is measured from the scratch line to the landing point of the medicine ball.[58]

Ellenbecker and Roetert demonstrated significant correlation between isokinetic trunk rotation peak torque and *stationary rotational medicine toss*. The athlete stands with his or her feet planted and uses both arms to throw a 6-lb medicine ball as with a two-handed tennis forehand and backhand. The longest of three trials on each side is taken as the maximal measure of rotational power.[59]

Single-Leg Hop Tests

Numerous researchers have studied single-leg hop tests as a means to evaluate lower extremity neuromuscular function and power. They are relatively simple to employ in any clinic and have been shown to be a reliable measure that is also a valid predictor of return to sports following anterior cruciate ligament and ankle injury.[60-69] For these reasons the authors strongly recommend their inclusion into any sports-specific rehabilitation evaluation.

> ### Clinical Application
> **Limb symmetry index (LSI)** is defined as the value of any single-leg hop test score divided by the score of the unaffected limb. An **LSI of less than 85%** with any of the single-leg hop tests indicates an abnormal test and the need for a plyometric/neuromuscular training program before return to full-speed sports participation.[60,62,66]

Table 12-16 describes the four most commonly employed single-leg hop tests. Some difference exists between the methodology of different researchers of single-leg hops. As such, the authors have attempted to provide easy-to-understand descriptions of the single-leg hop tests (Figure 12-23).

AGILITY TESTING

Agility is defined as "a skill-related component of physical fitness that relates to the ability to rapidly change the position of the entire body in space with speed and accuracy."[51] Thus clinical tests of agility can be appropriate function- and sports-specific tests for sports involving cutting, such as basketball, volleyball, football, lacrosse, and soccer. The reader should note that many of the tests for CORE power, such as the T-test, shuttle run, and single-leg hops, are also good tests of agility (Table 12-17).

BALANCE TESTING IN THE ATHLETE

Balance or postural stability is a motor skill, defined as the ability to maintain the position of the center of mass (COM) over the base of support (BOS). Athletes maintain their balance via the complex interaction of the nervous system and musculoskeletal systems.[70]

During slow-speed (120 ms or more) activities the body maintains balance via a closed feedback mechanism from the visual, proprioceptive, and vestibular sensory systems. The process begins when environmental forces are transduced by the sensory end organs into neural impulses, which travel via peripheral nerves to afferent spinal pathways to the central nervous system. Nuclei in the sensory cortex, brainstem, and cerebellum interact to process the information and produce a corrective efferent motor signal to the muscles, thus closing the feedback loop.[70,71]

Most high-speed activities do not allow sufficient time for the central balance processor to interpret data from the balance triad. In these situations balance is maintained more by feedforward mechanisms or the generalized motor righting responses triggered by specific stimuli.[70,71]

Table 12-16	Single-Leg Hop Tests	
Time	Lines or cones placed 6 m apart	Athlete must hop from one line to the other with only one leg. Therapist measures time.
Distance	Starting line and open space forward of line to jump into	Athlete begins with toes of leg behind line. Athlete must take off and land on the test limb. Distance from start line to front of toe is measured.
Triple Hop for Distance	Starting line with longer open space forward of line	As above, athlete must take off and land on only the test leg but is allowed 3 consecutive hops. Test can be measured for time to complete set distance or distance covered in 3 maximal jumps.
Triple Crossover Hop for Distance	As above with additional of longitudinal line for athlete to jump over.	Athlete starts on a single limb and jumps at a diagonal across the body, lands on the opposite limb with the foot pointing straight ahead, and immediately redirects himself or herself into a jump in the opposite diagonal direction.

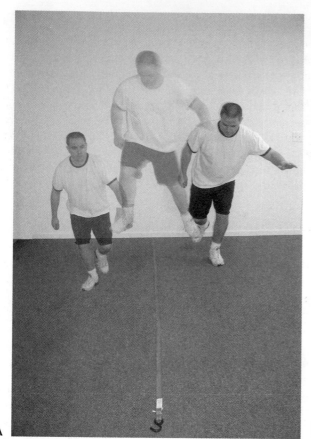

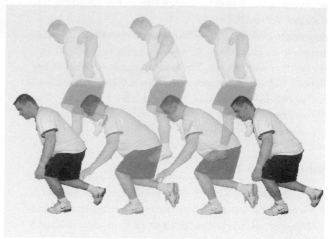

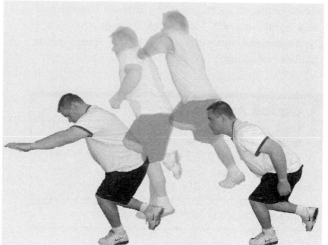

Figure 12-23 Single-leg hop tests. **A,** Cross over. **B,** Triple jump. **C,** Time and distance.

Table 12-17	Sample of Section of CORE Evaluation Sheet							

Power and Agility Testing

	Date		Date		Date		Date	
T-Test								
Shuttle Run								
Cycle Ergometer								
Back-Overhead Toss								
	R	L	R	L	R	L	R	L
Vertical Jump								
6 lb Rotational Throw								
6 m Hop for Time								
SL Hop Test for Dist								
Triple Hop for Distance								
Triple Crossover Hop								

SL, Single leg.

Numerous studies have documented a link between impaired balance and lower extremity injury.[60-69] Likewise, Basford et al[72] demonstrated lasting impairment in balance following traumatic brain injury. With the incidence of cerebral concussion (a form of traumatic brain injury) rising in contact, snow, and extreme sports, clearly there is a need to assess balance in all athletes.

Balance Triad

Visual Feedback

Light from the environment stimulates rods and cones located on the back of the retina. This stimulates the optic nerve, which carries the signal to the visual centers in the occipital lobe of the brain. Here the impulse or raw data are processed into useful visual information about the environment. For example, a windsurfer who sees a change in wave swell and alters his or her weight distribution on the board is using visual feedback to maintain balance.

Vestibular Feedback

The inner ear contains the delicate vestibular sensory end organs, so named because early anatomists could not understand the function of these organs and used the term *vestibule* or *anteroom* to describe the region.

The cupulae are tiny hair cells that move in response to the relative movement of endolymph in the anterior, posterior, and horizontal semicircular canals. This movement of the endolymph in the canals causes the hair cells to deform. Depending on the direction, deformation will either excite or inhibit the vestibular nerve from its resting firing rate. This neuroanatomical arrangement provides for a "push, pull" of vestibular stimulation with head rotation. For example, a gymnast who rapidly whips his or her head to the left during a floor routine will stimulate the firing rate in the left vestibular nerve while simultaneously inhibiting the firing rate in the right vestibular nerve.[70,71]

The otoliths are also composed of tiny hair cells embedded in sheets of gelatinous sheets, which are covered with microscopic calcium carbonate crystals known as *otoconia*. The sheets are aligned to vertical and horizontal. The weight of the otoconia on the gelatinous matrix allows the sheets to move in response to changes in linear acceleration, such as with head tilting or changes in elevation as with the motion of a surfboard on the ocean. Movement of the gelatin sheets causes deformation of the hair cells, causing them to depolarize. This signal is also carried to the central nervous system via the vestibular nerve.[70,71]

The central vestibular nuclei process this input and produce a combination of corrective motor outputs known as the *vestibulospinal* and *vestibulocular* reflexes. Damage to the peripheral vestibular sensory organs is not uncommon in sports injury and can lead to debilitating imbalance, abnormal vestibular ocular reflex output, and vertigo.

Proprioceptive Feedback

An excellent description of the proprioceptive pathways is provided in Chapter 15.

> ## Clinical Application
> The authors of this chapter want to reiterate Dr. Synder-Mackler's point that "proprioception" should not be used interchangeably with balance. Proprioception is only one of many inputs used by the CNS balance processor to detect error signals, which result in corrective motor output and maintain balance.
> For example, a baseball player with exceptional proprioception is hit in the head by a wild pitch. As a result he incurs an orbit fracture and damage to the vestibular organs of the inner ear. In this example the athlete's proprioception has not been affected by the injuries, but his balance would be abnormal as a result of the aberrant visual and vestibular input.

Central Balance Processor

The term *central balance processor* describes the complex interaction of the vestibular nuclei in the brainstem, the cerebellum, sensory cortex, motor cortex, and many other neurological tissues. With normal function these structures act seamlessly to integrate sensory information, compare it with a central reference to determine the error, and then generate a corrective motor output.[70,71]

BALANCE EVALUATION FOR THE ATHLETE

Assessment of balance in the athlete should include assessment of lower extremity motion, a strength that was discussed earlier. Evaluation should also include testing of sensation, static balance, and dynamic balance tests.

Sensory testing of lower extremity dermatomes and peripheral nerves is helpful in ruling out sensory deficit as a cause of imbalance, such as that seen with a peripheral neuropathy. Even a cursory sharp/dull discrimination test will provide the therapist some information as to the function of sensory receptors in the plantar surface of the foot.

The following standardized tests are useful in assessing balance in the athlete.

Single-Leg Stance Time

Single-leg stance time is a valid and reliable test (Figure 12-24).[73] Ekdahl et al[74] established normal values for single-leg stance times of healthy subjects and showed that the ability to maintain single-leg stance decreases with age. However, the typical protocol of timing for a maximal time of up to 30 seconds has been shown to be an artificial ceiling for young

Table 12-18	Modified Clinical Test of Sensory Integration and Balance		
Instructions: Maintain balance with feet together and arms at your sides for up to 30 seconds. Patient will perform 3 trials with each condition.			
Condition	Description		Interpretation
1	Firm surface, eyes open		
2	Firm surface, eyes closed		Increased postural sway or falls indicate "visual dependence"
3	Compliant (foam) surface, eyes open		
4	Compliant (foam) surface, eyes closed		Increased postural sway or falls indicate vestibular loss

athletes.[74] Most researchers agree that a healthy athlete should be able to maintain single-leg stance for at least 30 seconds and that times should be consistent between sides.

Modified Clinical Test of Sensory Integration and Balance

As discussed earlier, the central processor receives information from three basic classifications of sensory information: vision, somatosensory, and vestibular feedback. The modified clinical test of sensory integration and balance (MCTSIB) examine the athlete's ability to maintain balance in conditions that preferentially bias the type of sensory feedback available to the subject. This is accomplished with the use of four conditions, which sequentially take away types of sensory feedback (Figure 12-25).[75-78] The MCTSIB has been shown to have excellent test-retest reliability with elderly and young athletic subjects.[72,76] To perform this test in the clinic the therapist needs only a stopwatch and 24- × 24-inch piece of medium density Temper Foam of standardized density as described by Shumway-Cook and Horak.[77] The conditions of the MCTSIB

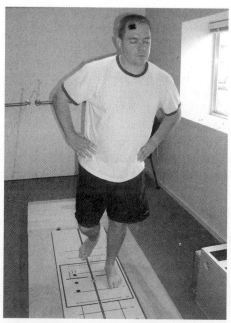

Figure 12-24 Single-leg stance.

are described in Table 12-18. The athlete is asked to maintain his or her balance for three trials of up to 30 seconds. Inability to maintain balance for 30 seconds is considered abnormal.

Patients who exhibit increased postural sway or falls with condition 2 are thought to be dependent on visual feedback. This is common after injury to the lower extremity and is thought to reflect the decrease in proprioceptive information coming from injured joints and tendons.[60,63,66-68] Patients with increased sway or falls in condition 4 demonstrate a vestibular loss, which warrants further vestibular function testing or referral to the appropriate health care provider if the therapist is unable to assess this function. Computerized systems, such as the Balance Master by Neurocom, allow comparison of patient performance to established normative values by age and height.

Reaction to Perturbation

With high-speed sports activities (<120 ms) the body cannot rely on closed-loop feedback to produce corrective righting motor responses. Instead, it uses a feed-forward mechanism by which sensory input generates a spinal reflex motor response.

Because most sports injuries occur at high speeds, it only makes sense to assess athletes' balance at these speeds. Along these lines, the majority of research on prevention of anterior cruciate ligament sprains suggests perturbation training produces the best results with neuromuscular training.[60-69] Thus an evaluation should include baseline measure of response to platform perturbation.

Until recently, clinical measures of reaction to perturbation were limited to costly computerized balance platforms. One device that holds great promise is the Shuttle Balance by Shuttle Sytems. With this device the athlete stands atop a platform suspended with chains and ropes from a sturdy frame. Perturbation is provided by rapidly moving the platform when the athlete has no knowledge of the direction, speed, and force of the perturbation. The stability and angle of the platform can be sequentially increased. Numbered markings on the platform also allow for standardization and replication of the athlete's stance with testing (Table 12-19). Established normal values have yet to be established for subjects maintaining balance in response to perturbation on this device. However, the scalability and reproducibility allowed by the "Shuttle Balance" warrant further research into its use as a balance assessment tool.

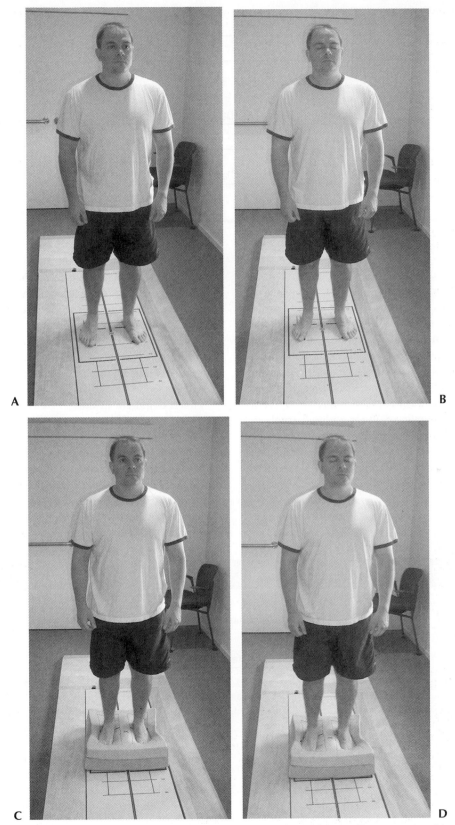

Figure 12-25 Modified clinical test of sensory integration and balance. **A,** Condition 1. **B,** Condition 2. **C,** Condition 3. **D,** Condition 4.

Table 12-19	Sample of Balance Testing Section of CORE Evaluation

Balance

	Date		Date		Date		Date	
	R	L	R	L	R	L	R	L
Sensory Testing								
SLS Eyes Open								
SLS Eyes Closed								

	Date				Date				Date				Date			
	1	2	3	4	1	2	3	4	1	2	3	4	1	2	3	4
MCTSIB																

	Date	Date	Date	Date
Perturbation				

SLS, Single leg stance.

SUMMARY

Evaluation of athletes presents special challenges to the rehabilitation professional. Athletes require tests and measures specific to their underlying CORE impairments and sensitive enough to detect relative weakness in otherwise strong patients. The evaluation described in this chapter reflects the tests and measures found by the authors to meet these special demands. Please refer to Table 12-20 for a sample trunk and hip CORE evaluation form. Using this evaluation format, the authors and other researchers have found the following cluster of signs extremely common in athletes and even not-so-athletic patients:

- Poor training habits
- Residual impairments from previous injury
- Abnormal trunk and hip biomechanical alignments
- Decreased rectus femoris length with accompanying impairment in hip extension active range of motion
- Decreased hip rotation
- Abnormal gait patterns
- Abnormal muscle activation patterns in trunk stabilizers
- Decreased endurance in the trunk stabilizers
- Decreased hip mobilizer strength (particularly in posterior fibers of gluteus medius)
- Insufficient CORE power and agility for sports tasks
- Impaired balance

Strong evidence exists to suggest impairments in the trunk and hip CORE predispose athletes to injury or reinjury, or both, in all areas of the body. On the basis of this evidence, the authors urge evaluation of the trunk and hip CORE with all athletes, regardless of the location of their injury.

Table 12-20	Trunk and Hip CORE Evaluation Sheet

Hip and Trunk CORE Evaluation

History/Pain Provocation

Observation

	Date	Date	Date	Date
Anterior Pelvic Tilt				
Posterior Pelvic Tilt				
Iliac Crest Asymmetry				
Feet together				
Feet apart				
Genu Recurvatum				
Genu Valgus				
Single-Leg Squat				
Drop-Jump Screening				
Gait				

Table 12-20	Trunk and Hip CORE Evaluation Sheet—cont'd

Trunk Motion (note motion, peripheralization, or centralization)

	Date	Date	Date	Date
Flexion				
Extension				
R Side Bending				
L Side Bending				
Knees to chest				
Prone Prop				

Trunk Special Tests

	Date	Date	Date	Date
Slump Test				
SLR				
Prone Instability				
Facet Scour				
SIJ				
Distraction				
Thigh Thrust				
Gaenslen's				
Compression				
Sacral Thrust				

Hip Motion

	Date		Date		Date		Date	
	R	L	R	L	R	L	R	L
Flexion								
Extension								
Abduction								
Adduction								
Sitting IR/ER								
Prone IR/ER								
Thomas Test								
Ober's Test								
Craig's Test								

Trunk Stabilization

	Date	Date	Date	Date
TrA Drawing In				
Multifidus Palpation				

	R	L	R	L	R	L	R	L
Active SLR								
Leg Loading Test								
Bird dog								
Side bridge								

Normal: R SB: M/F =83 seconds, M = 95 seconds, F = 75 seconds L SB: 86s M/F, M = 99 seconds, F = 78 seconds

Abdominal Bracing

Normal is M/F = 134 seconds, M = 136 seconds, F = 134 seconds

Back Extensor Test

Normal is M/F = 173 seconds, M = 160 seconds, F = 185 seconds

continued

Table 12-20 Trunk and Hip CORE Evaluation Sheet—cont'd

Hip Mobilizer Testing

Leg Drop Test—(abduction & extension for posterior fibers of gluteus medius)

	Date		Date		Date		Date		Date		Date	
	R	L	R	L	R	L	R	L	R	L	R	L
Unable to hold												
Unable to resist												

MMT

	Date		Date		Date		Date		Date		Date	
	R	L	R	L	R	L	R	L	R	L	R	L
Abduction												
Adduction												
Extension												
Flexion												
IR Sitting												
ER Sitting												

Power and Agility Testing

	Date	Date	Date	Date
T-Test				
Shuttle Run				
Cycle Ergometer				
Back-Overhead Toss				

	Date		Date		Date		Date	
	R	L	R	L	R	L	R	L
Vertical Jump								
6 lb								
Rotational Throw								
6 m Hop for Time								
SL Hop Test for Dist								
Triple Hop for Distance								
Triple Crossover Hop								

Balance

	Date		Date		Date		Date	
	R	L	R	L	R	L	R	L
Sensory Testing								
SLS Eyes Open								
SLS Eyes Closed								

	Date				Date				Date				Date			
	1	2	3	4	1	2	3	4	1	2	3	4	1	2	3	4
MCTSIB																

	Date	Date	Date	Date
Perturbation				

ER, External rotation; *IR,* internal rotation; *L SB,* left side bridge; *MCTSIB,* modified clinical test of sensory integration and balance; *R SB,* right side bridge; *SL,* single leg; *SLR,* straight leg raise; *SLS,* single leg stance; *TrA,* transversus abdominis.

REFERENCES

1. Nadler SF, Malanga GA, Feinberg JH, et al: Functional performance deficits in athletes with previous lower extremity injury, *Clin J Sport Med* 12(2):73-78, 2002.

2. Nadler SF, Malanga GA, Bartoli JH, et al: Hip muscle imbalance and low back pain in athletes: influences of core strengthening, *Med Sci Sports Exerc* 34(1):9-16, 2002.

3. Nadler SF, Malanga GA, DePrince M, et al: The relationship between lower extremity injury low back pain and hip muscle strength in male and female collegiate athletes, *Clin J Sport Med* 10(2):89-97, 2000.

4. Magee DJ: *Orthopedic physical assessment*, ed 3, Philadelphia, 1997, WB Saunders Company.

5. Lee D: *The pelvic girdle*, ed 3, Edinburgh, 2004, Churchill Livingstone.

6. American Physical Therapy Association: *Guide to physical therapist practice*, ed 2, Alexandria, Va, 2001, APTA.

7. McGill S: *Low back disorders: evidence-based prevention and rehabilitation*, Champaign, Ill, 2002, Human Kinetics.

8. Kendall FP, McCreary EK, Provance PG: *Muscles testing and function, ed 4*, Baltimore, 1993, Williams & Wilkins.

9. Sahrmann S: *Diagnosis and treatment of movement impairment syndromes*, St Louis, 2002, Mosby.

10. Sherry MA, Best TM: A comparison of 2 rehabilitation programs in the treatment of acute hamstrings strains, *JOSPT* 34(3):116-125, 2004.

11. Van Dillen LR, McDonnel MK, Flemming DA, et al: Effect of knee and hip position on hip extension range of motion in individuals with and without low back pain, *JOSPT* 30(6):307-316, 2000.

12. Razmjou H, Kramer JF, Yamada R: Intertester reliability of the McKenzie Evaluation in assessing patients with mechanical low-back pain, *JOSPT* 30(7):368-389, 2000.

13. Perry J: *Gait analysis normal and pathological function*, Thorofare, NJ, 1992, SLACK.

14. Ireland ML, Wilson JD, Ballantne BT, et al: Hip strength in females with and without patellofemoral pain, *JOSPT* 33(11):671-676, 2003.

15. Leetun DT, Lloyd, Ireland ML, et al: Core stability measures as risk factors for LE in athletes, *Med Sci Sports Exerc* 36(6):926-934, 2004.

16. Ballantyne BT, Leetun DT, Ireland ML, et al: Differences in core stability between male and female collegiate basketball athletes as measured by trunk and hip muscle performance, *Med Sci Sports Exerc* 33(5):S331, 2001.

17. Zeller B, McCrory J, Kibler B, et al: Differences in kinematics and electromyographic activity between men and women during the single-legged squat, *Am J Sports Med* 31(3):449-456, 2003.

18. Noyes FR, Barber-Westin S, Fleckenstein C, et al: The drop-jump screening test: difference in lower limb control by gender and effect of neuromuscular training in female athletes, *Am J Sports Med* 33(2):197-207, 2005.

19. Norkin CC, White DJ: *Measurement of joint motion: a guide to goniometry, ed 2,* Philadelphia, 1985, FA Davis.

20. Laslett M, Young SB, April CN, et al: Diagnosing painful sacroiliac joints: a validity study of McKenzie evaluation and sacroiliac provocation tests, *Aust J Physiother* 49:89-97, 2003.

21. Butler DA: *Mobilisation of the nervous system*, Melbourne, 1991, Churchill Livingstone.

22. Scham SM, Taylor T: Tensions signs in lumbar disc prolapse, *Clin Orthop* 75:195-204, 1971.

23. Cibulka MT, Aslin K: How to use evidence-based practice to distinguish between three different patients with low back pain, *JOSPT* 31(12):678-695, 2001.

24. Hicks GE, Fritz JM, Delitto A, et al: Interrater reliability of clinical examination measures for identification of lumbar segmental instability, *Arch Phys Med Rehab* 84:1858-1864, 2003.

25. Levangie PK: Four clinical tests results with innominate torsion among patients with and without low back pain, *Phys Ther* 79:1043-1057, 1999.

26. Freburger JK, Riddle DL: Measurement of sacroiliac joint dysfunction: a multicenter intertester reliability study, *Phys Ther* 79(12):1134-1141, 1999.

27. Richardson CA, Jull G, Hodges P, et al: *Therapeutic exercise for spinal segmental stabilization in low back pain: scientific basis and clinical approach*, Philadelphia, 1999, Churchill Livingstone.

28. Richardson CA, Jull GA, Richardson BA: A dysfunction of the deep abdominal muscles exists in low back pain patients. In Proceedings World Confederation of Physical Therapists, 1995, Washington, p. 932.

29. Richardson CA, Snijders CJ, Hides JA, et al: The relationship between the transversus abdominis muscles, sacroiliac joint mechanics, and low back pain, *Spine* 27(4):399-405, 2002.

30. Hodges PW, Richardson CA: Inefficient muscular stabilization of the lumbar spine associated with low back pain. A motor control evaluation of transverses abdominis, *Spine* 21(22):2640-2650, 1996.

31. Hodges PW, Richardson CA, Jull GA: Evaluation of the relationship between the findings of a laboratory and clinical test of transverses abdominis function, *Physiother Res Int* 1:30-40, 1996.

32. Hides JA, Stokes MJ, Saide M, et al: Evidence of lumbar multifidus muscles wasting in ipsilateral to symptoms patients with acute/subacute low back pain, *Spine* 19(2):165-177, 1994.

33. Hides J, Richardson C, Jull G: Multifidus muscle recovery is not automatic following resolution of acute first episode low back pain, *Spine* 21:2763-2769, 1996.

34. Mens JMA, Vleeming A, Snijders CJ, et al: The active straight leg raising test and mobility of the pelvic joints, *Eur Spine* 8:468-473, 1999.

35. Mens JMA, Vleeming A, Snijders CJ, et al: Validity and reliability of the active straight leg raise test in posterior pelvic pain since pregnancy, *Spine* 26(10):1167-1171, 2001.

36. Cowan S, Schache A, Brukner P, et al: Delayed onset of transverses abdominus in long-standing groin pain, *Med Sci Sports Exerc* 36(12):2040-2045, 2004.

37. Hides J, Richardson C, Jull G, et al: Ultrasound imaging in rehabilitation, Aust J Physiother 41(3):187-193, 1995.

38. Hodges PW, Pengel LHM, Herbert RD, et al: Measurement of muscle contraction with ultrasound imaging, *Muscle Nerve* 27:682-692, 2003.

39. Biering-Sorensen F: Physical measurements as risk indicators for low back trouble over a one-year period, *Spine* 9:106-119, 1984.

40. Juker D, McGill SM, Kropf P: Quantitative intramuscular myoelectric activity of lumbar portions of psoas and the abdominal wall during cycling, *J Applied Biomechanics* 12(4):428-438, 1998.

41. Saffer B, Jobe F, Perry J, et al: Baseball batting. An electromyographical study, *Clin Orthop* 292:285-293, 1993.

42. Watkins, Uppal J, Perry M, et al: Dynamic electromyographic analysis of trunk musculature in professional golfers, *Am J Sports Med* 24:535-538, 1996.

43. Hislop HJ, Montgomery J: *Daniels and Worthinghams's muscle testing: techniques of manual examination,* ed 6, Philadelphia, 1995, WB Saunders.

44. Bohanan RW, Andrews AW: Interrater reliability of handheld dynamometry, *Phys Ther* 67:931-933, 1987.

45. Wadsworth CT, Krishnan R, Sear M, et al: Intrarater reliability of manual muscle testing and hand-held dynametric muscle testing, *Phys Ther* 67(9):1342-1347, 1987.

46. Dunn JC, Iversen MD: Interrater reliability of knee muscle forces obtained by hand-held dynamometer from elderly subjects with degenerative back pain, *J Geriatr Phys Ther* 26(3):23-29, 2003.

47. Mont MA, Cohen DB, Campbell KR, et al: Isokinetic concentric versus eccentric training of shoulder rotators with functional evaluation of performance enhancement in elite tennis players, *Am J Sports Med* 22(4):513-517, 1994.

48. Donatelli R, Catlin PA, Backer GS, et al: Isokinetic hip abductor to adductor torque ratio in normals, *Isokinetics Exerc Sci* 1991; 1(2): 103-111.

49. Kraemer WJ, Fry AC: Strength testing: development and evaluation of methodology. In Maud P, Nieman C, editors: *Fitness and sports medicine: a health-related approach,* ed 3, Palo Alto, Calif, 1995, Bull Publishing.

50. Fleck S, Kraemer W: *Periodization breakthrough,* Ronkonkoma, NY, 1996, Advanced Research Press.

51. American College of Sports Medicine: *Principles of exercise prescription,* Baltimore, 1995, Williams & Wilkins.

52. American College of Sports Medicine: American College of Sports Medicine position stand on progression models in resistance training for healthy adults, *Med Sci Sports Exerc* 34(2):364-380, 2002.

53. Brzycki M: Strength testing: Predicting a one-rep max from a reps-to-fatigue, *J Phys Ed Recreat Dance* 64(1): 88-90, 1993.

54. Pauole K, Madole K, Garhammer J, et al: Reliability and validity of the T-test as a measure of agility leg power, and leg speed in college-aged men and women, *J Strength Cond Res* 14(4):443-450, 2003.

55. Maud PJ, Schultz BB: Percentile norms and descriptive statistics for fatigue index, *Res Q* 60:144-149, 1989.

56. Isaacs LD: Comparison of the Vertec and Just Jump system for measuring height of vertical jump for young children, *Percept Mot Skills* 86:659-663, 1998.

57. Patterson D, Peterson D: Vertical jump and leg power norms for young adults, *Measurement Phys Ed Exerc Sci* 8(1):33-41, 2004.

58. Stockbrugger B, Haennel R: Validity and reliability of Medicine ball explosive power test, *J Strength Cond Res* 15(4):431-438, 2003.

59. Ellenbecker T, Roertert E: An isokinetic profile of trunk rotation strength in elite tennis players, *Med Sci Sports Exerc* 36(11): 1959-1963, 2004.

60. Fitzgerald KG, Lephart SM, Hwang JH, et al: Hop tests as predictors of dynamic knee stability, *JOSPT* 31(10):588-597, 2001.

61. Myer GD, Ford KR, Palumbo JP, et al: Neuromuscular training improves performance and lower-extremity biomechanics in female athletes, *J Strength Cond Res* 19(1): 51-60, 2005.

62. Rudolph KS, Axe MJ, Synder-Mackler L: Dynamic stability after ACL injury: we can hop? *Knee Surg Sports Traumatol Arthrosc* 8:262-269, 2000.

63. Cerrulli G, Benoit DL, Caraffa A, et al: Proprioceptive training and preventing of anterior cruciate ligament injuries in soccer, *JOSPT* 31(11):655-660, 2001.

64. Hiemstra LA, Lo KY, Fowler PJ: Effect of fatigue on knee proprioception: implications for dynamic stabilization, *JOSPT* 31(10):598-605, 2001.

65. Risberg MA, Mork M, Jenssen HK, et al: Design and implementation of a neuromuscular training program following anterior cruciate ligament reconstruction, *JOSPT* 31(11):620-631, 2001.

66. Williams GN, Chmielewski T, Rudolph KS, et al: Dynamic knee stability: current theory and implications for clinicians and scientists, *JOSPT* 31(10):546-566, 2001.

67. Holm I, Fosdahol MA, Friis A, et al: Effect of neuromuscular training on proprioception, balance, muscle strength, and lower limb function in female team handball players, *Clin J Sport Med* 14(2):88-94, 2004.

68. Lephart SM, Abt JP, Ferris CM: Neuromuscular contributions to anterior cruciate ligament injuries in females, *Curr Opin Rheumatol* 14(2):168-173, 2002.

69. Ross MD, Langford B, Whelan PJ: Test-restest reliability of 4 single-leg horizontal hop tests, *J Strength Cond Res* 16(4):617-622, 2002.

70. Shumway-Cook A, Woolacoot M: *Motor control theory and practical applications,* Baltimore, 1995, Williams & Wilkins.

71. Herdman SJ: *Vestibular rehabilitation,* ed 2, Philadelphia, 2000, FA Davis.

72. Basford J, Chou L, Kaufman K, et al: An assessment of gait and balance deficits after traumatic brain injury, *Arch Phys Med Rehab* 84:343-349, 2004.

73. Bohanaon R, Larkin P, Cook A, et al: Decrease in timed balance test scores with aging, *Phys Ther* 64:1067-1070, 1984.

74. Ekdahl C, Jarnlo GB, Andersson SI: Standing balance in health subjects, *Scand J Rehab Med* 21(4):187-195, 1989.

75. Cohen H, Blatchly CA, Gombash LL: A study of the clinical test of sensory integration and balance, *Phys Ther* 73:346-351, 1993.

76. Anacker SL, DiFabio RP: Influence of sensory inputs on standing balance in community-dwelling elders with a recent history of falling, *Phys Ther* 72:575-584, 1992.

77. Shumway-Cook A, Horak FB: Assessing the influence of sensory integration on balance. Suggestions from the field, *Phys Ther* 66:1548-1550, 1986.

78. Horak FB: Clinical measurement of postural control in adults, *Phys Ther* 67:1881-1885, 1987.

CHAPTER

13

Robert A. Donatelli
and Donn Dimond

Strength Training Concepts in the Athlete

LEARNING OBJECTIVES

After studying this chapter, the reader will be able to do the following:

1. Describe the physiological adaptations within the muscle following strength exercises
2. Provide examples of the changes that occur with neural adaptations within muscle
3. List the major contributors to improving muscle strength
4. Explain the differences among strength, power, and endurance
5. Distinguish among how to train Type I, Type IIA, and Type IIB muscle fiber types
6. Identify the number of repetitions, sets, and amount of resistance necessary to increase muscle strength and hypertrophy
7. Describe the effects of aging on muscle
8. Describe the phases of periodization training
9. Describe the differences among eccentric, concentric, and isometric exercises
10. Provide examples of off-season, in-season, and maintenance programs for athletes

Strength training is an important part of any athlete's rehabilitation or performance enhancement program, or both. Optimal resistance training programs require consideration of numerous variables. The muscle and muscle groups to be exercised, the type of exercise, frequency, intensity, and duration are all important variables that determine the success of any strength training program. What are the physiological and neural adaptations that occur within the muscle and how long does it take to make changes? Can muscle fiber types be converted with strength training? Should eccentric, concentric, or isometric exercises, or a combination of all three, be used? Periodization strength training programs can result in significant changes in muscle strength. What are the different phases of a periodization program, and how long should each phase last? How does the therapist incorporate neuromuscular exercises into a strength-training program? Answers to these questions are essential to professionals responsible for prescribing resistance exercise for improvement of sports performance or for returning the athlete to normal function following injury and treatment.

Strength is the ability of the muscle to exert a maximum force at a specified velocity.[1] Power is defined as the force exerted multiplied by the velocity of movement.[1] Muscular power is a function of both strength and speed of movement. For most large muscle groups, maximal mechanical power is achieved at 30% to 45% of one's 1RM (one repetition at maximum effort). Endurance is the ability to sustain an activity for extended periods of time.[1] Local muscle endurance is best described as the ability to resist muscular fatigue.[1] The authors of this chapter believe that a good strength base is important to reestablishing function and improving performance. Often specific strengthening exercises have been labeled as nonfunctional because they are performed in the open kinetic chain (OKC). For the purposes of this chapter, a functional exercise is defined as an exercise specific to the muscle groups that are important to the activity the athlete wants to return to and that sufficient resistance, repetitions, and sets are used to stimulate the muscle to adapt by increasing strength. Several studies have demonstrated that when OKC exercises were used to strengthen the glenohumeral rotators, significant gains were made in the strength of the shoulder rotators and the velocity of the baseball in pitchers and the velocity of the tennis ball in a tennis serve.[2,3] Therefore strength training the rotators of the glenohumeral joint by moving the shoulder into internal and external rotation in an open kinetic chain position is a functional exercise (Figure 13-1).

This chapter describes the neural and physiological adaptations in muscle as a result of strength training programs. Time frames for developing strength gains, in addition to the amount of resistance, sets, and repetitions necessary to make these changes, are discussed. The effects of aging on muscle and

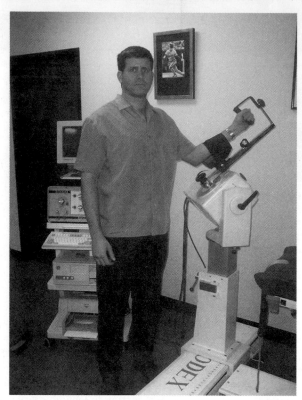

Figure 13-1 A functional exercise: Strengthening the glenohumeral rotators in the plane of the scapula.

exercise adaptations in the elderly are also discussed. Finally is a review of the differences among eccentric, concentric, and isometric exercises.

Understanding the cellular and molecular adaptations of skeletal muscle in response to strength training is important to provide the framework to improve performance in the athlete and the health and quality of life of the general population with or without chronic diseases.

PHYSIOLOGICAL ADAPTATIONS OF MUSCLE

Neural Adaptations

The first signs of muscle adaptation to strengthening exercises are neural adaptations. Several studies have demonstrated that early strength gains induced by resistance training are primarily due to modifications of the nervous system. Moritani and DeVires,[4] in a landmark study, found that "neural factors" accounted for the significant improvements observed during the first 4 weeks of an 8-week resistance-training program. Staron et al[5] demonstrated that only after 6 weeks of training was significant muscle fiber hypertrophy detected. Furthermore, Staron et al[6] demonstrated that with heavy resistance training the conversion of Type IIB fibers to Type IIA fibers occurred at 2 weeks in females and 4 weeks in males.

Views on the relative contribution of neural versus muscle adaptation with strength training lasting longer than 2 to 3 months are conflicting. Deschenes et al[1] indicate that with prolonged resistance training, the degree of muscle hyper-

trophy is limited and that significant hypertrophic responses can occur within a finite period of time, lasting no more than 12 months. A secondary neural adaptation explains the continued strength gains with prolonged resistance training. The secondary phase of neural adaptations takes place between the sixth and twelfth months. In contrast, Shoepe et al[7] demonstrated substantial muscle hypertrophy as a result of several years of resistance training, when compared with a group of sedentary individuals.

The neural adaptations elicited by resistance training include decreased co-contraction of antagonists and expansion in the dimensions of the neuromuscular junction, indicating greater content of presynaptic neurotransmitter and postsynaptic receptors.[8-10] Greater synchronicity of the discharge of motor units after strength training has also been reported.[11]

Contractile Adaptations

The contractile protein in muscle includes the actin and myosin filaments. (See Chapter 2 for great detail.) Beyond the first few weeks of resistance exercises, an increased contractile capacity that exists within the muscle accounts for strength gains.[12,13]

The turnover rate of muscle protein is one of the slowest in the body. Within skeletal muscle, synthesis and growth of contractile proteins lag behind that of other proteins, such as mitochondria and sarcoplasmic reticulum.[14,15] The synthesis and accretion of contractile proteins account for the hypertrophy that occurs with resistance training. This hypertrophy occurs mostly within the intracellular myofibrils (25% to 35%), in addition to hypertrophy within the whole muscle (5% to 8%).[1,16]

Hypertrophy versus Hyperplasia

Resistance exercise is a potent stimulus to increase the size of muscle. For a muscle to become larger, it must either increase in cross-sectional area (hypertrophy) or increase the number of muscle fibers (hyperplasia). The number of muscle fibers is generally believed to be innate and does not change during life.[17] In contrast, several researchers reported that muscle is capable of increasing its size as a result of an increase in fiber number.[18,19] The exact mechanism responsible for muscle hypertrophy is uncertain, but several theories have been expressed in the literature. Skeletal muscles are capable of remodeling under various conditions. The activation of myogenic stem cells within the muscle is one of the most important events that occurs during skeletal muscle remodeling.[19] The muscle (myogenic) stem cells remain dormant under the basement of the myofibers, and on stimulation they differentiate into satellite cells to form myofibers.[19] The muscle or myogenic stem cells start to generate, by a series of cell divisions, daughter cells that become satellite cells. Evidence suggests that strength training induces a significant increase in satellite cell content in skeletal muscle. Because the myonuclei in mature muscle fibers cannot divide, it is suggested that the incorporation of satellite cell nuclei into muscle fibers results in the maintenance of a constant nuclear/cytoplasmic ratio.

Therefore new muscle fibers are formed following strength training. When resistance or endurance exercises promote satellite cell proliferation and differentiation can be detected in injured fibers and those with no discernible damage, muscle hyperplasia occurs in human skeletal muscle.[18-21]

Resistance training has been shown to elicit a significant acute hormonal response, which is more critical to tissue growth and remodeling than chronic changes in resting hormonal concentrations. Anabolic steroids, such as testosterone and the growth hormones, have been shown to elevate during 15 to 30 minutes of exercise using high-volume, moderate-to-high-in-intensity, short rest periods and stressing a large muscle mass, when compared with low-volume, high-intensity protocols using long rest intervals.[22]

Other anabolic hormones, such as insulin and insulin-like growth factor-1 (IGF-1), are critical to skeletal muscle growth. Blood glucose and amino acid levels regulate insulin. However, following resistance exercise, elevations in circulating IGF-1 have been reported, presumably in response to growth hormone–stimulated secretion.[22]

Force developed by the myofilaments (actin and myosin) may stimulate the uptake of amino acids and thus result in muscle tissue growth.[23] Heavy forces encountered during resistance training lead to disruption in the Z lines. The disorganization after disruption of the Z disks may cause the myofibril to split and grow back full size.[24] Furthermore, the disruption and rebuilding of the muscle result in an increase in the connective tissue surrounding the muscle fibers. The ingestion use of amino acids before and after resistance training to promote hypertrophy is discussed at great length in Chapter 17.

In summary, as a result of strength training exercises, physiological adaptations of muscle result in an increase in strength. These adaptations include hypertrophy (within the first 6 to 8 weeks), hyperplasia, hormonal changes, increase in the connective tissue surrounding the muscle fibers, disruption of the myofilaments, and neuromuscular changes (within the first 2 weeks of training). In addition, metabolic adaptations occurring within the muscle fiber increase the ability of the muscle to generate adenosine triphosphate (ATP) for anaerobic metabolism. Anaerobic metabolism requires that the muscles increase phosphocreatine, glycogen stores, the enzyme creatine phosphokinase that breaks down PC, and the rate-limiting enzyme phosphofructokinase of glycolysis. Refer to Chapter 3 for a review of anaerobic metabolism.[25]

Muscle Fiber Type: Specific Adaptations

The fact that a prolonged program of resistance training brings about fiber type conversion with the muscle is well documented. The most common finding is an increase in the percentage of Type IIA fibers with a decrease in the percentage of Type IIB fibers.[6,26,27]

Apparently, as soon as a Type IIB muscle fiber is stimulated it starts a process of transformation toward the Type IIA, by changing the quality of proteins and expressing different types and amounts of myosin adenosine triphosphatase (mATPase).[28] Following a resistance-training program, few Type IIB fibers

remain, which is reversed during detraining. However, when resistance training starts again, the conversion from Type IIB to Type IIA is quicker. Although resistance training promotes hypertrophy in all three major muscle fiber types in humans— I, IIA, IIB—the amount of hypertrophy differs from each fiber type. On the basis of the examination of pretraining to post-training muscle samples, it has been established that muscle hypertrophy is greatest in Type IIA fibers, followed by Type IIB, with Type I fibers demonstrating the least amount of hypertrophy.[5,6,26,27,29] Sex differences are apparent in muscle cross-sectional examination before and after training; Type IIA fibers are the largest among men, whereas the Type I fiber is the greatest size among women.[30]

Exercise Variables

In order to achieve the physiological adaptations described earlier, several variables must be considered. The variables that need to be carefully planned for in the development of an exercise program include the choice of exercise, order of exercises, number of sets, number of repetitions, intensity of exercise, duration of rest between sets and exercises, and frequency of training.

The type of exercise should be specific to the specific muscle deficits revealed in the initial evaluation. Furthermore, the type of exercises should be specific to the muscle groups that are important to improving the performance of the athlete. For example, in the overhead-throwing athlete, the external rotators, infraspinatus and teres minor, provide a breaking action in the deceleration of the shoulder. Eccentric loading to the external rotators is a specific exercise to strengthen the external rotators, and eccentric activity of the external rotators is specific to the movement pattern and exercise performed by the athlete in competition. Furthermore, high-speed eccentric loading is damaging to the muscle. By increasing the eccentric strength of the external rotators, there is greater protection of the muscle from damage. This concept is discussed in greater detail later.

The order of the exercises performed by the athlete typically involves performance of large muscle group exercises before smaller muscle group exercises. Because the metabolic demand is greater for large muscle group exercises, exercises that recruit more than one muscle group, such as closed kinetic chain exercises, should be performed before isolation exercises.[28]

Once again, debate exists in the literature regarding the number of sets and frequency of strength training. For the athlete the number of sets within a workout is directly related to individual training goals. Multiple-set programs optimize the development of strength and local muscular endurance.[31] Gains in strength occur more rapidly with multiple-set programs compared with single-set protocols.[32] Single-set exercise programs may be effective for individuals who are untrained or those just beginning a resistance training program. One-set workouts are also useful for maintenance programs. Furthermore, strength changes over a short-term training period and nonperiodized multiple-set program may not be different among one, two, or three sets of 10 to 12RM.[33] However, when single-set protocol is compared with multiple-set periodized programs, significant superior results are observed with the multiset periodized programs that last longer than 1 month.[34] Gotshalk et al[35] demonstrated that higher volumes of total work produced significantly greater increases in circulating anabolic hormones during the recovery phase following multiset heavy-resistance exercise protocols.

McLester et al[36] demonstrated that training 1 day per week was an effective means of increasing strength, even in experienced recreational weight lifters. However, the previous study reported superior results with training 3 days per week when compared with 1 day per week when the total volume of the exercise was held constant.

Advanced training frequency varies considerably. Hoffman et al[37] demonstrated that football players training 4 to 5 days per week achieved better results that those who trained either 3 or 6 days per week. Frequencies as high as 18 sessions per week have been reported in Olympic weight lifters.[38]

The intensity of the exercise or the amount of resistance used for a specific exercise is the most important variable in resistance training. The most common method of determining the amount of resistance used in a strength-training program is the maximal load that can be lifted a given number of repetitions within one set. The greatest effects on strength measures or maximal power outputs are achieved when the strength training repetitions range between 6 and 12.[28] In other words, the maximum weight that can be lifted six times and six times only is the amount of resistance to start with. Addition of sets and repetitions occurs at subsequent workouts until 3 sets of 12 repetitions (reps) are reached. After reaching this reps and sets goal, the reps are reduced down to eight and weight is added, allowing only eight repetitions. Once 15 reps are achieved with a specific weight, the muscle will no longer continue to improve in strength. However, lighter loads allowing 15 to 20 reps are effective for increasing absolute local muscle endurance.[39,40]

Maximizing power requires a good strength base. Given that both force and time components are relevant to maximizing power, training to increase muscle power requires two general loading strategies. First, heavy resistance training recruits high-threshold fast-twitch muscle fibers that are necessary for strength. The second strategy is to incorporate lighter loads. Depending on the exercise, this may encompass 30% to 60% of 1RM.[41,42] Weight training for power has been referred to as "explosive strength training." Paavolainen et al[43] demonstrated that explosive strength training could improve 5-km running time by improving running economy and muscle power, although a large volume of endurance training was performed concomitantly. The maximum amount of resistance used in the explosive strength training exercises was 40% of 1RM. When performing explosive weight-training exercises, the athlete moves as fast as possible throughout the range of motion, resulting in losing contact with the ground in an explosive squat or losing contact with the bar in a bench press. During a traditional bench press and squat weight-training exercises performed at an explosive velocity, one study has shown that 40% to 60% 1RM and 50% to 70% 1RM, respectively, may be most beneficial in the development of power.[44]

The final variable that is important to muscle adaptation

from strength training is the time intervals between sets. The rest interval depends on the intensity of the training. For example, it has been shown that acute force and power production may be compromised with short rest periods of 60 seconds or less.[45] Longitudinal studies have shown greater strength increases resulting from long rest periods between sets, 2 to 3 minutes versus 30 to 40 seconds.[46,47]

Aging and Muscle Changes

Professional athletes have been performing longer and longer over the past decade. Demographics data clearly illustrate that, overall, the U.S. population is growing older. Aging causes a loss of functional capacity resulting from a decrease in muscle mass (sarcopenia).[48] Approximately one third of the total muscle mass is lost between 30 and 80 years of age.[49] This decrease in muscle loss is primarily as a result of selective loss and remodeling of motor units. By the seventh decade of life, some muscles may have only half the number of motor units and 75% of the total number of fibers compared with muscles of young adults.[50] Type II fibers appear to be the most affected, gradually decreasing in both size and number with advancing age. Loss of fiber begins at approximately 25 years of age and accelerates thereafter.[51] However, it appears that training can both reverse aging atrophy and maintain fiber-type distributions in elderly individuals similar to those found in the young. Several studies have determined that strength improvements in the elderly are coupled with cellular and whole muscle hypertrophy.[8,52,53] Also, muscle hypertrophy responses to resistance training have been found to be indistinguishable between young and elderly people.[8,54] The recommendations for the strength training variables noted as follows are beneficial to use with the elderly or the young athlete or patient, or both.

- Strength training reps 6 to 12
- Multiple sets 2 to 3
- At least 2 days per week and a maximum of 3 days per week of strength training
- 90 seconds' to 2 minutes' rest between sets
- Train the large muscle groups before the smaller muscle groups

The choice of the exercises should be based on an evaluation of muscle strength and the muscles that are important to the type of activity the patient wants to resume. The greater the intensity of activity the patient wants to return to, the greater the intensity the rehabilitation or training, or both, should be.

TYPES OF MUSCLE-STRENGTHENING ACTIONS

Eccentric Strengthening

Simply stated, an eccentric action occurs whenever opposing force acting on a muscle exceeds the force produced by that muscle.[55] This causes the muscle to lengthen while it is being activated. Eccentric actions are characterized by an ability to achieve high muscle forces and an enhancement of the tissue damage that is often associated with muscle soreness, and perhaps require unique control strategies.[56] Eccentric actions are used frequently throughout everyday life, especially in athletic competition. A common human movement strategy is to combine concentric and eccentric actions into a sequence called the *stretch-shorten cycle*.[56] This cycle typically involves a small-amplitude, moderate-to-high velocity eccentric contraction that is followed by a concentric contraction.[57] Eccentric contractions are mechanically efficient and can attenuate impact forces and maximize performance.[56]

When a muscle is trained eccentrically, a number of structural signs of muscle damage exist. Under electron microscope it has been shown that sarcomeres will become out of register and extended, and z-line streaming is evident, along with a regional disorganization of the myofilaments and t-tubule damage.[57] Mechanically, there are signs of a shift in the muscle's optimum length toward a longer muscle length, a decrease in active tension, an increase in passive tension, and muscle swelling and soreness.[57] This muscle swelling and soreness leads to delayed-onset muscle soreness (DOMS), which is thought to be purely mechanical and not an inflammatory response.[58] (See Chapter 6 for more information on muscle damage.)

After a bout of eccentric exercise, an adaptation occurs. This adaptation can be called the *repeated bout effect*. When one performs an eccentric bout of exercise, a repeated bout effect adaptation will protect the muscle against further damage from subsequent eccentric bouts.[59] This can help to improve performance and prevent injury. Recently the adaptations have been broken down into three categories: cellular, mechanical, and neural.[59] At the cellular level there is evidence of an increase in sarcomeres after bouts of eccentric exercise.[60] In fact, one study found an 11% increase in sarcomere number after eccentric loading.[57] At the mechanical level there is evidence of increases in dynamic and passive muscle stiffness.[61] Whitehead et al[61] state that the rise in passive muscle tension depends on the length range over which the muscle is worked. On the neural level there is still discussion whether adaptation is on the central or local level. Research shows that with a high enough velocity, there is cross education to the contralateral limb, which means there is definitely a central connection.[62] On the basis of this information, adaptations seemingly occur across the three categories and a unified theory has yet to exist.

With eccentric strengthening and adaptations, there are increases in strength, cross-sectional areas, and neural activation.[63] Along with muscle adaptation, there has been discussion of possible tendon adaptations, but no clear evidence exists yet. With biceps brachii eccentric loading, the muscle sense organs and the body's ability to sense joint position have shown both an increase and decrease in the flexed position. This seems to depend on whether there is actually a muscle spindle injury (increase flexed position) or if there is just sarcomere disruption (decreased flexed position) and the former happening with high-intensity strengthening.[57] An increased signal from a muscle spindle has been shown with heavy eccentric strength, while there have been no studies to show evidence of significant neural adaptation more so than concentric strengthening.

Eccentric contractions are one of three types of muscle contractions. When a muscle can overcome an opposing force and shorten while being activated, this is called a *concentric contraction*. When the force generated is equal to the opposing force and there is no movement, this is called an *isometric contraction*.

Typically, eccentric contractions can generate two to three times more force than concentric contractions.[64] This has led some authors to believe that by training someone eccentrically, one has a greater capability of overloading the muscle to a greater extent and enhancing muscle mass, strength, and power when compared with concentric strengthening.[64] This generalization may seem fair but may be too simple.

Many studies show an increase, decrease, or no change in functional performance, concentric strength, and eccentric strength after eccentric training.[65-76] The outcomes noted earlier can be attributed to different training protocols and methods of assessment.[65] Current research has shown that eccentric training is more effective than concentric training for developing eccentric strength and that concentric strengthening is more effective for developing concentric strength.[66] The specificity of training noted earlier is another application of the specific adaptations to imposed demands (SAID) principle.

The degree of that strength gain is relative to the volume/intensity and velocity of the eccentric exercise. In the majority of the studies the load used was appropriate to induce failure in the muscle. The actual volume does vary, but there is a study that supports the use of low-volume eccentric exercise.[76] Another study found that when compared with high-intensity eccentric training, low-intensity eccentric training has the same amount of muscle damage but without the large drop in muscle performance.[77] On the basis of these two studies, one may not need to use a high-intensity/volume model for eccentric strength gains. Other research has shown that to get the greatest hypertrophy and strength gains, one must work eccentrically 180 degrees per second over the range.[78] This study was performed with isokinetic equipment, so the carryover to isotonic is unknown.

Differences also seem to occur in relation to eccentric strength across genders and lifespan. Lindle et al[79] found that concentric peak torque decreased more with age than did eccentric peak torque for both men and women. In another study they found that women tended to better preserve muscle quality with age for eccentric peak torque.[80] In addition, older women seemed to have an enhanced capacity, about a decade longer, to store elastic energy better than similarly aged men and younger men and women.[80]

Concentric Strengthening

As discussed earlier, there are neural, contractile, and muscle fiber–type adaptations with strength training. Most athletes use a combination of eccentric, concentric, and isometric contractions. Because of the need to control a load when returning it to the starting position, most strengthening studies have used a combination of eccentric and concentric actions. As previously noted, the stretch shorten cycle is initiated by an eccentric action followed by a concentric contraction, while an eccentric contraction can happen by itself. Because of this, any time people work isotonically, they are working eccentrically even if they are concentrating on the shortening contraction. In the real world it is almost impossible to work only concentrically. This makes it so difficult to discuss the adaptations of concentric-only contractions. What follows is an attempt to discuss concentric strengthening, although the changes associated with concentric strength training are poorly understood.[81]

A concentric contraction occurs when the force produced by the muscle exceeds the external force or load.[56] This contraction causes the muscle to shorten and is the latter action of the stretch-shorten cycle. This cycle, as pointed out earlier, happens in most day-to-day activities and occurs without specialized training.[56] Enorka[56] considered that by performing a concentric contraction only without an eccentric action, muscle performance would be decreased.[56]

Concentric-only strengthening does not produce as much exercise-induced muscle injury as eccentric strengthening.[82] In fact, more muscle damage is produced when a muscle is loaded eccentrically than if it is loaded eccentrically and concentrically, regardless of whether this is done alternately or separated.[83] Whereas eccentric strengthening carryover seems to be specific to intensity, mode, and velocity of training, concentric strengthening may be more general with its carryover. One study found that velocity-specific, concentric-only strengthening resulted in increased peak torques above and below the training velocity.[84] Another study found that concentric training was less mode- and speed-specific than corresponding eccentric training.[85]

Isometric Strengthening

Isometric strengthening occurs when the force generated by muscle and the external force is the same and there is no lengthening or shortening of the muscle. Isometric strengthening has been shown to be joint angle specific, and there is not much carryover to other joint angles. Only about a 20-degree carryover exists either way from where the muscle was trained, although one study did show that there is greater carryover throughout the entire range when the muscle is trained isometrically in the lengthened position.[86] The question of what type of adaptations the muscle will undergo with isometric strengthening also exists. One study has reported that this depends on the type of rate of contraction. Progressive contractions produced modification of the nervous system at the peripheral level, whereas ballistic contractions affected the muscle's contractile properties.[87] Another study found increased isometric strength might be due to factors associated with hypertrophy, independent of neural adaptations.[88]

CLINICAL APPLICATION

With all this information, how does one apply it to a clinical situation? First, clinicians need to integrate eccentric strengthening into their practice. It needs to be more than just lowering the weight after a concentric contraction. On the basis of current research, it is known that in order to train an athlete for eccentric movements, they must perform eccentric movements. In the definition of a stretch-shorten cycle, an eccentric contraction is a low-amplitude and moderate- to high-velocity contraction. Therefore eccentric movements must be faster than concentric contractions. Eccentric isotonic training must produce forces two to three times greater than their concentric counterparts to have the proper intensity. This does not necessarily mean that istonic loads should be doubled or tripled. Force that is generated during an exercise is dependent on the amount of resistance used; the greater the resistance, the slower the speed. (Force equals mass times acceleration). Because an eccentric action should happen at a greater speed, one may have to only increase the load by 20% to 30% if one is moving the limb twice as fast as the concentric contraction. A rest period longer than 48 hours must be allowed. Athletes must be trained in a specific eccentric manner to get maximum gains from their rehabilitation and performance training. How to do that in a controlled clinical setting isotonically is the first question.

What injuries or muscle groups would benefit the most from eccentric strengthening? A number of studies discuss the use of eccentric strengthening in treating patients with Achilles tendinosis, patellar tendinopathy, iliotibial band syndrome in runners, and chronic isolated posterior cruciate ligament injured knees.[89-93] MacLean et al[92] demonstrated that in posterior cruciate ligament–deficit knees a significantly decreased eccentric-to-concentric ratio was noted compared with the contralateral hamstring. A study by Mafi et al[89] found that more patients with chronic Achilles tendinosis had a better overall satisfaction and decreased pain with eccentric strengthening training than concentric strengthening training. Another study by Young et al[93] showed that eccentric training with a decline squat protocol was superior to a traditional eccentric protocol with decreased pain and improved sporting function in elite volleyball players over 12 months who had suffered patellar tendinopathy. Ohberg et al[94] showed that with eccentric training in patients with Achilles tendinosis, there was an actual decrease in Achilles tendon width along with decreased pain. These studies indicate that eccentric strengthening should be a definite part of any tendinopathy treatment.

Other applications may include using eccentric actions and loading on muscle groups that primarily work concentrically but that have been immobilized. An example is a patient who has undergone anterior cruciate ligament repair. If the knee has been braced and the quadriceps group has been in a shortened position, muscular atrophy will occur along with a decrease in the number of sarcomeres. This remolding can occur within the first 5 days of immobilization.[57] If the quadriceps group is eccentrically loaded properly in the open chain, sarcomere lengthening exists along with an increase in the actual number of sarcomeres. This adaptation will help to speed up the return of a good quadriceps eccentric action and possibly the concentric contraction as well. With the eccentric loading of the tibia in the open chain position, the tibia will glide posteriorly, which will eliminate any anterior shear force on the anterior cruciate ligament. With a concentric open-chain quadriceps contraction, the force generated will be an anterior shear.

When working with athletes, one must consider what the specific function of a muscle is in relation to the athletes' sport. A track sprinter may be going through rehabilitation from a hamstring group strain. If the athlete's hamstring is properly loaded eccentrically, this may help to prevent further injury secondary to the repeated bout effect. The same is true with a baseball pitcher, who, by eccentrically training the rotator cuff muscles, may be able to adapt to higher eccentric forces and therefore decrease the chances of suffering from a deceleration injury. But in order to gain these benefits from eccentric training, the athlete would most likely need to be trained specifically by training the same muscle groups with the same intensity as needed by the sport. One study showed a decrease in the occurrence of hamstring strain injuries in elite soccer players after undergoing eccentric overload training.[95]

Examples of when not to use an eccentric loading action would be during the initial rehabilitation after a tendon repair or the initial stages of muscle healing. Because the force generated by an eccentric action can be two to three times greater than a concentric contraction, failure may be generated at the repair sight or the sight of tissue injury. For example, if a patient has just gone through a supraspinatus tendon repair and is status post 2 weeks, obviously eccentric loading should be avoided. However, if the same patient is working on active assistive range of motion with wall walks and at the top of the exercise starts to lower his or her arm, he or she will eccentrically load that tendon and may rerupture the tendon repair. Because concentric loading generates less force, it may be more beneficial when working with a repaired tissue to initially use concentric-only strengthening when the tissue has healed enough to withstand an external load.

Isometric contractions seem to be most beneficial when used to increase the endurance of those muscles that function as spinal stabilizers.[96] This will help to maintain low but continuous activation of the paraspinal and abdominal wall muscles that function as stabilizers.[97] According to recent research, isometric contractions lend themselves to more of a neural than contractile adaptation.[97]

CONCLUSION

In order to make progressive, efficient, and major strength gains in the athlete, one must apply numerous concepts. The athlete must be worked specifically toward his or her goals whether they are strength, hypertrophy, power, or endurance in the context of the sport. At the same time the athlete must vary his or her strengthening program with periodization if training will occur for extended periods. The basic concept of periodization is changing the intensity, velocity, and volume as needed. There also needs to be consideration of the type of muscle action (eccentric, concentric, and isometric) and the amount of focus that action will require to help the athlete in his or her sport. The authors of this chapter, when rehabilitating or training an athlete, or both, recommend the exercise variables listed as follows:

- Strength training repetitions of 8 to 12 repetitions for strength and hypertrophy, 4 to 6 repetitions for power, and 12 to 15 repetitions for endurance.
- Multiple sets for all types of strengthening.
- At least 2 days of strength training per week.
- 1- to 2-minute rest periods for smaller muscle groups and 2- to 3-minute rest periods for larger muscle groups.
- Start with multiple joint exercise and finish with single joint exercises.
- Intensity will start with 8 repetition (rep) max for strength and 10 rep max for hypertrophy, 6 rep max for power at either high or moderate velocity, and 15 rep max for muscular endurance.
- Velocity can be slow, moderate, or fast depending on specific goals.
- Eccentric strengthening needs to be focused on with deceleration muscles, and eccentric and concentric together need to focused on for the acceleration muscles.
- Any time an athlete's strength training goes beyond 4 weeks, his or her program needs to periodize.

The choice of exercises should be based on an evaluation of muscle strength and the muscles that are important to the type of activity in which the athlete competes. As previously noted, the greater the intensity of the activity, the greater the intensity of the training should be. Appendix B reviews three cases that exemplify strength training concepts and periodization principles.

REFERENCES

1. Deschenes M, Kraemer W: Performance and physiologic adaptations to resistance training, *Am J Phys Med Rehab* 81(11):3-16, 2002.
2. Monte M, Cohen D, Campbell K, et al: Isokinetic concentric versus eccentric training of shoulder rotators with functional evaluation of performance enhancement in elite tennis players, *Am J Sports Med* 22(4):513-517, 1994.
3. Wooden M, Greenfield B, Johanson M, et al: Effects of strength training on throwing velocity and shoulder muscle performance in teenage baseball players, *J Ortho Sports Phys Ther* 15(5):223-227, 1992.
4. Moritani T, Devires H: Neural factors versus hypertrophy in the time course of muscle strength gain, *Am J Phys Med* 58:115-130, 1979.
5. Staron RS, Leonardi MJ, Karapondo DL: Strength and skeletal muscle adaptations in heavy-resistance-trained women after detraining and retraining, *J Appl Physiol* 70: 631-640, 1991.
6. Staron RS, Karapondo DL, Kraemer WJ: Skeletal muscle adaptations in heavy resistance training in men and women, *J Appl Physiol* 76: 1247-1255, 1994.
7. Shoepe T, Stelzer J, Garner D, et al: Functional adaptability of muscle fibers to long-term resistance exercise, *Med Sci Sports Exerc* 35(6):944-951, 2003.
8. Hakkinen K, Alen M, Kallimen M: Neuromuscular adaptation during prolonged strength training, detraining,

and re-strength-training in middle-aged and elderly people, *Eur J Appl Physiol* 83:51-62, 2000.

9. Hakkinen K, Kallimen M, Izquierdo M: Changes in agonist-antagonist EMG, muscle CSA, and force during strength training in middle aged and older people, *J Appl Physiol* 84:1341-1249, 1998.

10. Dechenes MR, Judelson DA, Kraemer WJ: Effects of resistance training on neuromuscular junction morphology, *Muscle Nerve* 23:1576-1581, 2000.

11. Milner-Brown H, Stein R, Lee R: Synchronization of human motor units: possible roles of exercise and supraspinal reflexes, *Electroencephalogr Clin Neurophysiol* 38:245-254, 1975.

12. Stone M, O'Bryant H, Garhammer J: A theoretical model of strength training, *Nat Strength Cond Assoc J* 4:36-39, 1982.

13. Kraemer W, Patamess N, Fry A: Influence of resistance training volume and periodization on physiological and performance adaptations in collegiate tennis players, *Am J Sports Med* 28:626-633, 2000.

14. Balogopal P, Rooyacker O, Adey D: Effects of aging on in vivo synthesis of skeletal muscle myosin heavy-chain and sarcoplasmic protein in humans, *Am J Physiol* 273:E790-800, 1997.

15. Rooyackers O, Adey D, Ades P: Effect of age on in vivo rates of mitochondral protein synthesis in human skeletal muscle, *Proc Natl Acad Sci* 93:15364-15369, 1996.

16. McCall G, Byrnes W, Fleck S: Acute and chronic hormonal responses to resistance training designed to promote muscle hypertrophy, *Can J Appl Physiol* 24:96-107, 1999.

17. Malina R: Growth of muscle tissue and muscle mass. In Faulkner F, Tanner J, editors: *Human growth. A comprehensive treatise,* vol 2, pp. 77-99, New York, 1986, Plenum Press.

18. Larsson L, Tesch P: Motor unit fiber density in extremely hypertrophied skeletal muscle in men: muscle electrophysiological signs of fiber hyperplasia, *Eur J Appl Physiol* 55:130-136, 1986.

19. Yan Z: Skeletal muscle adaptation and cell cycle regulation, *Exerc Sport Sci Rev* 2801:24-26, 2000.

20. Irintchev A, Wernig A: Muscle damage and repair in voluntarily running mice: strain and muscle differences, *Cell Tissue Res* 249:509-521, 1987.

21. Rosenblatt JD, Parry DJ: Adaptation of rat extensor digitorum longus muscle to gamma irradiation and overlaid, *Pflugers Arch* 423:255-264, 1993.

22. Kadi F: Adaptation of human skeletal muscle to training and anabolic steroids, *Acta Physiol Scand Suppl* 168:4-53, 2000.

23. Goldberg A, Etlinger J, Goldspink D, et al: Mechanisms of work-induced hypertrophy of skeletal muscle, *Med Sci Sports* 7:248-261, 1975.

24. Goldspink G: Changes in striated muscle fibers during contraction and growth with particular reference to myofibril splitting, *J Cell Sci* 9:123-127, 1971.

25. Plowman S, Smith D: Muscular training principles and adaptations. In Plowman S, Smith D, editors: *Exercise physiology for health, fitness, and performance*, ed 2, pp. 549-565, San Francisco, 2003, Benjamin Cummings.

26. Kraemer W, Patton J, Gordon S: Compatibility of high intensity strength and endurance training on hormonal and skeletal muscle adaptations, *J Appl Physiol* 78:976-989, 1995.

27. Volek J, Duncan N, Mazzetti S: Performance and muscle fiber adaptations to creatine supplementation and heavy resistance training, *Med Sci Sports Exerc* 31:1147-1156, 1999.

28. Kraemer W, Duncan N, Volek J: Resistance training and elite athletes: adaptations and program considerations, *J Orth Sports Phy Ther* 28(2):110-119, 1998.

29. Johnson T, Klueber K: Skeletal muscle following tonic overload: functional and structural analysis, *Med Sci Sports Exerc* 23:49-55, 1991.

30. Staron R, Hagerman F, Hikida R: Fiber type composition of the vastus lateralis muscle of young men and women, *J Histochem Cytochem* 48:623-629, 2000.

31. McDougah M, Davies C: Adaptive response of mammalian skeletal muscle to exercise with high loads, *Eur J Appl Physiol* 52:139-155, 1984.

32. Baker J, Cooper S: Strength and body composition: single versus triple set resistance training programmes, *Med Sci Sports Exerc* 36(5)Suppl:S53, 2004.

33. Fleck S, Kraemer W: Designing resistance training programs, ed 2, Champaign, Ill, 1997, Human Kinetics Publishers.

34. Gotshalk L, Loebel C, Nindi B, et al: Hormonal responses of multiset versus single set heavy resistance exercise protocols, *Can J Appli Physiol* 22(3):244-255, 1997.

35. McLester J, Bishop P, Guilliams M: Comparsion of 1 day and 3 day per week of equal-volume resistance training in experienced subjects, *J Strength Conditioning Res* 14(3):273-281, 2000.

36. Hoffman J, Kraemer W, Fry A, et al: The effects of self-selection for frequency of training in a winter conditioning program for football, *J Appl Sport Sci Res* 3:76-82, 1990.

37. Kraemer W, Ratamess N: Fundamentals of resistance training: progression and exercise prescription, *Med Sci Sports Exerc* 36:674-688, 2004.

38. Campos G, Luecke H, Wendeln, et al: Muscular adaptations in response to three different resistance-training regimens: specificity of repetition maximum training zones, *Eur J Appl Physiol* 88:50-60, 2002.

39. Stone W, Coulter S: Strength/endurance effects from three resistance-training protocols with women, *J Strength Cond Res* 8:231-234, 1994.

40. Wilson G, Newton R, Murphy A, et al: The optimal training load for the development of dynamic athletic performance, *Med Sci Sports Exerc* 25:1279-1286, 1993.

41. Baker D, Nance S, Moore M: The load that maximizes the average mechanical power output during jump squats in power-trained athletes, *J Strength Cond Res* 15:92-97, 2001.

42. Paavolainen L, Hakkinen K, Hamalainen I, et al: Explosive-strength training improves 5km running time

by improving running economy and muscle power, *J Appl Physiol* 86:1527-1533, 1999.

43. Siegel J, Gilders R, Staron R, et al: Human muscle power output during upper and lower body exercises, *J Strength Cond Res* 16:173-178, 2002.

44. Kraemer W: A series of studies—the physiological basis for strength training in American football: fact over philosophy, *J Strength Cond Res* 11:131-142, 1997.

45. Pincivero D, Lephart S, Karunakara R: Effects of rest interval on isokinetic strength and functional performance after short-term high intensity training, *Br J Sports Med* 31:229-234, 1997.

46. Robinson J, Stone M, Johnson C, et al: Effects of different weight training exercise/rest intervals on strength, power, and high intensity exercise endurance, *J Strength Cond Res* 9:216-221, 1995.

47. Evans W, Campbell W: Sarcopenia and age related changes in body composition and functional capacity, *J Nutr* 123:465-468, 1993

48. Tzanoff S, Norris A: Effects of muscle mass decrease on age related BMR changes, *J Appl Physiol* 43:1001-1006, 1977.

49. Doherty T, Vandrervoot A, Taylor A, et al: Effects of motor unit losses on strength in older men and women, *J Appl Physiol* 74:868-874, 1993.

50. Larrson L, Sjodin B, Karlsson J: Histochemical and biochemical changes in human skeletal muscle with age in sedentary males, age 22-65 years, *Acta Phsiol Scand* 103:31-39, 1978.

51. Fromtera W, Meredith C, O'Reilly K, et al: Strength conditioning in older men: skeletal muscle hypertrophy and improved function, *J Appl Physiol* 64:1038-1044, 1988.

52. Taafe D, Marcus R: Dynamic muscle strength alterations to detraining and retraining in elderly men, *Clin Physiol* 17:311-324, 1997.

53. Esmarck B, Anderson J, Olsen S, et al: Timing of post-exercise protein intake is important for muscle hypertrophy with resistance training in elderly humans, *J Physiol* 535:301-311, 2001.

54. Newton R, Hakkinen K, Hakkinen A, et al: Mixed-methods of resistance training increases power and strength of young and older men, *Med Sci Sports Exerc* 34:1367-1375, 2002.

55. Lindstedt SL, Reich TE, Keim P, et al: Do muscles function as adaptable locomotor springs? *J Exper Biol* 205:2211-2216, 2002.

56. Enorka RM: Eccentric contractions require unique activation strategies by the nervous system, *J Physiol* 123:2339-2346, 1996.

57. Proske U, Morgan DL: Muscle damage from eccentric exercise: mechanism, mechanical signs, adaptation and clinical applications, *J Physiol* 537:333-345, 2001.

58. Yu JG, Malm C, Thornell: Eccentric contractions leading to DOMS do not cause loss of desmin nor fibre necrosis in human muscle, *Histochem Cell Biol* 118(1):29-34, 2002.

59. McHugh MP: Recent advances in the understanding of the repeated bout effect: the protective effect against muscle damage from a single bout of eccentric exercise, *Scand J Med Sci Sports* 13(2):88-97, 2003.

60. Yu JG, Furst DO, Thornell LE: The mode of myofibril remodeling in human skeletal muscle affected by DOMS induced by eccentric contractions, *Histochem cell Biol* 119(5):393-93, 2003.

61. Whitehead NP, Morgan DL, Gregory JE, et al: Rises in whole muscle passive tension of mammalian muscle after eccentric contractions at different lengths, *J Appl Physiol* 95:1224-1234, 2003.

62. Farthing JP, Chilibeck PD: The effect of eccentric training at different velocities on cross-education, *Eur J Appl Physiol* 89(6):570-577, 2003.

63. Higbie EJ, Cureton KJ, Warren III GL, et al: Effects of concentric and eccentric training on muscle strength, cross-sectional, and neural activation, *J Physiol* 19:2173-2181, 1996.

64. LeStayo PC, Woolf JM, Lewek MD, et al: Eccentric muscle contractions: their contribution to injury, prevention, rehabilitation, and sport, *J Ortho Sports Phys Ther* 33:557-571, 2003.

65. Tomberlin JP, Basford JR, Schwen EE, et al: Comparative study of kinetic eccentric and concentric quadriceps training, *J Orthop Sports Phys Ther* 14:31-36, 1991.

66. Colliander EB, Tesch PA: Effects of eccentric and concentric muscle actions in resistance training, *Acta Physiol Scand* 140:31-39, 1990.

67. Komi P, Buskirk ER: Effect of eccentric and concentric muscle conditioning on tension and electrical activity of human muscle, *Ergonomics* 15:417-434, 1972.

68. Colliander EB, Tesch PA: Responses to eccentric and concentric resistance training in females and males, *Acta Physiol Scand* 141:149-156, 1990.

69. Jones DA, Rutherford OM: Human muscle strength training: the effects of three different regimes and the nature of the resultant changes, *J Physiol Lond* 391:1-11, 1987.

70. Dudley GA, Tesch PA, Miller BJ, et al: Importance of eccentric actions in performance adaptations to resistance training, *Aviat Space Environ Med* 62:543-550, 1991.

71. Johnson BL, Adamczyk JW, Tennoe KO, et al: A comparison of concentric and eccentric muscle training, *Med Sci Sports Exerc* 8:35-38, 1976.

72. Duncan PW, Chandler JM, Cavanaugh DK, et al: Mode and speed specificity of eccentric and concentric exercise training, *J Orthop Sports Phys Ther* 11:70-75, 1989.

73. Johnson BL: Eccentric vs concentric muscle training for strength development, *Med Sci Sports Exerc* 4:111-115, 1972.

74. Ellenbecker TS, Davies GJ, Rowinski MJ: Concentric versus eccentric isokinetic strengthening of the rotator cuff: objective data versus functional test, *Am J Sports Med* 16:64-69, 1988.

75. Hortobagyi T, Katch FI: Role of concentric force in limiting improvement in muscular strength, *J Appl Physiol* 68:650-658, 1990.

76. Paddon-Jones D, Abernethy PJ: Acute adaptation to low volume eccentric exercise, *Med Sci Sports Exerc* 33 (7):1213-1219, 2001.

77. Paschalis V, Koutedakis Y, Jamurtas AZ, et al: Equal volumes of high and low intensity of eccentric exercise in relation to muscle damage and performance, *J Strength Cond Res* 19(1):184-188, 2005.

78. Farthing JP, Chilibeck PD: The effects of eccentric and concentric training at different velocities on muscle hypertrophy, *Eur J Appl Physiol* 89(6):578-586, 2003.

79. Porter MM, Myint A, Kramer JF, et al: Concentric and eccentric knee extension strength in older and younger men and women, *Can J Appl Physiol* 20(4):429-439, 1995.

80. Lindle RS, Metter EJ, Lynch NA, et al: Age and gender comparisons of muscle strength in 654 women and men aged 20-93 yr, *J Appl Physiol* 83(5):1581-1587, 1997.

81. Weir JP, Housch DJ, Housch TJ, et al: The effect of unilateral concentric weight training and detraining on joint angle specificity, cross training, and the bilateral deficit, *J Orthop Sports Phys Ther* 25(4):264-270, 1997.

82. Clarkson PM, Hubal MJ: Exercise-induced muscle damage in humans, *Am J Phys Med Rehabil* 81:S52-S69, 2002.

83. Nosaka K, Lavender AP, Newton MJ: Effect of alternating eccentric and concentric versus separated eccentric and concentric actions on muscle damage. American College of Sports Medicine 2004 Annual Meeting Abstracts: A-25: Athlete Care: Treatment and Prevention. Indianapolis, 2-5 June 2004.

84. Housch DJ, Housch TJ: The effects of unilateral velocity-specific concentric strength training, *J Orthop Sports Phys Ther* 17(5):252-256, 1993.

85. Seger JY, Thorsteensson A: Effects of eccentric versus concentric training in thigh muscle strength and EMG, *Int J Sports Med* 26(1):45-52, 2005

86. Bandy WD, Hanten WP: Changes in torque and electromyography activity of the quadriceps femoris muscles following isometric training, *Phys Ther* 73(7):455-465, 1993.

87. Maffiuletti NA, Martin A: Progressive versus rapid rate of contraction during 7 wk of isometric resistance training, *Med Sci Sports Exerc* 33(7):1120-1127, 2001.

88. Ebersole KT, Housch TJ, Johnson GO, et al: Mechanomyographic and electromographic responses to unilateral isometric training, *J Strength Cond Res* 16(2):192-201, 2001.

89. Mafi N, Lorentzon R, Alfredson H: Superior short term results with eccentric calf muscle training compared to concentric training in a randomized prospective multicenter study on patients with chronic Achilles tendinosis, *Knee Surg Sports Traumatol Arthrosc* 9(1):42-47, 2001.

90. Peers KH, Lysens RJ: Patellar tendinopathy in athletes: current diagnostic and therapeutic recommendations, *Sports Med* 35(1):71-87, 2005.

91. Fredericson M, Wolf C: Iliotibial band syndrome in runners: innovations in treatment, *Sports Med* 35(5):451-459, 2005.

92. MacLean CL, Taunton JE, Clement DB, et al: Eccentric and concentric isokinetic moment characteristics in the quadriceps and hamstrings of the chronic isolated posterior cruciate ligament injured knee, *Br J Sports Med* 33:405-408, 1999.

93. Young MA, Cook JL, Purdam CR, et al: Eccentric decline squat protocol offers superior results at 12 months compared with traditional eccentric protocol for patellar tendinopathy in volleyball players, *Br J Sports Med* 39(2):102-105, 2005.

94. Ohberg L, Lorentzon R, Alfredson H: Eccentric training in patients with chronic Achilles tendinosis: normalized tendon structure and decreased thickness at follow up, *Br J Sports Med* 38(1):8-11, 2004.

95. Askling C, Karlsson J, Thorstensson A: Hamstring injury occurrence in elite soccer players after preseason strength training with eccentric overload, *Scand J Med Sci Sports* 13(4):244-250, 2003.

96. Biering-Sorensen F: Physical measurements as risk indicators for low back trouble over a one year period, *Spine* 9:106-119, 1984.

97. McGill S: Low back disorders: evidence based prevention and rehabilitation, ed 1, Champaign, Ill, 2000, Human Kinetics.

14

Donald A. Chu
and Jay Shiner

Plyometrics in Rehabilitation

LEARNING OBJECTIVES

After studying this chapter, the reader will be able to do the following:

1. Understand the physiology of plyometric exercises
2. Design a functional progression of plyometric exercises
3. Determine the physiological requirements before starting a plyometric exercise program
4. Determine the importance of posture and jumping techniques in plyometric exercises
5. Identify the landing strategies in plyometric exercises
6. Design a plyometric training program
7. Integrate foot work into speed development programs
8. Give objectives for jumping patterns
9. Understand how to progress an athlete in work, intensity, and volume

Plyometric exercises are often included in rehabilitation programs to prepare athletes for the demands of their sport and a safe return to play. In a clinical setting, care plans are often developed on the basis of sound principles, such as functional progressions; SAID (*s*pecific *a*daptations to *i*mposed *d*emands); and manipulating routine variables ([FITTR] *f*requency, *i*ntensity, *t*ime/duration, *t*ype/mode, and *r*ate of progression). Progression from rehabilitation to performance conditioning for the injured athlete should be no different. The effectiveness of a plyometric workout should not be measured by "how tired" an athlete feels. It should focus on the "quality" of the movements. The "exercise-to-fatigue approach" may lead to overtraining, exercise-related pain, and even overuse injuries. Structure and accountability are necessary when including plyometric exercises in rehabilitation and strength and conditioning programs including progression in work volume and intensity.

FUNCTIONAL PROGRESSION

In Review

Functional progression is a series of basic movement patterns graduated according to the difficulty of the skill and an athlete's tolerance.[1] The primary objective of functional progression in rehabilitation is an athlete's timely and safe return to competition. From a prevention standpoint, it is the optimal preparation for the specific demands of a sport. At the heart of functional progression is the SAID principle (specific adaptations to imposed demands), which simply means that physical activities should be appropriate and strategic in preparing an athlete for the demands of his or her sport including such components as acceleration/deceleration of movement, specific velocities of movement, planes and ranges of motion, varied degrees of dynamic trunk stabilization, and coordinated whole body patterns of movement.

Tippett and Voight[1] provided guidelines governing the advancement of a functional progression program:

- Begin with static positions and progress to movement.
- Initiate skills at a slow speed and progress to faster speeds.
- Initiate skills that are simple and progress to more difficult skills.
- Initiate skills unloaded (bodyweight only) and progress to loaded (resisted) skills.

In this chapter, emphasis is placed on cardinal plane maneuvers performed in one place or covering short distances, or both, including 2- and 1-leg squatting, step-ups, and various jumping exercises, such as the four-square and staggered-ladder patterns. In these exercises the athlete moves within a cardinal plane or planes when traveling forward/backward. Movements in a sagittal or frontal plane occur with exercises, such as left-to-right jumps over a barrier. For the purposes of this chapter, these exercises are examples of simple skills that are building blocks in preparing an athlete for more difficult skills, such as running with quick starts and stops, changes of direction within varied sport-specific distances, and simulation of gamelike activities.

Following is an example of how to apply functional progression guidelines and graduate an athlete from one basic skill to the next. Two points on the exercise progressions are important to note:

1. The athlete learns to *attain* alignment and postural control before advancing to the next phase (i.e., static control in a squat position, followed by adding a dynamic movement).

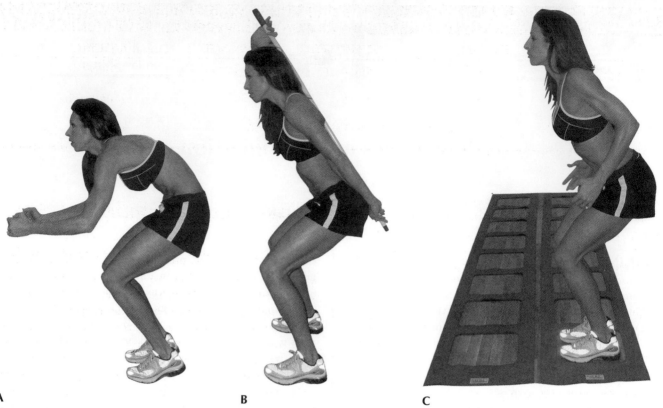

Figure 14-1 A, "Forward head" and "rounded shoulders" posture, which can increase ground contact time during landing due to the time needed to extend the spine before changing directions. **B,** A dowel is used as a cue for proper alignment from the head/neck, trunk, and low back/pelvis. **C,** The correct posture for the "freeze" positions described in the Landing Strategies section.

2. The athlete develops strength to *maintain* proper alignment, which builds a stronger base for dynamic actions (i.e., landing strategies before jump patterns).

The exercises should progress in the order listed:

1. *Strength phase:* Static squat-to-adding movement, two-leg squat to one-leg squat on bench, and forward/back (FW/BK) step-ups to lateral step-ups.
2. *Plyo-support* phase:* Landing strategies with simulated jump patterns.
3. *Performance phase:* Jump patterns as follows:
   FW/BK jumps and left/right jumps
   Add diagonals in four-square formations

Staggered-ladder formation—progressive locomotive patterns

Two-leg to one-leg jumps in patterns mentioned previously

In Figure 14-1, *B* a dowel is used as a cue for proper alignment from the head/neck, trunk, and low back/pelvis. In a squatting posture the spinal curves should change and adjust to the anterior tilt of the pelvis. As the pelvis tilts forward, the lumbar vertebrae are forced anteriorly, thereby increasing lumbar concavity (lordotic curve). The line of gravity (LOG) therefore is at a greater distance from the joint axes of the spinal segments, and the extension moment is increased at both the cervical and lumbar regions. The posterior convexity of the thoracic curve increases slightly and becomes kyphotic in order to balance the greater-than-normal lordotic lumbar curve. Referring to the dowel, the contact points of the body along the dowel are at the head, a midpoint along the thoracic spine, and base of the lumbar spine-pelvis, which assists the athlete in maintaining the three adjusted spinal positions—increased cervical, thoracic, and lumbar curves that accompany an increased anterior pelvic tilt. Figure 14-1, *C* also demonstrates the correct posture for the "freeze" positions, which are discussed later in the section on landing strategies. Therefore as an athlete jumps forward/back and "freezes," he or she needs to land while maintaining this posture. By maintaining the anterior pelvic tilt and proper curves of the spine and not

---

*The "plyo-support" phase is the period in which the athlete develops neurological control and dynamic stabilization of his or her body during the amortization phase, or during ground contact time (transition between eccentric muscle dampening and concentric muscle acceleration of the body) when performing jumps or change of direction, or both. If there is a breakdown in postural control and alignment, ground contact time will be delayed and the amortization phase will be longer than optimal. Figure 14-1, *A* demonstrates that a protracted and flexed cervical spine (forward head), protracted scapulae (rounded shoulders), flexed thoracic spine (bowing spine), and a posterior tilt of the pelvis will cause the individual to absorb the impact of landing. All of the stored energy during the eccentric phase will be dissipated as heat. In this case ground contact is also likely to be increased due to the time necessary to extend the spine before changing directions. The flexed spine position will also adversely affect correct joint positions and actions of the lower extremities.

Table 14-1	Total Foot Contacts Based on an Athlete's Level and Seasonal Periods			
	BEGINNER	**INTERMEDIATE**	**ADVANCED**	**INTENSITY**
OFF SEASON	60-100	100-150	120-200	LOW-MOD
PRESEASON	100-250	150-300	150-450	LOW-HIGH
IN-SEASON	———DEPENDS ON NEEDS OF THE SPORT———			LOW-MOD

flexing at the head/neck and trunk or losing lumbar lordosis, the athlete will be in the most effective position for subsequent takeoff. This is an example of dynamic postural control training, which is part of the plyo-support phase following the development of an adequate strength base.

PLYOMETRIC IN NATURE

The practical definition of plyometrics is a quick, powerful movement involving prestretching or countermovement that activates the stretch shortening cycle (SSC) of muscle.[2] Within this powerful movement is an eccentric phase or force reduction phase; amortization phase or *transition moment involving dynamic stabilization;* and concentric phase or *force production phase*.[3] Although it is common to view plyometrics as a by-product of muscle activity alone, the nervous system must be considered as well. Ultimately, the purpose of plyometric conditioning is to heighten the excitability of the nervous system for improved reactive ability of the neuromuscular system as a whole.[2] If one considers the parameters that go into describing a plyometric exercise including the use of the stretch reflex and taking advantage of the elastic rebound tendency of muscle tissue, then the definition can be broadened to include many exercises that are "plyometric in nature."[4]

The term *plyometrics* has been broadened to mean many different activities, from depth-jumps using a 48-inch box to aerobic dance exercise. Some aquatic programs even refer to certain exercises as being plyometric. Plyometrics, in its purist form, is meant to encompass maximal, all-out, quality efforts with gravity and body weight being the constants for each repetition of an exercise. This said, certain populations benefit from lower-intensity exercises that are plyometric in nature and performed with submaximal efforts. These include younger (prepubescent and adolescent) athletes and those recovering from injury. Younger athletes may lack the strength base or physical maturity to undergo the rigors of a maximal effort plyometric workout and would benefit by performing lower-intensity exercises designed to improve movement (kinesthetic awareness and body control). Athletes recovering from injury are involved in reestablishing the neural patterns and muscular reactivity that will allow them to perform at a higher level without the risk of reinjury or additional trauma. The nature of these exercises can definitely qualify under the heading of "plyometric in nature."

INTENSITY AND WORK VOLUME

Strategic and Appropriate: More Is Not Better!

The term *plyometric* is from the Latin plyo + metrics and is interpreted to mean "measurable increases." Inappropriate applications of plyometric exercises can happen if not monitored correctly. Part of the proper practice of using plyometrics is to simply measure performance and have a plan. In other words, if a scheduled workout has assigned 80 total foot contacts (2 exercises, 2 sets × 20R each exercise), the athlete is finished with the plyometrics portion of the session once that work is completed. An increased risk of overtraining and exercise-related injuries occurs when plyometric work is not measured and progressed appropriately, especially if a therapist, coach, or athlete uses a "feel-the-burn" approach and measures success by "how tired" he or she feels following the workout. When considering the workloads for those athletes who are rehabilitating from a lower extremity injury, the therapist must understand that, no matter their skill level, they are to be considered "beginners" at the high-end (final stages) of their rehabilitation. Their progress is merely on a longer continuum as compared with the noninjured athlete.

Table 14-1 adjusts work volume (total foot contacts) and intensity on the basis of seasonal periods and an individual's "readiness for plyometrics." The recommended volume of specific jumps in any one session will vary with intensity and each workout's objectives. Table 14-1 shows how work volume should vary for beginning, intermediate, and advanced workouts.[4] For example, a beginner in one workout during the off season could complete 60 to 100 foot contacts of low-intensity exercises, while the advanced exerciser might be able to do 120 to 200 foot contacts in one off-season workout. With low-intensity jump training, the work volume accumulates quickly. Note that an athlete performing two sets of each of the following exercises will complete 280 foot contacts in one workout using the four-square formation (Figure 14-2).

- 1,2 × 10 reps (2 foot contacts each repetition [rep], or 20 foot contacts per set)
- 2,3 × 10 reps (20 foot contacts per set)
- 1,2,3 × 10 reps (1 rep = 3 foot contacts, or 30 foot contacts per set)
- 4,3,2 × 10 reps (1 rep = 3 foot contacts, or 30 foot contacts per set)

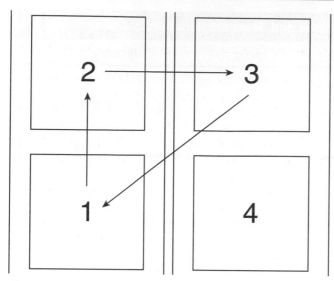

Figure 14-2 Four-square pattern. Sample "triangle" pattern (1, 2, 3). Count 1R each time the athlete hits "1." Following 20R, the athlete will then perform the opposite triangle pattern (4, 3, 2) for 20 R.

- 2,1,3,4 × 10 reps (1 rep = 4 foot contacts, or 40 foot contacts per set)

Consider: 1 set of each exercise above = 140 foot contacts, 2 sets = 280 foot contacts.

Considering the cumulative effect on work volume when combining low- and high-intensity exercises during "preseason" workouts for both intermediate- and advanced-level athletes is important. If an athlete at either level has a scheduled plyometric workout that includes 300 total foot contacts, the previous example of 280 foot contacts of low-intensity jumps using a four-square formation would only allow room for 2 sets of 10 reps of a high-intensity exercise, such as depth jumps. The proportion among low-, moderate-, and high-intensity work would depend on the objectives of the program and objectives of each session within a periodized (cycled training) model. *Periodization* is a method that divides the training year into specific phases, such as preparation, precompetition, competition, and transition phases. A schedule of periodization allows athletes to prepare for peak performance when they need it most, such as a qualifying event, competition, or competitive season. Once again, reiterating the importance of "measurement" and accountability, a therapist or strength and conditioning coach who carefully monitors work volume within his or her athletes' programs will be able to make more objective decisions regarding progression or even tapering work when necessary, following a periodized model. In addition to work volume, the *frequency* of plyometric work and *recovery* between sets are factors to measure and monitor as part of an objective-based strategic plan.

FREQUENCY AND RECOVERY

Allowing 48 to 72 hours between low-intensity plyometric sessions will ensure that adequate rest occurs and the athlete is ready for the next plyometric workout. For example, a common weekly schedule could include the submaximal jump patterns on lower-body strength days, such as Tuesday and Fridays, with upper-body sessions on Monday and Thursdays. An athlete might use a higher frequency (three to four times per week) of plyometric sessions if the exercises used are low in intensity (submaximal) efforts and volume (i.e., three to four exercises of low-intensity, "plyometric in nature" drills employed as part of a warm-up routine).

Adequate recovery between each set in a workout is equally as important as adequate rest between workouts. A common work-to-rest ratio is 1:5 (e.g., an exercise that takes 10 seconds to perform would have 50 seconds rest between sets). An important point to consider with low-intensity plyometric exercises, particularly the footwork patterns presented in this chapter, is that they are "submaximal" in nature. With this in mind, fatigue should not be a factor with this type of work. As stated earlier and also later in this chapter, proprioception, postural control, and dynamic stabilization are points of emphasis with this mode of exercise. Again, fatigue should not be an issue if an athlete follows a course of progression including development of an adequate strength base (i.e., squats and step-ups) and practices landing strategies with adequate body control before performing actual working sets of low-intensity jump training. An athlete will not reach a fatigue state given the submaximal intensity, short duration of activities, and appropriate work-to-rest ratios. As mentioned earlier, submaximal footwork patterns/jumps are often used as part of a warm-up in preparation for moderate- and high-intensity plyometrics.[4] Otherwise, they can be placed toward the end of a workout, following the primary work of the day (weight training, sprinting, and agility drills).

SAFETY CONSIDERATIONS

Low-intensity plyometrics should be performed in areas that allow both adequate space and a yielding training surface. Multipurpose rooms (e.g., group fitness classrooms), gymnasium floors, and outdoor fields are common places for performing footwork patterns. As in moderate- and high-intensity plyometrics, submaximal jump patterns should not be performed on cement or slippery surfaces.

Although it is common to use athletic or duct tape to set up the four-square and staggered ladder patterns discussed in this chapter, ladders may be preferable for the following reason. Ladders are portable and easy to set up, and they allow for consistency in the dimensions of the patterns. The foam ladders shown in this chapter are "foam ladders," which adds to performance safety should an athlete not clear the lines and land on the ladder. Another safety point is to use foam barriers, which are less likely to cause injury if landed on. In this chapter, 2-, 4-, and 6-inch foam blocks are used in the four-square and staggered ladder patterns shown.

Allowing time for an adequate warm-up is another important safety consideration in preparing for low-intensity jump training. "Jump rope" is one simple way to prepare for the low-intensity jump patterns, for example:

1. Jump rope 2 minutes. Perform 2 3 bouts with 60 seconds of dynamic stretching between bouts.
2. Dynamic stretching can include multidirectional lunging and standing quadriceps/hip, hamstring, and lower leg stretches.

READINESS FOR PLYOMETRICS

Medical and Orthopedic Considerations

Preexisting medical conditions need to be considered before beginning a plyometric program, particularly with adult and pediatric populations. For the collegiate and professional athlete, certain conditions, such as diabetes or a current viral illness, can have a significant detrimental effect on performance and recovery. With this in mind, it is important to keep an athlete's relevant-past medical history on file and current health status because it may be necessary in some cases to obtain formal medical clearance before starting the program.

Important orthopedic factors to consider when designing a specific conditioning program using plyometrics include age, gender, and physical maturity and experience level. What is appropriate for one 15-year-old may not be for another. For example, structural and physiological factors may predispose adolescent females to exercise-related pain or injury.

Any preexisting injury would have an important influence on the appropriateness of a plyometric program. For example, deep squats and resisted knee extension may be contraindicated in patients with significant patellofemoral symptoms. For some patients, specific strength training may be necessary before beginning a specific plyometric program, such as hamstring and triceps surae (gastrocnemius-soleus complex) strengthening and co-contraction strategies for patients with a history of anterior cruciate ligament insufficiency. Likewise, athletes who have undergone previous surgery may have specific contraindications or require special areas of emphasis.

At this point, emphasizing a crucial piece of the puzzle in successful plyometric training is necessary. Eccentric strength, or the ability to control the lengthening of a muscle under tension, is vital to becoming faster and jumping higher.[5] When the force exerted on a muscle exceeds the force developed by the muscle, work is done on the stretching muscle and in the process the muscle absorbs mechanical energy. If this energy is dissipated as heat, the muscle is acting as a shock absorber. If the temporarily stored energy is recovered as elastic recoil energy, it results in a muscle that then shortens in a concentric muscle contraction. This is known as the *stretch-shortening cycle* (SSC), and it results in improved economy of movement through a significant enhancement of the power output of subsequent contractions. In this way the muscles of the lower extremities are behaving as springs that cyclically absorb and recover elastic recoil energy. The other fundamental facts surrounding eccentric contractions are that the energy costs are unusually low and the magnitude of the force produced is unusually high. Therefore resistance training to improve eccentric strength is important to prepare the muscles and tendons for the stress and strains encountered in plyometric training.[6] The better prepared the muscles are in this area, the bigger the shock absorbers. Eccentric exercise performed as a regular part of the preparation of the athlete or as part of his or her rehabilitation program requires minimal energy/oxygen support and will increase strength and power in all individuals. The conclusion to be reached is that eccentric strength training should be part of all rehabilitation programs, as well as all performance-enhancement programs.

Body weight and strength ratios are also important factors to consider when initiating plyometric training. For instance, it is suggested for an athlete to be able to perform a back squat with 1.5 times his or her bodyweight (1RM) before beginning high-intensity plyometrics, such as depth jumps.[4] This can be a dilemma for a high school athlete who could otherwise benefit from a plyometric program but lacks this type of strength due to a lack of maturity or training background. When an athlete is running, he or she is already imposing up to three times his or her body weight in forces through the knees. Without the time, maturity, and preparation to obtain these types of strength levels, what alternatives might exist? As stated earlier, low-intensity plyometrics, such as submaximal footwork patterns, are a healthy alternative for young athletes who lack an adequate strength base to perform high-intensity plyometrics.[4] Continuing with the adolescent or prepubescent athlete as an example, the submaximal footwork patterns will teach a young athlete to control his or her center of gravity, land softly, change direction quickly, and spend as little time on the ground as possible. Low-intensity plyometrics can then be viewed as support work for healthier training in young athletes when combined with body weight resistance strength work and landing strategies, as well as development of eccentric strength.

Low-intensity plyometrics are also a healthy choice for larger athletes, such as those weighing more than 220 lb. For a tall, 260-lb basketball player, the four-square drill can be viewed as a dynamic ankle stabilization exercise and combined in a lower-leg circuit including wobble-board, "Bosu ball," or "Dyna-disk" exercises along with resisted dorsiflexion, eversion, and inversion of the ankle movements with a resistance band. In this case submaximal footwork patterns that are plyometric in nature are a healthy alternative for a heavier athlete, in whom high-intensity plyometrics may be contraindicated due to body weight and sport demands (e.g., basketball, a sport that innately includes high-volume/high-frequency jumping through a long season).

The concept of developing the base of strength within an athlete must never be lost during the training process. The types of strength necessary to improve or maintain performance can only be developed through adequate, monitored, and challenging resistance training programs. The fact that free weight lifting provides the exerciser with the resistance necessary to create greater force production, potential for power development, and faster speed of movement is a well-established concept. These movements are integral to the "functional training" or "sport-specific" philosophies followed by therapists and strength and conditioning coaches today. The following strength training exercises are examples of the progressive sequence that should be typically followed as one prepares to undergo the rigors of plyometric training.

SQUATTING AND STEP-UPS

The Basic Positions of Plyometric Training

"Squat" is a body position and posture; squatting is a movement. The squat position is part of most functional activities and a prominent part of most sports movements. The functional progression for squatting is as follows:

- Squat position—An athlete should practice the squat position as a prerequisite to performing the squatting movement. This is an example of "static-to-dynamic" progression. Controlling posture in a static squat position involves (1) aligning the head/neck (keeping the chin slightly "in"), (2) retracting the shoulder blades slightly, and (3) maintaining a slight lordotic posture at the low back in both two- and one-leg squat positions.
- Squatting—The actual squatting action should begin as a slow, controlled descent and progress to a faster ascent movement. This is a continuation of functional progression, from (1) static-to-dynamic, then (2) slow-to-fast movement(s). The manner in which an athlete performs a squat will depend on the objectives of the exercise. Variations of a squatting action can include less or more ankle dorsiflexion, with the tibia in a less or more vertical position and knee or hip dominant motion depending on what the movement is meant to accentuate. These actions will influence the body's position naturally through a kinetic link system, determining whether the trunk will be more upright or angled forward. Additional progressions include changing the body's base of support to condition the hip muscles globally (i.e., wide "sumo" squat as in Figure 14-3, *A*, squat with a staggered leg stance (asymmetrical) as in Figure 14-3, *B*, and the eccentric one-leg squat as in Figure 14-3, *C*.
- Eccentric one-leg squat—Variations of this movement may also include the addition of lateral or "across the body" reaches, or both, while one-leg squatting is a way to challenge frontal and transverse plane movements as well.[7]
- Step-ups—Perform FW/BK step-ups and then progress to lateral step-ups. Step-ups are a healthy alternative to barbell-resisted squats, particularly for prepubescent and adolescent athletes, as well as athletes in whom directly loading the spine is contraindicated. It should be noted that using a weighted vest is an excellent alternative to use of a barbell by beginners or rehabilitating athletes. In a step-up, the height of the bench is set according to the objectives of the exercise and the degree of desired hip action involved. For example, if an athlete's goal is to emphasize hip action and optimally engage the gluteal muscles, he or she can use a bench that allows the stepping leg to begin the step up in a 90-degree hip-flexed position once the foot steps onto the bench. Like a squatting movement, varying degrees of ankle motion, lower leg positions, and knee/hip flexion relationships will be based on the objectives for performing the exercise.

LANDING STRATEGIES

Landing strategies are the next progression from squats and step-ups. In essence, the landing position(s) of the body in low-intensity plyometrics is a partial-squat or what might be considered the "ready" position for an athlete. A partial-squat is a position with feet shoulder-width apart and the body weight centered over a stable base of support (BOS). Bearing weight symmetrically, a stable BOS includes the trunk being upright over the legs with slight flexion of the hips and knees, or a partial squat position. The partial-squat position may involve slightly more hip flexion (60 to 70 degrees) than knee flexion (30 to 45 degrees), keeping the knees posterior to the toes. By maintaining a more perpendicular position of the tibia to the ground, patellofemoral reaction forces are minimized and anterior translation of the tibia is minimized as well, particularly due to the normally occurring 7-degree posterior tilt of the tibial plateau.[5] In short, the partial-squat position is an important quality point in landing strategies, which will, in turn, have a carry-over effect to low-intensity jump training by doing the following:

1. Minimizing risk of *exercise-related* knee injuries (minimizing patellofemoral reaction forces and anterior tibial translation), and
2. Teaching an athlete to control the body's center of gravity within its base of support

Landing strategies bridge the gap between squats/step-ups and the actual low-intensity jump patterns by training an athlete to develop dynamic postural control in the partial-squat position and enhancing dynamic trunk stabilization at ground contact when the feet hit the ground. This type of training will have a direct transfer effect that carries over to jump training, particularly during the amortization phase(s) of each repetition in a jump training set. The objective is to enhance proprioception and kinesthetic awareness during ground contact time. Importantly, when an athlete is able to control posture at ground contact, he or she will be able to change direction quickly and easily, with minimal wasted effort. Each of the following movements ends with a static position. This "freeze" position is an effort to, once again, teach the athlete to control his or her landing using proprioception and eccentric strength to provide the dampening forces and control to hold a position after a dynamic movement precedes the freeze.

Examples of landing strategies should include the following jumps:

- FW and "freeze"
- FW/BK and "freeze"
- FW/BK/FW and "freeze"
- Lateral right (R) and "freeze"

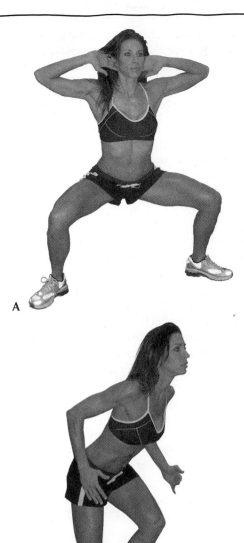

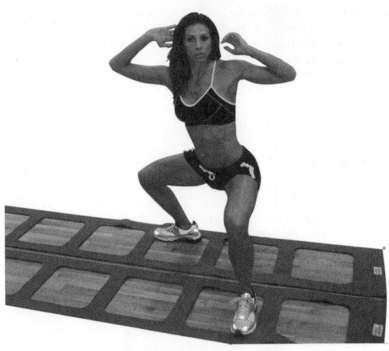

Figure 14-3 A, Wide "sumo" squat. **B,** Squat with a staggered-leg stance (asymmetrical). **C,** Eccentric one-leg squat.

- Lateral left (L) and "freeze"
- R/L/R and "freeze"
- L/R/L and "freeze"
- Adding a 6-inch box to the above patterns represents increases in the complexity and intensity of each exercise

Practicing landing strategies is one example of controlled, proactive exercises. The therapist or coach should be looking to ensure that the athlete is not relying on the medial ligaments of the knee to support his or her body weight during the landing phase. Increased valgus at the knee and instability are two key indicators that the strength levels of the athletes are not adequate to be performing these exercises. The therapist or coach should also make sure the athletes are landing with their knees in a flexed position. Athletes who land in less than 45 degrees of knee flexion are known as "quadriceps dominant" and are not using their hamstrings to support their landing position. This is thought to be an indicator of potential anterior cruciate ligament (ACL) injury. When an athlete demonstrates sufficient body control in the previously mentioned exercises and has concurrently developed an adequate strength base, he or she will then progress to the following:

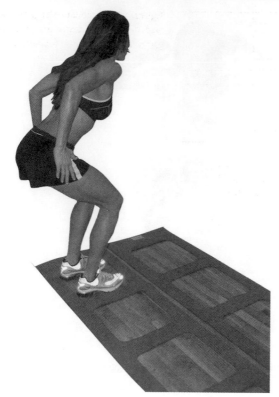

Figure 14-4 An athlete in position to begin a jump pattern in the 4-square formation.

- Advanced, controlled, proactive-type exercises—Repetitions of *preset* jump patterns (without "freeze" moments) that advance from FW/BK and L/R movement to adding diagonal patterns and foam barriers.
- Uncontrolled, reactive-type exercises—In this case the athlete progresses to situations in which he or she must control activity "reactively." The previously mentioned landing strategies and following jump patterns are examples of *controlled* movement patterns simply because the athlete initiates movement. In uncontrolled reactive exercises, the athlete reacts to a stimulus during eccentric, deceleration moments.[8] Using the four-square jump pattern as an example, the athlete would progress from preset jump patterns to random jump patterns "on command" by the coach. In this case the coach can combine both a visual and auditory stimulus to direct the athlete by "calling out" and pointing directions. *Note*: Other examples of controlled proactive versus uncontrolled reactive exercises would be balancing on a wobble board or mini-trampoline, then progressing to catching and throwing while two- and one-leg standing on the same apparatus, or progressing from lateral movement on a slide board to catching and throwing with lateral movement on the slide board.

OBJECTIVES FOR JUMP PATTERNS

Objectives for submaximal jump patterns include the following:

- Improved body control and movement in youth populations. These exercises are appropriate for young athletes who may lack the strength base or physical maturity to undergo the rigors of a maximal effort plyometric workout.
- In-season maintenance conditioning. These exercises are appropriate for collegiate and professional athletes "in season" who otherwise may lack adequate recovery time if performing maximal-effort plyometrics.
- Improve dynamic stabilization strength in knees, feet, and ankles. These exercises are prerequisites to agilities that require starts and stops, cuts, pivots, and changes of direction.

Footwork patterns with low-intensity plyometrics are common and found in special speed development programs. John Frappier, founder of Acceleration Products, created a program that includes the use of similar footwork patterns. Chu notes that the Frappier footwork patterns are based on the inverted funnel principle.[4] The inverted funnel principle is based on the premise that athletic movements require an individual to often move the feet out from under the body's center of gravity (COG) and then recover the position for a brief period so as to regain balance and stability. The essence of footwork drills is that they teach an athlete to maintain his or her body's COG in a relatively constant position, while the feet rapidly work out from under it in multiple directions. The result is improved proprioceptive awareness, or that sense of where the body is in relation to the environment.

INSTRUCTIONS FOR JUMP PATTERNS

The following jump patterns are low-intensity plyometrics that follow a natural progression to the exercises noted in *Landing Strategies*. Figure 14-4 shows an athlete in position to begin a jump-pattern in the four-square formation.

The body position in this figure is an example of the partial-squat position described earlier. Even though the athlete's feet will be traveling in and out of the boxes in prescribed patterns, the body's COG should remain constant. The partial squat position will allow an athlete to control the body's COG effectively during submaximal footwork drills. Refer to Figure 14-5 for an illustration of both the staggered-ladder and four-square patterns using two foam agility ladders, as well as the varied jump patterns in these formations. Note how the boxes are numbered (1 to 6 in the staggered-ladder and 1 to 4 in the four-square). The general rule for all patterns is to count "one" each time the athlete returns to the starting point. For example, when performing the staggered ladder pattern and going from box 1 to box 2, the scorer will count each time the athlete's foot or feet return to box 1. For box 1-2-3's pattern, again, count "1" each time the athlete's foot or feet return to box 1. In 1 to 6 for max-time (1, 2, 3, 4, 5, 6 formation), the athlete's COG should stay centered between the ladders as his or her feet jump from 1 to 6 and return 6 to 1 for max time. During the performance of these types of exercises, the therapist/coach can begin to note if any differences exist

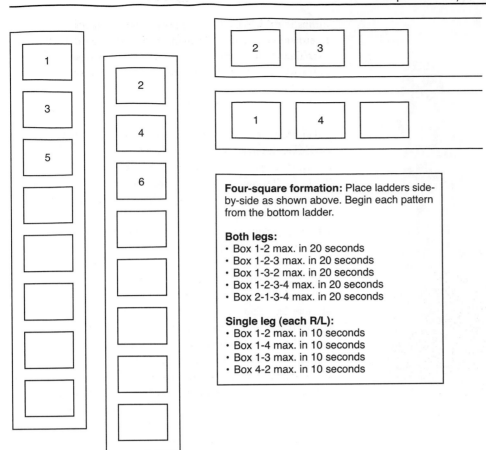

Figure 14-5 Both the staggered-ladder and 4-square patterns and the varied jump patterns in these formations.

Four-square formation: Place ladders side-by-side as shown above. Begin each pattern from the bottom ladder.

Both legs:
• Box 1-2 max. in 20 seconds
• Box 1-2-3 max. in 20 seconds
• Box 1-3-2 max. in 20 seconds
• Box 1-2-3-4 max. in 20 seconds
• Box 2-1-3-4 max. in 20 seconds

Single leg (each R/L):
• Box 1-2 max. in 10 seconds
• Box 1-4 max. in 10 seconds
• Box 1-3 max. in 10 seconds
• Box 4-2 max. in 10 seconds

Staggered ladder formation:
Ladders are side-by-side
2 inches apart. Perform 2 sets
of each of the following
exercises:
• Box 1-2 max. in 5 seconds
• Box 1-4 max. in 5 seconds
• Box 2-5 max. in 5 seconds
• Box 2-3-4 max. in 5 seconds
• Box 1-2-3 max. in 5 seconds
• Box 1-2-3-4-5-6 total time

between the legs. Consistent under performance on the right or left leg is yet another indicator of needed work or compensation to correct potential injury risk. The body is a system of balance, and both right and left legs should share fairly equal scores between them (within 90%) in order to ensure that an athlete is working as a balanced system.

When jumping foam barriers, the method of counting changes. Each "foot contact" is counted. Using the staggered ladders and box 1 to 2 jumps with a foam barrier, count "1" when the athlete contacts box 2 on the initial jump, count 2 when the athlete touches box 1 on the return trip, and continue in this manner for the remainder of the drill time (10 to 20 seconds). Figure 14-6 shows an athlete performing jump patterns using the staggered ladders.

Different-sized foam blocks can be used to increase the intensity of a "staggered" footwork pattern. This is particularly helpful in teaching an athlete to simply pick his or her feet

up in an "off-time" rhythm, or syncopated pattern. Using the staggered ladder pattern and (1, 2, 3, 4) as an example, an athlete develops a natural rhythm and pattern of movement while his or her feet move from box to box. After the athlete becomes familiar with the 1, 2, 3, 4 pattern under normal conditions (consistent spacing and jump heights between boxes), a 4-inch foam block can be placed between boxes 3 and 4, which will augment the athlete's previously learned pattern of movement and rhythm. Picture the athlete jumping a similar height and angular distance from 1 to 2 to 3, then having to quickly pick up his or her feet to clear a different height (of the foam block) from 3 to 4, and upon landing in box 4, "picking up" the feet again to change direction, landing in box 3, then continuing the return to box 1 under the normal dimensions of the jump pattern. Using the same pattern (1, 2, 3, 4), a 2-inch block can be placed between 1 and 2 and a 6-inch block between 3 and 4, which is another example of staggering

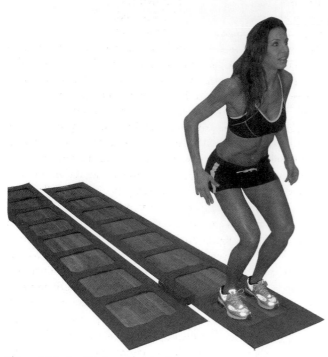

Figure 14-6 An athlete performing jump patterns using the staggered-ladder pattern.

jumps/footwork patterns and training in a syncopated rhythm. In either case, an athlete can improve body control by learning to maintain a rhythm during normal jump patterns, then progress to varied syncopated patterns using the foam blocks.

INTEGRATING FOOTWORK PATTERNS INTO SPEED DEVELOPMENT PROGRAMS

Table 14-2 shows examples of how to integrate low-intensity plyometrics into a strength and conditioning program designed for speed development over a 6-week period. In this sample program lower body (LB) strength training and plyometrics (PLYOS) are performed on Monday and Thursday, and upper body (UB) weight training and plyometrics are performed on Tuesday and Friday.

In Table 14-3 note the order and sequence of exercises on Monday and Thursday workouts. This sample program has LB strength training preceding LB plyometrics, followed by sprinting or multidirectional speed drills, or both, for three workouts (Monday, Thursday, and the following Monday). In this schedule, every other Thursday is a "measurement" day. On that day, the workout will *begin* with maximal-effort speed drills including sprinting, following a proper warm-up. In other words, every other Thursday is the day to measure progress and note improvements in speed including straight-ahead (sprinting over a specified distance) or lateral change of

Table 14-2	Weeks 1 and 3*			
Monday	**Tuesday**	**Wednesday**	**Thursday**	**Friday**
LB STRENGTH	UB WTS	SPORTS	LB STRENGTH	UB WTS
LB PLYOS	UB PLYOS	BALANCE	LB PLYOS	UB PLYOS
MAX SPEED & SPRINTING	AEROBIC	CORE 3	MAX SPEED & SPRINTING	AEROBIC
CORE 1	CORE 2		CORE 1	CORE 2

LB, Lower body; *UB,* upper body; *WTS,* weights.
*Follows the exercise order of strength, plyometrics, and sprinting.

Table 14-3	Weeks 2 and 4			
Monday	**Tuesday**	**Wednesday**	***Thursday**	**Friday**
LB STRENGTH	UB WTS	SPORTS	*MAX SPEED & SPRINTING	UB WTS
LB PLYOS	UB PLYOS	BALANCE	LB STRENGTH	UB PLYOS
MAX SPEED & SPRINTING	AEROBIC	CORE 3	LB PLYOS	AEROBIC
CORE 1	CORE 2		CORE 1	CORE 2

LB, Lower body; *UB,* upper body; *WTS,* weights.
*Tests and measurements day.

direction speed, such as the Edgren Side-Step test. The equipment required to administer the Edgren test are three cones and a stopwatch. Two cones should be placed 12 feet apart, and one cone should be in the center (Figure 14-7).

The Edgren test is performed as follows:
1. The athlete shuffles right and touches the base of the cone with his or her right hand.
2. Then he or she shuffles left past the center cone and touches the base of cone 2 with his or her left hand.
3. Then he or she shuffles right and finishes at the center cone (cone 3).

The athlete's foot needs to pass the lateral cones when shuffling L/R. The clock starts on the first move and stops when his or her foot passes the center cone at the finish. This test should be initiated in both right and left directions. The difference should not be greater than 0.2 second.

In this example the athlete *starts by shuffling right* from the center cone. This means the athlete only covers a 6-ft distance before changing direction and shuffling left to cone 2. The greater challenge will be to change direction at cone 2 after shuffling the full 12-ft distance. Testing the athlete starting in both directions and noting any differences is important. Differences could be quantitative (e.g., number based [time]) or qualitative (e.g., "awkward arm movements" or poor control of the body's COG, or both).

Rate	Score
Excellent	≤ 2 seconds
Average	≤ 2.5 seconds
Needs Improvement	> 2.6 seconds

Multiple methods can be used to test speed in linear, lateral-change-of-direction, and various multidirectional speed drills. This sample program provides for a test day to formally track data within a 4-week training period. The practitioner can choose which test seems appropriate for the conditions.

Following proper progression and a strategic plan based on an athlete's functional capacity and manipulating variables, such as intensity and work volume (refer to the earlier section on intensity and work volume), are important. Tables 14-2 and 14-3 show a sample off-season schedule in a cycled conditioning program. In the off season an athlete is not competing, and recovery between sessions is not a critical concern. In the off season performance enhancement can become a primary objective due to the extra time an athlete has to recover between workouts. When an athlete is in season, injury prevention becomes the primary objective of a strength and conditioning program. Additional information on this sample program is presented at the end of this chapter in Boxes 14-1 through 14-4. Box 14-1 details the aerobic and anaerobic work on Tuesday and Friday of the weekly program, and Box 14-2 provides a list of the strength training and plyometric exercises

Equipment: Three cones and a stopwatch. Place two cones 12-feet apart and one cone in the center.

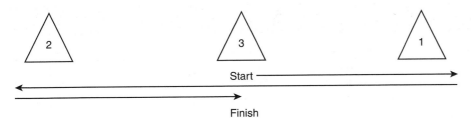

Figure 14-7 The Modified Edgren Test is a great exercise for measuring lateral change of direction.

In this example, the athlete *starts by shuffling right* from the center cone. This means he or she covers only a 6-foot distance before changing direction and shuffling left to cone 2. In the above example, the greater challenge will be to change direction at cone 2 after shuffling the full 12-foot distance. It is important to test the athlete starting in both directions and note any differences. Differences could be quantitative, or numbers-based (time) or qualitative, such as "awkward arm movements" or poor control of the body's center of gravity. The Edgren Side-Step test is performed as follows:

1. The athlete shuffles right and touches the base of the cone with his or her right hand.
2. Then the athlete shuffles left past the center cone and touches the base of cone 2 with his or her left hand.
3. Then the athlete shuffles right and finishes at the center cone (cone 3).

The athlete's foot needs to pass the lateral cones when shuffling left/right. The clock starts on his or her first move and stops when his or her foot passes the center cone at the finish. Perform this test initiating both right and left directions. The difference should not be greater than 0.2 second.

Rate	Score
Excellent	≤2.0 seconds
Average	≤2.5 seconds
Needs Improvement	>2.6 seconds

for lower body on Monday/Thursday and upper body on Tuesday/Friday. Trunk conditioning exercises and sports balance training can be found in Boxes 14-3 and 14-4.

CONCLUSION

Plyometric training can be a wonderful adjunct to the athlete who is rehabilitating from injury and attempting to return to play. The expected demands on high-end athletes today are exceptional. Reduced down time from injury, early return to play, minimizing opportunities for reinjury, and performance at a consistent level equal to or higher than before the onset of the injury are all expectations that are placed on today's athletes. When properly introduced to younger athletes, plyometrics can be the tool that leads to increased confidence and satisfaction with sport activity through the positive feedback that occurs with accomplishing new tasks, setting higher scores for oneself, and correcting imbalances within the musculoskeletal system. All of these can have a motivating effect on young athletes attempting to engage in competitive sports for the first time.

A general strength base can and should be developed through exercises, such as step-ups and different types of squats, in which practicing landing strategies and dynamic postural control exercises can develop greater body control.

The balance between qualitative and quantitative measures of performance is important. Using the staggered-ladder formation or maintaining a relatively centered COG as the feet move quickly from box to box is a "qualitative" measure in low-level plyometrics (i.e., inverted funnel principle). Quantitative measures with low-level plyometrics include monitoring work volume per session and following a logical and strategic progression throughout a training period. Work volume can be measured through actual "foot contacts," and the number of foot contacts prescribed can be based on the athlete's skill level, the intensities of combined plyometrics in one workout (low, moderate, high), and seasonal period (in season vs. off season).

Foam ladders and blocks also contribute to a safe environment, should an athlete land on the blocks/ladders. Adequate space and a yielding surface are additional safety points to consider when performing jump patterns.

Finally, the effectiveness of a plyometric workout should not be measured by "how tired" an athlete feels. The "quality" of the movement is still the most crucial factor in development of the neuromuscular system as a whole. The "quantity" above "quality" approach may lead to overtraining, exercise-related pain, and even overuse injuries. Structure and accountability are necessary when including plyometric exercises in rehabilitation and strength and conditioning programs, but the overall impression should be the satisfaction of the client/athlete as the end result.

BOX 14-1   Sample Program: Aerobic and Anaerobic Conditioning Defined

Weeks 2 and 4

Monday	Tuesday	Wednesday	Thursday	Friday
LB STRENGTH	UB WTS	SPORTS	LB STRENGTH	UB WTS
LB PLYOS	UB PLYOS	BALANCE	LB PLYOS	UB PLYOS
MAX SPEED & SPRINTING	AEROBIC	CORE 3	MAX SPEED & SPRINTING	AEROBIC
CORE 1	CORE 2		CORE 1	CORE 2

Monday/Thursday—Max Speed and Sprinting

Monday—Quality work: start-speed, speed acceleration, form running, lateral speed
1. Treadmill protocol (high-speed treadmill, sample workout)
    a. 10 mph @ 5% incline, 30 sec work: 30 sec rest × 2R
    b. 10 mph @ 10% incline, 20 sec work: 40 sec rest × 4R
    c. 12 mph @ 10% incline, 12 sec work: 40 sec rest × 4R
    d. 14 mph @ 12% incline, 8 sec work: 35 to 40 sec rest × 4R
    e. Stretch briefly and finish with retrograde treadmill walking, 2.5 mph @ 15% incline, 60 sec work: 60 sec rest × 3 to 4R
2. "Starts" on the ground—20 yd "starts" × 6 to 10R
3. Edgren side-step—8R, 4R each direction (start right × 4R, start left × 4R)
Thursday—Sport-Specific Speed (using an infielder in baseball as an example)
1. 90-ft sprints × 5R (a "single"—distance to first base)
2. 180-ft sprints × 5R (a "double"—two-base run)
3. Edgren side-step—8R, 4R each direction (start right × 4R, start left × 4R)

Tuesday/Friday—Aerobic Conditioning

Tuesday—Stationary bike 20 minutes
Friday—Indoor "triathlete" workout (Run, Bike, Row—10 minutes each) 30 minutes total

R, Repetitions.

BOX 14-2   Strength Training and Plyometrics Defined

Weeks 2 and 4

Monday	Tuesday	Wednesday	Thursday	Friday
LB STRENGTH	UB WTS	SPORTS	MAX SPEED & SPRINTING	UB WTS
LB PLYOS	UB PLYOS	BALANCE	LB STRENGTH	UB PLYOS
MAX SPEED & SPRINTING	AEROBIC	CORE 3	LB PLYOS	AEROBIC
CORE 1	CORE 2		CORE 1	CORE 2

Monday/Thursday–Lower Body Strength and Plyometrics

1. Functional leg circuit (walking lunge, lateral lunge, one-leg squat): 1 × 10R each
2. Complex training—Barbell squat with squat jumps: 2 × 10R each
3. One-leg dead lift with split squat jumps: 2 × 10R each
4. Leg curl (two legs up on concentric/one leg down on eccentric): 2 × 10R
5. Low-intensity plyometrics—four-square pattern: "Full Circuit"

Tuesday/Friday–Upper Body Strength and Plyometrics

1. Lat pull down: 2 × 10R
2. Seated row: 2 × 10R
3. Complex training set—bench press with med-ball chest pass: 2 × 10R each
4. Deltoid and rotator cuff circuit
   a. Off-set pushups on med-ball, plyo-pushups on med-ball: 2 × 10R each
   b. Lateral raise, full can (scaption), D2 pattern: 2 × 10R each
   c. Prone fly on phys-ball, sidelying external rotation: 2 × 10R each
   (use "cuff weights," or wrist weights for b. and c. exercises)
5. Biceps curl with dumbbells/triceps extension with cable: 2 × 10R each
6. Forearm circuit—(flexion/extension, supination/pronation radial/ulnar deviation): 2 × 10R each

BOX 14-3   Trunk Conditioning Defined

CORE 1, 2, and 3 Workouts

Monday	Tuesday	Wednesday	Thursday	Friday
LB STRENGTH	UB WTS	SPORTS	LB STRENGTH	UB WTS
LB PLYOS	UB PLYOS	BALANCE	LB PLYOS	UB PLYOS
MAX SPEED & SPRINTING	AEROBIC	CORE 3	MAX SPEED & SPRINTING	AEROBIC
CORE 1	CORE 2		CORE 1	CORE 2

CORE 1 = Phys-ball trunk exercises

1. Trunk curl: 2 × 20R
2. Trunk curl w/twist: 2 × 20R
3. Reverse curl (on floor, legs "gripping" ball): 2 × 20R
4. Prone pushup position on phys-ball—hands on ball, attain and maintain neutral spine/pelvis, therapist performs "rhythmic beats" on phys-ball/perturbations

CORE 2 = Med-ball trunk exercises on the floor

1. Trunk curl w/med-ball, legs elevated: 1 × 20R
2. Pullover with med-ball–to-cycling legs: 1 × 20R
3. Situp with twist (pullover with med-ball and twist, slow eccentric): 1 × 20R
4. Reverse curl (med-ball between knees): 1 × 20R
5. Russian twists with med-ball: 1 × 20R

CORE 3 = Standing med-ball exercises (e.g., chops, throws)

1. Step-to-lunge with chest pass: 2 × 10R
2. Step-to-lunge, "catch," diagonal chop and throw: 2 × 10R
3. Trunk twists with throw (off wall or rebounder): 2 × 10R

BOX 14-4	Sports Balance Training Defined

Wednesday (and Saturday optional)

Monday	Tuesday	Wednesday	Thursday	Friday
LB STRENGTH	UB WTS	*SPORTS	MAX SPEED & SPRINTING	UB WTS
LB PLYOS	UB PLYOS	BALANCE	LB STRENGTH	UB PLYOS
MAX SPEED & SPRINTING	AEROBIC	CORE 3	LB PLYOS	AEROBIC
CORE 1	CORE 2		CORE 1	CORE 2

Wednesday–Sports Balance Training

Note: Wednesday is scheduled for sports balance training and core work only. "CORE 3" is repeated to give a greater perspective on the work for that day.

1. Balance beam circuit:
   a. Step-lunge on beam: 1 × 10R
   b. Lateral squat walk on beam: 1 × 10R
   c. One-leg stance—reaches on beam: 1 × 10R
   d. Heel-raise on beam—2-legs-to-1-leg: 1 × 10R
   e. One-leg stance on mini-trampoline—multidirectional "ball toss" (catch and throw): 2 × 10R
   f. Kneel on phys-ball (neutral spine/pelvis), multidirectional "ball toss" (catch and throw): 2 × 10R
2. *CORE 3 = Standing med-ball exercises (e.g., chops, throws)
   a. Step-to-lunge with chest pass: 2 × 10R
   b. Step-to-lunge, "catch," diagonal chop and throw: 2 × 10R
   c. Trunk twists with throw (off wall or rebounder): 2 × 10R

REFERENCES

1. Tippett SR, Voight ML: *Functional progressions for sport rehabilitation*, Champaign, Ill, 1995, Human Kinetics.
2. Voight ML, Draovitch P: Plyometrics. In Albert M, editor: *Eccentric muscle training in sports and orthopedics*, New York, 1991, Churchill Livingstone.
3. Clark MA, Wallace TWA: Plyometric training with elastic resistance. In Page P, Ellenbecker T, editors: *The scientific and clinical application of elastic resistance*, Champaign, Ill, 2003, Human Kinetics.
4. Chu DA: *Jumping into plyometrics*, ed 2, Champaign, Ill, 1998, Human Kinetics.
5. Lindstedt SL, LaSatyo PC, Reich TE: When active muscles lengthen: properties and consequences of eccentric contractions, *News Physiological Sci* December:256-261, 2001.
6. LaStayo PC, Woolf JM, Lewek MD, et al: Eccentric muscle contractions: their contribution to injury, prevention, rehabilitation, and sport, *J Orthop Sports Phys Ther* 33(10):57-571, 2003.
7. Button SL: Closed kinetic chain training. In Hall C, Brody L, editors: *Therapeutic exercise: moving toward function*, Philadelphia, 1999, Lippincott Williams & Wilkins.
8. Ellenbecker TS, Davies GJ: Closed kinetic chain exercises, Champaign, Ill, 2001, Human Kinetics.

15

Wendy J. Hurd
and Lynn Snyder-Mackler

Neuromuscular Training

LEARNING OBJECTIVES

After studying this chapter, the reader will be able to do the following:

1. Discuss the importance of proprioception in the lower limb and upper limb
2. Describe the components of the sensorimotor system
3. Discuss the role of the sensorimotor system in neuromuscular control
4. Define postural control and describe how postural control is achieved in stance and gait
5. Identify techniques used for assessment of neuromuscular function
6. Discuss the various effects an injury may have on neuromuscular function
7. Summarize the purpose(s) and components of a neuromuscular training program

Neuromuscular control involves the subconscious integration of sensory information that is processed by the central nervous system, resulting in controlled movement through coordinated muscle activity.[1] Dynamic joint stability and postural control are the result of coordinated muscle activity achieved through neuromuscular control. Any injury that disrupts the mechanoreceptors, alters normal sensory input, or interferes with the processing of sensory information may result in altered (also referred to as *decreased* or *dysfunctional*) neuromuscular control. Consequently, impairments of the neuromuscular system often result in dysfunctional dynamic joint stability and postural control. Neuromuscular control impairments can also change movement patterns and increase the risk for musculoskeletal injury. Conversely, musculoskeletal injury, by disrupting the interactions within the neuromuscular system, can be a cause of altered neuromuscular control. The authors believe an understanding of the neuromuscular control system and the functional manifestations of neuromuscular control are fundamental to designing effective treatment programs and meaningful research studies related to dynamic joint stability.

PROPRIOCEPTION

Why can one baseball pitcher exhibit excessive glenohumeral motion yet never experience injury, while another pitcher with the same glenohumeral motion require surgery in order to throw effectively without pain? Why does one athlete experience a single-episode lateral ankle sprain, while the next athlete develops chronic ankle instability? The answer to both questions is most commonly proprioception. For the healthy athlete, high levels of proprioception can contribute to enhanced neuromuscular control and functional joint stability, thus decreasing the risk for injury. For the injured athlete, restoration of proprioception is critical to ward off repetitive injury (Figure 15-1). Therefore proprioceptive training plays a key role for the athlete in both injury prevention and rehabilitation.

Proprioception may be inferred from Sherrington's 1906 description of the "proprioceptive-system" as the afferent information from proprioceptors (e.g., mechanoreceptors) located in the proprioceptive field that contributes to conscious sensations, total posture, and segmental posture.[2,3] Proprioception is a product of sensory information gathered by mechanoreceptors.[2] This definition views proprioception primarily as a sensory activity. More recently, authors have expanded the definition of the proprioceptive system to include the complex interaction between the sensory pathways and the motor pathway (efferent system).[4] One assumption underlying both definitions of proprioception is that incoming sensory information processed by the central nervous system (CNS) has not been compromised. In the presence of an injury that disrupts mechanoreceptor input, proprioceptive function will be compromised and may lead to movement dysfunction.

Over the years, many terms have been used either synonymously with proprioception or to describe proprioception including *kinesthesia, joint position sense, joint stability,* and *postural control.* Kinesthesia and joint position sense may both be viewed as submodalities of proprioception.[3] *Kinesthesia* refers to the sensation of joint movement (both active and passive), while joint position sense refers to the sensation of joint

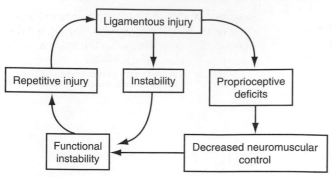

Figure 15-1 Functional stability paradigm depicting the progression of functional instability due to the interaction between mechanical stability and decreased neuromuscular control. (From Lephart S, Reimann B, Fu F: *Proprioception and neuromuscular control in joint stability*, Champaign, Ill, 2000, Human Kinetics.

position.[3] Joint stability is accomplished through both passive (osseous congruity and ligamentous restraints) and dynamic (coordinated muscle contractions) mechanisms. Dynamic joint stability is the result of neuromuscular control and proprioception, while postural control is the result of integrated visual, vestibular, and proprioceptive inputs.[5,6] Consequently, any disruption in mechanoreceptor input that affects proprioception will negatively affect dynamic joint stability and posture.

SENSORIMOTOR SYSTEM

The sensory organs in the neuromuscular system are referred to as *mechanoreceptors*. Sensitive to various forms of mechanical deformation including tension, compression, and loading rate, these small sensors are located in various connective tissues throughout the body. The three classifications of mechanoreceptors are based on tissue location: joint receptors, cutaneous (skin) receptors, and muscle receptors.

Joint Receptors

Ruffini receptor endings are described as slowly adapting mechanoreceptors because they continue their discharge in response to a continuous stimulus.[7] These receptors have a low activation threshold and are active during both static and dynamic joint conditions. Consequently, Ruffini endings may signal static joint position, intraarticular pressure, and amplitude and velocity of joint rotations.[7-10]

Golgi tendon organ-like receptors are the largest of the articular mechanoreceptors. They are also slow to adapt to stimuli, have a high activation threshold, and are active only during dynamic joint states. Some researchers have suggested that the high threshold of the Golgi tendon organ-like ending makes this receptor ideally suited for sensing the extremes of the joint's normal movement range.[11] The Golgi and Ruffini endings belong to a group called *spray endings*. Collectively, these mechanoreceptors represent a virtually continuous morphological spectrum of receptors.[12] Whether the spray endings should be divided into distinct receptor types has not been resolved.

Pacinian corpuscles are the only rapidly adapting joint receptor. Sensitive to low levels of mechanical stress, the Pacinian corpuscle is active only during dynamic joint states. Therefore this receptor is silent during static conditions and constant velocity situations but is sensitive to joint acceleration and deceleration.[13]

Free nerve endings constitute the fourth type of joint receptor. Free nerve endings are widely distributed throughout most joint structures. These receptors are typically inactive during normal activities, but when activated by high levels of noxious stimuli they are slow to adapt during both static and dynamic states.

Cutaneous Receptors

Sensory information from cutaneous (skin) receptors is processed by the CNS in conjunction with joint and muscle receptors. The role of cutaneous receptors in initiating reflexive responses, such as the flexion withdrawal reflex in response to potentially harmful stimuli, is well established.[15] Cutaneous receptors may also signal information regarding joint position and kinesthesia when the skin is stretched.[15,16] However, no evidence indicates that these receptors contribute significantly to these sensations[17] or that cutaneous receptors contribute to joint stability.[18]

Muscle Receptors

The muscle spindle and the Golgi tendon organ (GTO) are the two primary types of muscle receptors.[15] The muscle spindle lies in parallel with extrafusal muscle fibers and has three main components: (1) intrafusal muscle fibers, (2) sensory axons that wrap around the intrafusal fibers and project afferent information to the CNS when stimulated, and (3) motor axons that innervate the intrafusal fibers and regulate the sensitivity of the muscle spindle[1,15,19,20] (Figure 15-2). The primary sensory axons from the spindle make monosynaptic connections with alpha motoneurons in the ventral roots of the spinal cord that, in turn, innervate the muscle where the muscle spindle is located.[1] Collectively, this feedback loop is called the *muscle stretch reflex*.[15] Although extrafusal muscle fibers comprise the bulk of the muscle responsible for generating force and are innervated by alpha motoneurons, intrafusal fibers are composed of a small bundle of modified muscle fibers that function to provide feedback to the CNS and are innervated by gamma motoneurons.[21] Sensitivity of the muscle spindle is continually modulated by the gamma motor system. This allows the spindle to be functional at all times during a contraction[21] and modulate muscle length.[15,22-24] Sensory output from the muscle spindle is triggered at low thresholds, is slowly adapting, and senses joint position throughout the range of motion.[15,20]

The GTO is located at the musculotendinous junction and is positioned in series with extrafusal muscle fibers and tendon. A single axon enters the GTO and then branches into many unmyelinated endings that are woven in and between the collagen fibers at the musculotendinous junction. Thus during a muscle contraction the tendon is stretched, straightening the

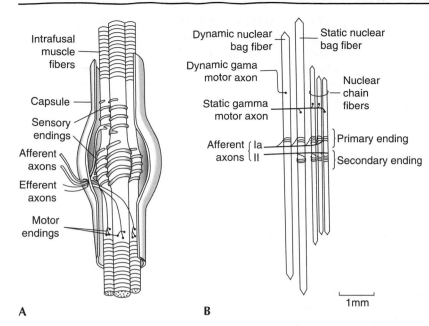

Figure 15-2 A, Gross structure. **B,** Structure and innervation of the intrafusal fibers of the muscle spindle. (From Williams GN, Chmielewski T, Rudolph K, et al: *J Orthop Sports Phys Ther* 31:546-566, 2001.)

collagen fibers and distorting the receptor endings of the GTO afferent neurons.[25] Increased activity of the GTO afferents results in inhibition of the motor neurons innervating the muscles that were stretched while exciting the motor nerves of the antagonistic muscles. This feedback loop is often referred to as the *inverse myotatic reflex*. Because each organ is connected to a small number of muscle fibers and can respond to low levels of force (as little as 0.1 g),[22] the GTO can provide the CNS with specific force feedback.[22-24]

Motor Response Pathways

Sensory information gathered by mechanoreceptors is sent to the spinal cord via afferent pathways for processing and ultimately results in a regulation of reflexes and muscle activity. In addition to being influenced by incoming afferent information, the resulting motor response also depends on the level of processing of afferent inputs within the CNS. The processing can occur at three different levels: the spinal cord, the brainstem and cerebellum, and the cerebral cortex (Table 15-1).

Spinal reflexes represent the shortest neuronal pathways, and consequently the most rapid responses to afferent stimuli. These responses are typically uniform in nature and modified by the intensity of the afferent signals.[15] Spinal reflexes range from simple monosynaptic reflexes to complex multisynaptic circuits resulting in coordinated activity of groups of muscles.[13,15,26] The speed of spinal reflexes is faster than ligamentous failure, yet is not considered modifiable through training to aid in dynamic joint stability.[27,28]

Sensory information mediated at the brainstem and cerebellum is typically referred to as a *long-loop reflex*.[27-29] Because sensory information travels a greater distance before being processed, these responses are typically longer than spinal reflexes. However, because these pathways are multisynaptic with potentially more sources of sensory input, long-loop reflexes are flexible and may adapt when feed-forward informa-

Table 15-1 Motor Response Intervals

Motor Response Type	Level of Mediation	Able To Be Modified
Spinal reflexes	Segmental level of spinal cord	No
Long-loop reflexes	Brainstem and cerebellum	No
Triggered reactions	Cortical centers	Yes
Voluntary reactions	Cortical centers	Yes

tion is provided to the system.[27,28,30] As a result of both the adaptability and the relative quickness with which they occur, these pathways are thought to be important in the maintenance of dynamic joint stability.[1,31]

Both voluntary reactions and triggered reactions are processed at the cortical level of the brain and represent the longest motor response times. Voluntary reactions involve the processing of multiple variables and are highly flexible.[27,28,32] In contrast, "triggered" reactions represent preprogrammed, coordinated reactions that occur in response to afferent stimuli that trigger them into action.[1,28] One example of a triggered reaction has been termed *the wine glass effect*[28]: When one holds an expensive wine glass, one instinctively tightens the grip on it if the glass begins to slip. The cutaneous message that the object is slipping comes from the fingertips, but the muscle response to increase grip pressure comes from the forearm. In this case the reaction occurs quickly, is probably not conscious in nature, and appears to have the overall purpose of reorganizing the system slightly to complete an action successfully. Because of their preprogrammed nature, triggered reactions occur slightly more quickly than voluntary reactions but may be unable to accommodate to circumstances in atypical situations.[1]

POSTURAL CONTROL

Postural control involves controlling the body's position in space for the dual purposes of stability (balance) and orientation (maintaining an appropriate relationship between the body segments and between the body and the environment for a task).[6,33] The postural control system uses complex processes involving both sensory and motor components and results from the combined integration of visual, vestibular, and proprioceptive afferent inputs.[5,6] The combined effort of these sensory modalities lays the framework for dynamic balance (stability). If feedback from any one of these modalities is impaired, then postural stability suffers.[1]

Investigators have identified several postural control strategies that result from different types of perturbations applied during stance. Typically, if forward sway is induced as a result of a posterior horizontal perturbation, muscles on the posterior aspect of the body are recruited.[34] Conversely, if backward sway is induced from an anterior horizontal perturbation, muscles on the anterior aspect of the body are recruited.[34] Additionally, small perturbations applied during standing result in sway at the ankle joint; this is called an ankle strategy.[35] On the other hand, large perturbations result in large movements at the hip; this is called a *hip strategy*.[35] The hip strategy is also implemented when the individual cannot generate enough force with the ankle strategy. A third strategy called the *stepping strategy* is implemented when the perturbation displaces the center of mass outside the individual's base of support.[6] Postural control strategies can be modified and are adaptive to the circumstances of the moment; however, in the absence of other instructions they are predictable.[6] Evidence suggests that a person's expectations of impending perturbations and training can have a significant impact on the magnitude and variability of the responses.[6] These postural control strategies provide stability in stance and therefore are applicable to the maintenance of joint stability in the lower extremity during stance.[1]

The motor skills that people perform daily including walking pose a complicated problem for the neuromuscular system because many muscles crossing multiple joints must be coordinated to produce a given outcome. Bernstein[36] called this the "degrees of freedom problem." One theory for controlling the degrees of freedom problem is based on the concept of motor programs (a set of commands that are prestructured at higher brain centers and define the essential details of a skilled action). The most recent update to this theory, put forth by Schmidt,[28] contends that features that do not vary among different skills—the relative timing, force, or sequence of components—are stored in memory as motor programs, while the parameters that do vary (e.g., speed or duration) are specified according to the task at hand. These programs are under central control and are generally not dependent on feedback from the periphery.[28] Feedback is, however, used to select the appropriate motor program, monitor whether the movement is in keeping with the program, and reflexively modulate the movement when necessary.[27,28]

The idea of a central pattern generator is similar in concept to a motor program. These control mechanisms located in the spinal cord produce mainly genetically defined, repetitive actions, such as gait.[37] The concept of the central pattern generator is supported by animal studies including spinalized models, which have shown that the rhythmic pattern of gait can continue in the absence of feedback from the limbs or descending control from the brain.[38-40] Central pattern generators may be turned on or off by a variety of stimuli, although they are primarily stimulated or inhibited by signals originating in the brainstem.[39-41] Although gait is centrally controlled at the lower brain and spinal cord level, descending influences from higher brain centers including the cerebellum, visual cortex, hippocampus, and frontal cortex, along with peripheral sensory input, permit effective gait even when unexpected changes in the environment are encountered.[6,27,28] Thus gait is controlled through the complex interaction of central pattern generators, descending input from higher brain centers, and feedback from peripheral sensory receptors. Through this complex interaction and similar processes that occur with other motor programs, the neuromuscular system acts to maintain joint stability during dynamic situations.[1]

ASSESSMENT OF NEUROMUSCULAR FUNCTION

Following injury, assessment of neuromuscular function is necessary to determine if impairments are present, aid in the development of an appropriate treatment intervention, and assess the effectiveness of the intervention.[1] Various analysis techniques are available for testing neurosensory components (e.g., kinesthesia) and neuromuscular performance (e.g., biomechanical gait analysis). Readily available clinical assessment techniques include joint position (JPS) testing; observational analysis; functional testing, such as hop testing; and threshold to detection of passive motion (TTDPM) testing. Stabilometry and strength testing are common clinical assessment techniques that are performed with the aid of commercially available equipment.

Other techniques for identifying neuromuscular control deficits include kinetic and kinematic evaluation with motion analysis, force plates, and electromyography. These measures are more commonly used in the laboratory versus the clinical setting. An advantage to these laboratory testing techniques includes a high level of precision and sensitivity, allowing the investigator to identify complex yet often subtle neuromuscular dysfunction. Because of the variety of testing methods and strategies available, it is important that clinicians and scientists carefully consider the question they are trying to answer when selecting neuromuscular assessment methods.[1]

EFFECT OF INJURY ON NEUROMUSCULAR FUNCTION

The effects of injury on the neuromuscular system have been assessed in many studies. Receiving the most attention in the

Table 15-2	Screening Tool Selection Criteria for Rehabilitation Candidate Classification

Episodes of Giving Way since Initial Injury ≤1
Timed Hop Test score ≥80%
KOS-ADL score ≥80%
Global Rating score ≥60%

KOS-ADL, Knee Outcome Survey–Activities of Daily Living.

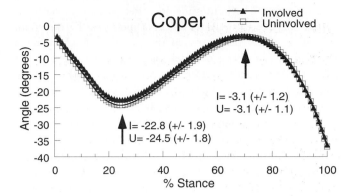

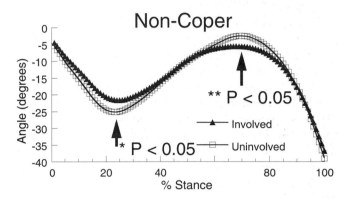

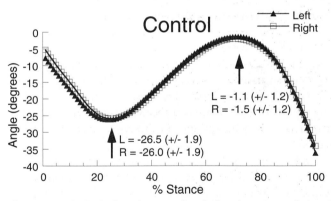

Figure 15-3 Sagittal plane knee angles during the stance phase of walking in copers *(top)*, noncopers *(middle)*, and uninjured *(bottom)* subjects. (*I,* Involved; *U,* uninvolved). The noncopers demonstrate a reduced knee angle, although the copers maintain knee angles that are similar to both the uninvolved side and the knee angles of the uninjured subjects. *Significant differences at peak knee flexion. **Differences in peak knee extension on the injured vs. the uninjured limb.

literature is what neuromuscular adaptations occur in order to maintain dynamic joint stability following ligament injury. Injury to the anterior cruciate ligament (ACL) is a common ligament injury and typically requires surgical reconstruction and prolonged rehabilitation for a return to preinjury activity levels. This section focuses on specific neuromuscular adaptations that occur following ACL injury. The subsequent section addresses the design and implementation of a training program to improve neuromuscular function following ACL injury.

Some individuals can stabilize their knees following ACL rupture, even during activities involving cutting and pivoting, although most experience instability with daily activities.[42] Because there can be vast differences in functional outcome following ACL injury, we have developed a classification scheme at the University of Delaware to improve studies of knee stabilization strategies in patients following ACL rupture. Those patients with ACL rupture who returned to activities involving cutting, jumping, or pivoting for a minimum of 1 year and had not experienced knee instability were classified as "copers," and those who experienced episodes of giving way were classified as "noncopers."[42] Potential copers are individuals identified early after injury through a screening process (Table 15-2) who have the potential to develop dynamic knee stability.[43] Once a potential coper returns to preinjury, high-level activities for a minimum of 1 year without experiencing episodes of giving way, the potential coper is classified as a coper.

The authors have conducted research to delineate knee stabilization strategies of copers, potential copers, and noncopers. Copers use strategies involving more coordinated muscle activation that stabilize the knee without compromising knee motion.[44,45] An analysis of movement patterns during walking and jogging shows that copers have sagittal plane knee motions and moments during weight acceptance that are similar to uninjured individuals[44,45] (Figure 15-3). Copers do have differences in onset timing and magnitude of muscle activity when compared with uninjured subjects. These alterations in muscle activity allow copers to stabilize their knees while maintaining normal movement patterns.[45] However, no single pattern has been adopted by the copers; individuals adopt idiosyncratic compensation patterns that are related to rate of muscle activation and *unrelated* to quadriceps strength[42,44] or knee laxity.[42]

Conversely, noncopers adopt a remarkably limited strategy to stabilize their knees across activities with widely differing demands on the knee.[44-46] The pattern is a robust stiffening strategy that includes reduced knee motion, reduced internal knee extension moment, distribution of support moment away from the knee, slower muscle activation, and generalized co-contraction of the muscles that cross the knee. This pattern is present in activities ranging from walking to jumping.[45-47] Rudolph hypothesized that this reduced knee motion and internal knee extensor moment during weight acceptance, which has been observed by other researchers,[48] is the hallmark of a noncoper. The joint stiffening strategy seen in the noncopers may reflect the early stages of motor skill acquisition. Vereijken et al[49] demonstrated that individuals often freeze the degrees of freedom of a task via massive co-contraction of muscles. As the skill level improves, joint stiffening gives way to a larger variety of movements and more selective motor responses during the activity. The muscle co-contraction strategy seen in the noncopers reflects an unsophisticated adaptation to the ACL rupture for which appropriate muscle activation strategies to dynamically stabilize the injured knee have not yet developed. The authors speculate that the noncopers' stiffening strategy bodes poorly for long-term joint integrity and that it could contribute to the high incidence of early-onset knee osteoarthritis in individuals following ACL rupture.

Recent research at the University of Delaware has illuminated a short-term differential response to acute ACL injuries, which the authors believe is based on the potential for the neuromuscular system to reorganize appropriate responses soon after injury in order to better stabilize the knee. Potential copers are identified through a screening process to determine which patients are appropriate candidates for nonoperative rehabilitation.[43] The screening tool was validated on 93 consecutive patients with acute ACL rupture.[50] Thirty-nine subjects (42%) met the criteria for classification as appropriate rehabilitation candidates, and 28 of these elected to pursue nonoperative management. Of those subjects participating in nonoperative rehabilitation, 79% were successful in returning to preinjury activity levels for a short time. Success was defined as the absence of giving way on return to activity. The results demonstrate that the high success rate of nonoperative management appears to be contingent on appropriate rehabilitation candidates.

Evidence Based Clinical Application: Screening Examination to Identify Rehabilitation Candidates after Anterior Cruciate Ligament Screening

ACL screening can identify individuals who have the potential to develop good dynamic knee stability after participating in a neuromuscular training program and return to preinjury activity levels without surgical reconstruction. Before patients can be screened, they must have full active knee range of motion, greater than or equal to 70% quadriceps strength on bilateral comparison, and no swelling. Exclusion from a nonoperative course includes no concomitant ligament injuries, no repairable meniscal tears, no pain with hopping, and no full-thickness articular cartilage lesions. Screening components and passing criteria may be found in Table 15-2.

Subsequent studies have since identified characteristics of the potential coper before and after specialized rehabilitation to determine which neuromuscular adaptations are occurring to aid in the development of dynamic joint stability. If the hallmark of the noncoper is reduced knee motion and reduced internal knee extension moment during weight acceptance, the potential copers appear to be intermediate to noncopers and uninjured subjects.[51] Before training, potential copers stiffen their knees with significantly higher muscle co-contraction and slightly lower peak knee flexion angles. These altered movement patterns indicate an undeveloped knee stabilization strategy. After perturbation training, potential copers can increase knee flexion during weight acceptance and reduce the level of muscle co-contraction; they became more similar to uninjured subjects.[51] An increase in knee flexion after training in conjunction with a decrease in rigid muscle co-contraction indicates the adoption of a movement pattern that is consistent with clinical findings of improved dynamic knee stability.

NEUROMUSCULAR TRAINING PROGRAMS

Like the injury research, studies assessing the effectiveness of neuromuscular training programs have predominantly investigated individuals with ACL injuries as their subjects.[50,52-55] The purpose of the training program may be to prevent injury or to return the injured patient to preinjury activities either nonoperatively or postoperatively. Several training techniques have been used including balance training, functional training (jump and agility drills), technique instruction, and perturbation training.[50,52,54,56,57]

Injury-Prevention Training Programs

Multiple training programs have been shown to be effective in reducing injury rates.[56-60] Retrospective analysis has suggested that body positioning during noncontact ACL injury includes external rotation of the tibia, the knee in close-to-full extension, the foot planted, and limb deceleration followed by a valgus collapse.[61] Hewett et al[62] have termed this collective positioning of the lower extremity *dynamic valgus*. Both male and female athletes commonly adopt similar dynamic valgus body alignment during competitive play,[63] and with sufficient neuromuscular control, knee stability can be maintained without ACL injury.[64] Female athletes often demonstrate insufficient neuromuscular control during performance of high-risk maneuvers, which may result in valgus collapse (Figure 15-4) and ACL rupture.[61,63,65] Neuromuscular imbalances that women may demonstrate include ligament dominance, quadriceps dominance, and leg dominance.[62] Evidence that neuromuscular training is effective in reducing neuromuscular imbalances and preventing ACL injuries is increasing.

Secondary to the high rate of noncontact ACL injuries among physically mature female athletes, many injury-prevention studies have focused on decreasing injury rates within this highly select population.[66] Henning identified potentially dangerous maneuvers in sports and recommended modifications of these potentially dangerous athletic maneuvers that may contribute to ACL injury.[67] These recommendations included landing from a jump in a more bent-knee position and decelerating before a cutting maneuver. Early results have suggested that technique modifications are successful in decreasing injury rates among trained subjects. Hewett et al[57] later developed a

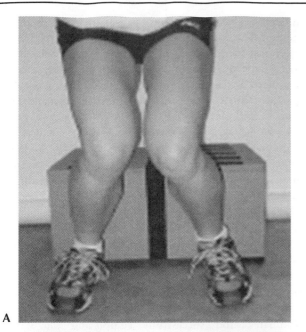

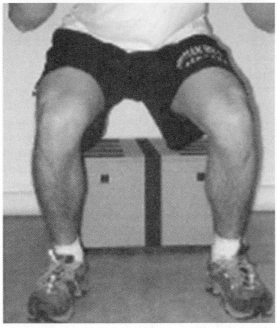

Figure 15-4 A, Valgus collapse position for a female athlete on jump landing secondary to poor neuromuscular control compared with **B,** good lower extremity limb positioning when landing from a jump for a male athlete. (From Hewett TE, Paterno MV, Myer GD: *Clin Orthop Relat Res* 402:76-94, 2002.)

training program that was based on a thorough review of the literature and prior athletic experience. Hewett's training program included an initial phase devoted to correcting jump and landing techniques in female athletes. Four basic techniques were stressed: (1) correct posture throughout the jump, (2) jumping straight up with no excessive side-to-side movement, (3) soft landings including toe-to-heel rocking and bent knees, and (4) instant recoil preparation for the next jump. Hewett's program was successful in reducing noncontact ACL injuries among trained women. The studies by both Henning[67] and

Hewett[57] demonstrate the importance of incorporating dynamic, biomechanically correct movements into training protocols aimed at injury prevention.[62]

In a prospective study of 300 semiprofessional male soccer players, Caraffa[56] demonstrated a significant reduction of ACL injury rates following participation in a balance-board program. The training consisted of 20 minutes of balance-board exercises divided into five phases. Athletes who participated in proprioception training before their competitive season had a significantly decreased rate of knee injuries. In an attempt to validate Caraffa's injury prevention program among a comparable cohort of female athletes, Soderman[68] implemented Caraffa's wobble board balance program with 221 female soccer players. In contrast to Caraffa's results, Soderman found no difference between the control and intervention groups with respect to the number, incidence, or type of traumatic injuries of the lower extremities. Subsequently, Myklebust[59] examined the effects of a more comprehensive and dynamic neuromuscular training program on female athletes. Their program incorporated the wobble board protocol of Caraffa[56] and the techniques of Hewett[57] by adding a focus to improve awareness and knee control during standing, cutting, jumping, and landing. Myklebust was able to reduce the incidence of ACL injury in women's elite handball players over two consecutive seasons. These studies demonstrate the ability of a neuromuscular/balance component to reduce knee injury risk for athletes when incorporated into an injury prevention protocol.[62]

Evidence Based Clinical Application: Dynamic Neuromuscular Analysis

The Biodynamics Center at Cincinnati Children's Hospital has described a rationalized approach to address specific factors that may be evident in at-risk (for ACL injury) athletes.[62] Dynamic neuromuscular analysis is a synthesis of the most important findings derived from existing research studies and prevention techniques developed through more recent empirical and analytical evaluations of neuromuscular training and on-field play.[62] The three essential components of the comprehensive training program are *dynamic*: biomechanically correct movement skills; *neuromuscular*: patterning based on the identification of underlying neuromuscular imbalances; and constant biomechanical *analysis* by the instructor with feedback to athletes both during and after training. These training principles and techniques provide a general framework for clinicians who want to design and administer injury-prevention programs targeted to this population.

Nonoperative and Postoperative Training Programs

Training objectives for the ACL-injured patient include improving the nervous system's ability to generate fast and optimal muscle firing patterns, to increase dynamic joint stability, to decrease joint forces, and relearn movement patterns and skills.[69] Limited work has been done to evaluate the effectiveness of neuromuscular training in achieving these objectives among ACL-injured or reconstructed patients. Risberg[69] developed a neuromuscular training program for the ACL-reconstructed patient. The main areas considered when developing this program were ACL graft healing and ACL strain values during exercises, proprioception and neuromuscular control, and clinical studies on the effect of neuromuscular training programs. The program consists of balance exercises, plyometric exercises, agility drills, and sport-specific exercises. The program is divided into six phases, each 3 to 5 weeks in length. Progression through the program is criteria based and includes no increase in pain or swelling and the ability to maintain postural control of the position before movements are superimposed on the position. The scientific rationale underlying the program design, as well as the clinical assessment of patient performance and progression, are key components to the Risberg program. The effectiveness of this rehabilitation program is not known at this time; however, ongoing work is evaluating the effect of training on proprioception, balance, muscle activity patterns, muscle strength, and knee joint laxity.

Ihara and Nakayama[70] were the first to assess a neuromuscular training program consisting of balance and perturbation exercises among an ACL-deficient group. The experimental group consisted of four ACL-deficient female athletes who had suffered the sensation of "giving way" during sports activity. Training for the experimental group consisted of four training sessions per week for 3 months. Patients were compared with a control group of five subjects who did not participate in a training program. After training, the experimental group demonstrated significant improvement in peak torque time and rising torque value of the hamstrings compared with the control group. The authors concluded that simple muscle training does not increase the speed of muscular reaction, but dynamic joint control training has the potential to shorten the time lag of muscular reaction.

Beard[54] also studied the effects of neuromuscular training among ACL-deficient subjects. In this study 50 ACL-deficient patients were randomly assigned to either a neuromuscular and weight-training program, or a weight-training–only program. Neuromuscular training consisted of balance, dynamic stability, and perturbation training all performed in a weight-bearing position; the program was 1 hour in length and performed twice a week for 12 weeks. Results for the neuromuscular training group included significant improvement in Lysholm scoring and mean hamstring contraction latency compared with the weight-training–only group.

The studies by both Ihara[70] and Beard[54] underscore the importance of neuromuscular training in promoting components of dynamic joint stability. Neither study, however, assessed the effectiveness of neuromuscular training in returning patients to preinjury activities. Fitzgerald[50] used return to sport as the primary outcome measure after a select group of ACL-deficient patients (potential copers identified through a screening process) had participated in either a traditional or perturbation-enhanced training program. The traditional training performed by both groups included lower extremity resistance training and agility drills performed while in a brace. Perturbation training consisted of a series of progressively challenging drills performed on unstable support surfaces. Fitzgerald found that 93% of the subjects who received the additional perturbation training could return to sports for at least 6 months without episodes of giving way. Only 50% of those who participated in traditional training alone returned to sporting activities. The results of this study indicate that the subjects receiving perturbation training were able to improve their dynamic knee stability, which manifested in improved functional levels.

At the University of Delaware the authors use the perturbation training program developed by Fitzgerald[71] as their primary treatment intervention for ACL-deficient patients. Nonoperative rehabilitation candidates at this time consist of high-level athletes who are identified as good nonoperative candidates after successfully completing the screening process.[43] Ongoing work is being conducted to determine the efficacy of perturbation training among patients who have lower functional activity levels, as well as those who do not pass the screening process.

Fitzgerald's perturbation training protocol[71] is a multifaceted, 10-session neuromuscular training program that incorporates strength training, agility drills, and three perturbation tasks (Figure 15-5) (Table 15-3). A variety of progressive resistance exercises are implemented and systematically advanced to address lower extremity muscle weakness. Agility and perturbation drills are also included and progressed based on the basis of the successful completion of each task. Verbal cues, such as "keep your knees soft," "keep your trunk still," and "relax between perturbations" are provided during perturbation training early in the program to provide patients with a framework for successful task completion. The focus of training is not on developing specific muscle activation patterns. Instead, patients are allowed to develop individualized patterns as long as the task is successfully completed (i.e., maintain balance and dynamic joint stability without rigid muscle co-contraction). During the first five sessions, perturbations are initiated in a block manner in anterior/posterior, medial/lateral, or rotational planes, and verbal cues are gradually decreased as the patient becomes more proficient with the task. During the last five treatments, the perturbation directions are applied randomly while the patient performs a sport-specific task (e.g., kicking a ball). Intensity, speed, and force of perturbations are advanced throughout the program.

Patients can usually begin a partial return to sport by the eighth perturbation training session. Patients are generally discharged to competition after the tenth session as long as they successfully pass a posttreatment ACL screening by scoring greater than or equal to 90% on the screening criteria (timed hop test, Knee Outcome Survey–Activities of Daily Living scale, global rating) and demonstrate greater than or equal to 90% contralateral quadriceps maximum voluntary isometric contraction strength.

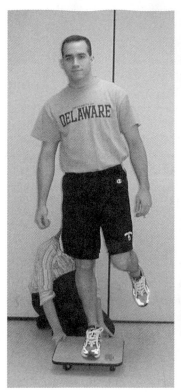
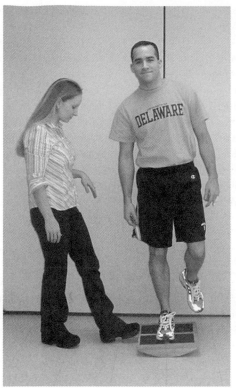
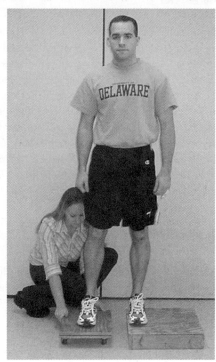

A   B   C

Figure 15-5 Perturbation training involves maintaining balance on three unstable support surfaces: **A,** a rollerboard; **B,** a rockerboard; and **C,** a rollerboard with block.

Table 15-3	Perturbation Training Protocol		
Rockerboard	2-3 sets/1 min each	A/P, M/L	Begin in bilateral stance for first session. Perform in single-leg stance for remaining sessions.
Rollerboard/Platform	2-3 sets/1 min each, perform bilaterally	Initial: A/P, M/L Progression: Diagonal, rotation	Subject force is counter-resistance opposite of rollerboard, matching intensity, and speed of application so that rollerboard movement is minimal. Leg muscles should not be contracted in anticipation of perturbation, nor should response be rigid co-contraction.
Rollerboard	2-3 sets/30 sec to 1 min each	Initial: A/P, M/L Progression: Diagonal, rotation	Begin in bilateral stance for first session. Perform in single-leg stance for remaining sessions. Perturbation distances are 1-2 inches.

Early Phase (Sessions 1-4)
Treatment Goals:
- Expose athlete to perturbations in all directions
- Elicit an appropriate muscular response to applied perturbations (no rigid co-contraction)
- Minimize verbal cues

Middle Phase (Sessions 5-7)
Treatment Goals:
- Add light sport-specific activity during perturbation techniques
- Improve athlete accuracy in matching muscle responses to perturbation intensity, direction, and speed

Late Phase (Sessions 8-10)
Treatment Goals:
- Increase difficulty of perturbations by using sport-specific stances
- Obtain accurate, selective muscular responses to perturbations in any direction and of any intensity, magnitude, or speed

A/P, Anterior/posterior plane; *M/L,* medial/lateral plane.

SUMMARY

Neuromuscular control represents the complex interaction among sensory input, central processing, and efferent output. Dysfunction at any level can result in altered neuromuscular control and consequently lead to injury or reduced functional levels. An appreciation of how injury influences the sensorimotor system, as well as proprioception, dynamic joint stability, and postural control will aid in the identification of altered neuromuscular control. Once specific alterations in neuromuscular control are identified, implementation of appropriate treatment strategies will assist in returning the athlete to competition.

REFERENCES

1. Williams GN, Chmielewski T, Rudolph K, et al: Dynamic knee stability: current theory and implications for clinicians and scientists, *J Orthop Sports Phys Ther* 31:546-566, 2001.

2. Sherrington CS: *The integrative action of the nervous system,* New Haven, Conn, 1906, Yale University Press.

3. Lephart S, Reimann B, Fu F: *Proprioception and neuromuscular control in joint stability,* Champaign, Ill, 2000, Human Kinetics.

4. Hewett TE, Paterno MV, Myer GD: Strategies for enhancing proprioception and neuromuscular control of the knee, *Clin Orthop* 492:76-94, 2002.

5. Ghez C: Posture. In Kandel E, Schwartz J, Jessell T, editors: *Principles of neural science,* pp. 533-547, New York, 1991, Elsevier.

6. Shumway-Cook A, Woollacott M: *Motor control: theory and practical applications,* Baltimore, 1995, Williams & Wilkins.

7. Grigg P, Hoffman AH: Ruffini mechanoreceptors in isolated joint capsule: responses correlated with strain energy density, *Somatosens Res* 2:159-162, 1984.

8. Eklund G, Skoglund S: On the specificity of the Ruffini like joint receptors, *Acta Physiol Scand* 49:184-191, 1960.

9. Grigg P: Peripheral neural mechanisms in proprioception, *J Sport Rehab* 3:1-17, 1994.

10. Ferrell WR: The effect of acute joint distension on mechanoreceptor discharge in the knee of the cat, *Q J Exp Physiol* 72:493-499, 1987.

11. Zimny ML: Mechanoreceptors in articular tissues, *Am J Anat* 182:16-32, 1988.

12. Stilwell DL Jr: The innervation of deep structures of the hand, *Am J Anat* 101:75-99, 1957.

13. Boyd IA: The histological structure of the receptors in the knee-joint of the cat correlated with their physiological response, *J Physiol* 124:476-488, 1954.

14. Gordon J, Ghez C: *Muscle receptors and spinal reflexes: the stretch reflex,* pp. 564-580, New York, 1991, Elsevier Science.

15. Hulliger M, Nordh E, Thelin AE, et al: The responses of afferent fibres from the glabrous skin of the hand during voluntary finger movements in man, *J Physiol* 291:233-249, 1979.

16. Edin BB, Johansson N: Skin strain patterns provide kinaesthetic information to the human central nervous system, *J Physiol* 487(Pt 1):243-251, 1995.

17. Prete ZD, Grigg P: Responses of rapidly adapting afferent neurons to dynamic stretch of rat hairy skin, *J Neurophysiol* 80:745-754, 1995.

18. Burgess PR, Wei JY, Clark FJ, et al: Signaling of kinesthetic information by peripheral sensory receptors, *Annu Rev Neurosci* 5:171-187, 1982.

19. Matthews PB: Recent advances in the understanding of the muscle spindle, *Sci Basis Med Annu Rev:* 99-128, 1971.

20. Matthews PB: Evolving views on the internal operation and functional role of the muscle spindle, *J Physiol* 320:1-30, 1981.

21. Lephart SM, Pincivero DM, Giraldo JL, et al: The role of proprioception in the management and rehabilitation of athletic injuries, *Am J Sports Med* 25:130-137, 1997.

22. Houk J, Henneman E: Responses of Golgi tendon organs to active contractions of the soleus muscle of the cat, *J Neurophysiol* 30:466-481, 1967.

23. Houk JC: Regulation of stiffness by skeletomotor reflexes, *Annu Rev Physiol* 41:99-115, 1979.

24. Nichols TR, Houk JC: Improvement in linearity and regulation of stiffness that results from actions of stretch reflex, *J Neurophysiol* 39:119-42, 1976.

25. Moffett DF, Moffett SB, Schauf CL: *Human physiology: foundations and frontiers,* St Louis, 1993, Mosby-Year Book.

26. Nichols TR, Cope TC, Abelew TA: Rapid spinal mechanisms of motor coordination, *Exerc Sport Sci Rev* 27:255-284, 1999.

27. Brooks VB: *The neural basis of motor control,* New York, 1986, Oxford University Press.

28. Schmidt R, Lee T: *Motor control and learning: a behavioral emphasis,* Champaign, Ill, 1999, Human Kinetics.

29. Lee R, Tatton W: Long loop reflexes in man: clinical applications. In Desmedt J, editor: Cerebral motor control in man: long loop mechanisms, *Prog Clin Neurophys* 4:320-333, 1978.

30. Evarts EV: Motor cortex reflexes associated with learned movement, *Science* 179:501-503, 1973.

31. Di Fabio RP, Graf B, Badke MB, et al: Effect of knee joint laxity on long-loop postural reflexes: evidence for a human capsular-hamstring reflex, *Exp Brain Res* 90:189-200, 1992.

32. Ghez C: Voluntary movement. In Kandel E, Schwartz J, Jessell T, editors: Principles of neural science, pp. 533-547, New York, 1991, Elsevier.

33. Horak F, Macpherson J: Postural orientation and equilibrium. In Shepard J, Rowell L, editors: *Handbook of physiology,* pp. 255-292, New York, 1996, Oxford University.

34. Nashner LM: Fixed patterns of rapid postural responses among leg muscles during stance, *Exp Brain Res* 30:13-24, 1977.

35. Horak FB, Nashner LM: Central programming of postural movements: adaptation to altered support-surface configurations, *J Neurophysiol* 55:1369-1381, 1986.

36. Bernstein NA: *The coordination and regulation of movements,* London, 1967, Pergamon Press.

37. Schmidt R, Wrisberg C: *Motor learning and performance. A problem-based learning approach,* Champaign, Ill, 2004, Human Kinetics.

38. Duysens J, Van de Crommert HW: Neural control of locomotion; the central pattern generator from cats to humans, *Gait Posture* 7:131-151, 1998.

39. Grillner S: Locomotion in vertebrates: central mechanisms and reflex interaction, *Physiol Rev* 55:247-304, 1975.

40. Grillner S, Wallen P: Central pattern generators for locomotion, with special reference to vertebrates, *Annu Rev Neurosci* 8:233-261, 1985.

41. Van de Crommert HW, Mulder T, Duysens J: Neural control of locomotion: sensory control of the central pattern generator and its relation to treadmill training, *Gait Posture* 7:251-263, 1998.

42. Eastlack ME, Axe MJ, Snyder-Mackler L: Laxity, instability, and functional outcome after ACL injury: copers versus noncopers, *Med Sci Sports Exerc* 31:210-215, 1999.

43. Fitzgerald GK, Axe MJ, Snyder-Mackler L: A decision-making scheme for returning patients to high-level activity with nonoperative treatment after anterior cruciate ligament rupture, *Knee Surg Sports Traumatol Arthrosc* 8:76-82, 2000.

44. Rudolph KS, Axe MJ, Buchanan TS, et al: Dynamic stability in the anterior cruciate ligament deficient knee, *Knee Surg Sports Traumatol Arthrosc* 9:62-71, 2001.

45. Rudolph KS, Eastlack ME, Axe MJ, et al: 1998 Basmajian Student Award Paper: movement patterns after anterior cruciate ligament injury: a comparison of patients who compensate well for the injury and those who require operative stabilization, *J Electromyogr Kinesiol* 8:349-362, 1998.

46. Rudolph KS, Axe MJ, Snyder-Mackler L: Dynamic stability after ACL injury: who can hop? *Knee Surg Sports Traumatol Arthrosc* 8:262-269, 2000.

47. Ramsey DK, Lamontagne M, Wretenberg PF, et al: Assessment of functional knee bracing: an in vivo three-dimensional kinematic analysis of the anterior cruciate deficient knee, *Clin Biomech (Bristol, Avon)* 16:61-70, 2001.

48. Berchuck M, Andriacchi TP, Bach BR, et al: Gait adaptations by patients who have a deficient anterior cruciate ligament, *J Bone Joint Surg Am* 72:871-877, 1990.

49. Vereijkin B, van Emmerik REA, Whiting HTA, et al: Freezing degrees of freedom in skill acquisition, *J Motor Behavior* 24:133-152, 1992.

50. Fitzgerald GK, Axe MJ, Snyder-Mackler L: The efficacy of perturbation training in nonoperative anterior cruciate ligament rehabilitation programs for physical active individuals, *Phys Ther* 80:128-140, 2000.

51. Chmielewski T, Hurd W, Rudolph K, et al: Perturbation training decreases knee stiffness and muscle co-contraction in the ACL injured knee, *Phys Ther* 85:740-749, 2005.

52. Zatterstrom R, Friden T, Lindstrand A, et al: The effect of physiotherapy on standing balance in chronic anterior cruciate ligament insufficiency, *Am J Sports Med* 22:531-536, 1994.

53. Barrett DS: Proprioception and function after anterior cruciate reconstruction, *J Bone Joint Surg Br* 73:833-837, 1991.

54. Beard DJ, Dodd CA, Trundle HR, et al: Proprioception enhancement for anterior cruciate ligament deficiency. A prospective randomised trial of two physiotherapy regimens, *J Bone Joint Surg Br* 76:654-659, 1994.

55. Carter ND, Jenkinson TR, Wilson D, et al: Joint position sense and rehabilitation in the anterior cruciate ligament deficient knee, *Br J Sports Med* 31:209-212, 1997.

56. Caraffa A, Cerulli G, Projetti M, et al: Prevention of anterior cruciate ligament injuries in soccer. A prospective controlled study of proprioceptive training, *Knee Surg Sports Traumatol Arthrosc* 4:19-21, 1996.

57. Hewett TE, Lindenfeld TN, Riccobene JV, et al: The effect of neuromuscular training on the incidence of knee injury in female athletes. A prospective study, *Am J Sports Med* 27:699-706, 1999.

58. Heidt RS Jr, Sweeterman LM, Carlonas RL, et al: Avoidance of soccer injuries with preseason conditioning, *Am J Sports Med* 28:659-662, 2000.

59. Myklebust G, Engebretsen L, Braekken IH, et al: Prevention of anterior cruciate ligament injuries in female team handball players: a prospective intervention study over three seasons, *Clin J Sport Med* 13:71-78, 2003.

60. Wedderkopp N, Kaltoft M, Lundgaard B, et al: Prevention of injuries in young female players in European team handball. A prospective intervention study, *Scand J Med Sci Sports* 9:41-47, 1999.

61. Boden BP, Dean GS, Feagin JA Jr, et al: Mechanisms of anterior cruciate ligament injury, *Orthopedics* 23:573-578, 2000.

62. Myer GD, Ford KR, Hewett TE: Rationale and clinical techniques for anterior cruciate ligament injury prevention among female athletes, *J Athl Train* 39:352-364, 2004.

63. Teitz CC: Video analysis of ACL injuries. In Griffin LY, editor: *Prevention of non-contact ACL injuries,* pp. 93-96, Rosemont, Ill, 2001, American Academy of Orthopaedic Surgeons.

64. Myer GD, Ford KR, Hewett TE: The effects of gender on quadriceps muscle activation strategies during a maneuver that mimics a high ACL injury risk position, *J Electromyogr Kinesiol* 15:181-189, 2005.

65. Ford KR, Myer GD, Hewett TE: Valgus knee motion during landing in high school female and male basketball players, *Med Sci Sports Exerc* 35:1745-1750, 2003.

66. Hewett TE, Myer GD, Ford KR: Decrease in neuromuscular control about the knee with maturation in female athletes, *J Bone Joint Surg Am* 86-A:1601-1608, 2004.

67. Griffin LY: *The Henning program,* pp. 93-96, Rosemont, Ill, 2001, American Academy of Orthopaedic Surgeons.

68. Soderman K, Werner S, Pietila T, et al: Balance board training: prevention of traumatic injuries of the lower extremities in female soccer players? A prospective randomized intervention study, *Knee Surg Sports Traumatol Arthrosc* 8:356-363, 2000.

69. Risberg MA, Mork M, Jenssen HK, et al: Design and implementation of a neuromuscular training program following anterior cruciate ligament reconstruction, *J Orthop Sports Phys Ther* 31:620-631, 2001.

70. Ihara H, Nakayama A: Dynamic joint control training for knee ligament injuries, *Am J Sports Med* 15:309-315, 1986.

71. Fitzgerald GK, Axe MJ, Snyder-Mackler L: Proposed practice guidelines for nonoperative anterior cruciate ligament rehabilitation of physically active individuals, *J Orthop Sports Phys Ther* 30:194-203, 2000.

Manual Therapy in Sports Rehabilitation

LEARNING OBJECTIVES

After studying this chapter, the reader will be able to do the following:

1. Understand the role of manual therapy in rehabilitation following injury
2. Identify repair process and adaptation process
3. Understand the multidimensional nature of repair and adaptation
4. Identify the signals and stimuli needed to assist repair and adaptation
5. Identify the manual techniques that provide these stimuli
6. Use the dimensional model to match suitable manual techniques to underlying processes
7. Identify when to use stretching, pumping, or neuromuscular techniques
8. Understand how to develop a treatment plan

Manual therapy (MT) has a unique clinical role in the overall management of sports rehabilitation. This role becomes apparent in practice where the athlete/patient is unable to self-provide the adequate physical stimulation necessary for repair and adaptation. MT provides these physical stimuli, assisting the smooth transition from the disability of injury to the high physical demands of sport activities.

In order to understand how MT can be used in sports rehabilitation, MT must be viewed as providing the necessary physical signals for repair and adaptation. This chapter examines what these signals are and which MT techniques provide them. The aim of this process is to address two important clinical goals. The most suitable MT techniques can be matched to the patient's condition and, furthermore, long-term clinical strategies can be developed using distinct MT approaches at different phases along the time-line of rehabilitation/treatment.

OVERALL THERAPEUTIC AIMS

The place to start one's understanding of the therapeutic potential of MT in sports rehabilitation is to identify the overall therapeutic aims.[1] The ultimate goal is to assist two principal body processes:

- Repair process
- Adaptation process

The athlete who presents with a painful joint or muscle has an ongoing repair process in the damaged tissues. The therapeutic aim is to assist and direct this repair process for its optimal resolution.

Adaptation and its opposite dysfunctional adaptation can take many forms. One form is dysfunctional adaptation due to poor quality repair. Once the inflammatory phase is nearing completion, an adaptive remodeling process commences.[2-6] This process is highly dependent on the stresses that are imposed on the tissue.[7-11] A dysfunctional adaptation may ensue if, for any reason, the normal mechanical environment for repair is not provided. The most striking example is the atrophy seen when tissues are immobilized in a plaster cast.[12-18] Such immobilization leads to muscle wasting, excessive connective tissue proliferation, and loss of sarcomeres in series resulting in general shortening.[19-21] This change in the tissues is an adaptation process, albeit a dysfunctional one. The therapeutic aim under these circumstances is to create a "mechanical environment" in which the MT techniques and exercise provide the needed physical stimulation to "redirect" the adaptation process.

Adaptation and repair can also be seen in the motor system. Adaptation to physical experiences in the form of plasticity has been shown to occur throughout the neuromuscular continuum including the brain,[18,22-31] spinal cord,[32-35] motoneuron pools,[36-38] and finally the servant of the nervous system—the muscle.[39,40] Repair takes different forms in the nervous system depending on whether the system is damaged or intact. Structural repair of damaged neural tissue is seen in such conditions as head injuries.[41-43] Another form of "functional repair" is seen in the nervous system following musculoskeletal injuries. In these conditions the nervous system is intact but associated with reorganization of motor control to protect the injured area.[44] Repair can be viewed as a change from a dysfunctional motor pattern of injury to a normal function seen following full recovery. Postural instability often observed following ankle injury is an example of such dysfunctional motor pattern.[45] In this condition functional training is known to assist the recovery of motor control from an injury state to a more functional state, resulting in stability improvements. In both the damaged and intact nervous system the therapeutic aim is to assist the transition of the neuromuscular system from a dysfunctional to a functional state. These conditions will require manual approaches that provide a particular physical environment in which neural repair and adaptation can take place.

The examples given earlier demonstrate that repair and adaptation are multidimensional processes, and to activate them different therapeutic approaches are necessary. Accordingly, the manual techniques used at each dimension and with each process will change dramatically. This brings up an important clinical question: If techniques change with each dimension and process, how does one choose which technique to use? This clinical conundrum can be resolved by using the Dimension Model of Manual Therapy.[1] This useful model enables one to match the most effective MT techniques and the patient's condition/process.

DIMENSIONAL MODEL OF MANUAL THERAPY

The dimensional model of MT is a practical tool for developing clinical strategies that allow one to maximize the efficacy of the therapeutic intervention. In this model, MT techniques and their effects can be described in three dimensions (Figure 16-1):

- Tissue dimension
- Neurological dimension
- Psychological dimension

Tissue Dimension

The tissue dimension is where the direct physical effects of MT take place. This dimension is directly under the therapist's hands—skin; muscles; tendons; ligaments; joint structures; and different fluid systems, such as vascular, lymphatic, and synovial. In this dimension the therapist can expect the mechanical forces transmitted by the manual techniques to influence three principal processes:

- Assist tissue repair
- Assist fluid flow
- Assist tissue (length) adaptation

Techniques that stimulate repair play an important role in the rehabilitation of sports injury. These techniques are often used in combination with "pump" techniques that aim to stimulate fluid flow. Together, these techniques impose positive mechanical stresses on the tissue necessary for regeneration and remodeling, as well as stimulating local fluid flow. Such effects on fluid dynamics may help tissue reperfusion, improve tissue nutrition (in time of increased metabolic needs),[46] reduce swelling, and improve tissue washout of inflammatory byproducts. This could assist repair, as well as influence local pain mechanisms.

Improving fluid flow may also help ischemic musculoskeletal conditions often seen in sports, such as compartment syndromes,[47] chronic myalgias,[48,49] and nerve root irritation.[50,51]

Another common clinical presentation is reduced range of movement as a result of injury or long-term nontraumatic events, such as postural sets, patterns of behavior,[52] sports,[53] aging,[54,55] and central nervous system damage.[56-58] Accordingly, a large group of manual stretching techniques is aimed at improving tissue length and flexibility.

Neurological Dimension

MT has effects that reach beyond the tissue dimension to influence neurological processes; in particular, therapists are interested in the effects of MT on the following:

- The neuromuscular (motor) system
- Neurological pain mechanisms

These changes in the neurological dimension underlie a wide range of conditions both in the intact and damaged nervous

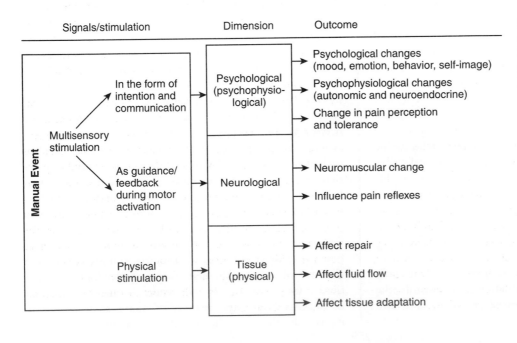

Figure 16-1 The dimensional model of manual therapy. (Modified from Lederman E: *The science and practice of manual therapy*, ed 2, London, 2005, Churchill Livingstone.)

systems.[1] These can present as postural and movement dysfunction often associated with sports injuries, as well as conditions associated with central nervous damage, such as spinal cord and head trauma.

In both the intact and damaged nervous systems the initial neuromuscular rehabilitation is manual in nature. The nervous system is well buffered against external influences, and previous manual approaches had been largely ineffective at influencing this system. A new, more active approach has been developed in MT over the past 10 years.[1] Some of these techniques are described as follows and in Table 16-1.

Psychological Dimension

The effects of MT technique at the psychological dimension rely on the potent psychodynamic effects of touch and the quality of the therapeutic relationship. These effects on mind and emotion play an important but often forgotten part in the overall therapeutic process. Touch is a potent stimulus to psychological processes that may result in a wide spectrum of physiological responses affecting every system in the body. Recent studies have demonstrated the psychological and psychophysiological effects of MT:

- Psychological manifestations
  - ◆ Behavioral changes[59-64]
  - ◆ Mood changes[59-64]
  - ◆ Changes in body image[1,63,64]
  - ◆ Altered pain tolerance/perception[19-21,65-68]
  - ◆ Psychophysiological manifestations
- Nonspecific, generalized changes in muscle tone[1]
  - ◆ Generalized autonomic, neuroendocrine, and autoimmune changes[69-75]
  - ◆ Self-regulation[19-21,59-77]

People often associate sports injuries with physical trauma. However, an athlete, like any other person, may develop psychosomatic or psychomotor conditions associated with psychological stress. Although the aim of MT is not necessarily directed at the emotional process, the treatment outcome may have an impact on psychological processes.

Considering the psychological and psychophysiological effects of touch, it is of no surprise that athletes often seek MT, often in the form of sports massage, before or after a competition. The hands-on contact may have important psychological implications in sports therapy.

CLINICAL EXAMPLES OF DIMENSIONAL MODEL

This section examines the dimensional model by using several clinical presentations. The first example is the athlete who has just had a fall and is presenting with a swollen painful ankle. Providing the injury is mild and the overall architecture of the tissue is intact, this could be considered a straightforward injury with an active repair process taking place in the tissue dimension. In addition, changes in the neuromuscular dimension will occur in the form of reorganization of motor control to the area of injury. This could be reflected in changes to synergistic control of muscle to the lower limb (and beyond). In this condition the MT is aimed at working in the tissue and neurological dimension; however, the MT techniques will change dramatically when working within a specific dimension, as well as along the time-line of repair (see later).

The next example is of an athlete who has been immobilized in a plaster cast. Once the cast has been removed, the joint's range of movement is reduced due to muscle and connective tissue shortening/adhesions. This is a condition occurring in the local tissue dimension but with repercussions in the neuromuscular dimension. Such immobilization can cause adaptation throughout the neuromuscular continuum, with changes observed centrally in the brain and spinal motoneuron centers and peripherally as muscle atrophy. In this example, too, the MT approach would aim to work in both dimensions with techniques that stimulate length adaptation in the tissue dimension and techniques that assist neuromuscular adaptation.

Another scenario is the athlete who has had an ankle injury and is no longer in pain. However, several months later the athlete finds that the injury is repeated frequently by "going over the ankle." This patient has functional instability (postural instability). The injured tissues are now repaired, but the motor system still "remembers" and functions in an injury mode (i.e., repair in the tissue dimension has been fully resolved, but the injury is being maintained by a dysfunction in the neuromuscular dimension). The difference between this condition and the previous one is that here the focus of the treatment is toward the neurological dimension (without the need to work in the tissue dimension). In this example one can see that the dimensional model allows therapists to focus the treatment and become more specific with their techniques.

Another clinical example is a tennis player who presents with severe neck and suprascapular pain, which is affecting playing performance. The onset of symptoms coincided with an emotionally stressful event in the patient's personal life. This is an example of a patient whose physical symptoms could be psychosomatic in nature. Using the dimensional model, one can analyze the condition as a sequence that started in the psychological dimension in response to a particular stressful event. The next stage in the sequence is the abnormal and subconscious increase in neuromuscular activity to the now painful muscles (inability to motor relax; see later discussion on motor abilities).[78-83] This phenomenon occurs in the neuromuscular dimension. This process culminates in the local tissue dimension as overuse damage to the muscle fibers, manifested as painful and tender areas in the muscles of the neck and scapular muscles. This clinical example involves a condition that "resides" in three dimensions, with each dimension requiring a different therapeutic approach and specific manual techniques (i.e., manual approaches that will help calm and relax the patient in the psychological dimension; manual techniques that will address the increased neuromuscular activity in the neurological dimension; and, finally, techniques that will address long-term changes in the muscle, such as chronic repair process and shortening).

MANUAL THERAPY—A SIGNAL FOR CHANGE

Each dimension in the dimensional model can be pictured as a door with a combination lock. The doors are the natural buffers of the body against unwanted external influences. In daily life these buffers allow only particular events to influence one's system, while others are deflected (Figure 16-2). For example, the neuromuscular system adapts to certain events, such as repetitive exercise, but not to single motor events, consequently "forgetting" many insignificant daily actions. The signals that do activate the processes and behavior of the system can be likened to the code in the combination lock. Each of the three dimensions has a door with its own particular (and highly specific) combination code. Events that have the right code will be more successful in bypassing these buffers. This principle applies to manual events. Techniques that contain these code elements are more likely to have long-lasting therapeutic effects and vice versa. The research task that therapists have at hand is to identify the code elements for each dimension/process and incorporate them into their manual techniques.

CHARACTERISTIC OF SIGNALS/STIMULI IN THE TISSUE DIMENSION

The signals that are required to activate the different processes therapists associate in the tissue dimension are described next.

Repair

Research in the past few years has demonstrated why MT can have such profound effects on repair and adaptation. This is related to a physiological phenomenon called *mechanotransduction,* a process whereby mechanical signals are converted into biochemical signals by fibroblasts and muscle cells, culminating in synthesis of different building blocks of connective tissue matrix and muscle proteins.[84-95] This process is at the heart of repair and adaptation and is probably the mechanism for change activated by MT. When one stretches a muscle, the

mechanical tension is a signal for the myocytes to synthesize the contractile proteins. These will be deposited in series, like beads on a chain, resulting in long-term muscle elongation.

Repair is a highly adaptive process, and the regeneration and remodeling of tissue depend heavily on the mechanical environment of the tissue (mechanotransduction). A well-established fact is that repair responds well to mechanical stimulation in the form of movement.[6-18] Movement provides a blueprint from which the regenerating connective tissue scaffolding is reconstructed. Movement has been shown to be highly effective in improving the rate of recovery, improving the quality of the regenerating tissue, reducing hospital stays, improving the quality of cartilage repair, improving circulation, and reducing edema in the tissues.[96-112]

Repair will fail if the tissues are not provided with mechanical stresses. This will manifest in excessive connective tissue proliferation, adhesion formation, and a low-quality matrix that is mechanically weaker. In the muscle-tendon unit this will result in atrophy shortening and abnormal revascularization.[12-18]

Research in movement suggests that during repair manual techniques should provide the following mechanical signals/stimulations:

- Adequate mechanical stress
- Dynamic/intermittent/cyclical force
- Repetition

Adequate mechanical tension is movement within the slack to early elastic region of the tissue. The tensional forces should be within the pain-free range and should be about movement rather than stretching. Generally, movement should be passive in the early stages of repair and become active later in the repair process. The reason for this is that during active movement, greater mechanical stresses are imposed on the tissues (including joints), which may cause further tissue damage.

The mechanical force should be dynamic/cyclical, repetitive,[97-117] and within the normal physiological ranges. Human and animal studies have shown a trend in which dynamic and cyclical events are more effective than static mechanical events in stimulating repair. Movement can be either in the form of passive joint oscillation or active by assisted movement.

Some research on joint repair suggests that passive movement, in comparison with active movement, is ideal in the early stages of repair because it provides a better control of the stresses imposed on the tissues.[115,116] Movement is also important in stimulating fluid flow at the site of damage necessary for successful repair (see later).

Different MT techniques can be selected according to their content of code elements. The greater code elements a technique has, the more effective it is likely to be at assisting repair and vice versa. The manual techniques that contain these mechanical code elements are harmonic techniques,[118] oscillatory techniques, joint articulation, and soft tissue massage techniques (for more superficial tissues).

Harmonic techniques were developed by Lederman[118] with the particular aim of providing repair-assisting manual techniques. Harmonic technique is a form of oscillatory technique

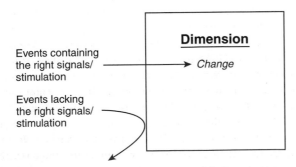

Figure 16-2 All experiences including manual therapy events need to contain certain signals/stimulation in order to activate different processes at each dimension. (Modified from Lederman E: *The science and practice of manual therapy,* ed 2, London, 2005, Churchill Livingstone.)

that provides continuous passive motion (depending on the area of the body, the frequency is about 60 cycles per minute and can be applied for periods up to 20 minutes).

Techniques that provide passive movement will also have an effect on the transsynovial pump, a physiological system in joints responsible for stimulating fluid flow in and out of the joint space.[119-121] These techniques are important in treating joint injuries where there is inflammation, effusion, and edema.

Fluid Flow

Gross fluid flow in the body is generated by mechanical pump systems (heart, vascular pump, muscle including peristalsis, respiratory pump, and movement). All these systems share similar mechanical properties. They work on the principle of the pulsatile pump, which generates fluctuating pressure gradients within and between the different fluid compartments (fluid moving from high-pressure to low-pressure areas).[122] From these systems important clues can be obtained as to the mechanical nature of manual pumping techniques. To stimulate fluid flow these techniques should provide

- Adequate compression force
- Intermittent/rhythmic force
- Repetitive force

In this group of techniques manual compressive force is applied to the target tissue. The compression should be of sufficient force to bring about the collapse of the vessels' lumen (venous and initial lymphatics) within the target tissue. Higher forces of compression are required to drain deeper tissue, such as muscle, whereas light compression may be sufficient for stimulating lymph drainage in the skin and subcutaneous tissues.

The compression should be in a cyclical pattern alternating between compression and decompression. This alternating manual pressure should be rhythmic and repetitive, comprising many cycles during single and subsequent treatments.[123-126]

The potency of different manual therapy techniques in stimulating flow can be estimated by their content of pump code element. In order of efficacy are harmonic pump techniques, massage (if performed with compression rather than stretching), and effleurage for superficial drainage. Techniques that provide rhythmic movement will also activate fluid flow (see previous discussion on repair).[118]

Length Adaptation

The physical signals necessary for length adaptation have been identified from the extensive research into physiology stretching. These manual techniques should provide[127-141]

- Adequate tension
- Rate of stretching (low velocity)
- Sufficient duration
- Repetition

Generally an adequate force for stretching is somewhere around the end-elastic and early-plastic ranges. At this point micro-

scopic damage seems to act as a trigger for length adaptation (see previous section on mechanotransduction).

Stretching should be performed at slow rather than high velocities and kept stretched sufficiently long (anywhere from 6 to 60 seconds; however, duration will be affected by variables, such as the force used, the diameter and length of the tissue, the level of tissue damage, inflammation, and scar formation).[133-141] Slow and sustained stretching allows the tissue to gradually elongate, bringing it more rapidly to the end-elastic range.[133-141]

Generally the fibroblast and myocytes are more responsive to dynamic rather then static stimuli.[92-95] Therefore introducing repetition can greatly enhance the long-term effects of stretching. This can be applied in different time scales—as rhythmic low amplitude oscillation at the end-elastic range, as repetition several times a day, and as repetition that is carried out over several weeks.

From the previous code one can identify the manual therapy techniques that are likely to be more effective in promoting length adaptation. They are static and rhythmic stretching and can be either passive or active (e.g., muscle energy techniques). Important differences between passive and active stretching are discussed fully in Lederman.[1]

CHARACTERISTIC OF SIGNALS/STIMULI IN THE NEUROLOGICAL DIMENSION

Motor processes are well buffered against external influences. In order to assist a change in motor control, challenging motor experiences must be created and applied during the treatment. These experiences must be of a particular nature in order to assist a neuromuscular adaptation. Such adaptation is known to rely on motor learning principles. Five key elements of motor learning should be incorporated into the manual approach:

- Cognition
- Active
- Feedback
- Repetition
- Similarity

The patient must be aware of and attentive to the therapeutic process and take an active conscious part in it. Cognition is probably one of the most important elements in motor learning and neuromuscular rehabilitation.[142-146] The athlete must be aware of and engaged in the rehabilitation process.

In the past MT has been dominated by passive manual approaches. However, in the past 2 decades research has shown that active manual approaches are more likely to bring about neuromuscular changes[147-161] (see discussion in Lederman[1]).

Feedback provides ongoing information for immediate adjustments to movement (short-term contribution). It also provides the feedback necessary for motor learning, replenishing existing motor programs (long-term contribution).[146] Sensory loss due to peripheral or central nervous system damage may severely impair the ability to perform normal movement or rehabilitate it.[162-164] For example, therapists know that joint injuries are often accompanied by proprioceptive losses. Such losses and their recovery may play a crucial role in determining the successes of motor rehabilitation. Generally the more dynamic and active the movement is, the greater the feedback from proprioception. In clinical conditions in which such losses are present, proprioceptive stimulation can be provided by dynamic manual technique, which should gravitate toward an active approach.

Another form of feedback is guidance. This term is used in training and teaching when subjects are provided with knowledge of their results. This enables them to modify their actions and assists learning.[164] Clinical situations in which the therapist manually assists and guides the patient's movement is a form of (manual) guidance.

"Practice makes better," a saying drummed into people by their parents and teachers, is regrettably true. Repetition is another key element in promoting motor learning and is applicable to manual rehabilitation—when working in the neurological dimension the pattern used during the treatment should be repeated many times. Manual events that elicit a single motor response will be ineffective in promoting long-term neuromuscular adaptation.[165-169]

The similarity principle is that people learn what they practice.[165-170] This principle applies to rehabilitation following injury. The manual event must be similar to normal functional movement: the closer the manual pattern is to daily patterns, the greater the potential that this movement will transfer to daily activities. Movement that is nonphysiological or nonfunctional will fail to transfer to normal daily use. If the patient is unable to balance, rehabilitation should be focused at balance. If strength is affected, rehabilitation should be toward force ability. If the patient cannot raise an arm to eat, rehabilitation should simulate this movement. If walking is affected, treatment should imitate the neuromuscular patterns of walking.[170-172]

These five motor learning elements are the therapeutic drive underlying any treatment in the neuromuscular dimension. Manual approaches that are rich in these elements will be highly effective in influencing motor processes in the long term. Techniques that are missing any number of these code elements are unlikely to be therapeutically effective in this dimension.

From Similarity to "Re-abilitation"

From the previous motor learning principles, one can see an MT approach that engages the patient cognitively and is an active process. Furthermore, it promotes activity that is functional in nature and similar in pattern to the athletic pursuit of the individual.

The question that arises next is what are therapists rehabilitating when working within the neurological/neuromuscular dimension? For example, the athlete who has sprained an ankle may keep up his or her exercise and sports pursuits and yet, when tested, still demonstrate motor losses (these losses are known to be the maintaining factors behind reinjury and reduced athletic performance).[173-176] One would have expected that the athlete's motor losses would spontaneously recover by his or her training. This clinical observation leads to two principal strategies that can be used for treating neuromuscular conditions. One strategy is rehabilitation imitating normal functional activities (e.g., retrain walking if walking is affected). However, this approach does not always seem to work. It seems that individuals can learn to compensate and circumvent their motor losses (at the expense of poorer performance and reinjury). For example, if balance losses are the cause for the walking difficulty, the individual may compensate by walking with a wider base.

This observation leads to another rehabilitation strategy called *neuromuscular re-abilitation* (or *manual neuromuscular re-abilitation*).[1,172] Any movement can be broken down into underlying functional building blocks called sensory-motor abilities. When the athlete presents with a musculoskeletal injury, one or several of these abilities may be affected. In neuromuscular re-abilitation these abilities are tested, "disabilities" identified, and treatment focused on re-abilitating these losses. Using the example of the athlete with the ankle sprain, reciprocal activation (one of the motor abilities, see later) may be affected in the lower leg and impede normal locomotive activities. In this case re-abilitation would focus on reestablishing functional synergistic control in the lower leg. Eventually, this focus would be incorporated into functional activities, such as walking at a later stage in the treatment. Such treatment often starts on the table, where the synergistic control is challenged manually by the therapist. Synergistic control is then challenged dynamically and statically in weight bearing once the athlete shows improvements in motor control.

Motor and sensory abilities can be grouped according to their level of complexity (Figure 16-3). From lower to higher levels of complexity, the motor abilities are as follows:

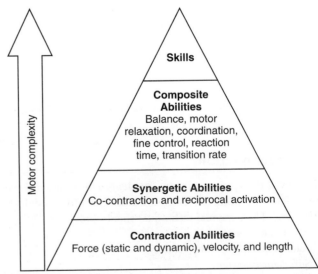

Figure 16-3 Motor abilities arranged according to their level of complexity. (Modified from Lederman E: *The science and practice of manual therapy*, ed 2, London, 2005, Churchill Livingstone.)

- Contraction abilities—control of force, velocity, and length of muscle
- Synergistic abilities—control of co-contraction (for stability, which can be dynamic or static) and reciprocal activation (for production of movement). Synergistic abilities are also about onset timing between muscle groups and the duration of contraction.
- Composite abilities—coordination, reaction time, fine control, balance, motor relaxation, and motor transition rate

The sensory abilities are as follows:

- Position sense (static and dynamic)—the ability to identify the position and change of position of a single joint
- Spatial orientation—the ability to identify the position and change of position of a whole limb (several joints)
- Composite sensory ability—the ability to integrate sensory information from exteroceptive and proprioceptive sources for the execution of movement, such as balance

Over the past decade, tests have been developed to assess these sensory-motor abilities. The tests and the treatment of specific abilities are mostly manual in nature. Some of the abilities and their tests are described in Table 16-1.

Table 16-1	Sensory-Motor Abilities: Description, Tests, and Their Re-abilitation		
Sensory-Motor Ability	Description	Tests	Re-abilitation
Motor Abilities			
Force (dynamic or static)	The ability to produce and control sufficient contraction force and control its level.	For static force use standard muscle testing methods to gauge muscle strength. For dynamic force ask the patient to perform an arc of movement while resisting that movement. In both tests endurance can also be tested by a longer duration of muscle contraction in the static test and several repetitions of the movement in the dynamic test.	Static force can be re-abilitated by straightforward resistive-type movement. This can be applied for both static and dynamic contractions. Resistance can be applied manually by the practitioner alternating between static and dynamic movement, continuously varying the starting angles of the forces applied. For example, in the arm, instruct the patient to elevate the arm against resistance (dynamic phase). At different angles instruct the patient to stop and hold a static contraction. This can be combined with continuously changing the position of the whole of the upper limb. The movement patterns should be within normal functional arm movement (e.g., hand to mouth, tennis serve patterns).
Velocity	The ability to control the rate of contraction.	The patient uses the affected side to move rapidly from one spatial position to another, marked by the therapist's hands. The patient is instructed to repeat the movement but at a progressively increasing rate.	Perform like the test, but increase repetition. Change variables, such as limb position, by therapist moving hands apart to new positions.
Length	The ability to produce movement and sufficient forces at the end ranges of movement.	Instruct patient to perform the movement at end ranges. Test range and force production.	Perform like the test, but increase repetition. Change variables, such as limb position, resistive force (either dynamic or static), and velocity.
Co-contraction (dynamic or static stabilization)	The ability to control the active stability of joints including onset timing and duration of activation of synergistic muscles. Also the ability to control the relative force, velocity, and length between synergists during movement.	Static control: Instruct the patient to "stiffen the joint" and apply fine perturbations to the limb at increasing rates and in different directions. Dynamic control: Instruct the patient to move the limb in one plane. The therapist challenges this movement by sudden lateral pushes to the moving limb.	Perform like the test, but start a low force and speed perturbation and gradually increase as the patient improves. Vary the joint position (static control) or planes of movement (for dynamic control).

continued

Table 16-1	Sensory-Motor Abilities: Description, Tests, and Their Re-abilitation—cont'd		
Sensory-Motor Ability	**Description**	**Tests**	**Re-abilitation**
Reciprocal activation	The ability to control local movement production at a joint including onset timing and duration of activation of synergistic muscles. Also the ability to control the relative force, velocity, and length between synergists during movement.	Test 1: Instruct patient to maintain the joint in a particular position. Apply force in one plane of movement (e.g., flexion-extension). Increase the rate at which the forces are imposed. Test 2: Instruct the patient to dynamically move his or her limb in one plane against your resistance.	Perform like the test, but start a low force and speed perturbation and gradually increase as the patient improves. Vary the joint position.
Reaction time	Response time to a stimulus.	Instruct patient to produce a static force against your resistance. Tell the patient to try to keep the limb in the same position when you suddenly remove the hand (patient should close eyes).	Use the method described earlier in synergistic re-abilitation.
Balance	The ability to maintain an upright position with minimal effort and mechanical stress.	Numerous tests.	See text for description.
Motor relaxation	The ability to perform movement with minimal muscle activity. The ability to fully relax muscles in resting positions.	Test using palpation for tense muscles in resting positions. Also palpate/observe muscle activities during different tasks.	Using palpation, scan areas where patient complains of muscle tension and pain. Guide patient on how to relax using verbal and palpatory feedback.
Fine control	The ability to control small amplitude and precise movement.	Observe patient handling of objects, etc.	Encourage use of affected part/limb.
Coordination	The harmonious control of muscles over several joints, limbs, and body masses.	Instruct patient to perform different tasks. Observe the ability to control the movement within the same limb and in relation to other limbs.	Encourage functional movement within single or multiple limbs. Vary limb positions, angles, force, and velocity.
Transitional ability	Transition rate is the speed and flexibility at which the patient can move from one ability to another (i.e., how fast the patient can organize motor patterns).	Take two abilities, such as reciprocal activation and co-contraction, and instruct the patient to change rapidly between them.	Once specific contraction or composite abilities improve, introduce the transition rate by mixing the contraction abilities (e.g., moving quickly at low force to suddenly shifting to a high force and slow movement).
Sensory Abilities			
Static position sense	Ability to perceive the static angle of the joint.	With the patient's eyes shut, move one limb to a position. The patient must move the affected limb to the same position. Test in different angles.	Repeat the test.
Dynamic position sense	Ability to perceive the angle of the joint during movement.	With the patient's eyes shut, move one limb. Instruct the patient to follow the movement with the other limb. Test in different velocities.	Repeat the test.
Spatial orientation (proprioceptive)	Ability to perceive the position of limbs or trunk in space and direction of movement.	Instruct the patient to shut his or her eyes. Take the unaffected limb, and move it slowly in space in different directions. The patient must actively follow these movements with the affected arm.	Repeat the test. Increase the rate of the movement.

Modified from Lederman E: *The science and practice of manual therapy*, ed 2, London, 2005, Churchill Livingstone.

CHARACTERISTIC OF SIGNALS/STIMULI IN THE PSYCHOLOGICAL DIMENSION

In the tissue dimension the signals for change are physical in nature, and in the neurological dimension they are associated with patterns of motor activation. The signals in the psychological dimension are less defined or quantifiable. In the psychological dimension it is the way the touch is applied and the intention of the therapist that influence the psychological processes. For example, a patient who is anxious may benefit from a form of touch that is relaxing in nature. The therapist's intention will be that of calming, expressed manually by applying a broad and slow hand contact (see full discussion on expressive touch in Lederman[1]).

The Dimensional Model in Practice

Using the dimensional model, one can now match the most effective manual approach and techniques to the patient's condition (Figure 16-4). For example, an athlete with an acute ankle sprain is presenting with a condition that is predominantly in the tissue dimension, with repercussions in the neuromuscular dimension. The repair process requires particular mechanical signals—adequate, cyclical, and repetitive mechanical stress. Furthermore, such tissue damage is associated with edema and possibly joint effusion. This, too, occurs

in the tissue dimension and is likely to respond to rhythmic intermittent compression and movement. From the manual toolbox, one can pick techniques that contain these physical characteristics. Massage techniques that comprise intermittent compression can be used around the swollen area to reduce superficial edema. This would be in combination with passive joint articulation to activate the transsynovial pump and reduce joint effusion. Although this condition has repercussions in the neurological dimension, this will be dealt with later in the treatment, once repair has taken place and pain is reduced (discussed in the next example).

Regarding the athlete who was immobilized in a plaster cast, this was also identified as a condition occurring in the tissue and neurological dimensions and being largely a process of shortening adaptation and adhesions. This process would respond well to mechanical stimulation that produces slow, sustained, tensional force. Going back to the manual toolbox, the therapist's choice would be passive and active forms of stretching techniques.

In the neurological dimension the patient would be expected to have a range of abilities affected. There would be force, velocity, and length control losses, as well as synergistic control losses. However, the manual techniques used to work in the tissue dimension will be ineffective in influencing these motor changes. Using the dimensional model, one can see that at the neuromuscular dimension the manual techniques should incorporate the five motor learning principles—cognition,

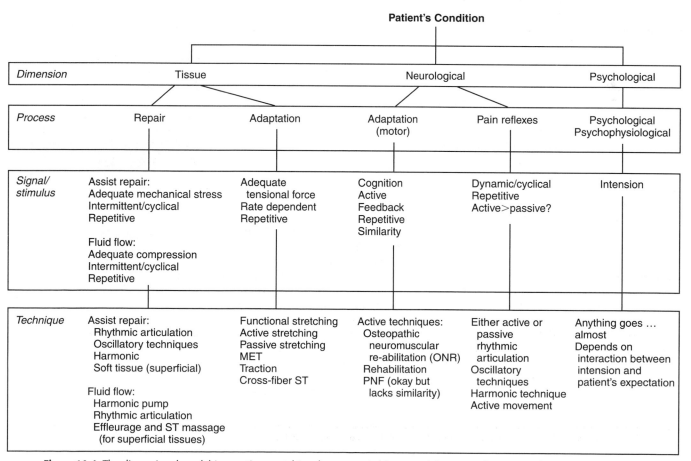

Figure 16-4 The dimensional model in practice: matching the most suitable manual therapy techniques to the patient's condition.

active movement, feedback, repetition of the movement patterns, and using the similarity principle. Hence the manual techniques will be active rather than passive, with an emphasis on challenging specific motor losses. Initially these would be the contraction and synergistic abilities and eventually the more complex, composite abilities, such as reaction time and transitional rate. In this particular case, because the patient was immobilized, the focus will be on challenging force, length, and velocity control at the newly recovered ranges.

The treatment of the acute and postimmobilization ankle (in previous examples) is fairly similar in the neurological dimension. However, two important differences exist. In the case of the acute ankle patient, the sensory-motor abilities will be tested and treated only toward the end of the treatment when pain subsides (Figure 16-5). The postimmobilization patient would receive neuromuscular rehabilitation immediately on the first treatment (providing the patient is not in too much pain). Another difference is that treatment will focus on specific abilities in each condition. As suggested earlier in the postimmobilization patient, this would be on motor activities that challenge length, whereas in the acute ankle condition, length is not an issue and the treatment would be more generalized, challenging the contraction and synergistic abilities. In both conditions the treatment would gravitate

toward challenging the abilities at progressively higher velocities to account for the demands placed on the motor system during athletic pursuits. Much of the initial treatment is manual, focusing on specific motor losses and later as dynamic weight-bearing exercise (similarity principle).

Differences and similarities of approach can be seen in the example of the athlete who was displaying postural instability. The difference from the immobilized and acute ankle conditions is that the manual approach would be exclusively in the neurological dimension. Similarities of the approaches would be in using the motor learning principles and abilities described earlier.

The last clinical case was the tennis player who was exhibiting a musculoskeletal condition, which was potentially brought about by emotional stress. As has been discussed, this condition "resides" in three dimensions. Using the dimensional model, one can identify the most suitable manual approach (i.e., *intension* in the psychological dimension and the motor learning and abilities principles in the neurological dimension).

In this case one must unify the psychological and neurological dimensions and apply a cognitive behavioral approach. The therapist's hands are used to scan the patient's neck and shoulder muscles, identifying painful and tense areas. The

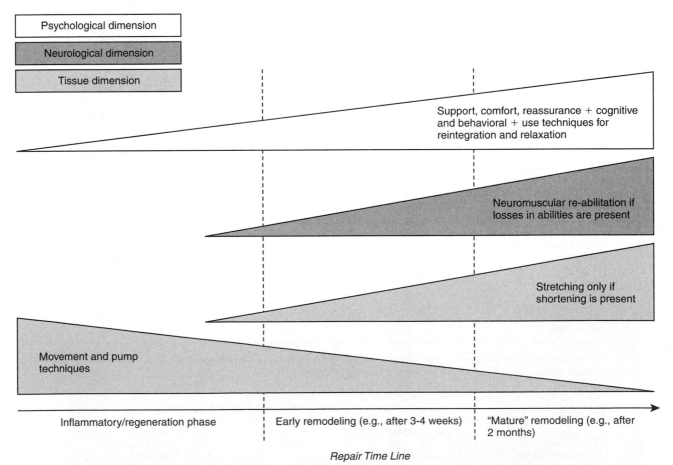

Repair Time Line

Figure 16-5 Using the dimensional model during the different phases of repair: In each phase of repair the manual approach changes according to the underlying process being targeted. Initially the treatment is focused on assisting repair. Later in the time line of repair, the focus should change toward assisting adaptation. This would be in the form of neuromuscular rehabilitation and stretching. Psychological factors should be considered throughout the treatment period. (Modified from Lederman E: *The science and practice of manual therapy*, ed 2, London, 2005, Churchill Livingstone.)

patient is given verbal guidance to relax these specific muscles. The motor learning principles and abilities are applied in this case, but the focus is on relaxation ability (i.e., the patient is aware of the process, engaged in the process by actively relaxing while the therapist gives the patient feedback on the level of relaxation). This is repeated several times during the treatment (repetition principle). A calming form of touch is used throughout the treatment to help the patient relax (see previous discussion on signals in psychological dimension).

When the patient can relax more successfully, he or she can begin to bring awareness into their activities. This "active" form of relaxation can be practiced in upright postures, such as sitting and standing, and eventually covers relaxation during the use of the tennis racket (similarity principle).

In the tissue dimension the underlying process is that of repair and shortening adaptation in the affected muscles. Using the dimensional model, the ideal mechanical environment for repair is low force, cyclical tension, and intermittent compression. The technique choice at this stage would be rhythmic, intermittent, manual compression of the affected muscles. This could be in the form of compressive soft tissue/massage. As pain reduces, the treatment would shift toward treating the shortening changes. Now, a different mechanical stimulation is necessary—sustained or rhythmic tensional forces (i.e., different forms of manual stretching).

MANUAL THERAPY: CREATING AN ENVIRONMENT FOR REPAIR AND ADAPTATION

In essence, the MT session is about creating ideal environments in which repair and adaptation can take place. Treatment should be seen as the initiation of these processes, and the patient should be encouraged to maintain the repair and adaptation environment outside the treatment sessions (see Fig. 16-4). This can be achieved by daily activities and exercise that stimulate these processes.

In the tissue dimension a repair environment can be created in the clinic by the use of passive joint movement. This envi-

ronment can be extended into functional daily activities. The athlete can be encouraged to maintain low-force, active movement, such as pendulum swinging of the affected limb. An adaptation environment can also be created in the clinic by using stretching techniques. This lengthening environment can be extended into daily activities by encouraging the patient to perform functional activities that challenge length. For example, the postimmobilization athlete could be encouraged to lower his or her foot over a step into dorsiflexion or walk on his or her heels (with foot in dorsiflexion) several times throughout the day.

In the neurological dimension repair and adaptation are driven by similar stimuli—challenging physical experiences. Such an environment can be created in the clinic by extensive motor stimulation provided by another person (therapist) and extended into daily activities. For example, when reabilitating postural stability the patient can perform single-leg balancing exercise or hop on the affected side when watching TV, washing up, etc.

The principles discussed throughout this chapter are demonstrated by a case history in Table 16-2.

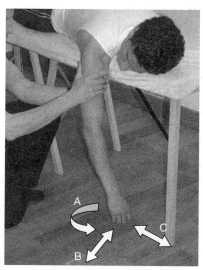

Figure 16-7 Passive oscillation at shoulder height and above. **A,** Oscillation in circumduction. **B,** Oscillation in abduction/adduction. **C,** Oscillation in flexion/extension. During the oscillations the therapist's hands are clasped around and close to the glenohumeral joint, applying intermittent compression.

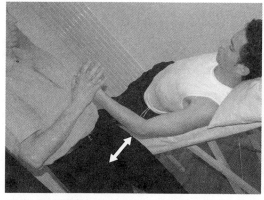

Figure 16-6 Glenohumeral adduction-abduction oscillations (*arrow* indicates direction of elbow swinging). Patient is fully relaxed, while the therapist initiates passive oscillation of the shoulder. As the condition of the shoulder improves, the range of motion increases and the arm can be taken into further flexion or extension.

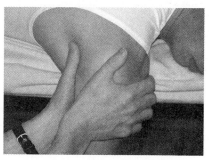

Figure 16-8 Applying intermittent compression around the glenohumeral joint during the oscillations.

Table 16-2　Example of Treatment of a Tennis Player Using Manual Therapy Principles

A therapist is currently treating a medical consultant who is a keen tennis player. The medical consultant is 65 years old and has been playing tennis since childhood. The consequences of playing tennis for so many years, combined with natural changes associated with aging, have resulted in a shoulder condition that included a large acromial spur, which has cut into the superior part of the joint capsule, resulting in a large superior capsular tear and a 10-cm longitudinal tear in the supraspinatus tendon. In addition, he seems to have had every known shoulder condition including subacromial bursitis, various tendinosa, capsular wasting, and acromioclavicular arthritis. These conditions were corrected recently by extensive surgery to the shoulder, which included shaving off the acromial spur and suturing the capsular and supraspinatus tears.

Within 3 days of surgery the medical consultant was in the therapist's clinic for treatment. The initial aim of the treatment was to assist and direct the repair process in the postsurgery shoulder. This was done by the introduction of manually applied passive motion within pain-free ranges (see below). Successful surgery also depends on the draining of the tissue from edema. This was partly achieved by the movement itself and partly by manual pump techniques (applying intermittent compression directly to edematous tissue).

The result was quite dramatic; within 3 days of treatment the patient was pain free (except for night discomfort) and had almost full range of passive motion in the shoulder. By gaining confidence from the ranges achieved during the manual phase and by the direction they provided, the patient was learning about low-force active movement. He could perform low-force pendulum swings of the shoulder in different ranges of movement. Later in the week low-level neuromuscular stimulation was introduced by applying low-level resistance force while the patient actively swung his arm. This established that the patient could carry out low-force active movement. This was introduced in the beginning of the second week in the form of exercise consisting of drawing an imaginary number, in space, with an outstretched arm. By the fifth week the treatment had dramatically changed. It was estimated that the patient was well out of the early repair phase and now in remodeling, adaptive phase. The treatment was progressively shifting from passive to active manual approaches (neurological dimension). This phase focused on motor abilities using specific active manual techniques that challenge these abilities. The manual approach was complemented by the patient carrying out functional exercise (without the use of a gym—see later). Within 3 weeks of commencing the active phase, the patient regained many of the lost motor abilities to the extent that it was difficult to distinguish between the operated and nonoperated arm. The manual contribution to the repair and adaptation has been achieved, and the patient was encouraged to resume normal activities.

| | | Repair and Adaptation Environment | |
	Signals/Stimulation Necessary	Manual Therapy Techniques	Functional Exercise
Time dimension	Stimulate repair: Adequate mechanical force Rhythmic/cyclical Repetitive Stimulate flow: Intermittent compression Dynamic/cyclical Repetitive Stimulate length adaptation: Not needed—all improvements in range achieved by passive motion at end-range/pain-free ranges.	Rhythmic joint articulation using harmonic techniques: patient lying supine, arm oscillation into adduction/abduction (Figure 16-6). Patient lying prone, joint oscillation into external/internal rotation. In this position circumduction of the glenohumeral joint can be added (Figure 16-7). Throughout the manipulation, the therapist's hands apply massage/soft tissue manipulation using intermittent compression of edematous tissue around the joint (Figure 16-8).	Frequent pendulum swings of the arm in pain-free ranges during the day. This can be done in flexion/extension by the side of the body or adduction/abduction and circumduction in front of the body
Neurological dimension	Motor adaptation: Cognition Active Feedback Repetition Similarity	Working with motor abilities, the contraction and synergistic abilities are put together. *Co-contraction:* Static co-contraction—Instruct the patient to stiffen the shoulder and keep the arm in the same position (Figure 16-9). The therapist attempts to move it while the patient resists. This is done at different glenohumeral angles and around different axes. The contraction abilities can be changed while the patient is holding his or her position. The therapist applies different force and velocity while the patient resists. Dynamic co-contraction—Instruct patient to move arm rhythmically in one plane (e.g., reaching forward motion). The therapist adds sudden, lateral, and medial perturbations while the patient tries to maintain the movement in one plane (Figure 16-10). Force and velocity of perturbations increase as the patient improves.	*Co-contraction (stability):* Static cocontraction— Instead of the therapist, the patient is applying the perturbation with the unaffected arm (i.e., he or she stiffens the affected side and tries to move it with the normal arm). Dynamic co-contraction— The patient is moving his or her injured arm in one plane while applying the lateral and medial shift with the good arm. Both static and dynamic co-contraction are done in different joint ranges and at increasing force and velocities.

Table 16-2	Example of Treatment of a Tennis Player Using Manual Therapy Principles—cont'd	

| | Repair and Adaptation Environment | |
Signals/Stimulation Necessary	Manual Therapy Techniques	Functional Exercise
	Reciprocal activation: Essentially movement against resistance in all ranges. At the beginning the movement may be assisted and rapidly change into resisted as the condition improves. This is achieved by the patient pulling and pushing the therapist in different directions (Figure 16-11). In another method the therapist holds his hands apart in space, and the patient has to alternately tap each hand with his own hand (Figure 16-12, *A*). Velocity of movement can be challenged by faster tapping and by the therapist changing his or her hand positions. Force and velocity are increased as the patient improves. Composite abilities: *Reaction time:* Using the method described earlier with the two hands, the therapist surprises the patient by suddenly changing the position of his hands. In another method the therapist holds his or her hand in front and the patient, touching the hand, has to follow the therapist arm movement in space. The therapist's movements are gradually increased in speed and randomness, and the patient must quickly adjust to them. These methods will also challenge coordination ability. *Fine control:* Same as for reaction time but the hands are brought together closely, while the patient must tap them rapidly using small amplitude of movement (Fig. 16-11, *B*). *Transitional ability:* Switch rapidly between the abilities being challenged. For example, instruct the patient to follow your hand, then suddenly stop and instruct him or her to stiffen the shoulder in this position, hold it for a few seconds challenging static co-contraction, and then ask the patient to pull and push (reciprocal activation). Eventually, many of these abilities are challenged in movement patterns that simulate a tennis serve. This is done to address the similarity principle.	*Reciprocal activation:* Use the exercise described earlier, with the good side training the injured side, but here the injured arm is pulling and pushing against resistance of the good arm, in large-amplitude movement (e.g., into flexion/extension, internal/external, and abduction/adduction movements). Increase force and angles as the condition improves. In another exercise the patient is instructed to draw an imaginary number in the air, in front and at the side of the body. Increase the size of the numbers. This can be done lying supine counting on the ceiling or behind the head. Add velocity by doing the number faster or by drawing small numbers quickly. Add force by holding a book or a can (nonalcoholic) while counting. These exercises can be performed throughout the day without the need for a gym.

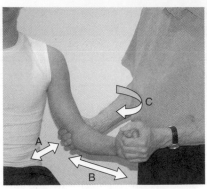

Figure 16-9 Challenging static co-contraction: the patient is instructed to "stiffen his or her shoulder" and keep it in the same position, while the therapists pushes and pulls it in different directions. *A,* Abduction/adduction. *B,* Flexion/extension. *C,* Internal/external rotation of glenohumeral joint. The angles, force, and velocity of perturbations imposed by the therapist can increase as the patient's co-contraction ability improves. Another challenge is to surprise the patient by sudden and rapid changes in the directions of perturbations and their velocity.

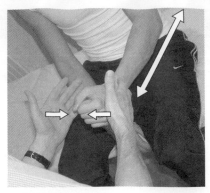

Figure 16-10 Challenging dynamic co-contraction: The patient is instructed to move in one plane (e.g., flexion/extension), while the therapist applies sudden lateral and medial disturbances to the movement. The patient must maintain this movement and overcome the lateral disturbances.

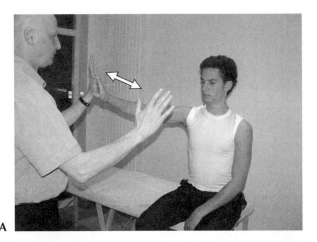

A

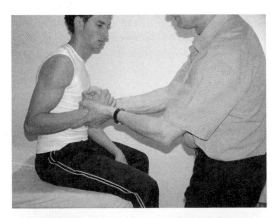

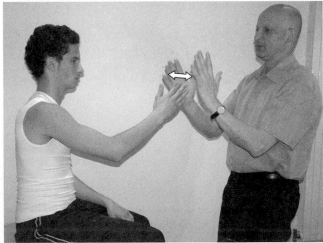

B

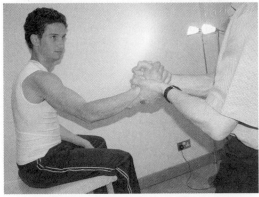

Figure 16-11 Challenging reciprocal activation: The patient is instructed to push and pull against the therapist's resistance. Force, velocity, and angles of shoulder movement are continuously changed.

Figure 16-12 This hand position is useful for challenging various abilities. **A,** Velocity of movement (the therapist instructs the patient to alternately touch each hand at increasing speed), length control (therapist continuously changes hand position, holding the hands farther apart and at different positions), and reaction times (therapist introduces sudden changes of hand positions). **B,** The therapist holds the hand closer to challenge fine movement of the shoulder. The patient is instructed to produce rapid movement with the outstretched arm between the two hands.

SUMMARY

This chapter examined the role of MT in sports rehabilitation. The aim of MT is to assist repair and adaptation processes associated with sports injuries. Repair and adaptation respond to specific signals, which can be provided by identifiable manual techniques/approaches.

The Dimensional Model of MT was introduced in this chapter as an important clinical tool for matching the most suitable manual technique to the patient's condition. In this model the effects of MT are observed in three dimensions—tissue, neurological, and psychological dimensions. At each dimension the manual approach changes in order to provide the necessary stimulation and signals to activate the processes associated with each dimension.

REFERENCES

1. Lederman E: *The science and practice of manual therapy*, ed 2, Edinburgh, 2005, Elsevier.
2. Tillman LJ, Cummings GS: Biology mechanisms of connective tissue mutability. In Currier DP, Nelson RM, editors: *Dynamics of human biological tissue*, pp. 1-44, Philadelphia, 1993, FA Davis.
3. Baur PS, Parks DH: The myofibroblast anchoring strand: the fibronectin connection in wound healing and possible loci of collagen fibril assembly, *J Trauma* 23:853-862, 1983.
4. Madden JW, Peacock EE: Studies on the biology of collagen during wound healing. I. Rate of collagen synthesis and deposition in cutaneous wounds of the rat, *Surgery* 64(1):288-294, 1968.
5. Hunt TK, Van Winkle W: Normal repair. In Hunt TK, Dunphy JE, editors: *Fundamentals of wound management*, pp. 2-67, New York, 1979, Appleton-Century-Crofts.
6. Hargens AR, Akeson WH: Stress effects on tissue nutrition and viability. In Hargens AR, editor: *Tissue nutrition and viability*, New York, 1986, Springer-Verlag.
7. Gelberman RH, Menon J, Gonsalves M, et al: The effects of mobilization on vascularisation of healing flexor tendons in dogs, *Clin Orthop* 153:283-289, 1980.
8. Tohyama H, Yasuda K: Significance of graft tension in anterior cruciate ligament reconstruction. Basic background and clinical outcome, *Knee Surg Sports Traumatol Arthrosc* 6(Suppl 1):S30-37, 1998.
9. Buckwalter JA, Grodzinsky AJ: Loading of healing bone, fibrous tissue, and muscle: implications for orthopaedic practice, *J Am Acad Orthop Surg* 7(5):291-299, 1999.
10. Kiviranta I, Tammi M, Jurvelin J, et al: Articular cartilage thickness and glycosaminoglycan distribution in the young canine knee joint after remobilization of the immobilized limb, *J Orthop Res* 12(2):161-167, 1994.
11. Dhert WJ, O'Driscoll SW, van Royen BJ, et al: Effects of immobilization and continuous passive motion on postoperative muscle atrophy in mature rabbits, *Can J Surg* 31(3):185-188, 1988.
12. Akeson WH, Amiel D, Woo SL: Immobility effects on synovial joints: the pathomechanics of joint contracture, *Biorheology* 17:95-110, 1980.
13. Akeson WH, Amiel D, Mechanic GL, et al: Collagen cross-linking alterations in joint contractures: changes in the reducible cross-links in periarticular connective tissue collagen after nine weeks of immobilization, *Connect Tissue Res* 5:15-19, 1977.
14. Amiel D, Woo SL-Y, Harwood F, et al: The effect of immobilization on collagen turnover in connective tissue: a biochemical-biomechanical correlation, *Acta Orthop Scand* 53:325-332, 1982.
15. Harwood FL, Amiel D: *Differential metabolic responses of periarticular ligaments and tendons to joint immobilization*, pp. 1687-1691, Bethesda, Md, 1990, American Physiological Society.
16. Gossman MR, Sahrmann SA, Rose SJ: Review of length associated changes in muscle, *Phys Ther* 62(12):1799-1808, 1982.
17. Evans EB, Eggers GWN, Butler JK, et al: Experimental immobilisation and remobilisation of rat knee joints, *J Bone Joint Surg Am* 42(5):737-758, 1960.
18. Williams PE: Use of stretch in the prevention of serial sarcomere loss in immobilised muscle, *Ann Rheum Dis* 49:316-317, 1990.
19. Hernandez-Reif M, Field T, Krasnegor J, et al: Low back pain is reduced and range of motion increased after massage therapy, *Int J Neurosci* 106:131-145, 2001.
20. Field T, Hernandez-Reif M, Taylor S, et al: Labor pain is reduced by massage therapy, *J Psychosom Obstet Gynecol* 18:286-291, 1997.
21. Hirayama F, Kageyama Y, Urabe N, et al: The effect of postoperative ataralgesia by manual therapy after pulmonary resection, *Man Ther* 8(1):42-45, 2003.
22. Rowe LB, Frackowiak RSJ: The impact of brain imaging technology on our understanding of motor function and dysfunction, *Curr Opin Neurobiol* 9(6):728-734, 1999.
23. Cramer SC, Finklestein SP, Schaechter JD, et al: Activation of distinct motor cortex regions during ipsilateral and contralateral finger movements, *J Neurophysiol* 81:383-387, 1999.
24. Karni A, Meyer G, Rey-Hipolito C, et al: The acquisition of skilled motor performance: fast and slow experience-driven changes in primary motor cortex, *PNAS* 95(3):861-868, 1998.
25. Liepert J, Tegenthoff M, Malin JP: Changes of cortical motor area size during immobilization, *Electroenceph Clin Neurophysiol* 97:382-386, 1995.
26. Kaneko F, Murakami T, Onari K, et al: Motor imagery after disuse of an upper limb in humans, *Clin Neurophysiol* 114(12):2397-2403, 2003.
27. Elbert T, Sterr A, Flor H, et al: Input-increase and input-decrease types of cortical reorganization after upper extremity amputation in humans, *Exp Brain Res* 117(1):161-164, 1997.

28. Elbert T, Pantev C, Wienbruch C, et al: Increased use of the left hand in string players associated with increased cortical representation of the fingers, *Science* 220:21-23, 1995.

29. Cohen LG, Bandinelli S, Findley TW, et al: Motor reorganization after upper limb amputation in man. A study with focal magnetic stimulation, *Brain J Neurol* 114(1B):615-627, 1991.

30. Kidd G, Lawes N, Musa I: *Understanding neuromuscular plasticity: a basis for clinical rehabilitation*, London, 1992, Edward Arnold.

31. Pascual-Leone A, Cohen LG, Hallet M: Cortical map plasticity in humans, *Trends Neuro Science* 15(1):13-14, 1992.

32. Wolpaw JR: Adaptive plasticity in the spinal stretch reflex: an accessible substrate of memory? *Cell Mol Neurobiol* 5(1/2):147-165, 1985.

33. Wolpaw JR, Lee CL: Memory traces in primate spinal cord produced by operant conditioning of H-reflex, *J Neurobiol* 61(3):563-573, 1989.

34. Evatt ML, Wolf SL, Segal RL: Modification of the human stretch reflex: preliminary studies, *Neurosci Lett* 105:350-355, 1989.

35. Hodgson JA, Roland RR, de-Leon R, et al: Can the mammalian lumbar spinal cord learn a motor task? *Med Sci Sports Exerc* 26(12):1491-1497, 1994.

36. Seki K, Taniguchi Y, Narusawa M: Effects of joint immobilization on firing rate modulation of human motor units, *J Physiol* 530(3):507-519, 2001.

37. Patten C, Kamen G: Adaptations in motor unit discharge activity with force control training in young and older human adults, *Eur J Appl Physiol* 83(2-3):128-143, 2000.

38. Duchateau J, Hainaut K: Effects of immobilization on contractile properties, recruitment and firing rates of human motor units, *J Physiol* 422:55-65, 1990.

39. McComas AJ: Human neuromuscular adaptations that accompany changes in activity, *Med Sci Sports Exerc* 26(12):1498-1509, 1994.

40. Henneman E: Skeletal muscle: the servant of the nervous system. In Mountcastle VB, editor: *Medical Physiology*, St Louis, 1980, Mosby. pp. 674-702.

41. Brion JP, Demeurisse G, Capon A: Evidence of cortical reorganization in hemiparetic patients, *Stroke* 20(8): 1079-1084, 1989.

42. Cao Y, D'Olhaberriague L, Vikingstad EM, et al: Pilot study of functional MRI to assess cerebral activation of motor function after poststroke hemiparesis, *Stroke* 29(1):112-122, 1998.

43. Cramer SC, Nelles G, Benson RR, et al: A functional MRI study of subjects recovered from hemiparetic stroke, *Stroke* 28:2518-2527, 1997.

44. van Die'n JH, Selen LPJ, Cholewicki J: Trunk muscle activation in low-back pain patients, an analysis of the literature, *J Electromyogr Kinesiol* 13(4):333-351, 2003.

45. Freeman MAR, Dean MRE, Hanham IWF: The etiology and prevention of functional instability of the foot, *J Bone Joint Surg Br* 47(4):678-685, 1965.

46. Geeraedts LM Jr, Vollmar B, Menger MD, et al: Striated muscle microvascular response to zymosan-induced generalized inflammation in awake hamsters, *Shock* 10(2):103-109, 1998.

47. Garfin SR, Tipton CM, Mubarak SJ, et al: Role of fascia in maintenance of muscle tension and pressure, *J Appl Physiol* 51(2):317-320, 1981.

48. Larsson SE, Bodegard L, Henriksson KG, et al: Chronic trapezius myalgia. Morphology and blood flow studied in 17 patients, *Acta Orthop Scand* 61(5):394-398, 1990.

49. Larsson SE, Larsson R, Zhang Q, et al: Effects of psychophysiological stress on trapezius muscles blood flow and electromyography during static load, *Eur J Appl Physiol Occup Physiol* 71(6):493-498, 1995.

50. Hoyland JA, Freemont AJ, Jayson MIV: Intervertebral foramen venous obstruction: a cause of periradicular obstruction? *Spine* 14(6):558-568, 1989.

51. Toyone T, Takahashi K, Kitahara H, et al: Visualisation of symptomatic nerve root: prospective study of contrast enhanced MRI in patients with lumbar disc herniation, *J Bone Joint Surg Br* 75(4):529-533, 1993.

52. Magnusson SP, Simonsen EB, Aagaard P, et al: A mechanism for altered flexibility in human skeletal muscle, *J Physiol* 497(1):291-298, 1996.

53. Gleim GW, McHugh MP: Flexibility and its effects on sports injury and performance, *Sports Med* 24(5): 289-299, 1997.

54. Alnaqeeb MA, Goldspink G: Changes in fibre type, number and diameter in developing and ageing skeletal muscle, *J Anat* 153:31-45, 1987.

55. Alnaqeeb MA, Al Zaid NS, Goldspink G: Connective tissue changes and physical properties of developing and ageing skeletal muscle, *J Anat* 139(Pt 4):677-689, 1984.

56. Lehmann JF, Price R, deLateur BJ, et al: Spasticity: quantitative measurements as a basis for assessing effectiveness of therapeutic intervention, *Arch Phys Med Rehabil* 70(1):6-15, 1989.

57. Hufschmidt A, Mauritz K-H: Chronic transformation of muscle in spasticity: a peripheral contribution to increased tone, *J Neurol Neurosurg Psychiatry* 48(7):676-685, 1985.

58. Singer B, Dunne J, Singer KP, et al: Evaluation of triceps surae muscle length and resistance to passive lengthening in patients with acquired brain injury, *Clin Biomech* 17(2)152-161, 2002.

59. Field T, Morrow C, Valdeon C, et al: Massage therapy reduces anxiety in child and adolescent psychiatric patients, *J Am Acad Child Adolesc Psychiatry* 31:125-130, 1992.

60. Diego M, Field T, Hernandez-Reif M, et al: Aggressive adolescents benefit from massage therapy, *Adolescence* 37:597-607, 2002.

61. Field T, Ironson G, Scafidi F, et al: Massage therapy reduces anxiety and enhances EEG pattern of alertness and math computations, *Int J Neurosci* 86:197-205, 1996.

62. Field T, Quintino O, Hernandez-Reif M, et al: Adolescents with attention deficit hyperactivity disorder benefit from massage therapy, *Adolescence* 33:103-108, 1998

63. Hart S, Field T, Hernandez-Reif M, et al: Anorexia symptoms are reduced by massage therapy, *Eat Disord* 9:289-299, 2001.

64. Field T, Shanberg S, Kuhn C, et al: Bulimic adolescents benefit from massage therapy, *Adolescence* 131:555-563, 1997.

65. Delaney JP, Leong KS, Watkins A, et al: The short-term effects of myofascial trigger point massage therapy on cardiac autonomic tone in healthy subjects, *J Adv Nurs* 37(4):364-371, 2002.

66. Goffaux-Dogniez C, Vanfraechem-Raway R, Verbanck P: Appraisal of treatment of the trigger points associated with relaxation to treat chronic headache in the adult. Relationship with anxiety and stress adaptation strategies, *Encephale* 29(5):377-390, 2003.

67. De Laat A, Stappaerts K, Papy S: Counseling and physical therapy as treatment for myofascial pain of the masticatory system, *J Orofac Pain* 17(1): 42-49, 2003.

68. Furlan AD, Brosseau L, Imamura M, et al: Massage for low-back pain: a systematic review within the framework of the Cochrane Collaboration Back Review Group, *Spine* 27(17):1896-910, 2002.

69. Ironson G, Field T, Scafidi F, et al: Massage therapy is associated with enhancement of the immune system's cytotoxic capacity, *Int J Neurosci* 84:205-218, 1996.

70. Hernandez-Reif M, Ironson G, Field T, et al: Breast cancer patients have improved immune and neuroendocrine functions following massage therapy, *J Psychosom Res* 57(1):45-52, 2004.

71. Deigo MA, Hernandez-Reif M, Field T, et al: Massage therapy effects on immune function in adolescents with HIV, *Int J Neurosci* 106:35-45, 2001.

72. Hernandez-Reif M, Field T, Krasnegor J, et al: High blood pressure and associated symptoms were reduced by massage therapy, *J Bodywork Move Ther* 4:31-38, 2000.

73. Morrow C, Field T, Scafidi FA, et al: Differential effects of massage and heelstick procedures on transcutaneous oxygen tension in preterm neonates, *Infant Behav Dev* 14:397-414, 1991.

74. Field T, Peck M, Krugman S, et al: Burn injuries benefit from massage therapy, *J Burn Care Rehabil* 19:241-244, 1997.

75. Field T, Hernandez-Reif M, LaGreca A, et al: Massage therapy lowers blood glucose levels in children with diabetes mellitus, *Diabetes Spectrum* 10:237-239, 1997.

76. Field T, Scafidi F, Schanberg S: Massage of preterm newborns to improve growth and development, *Pediatr Nursing* 13:385-387, 1987.

77. Field T, Hernandez-Reif M: Sleep problems in infants decrease following massage therapy, *Early Child Dev Care* 168:95-104, 2001.

78. Larsson B, Bjork J, Henriksson KG, et al: The prevalences of cytochrome c oxidase negative and superposi-tive fibres and ragged-red fibres in the trapezius muscle of female cleaners with and without myalgia and of female healthy controls, *Pain* 84(2-3):379-387, 2000.

79. Kadi F, Waling K, Ahlgren C, et al: Pathological mechanisms implicated in localized female trapezius myalgia, *Pain* 78(3):191-196, 1998.

80. Kadi F, Hagg G, Hakansson R, et al: Structural changes in male trapezius muscle with work-related myalgia, *Acta Neuropathol (Berl)* 95(4):352-360, 1998.

81. Lindman R, Hagberg M, Angqvist KA, et al: Changes in muscle morphology in chronic trapezius myalgia, *Scand J Work Environ Health* 17(5):347-355, 1991.

82. Larsson SE, Bengtsson A, Bodegard L, et al: Muscle changes in work-related chronic myalgia, *Acta Orthop Scand* 59(5):552-556, 1988.

83. Larsson B, Bjork J, Elert J, et al: Fibre type proportion and fibre size in trapezius muscle biopsies from cleaners with and without myalgia and its correlation with ragged red fibres, cytochrome-c-oxidase-negative fibres, biomechanical output, perception of fatigue, and surface electromyography during repetitive forward flexions, *Eur J Appl Physiol* 84(6):492-502, 2001.

84. Arnoczky SP, Tian T, Lavagnino M, et al: Activation of stress-activated protein kinases (SAPK) in tendon cells following cyclic strain: the effects of strain frequency, strain magnitude, and cytosolic calcium, *J Orthop Res* 20(5):947-952, 2002.

85. Graf R, Freyberg M, Kaiser D, et al: Mechanosensitive induction of apoptosis in fibroblasts is regulated by thrombospondin-1 and integrin associated protein (CD47), *Apoptosis* 7(6):493-498, 2002.

86. Bosch U, Zeichen J, Skutek M, et al: Effect of cyclical stretch on matrix synthesis of human patellar tendon cells, *Unfallchirurg* 105(5):437-442, 2002.

87. Salter DM, Millward-Sadler SJ, Nuki G, et al: Differential responses of chondrocytes from normal and osteoarthritic human articular cartilage to mechanical stimulation, *Biorheology* 39(1-2):97-108, 2002.

88. Grinnell F: Fibroblast-collagen-matrix contraction: growth-factor signalling and mechanical loading, *Trends Cell Biol* 10(9):362-365, 2000.

89. Parsons M, Kessler E, Laurent GJ, et al: Mechanical load enhances procollagen processing in dermal fibroblasts by regulating levels of procollagen C-proteinase, *Exp Cell Res* 252(2):319-331, 1999.

90. Jarvinen TA, Jozsa L, Kannus P, et al: Mechanical loading regulates tenascin-C expression in the osteotendinous junction, *J Cell Sci* 112:3157-3166, 1999.

91. Buckwalter JA, Grodzinsky AJ: Loading of healing bone, fibrous tissue, and muscle: implications for orthopaedic practice, *J Am Acad Orthop Surg* 7(5):291-299, 1999.

92. Goldspink G, Williams P, Simpson H: Gene expression in response to muscle stretch, *Clin Orthop* (403 Suppl):S146-152, 2002.

93. Goldspink G: Gene expression in skeletal muscle, *Biochem Soc Trans* 30(2):285-290, 2002.

94. Goldspink G, Yang SY: Effects of activity on growth factor expression, *Int J Sport Nutr Exerc Metab* 11:S21-27, 2001.

95. Williams P, Watt P, Bicik V, et al: Effect of stretch combined with electrical stimulation on the type of sarcomeres produced at the end of muscle fibers, *Exp Neurol* 93:500-509, 1986.

96. Fronek J, Frank C, Amiel D, et al: The effect of intermittent passive motion (IMP) in the healing of medial collateral ligament, *Proc Orthopaed Res Soc* 8:31(abstract), 1983.

97. Takai S, Woo SL, Horibe S, et al: The effects of frequency and duration of controlled passive mobilization on tendon healing, *J Orthopaed Res* 9(5):705-713, 1991.

98. Vailas AC, Tipton CM, Matthes RD, et al: Physical activity and its influence on the repair process of medial collateral ligament, *Connect Tissue Res* 9:25-31, 1981.

99. Strickland JW, Glogovac V: Digital function following flexor tendon repair in zone 2: a comparison of immobilization and controlled passive motion techniques, *J Hand Surg* 5(6):537-543, 1980.

100. Gelberman RH, Woo SL, Lothringer K, et al: Effects of early intermittent passive mobilization on healing canine flexor tendons, *J Hand Surg {Am}* 7(2):170-175, 1982.

101. Pneumaticos SG, McGarvey WC, Mody DR, et al: The effects of early mobilization in the healing of achilles tendon repair, *Foot Ankle Int* 21(7):551-557, 2000.

102. Woo SL, Gelberman RH, Cobb NG, et al: The importance of controlled passive mobilization on flexor tendon healing. A biomechanical study, *Acta Orthop Scand* 52(6):615-622, 1981.

103. Loitz BJ, Zernicke RF, Vailas AC, et al: Effects of short-term immobilization versus continuous passive motion on the biomechanical and biochemical properties of the rabbit tendon, *Clin Orthop* 244:265-271, 1989.

104. Savio SL-Y, Gelberman RH, Cobb NG, et al: The importance of controlled passive mobilization on flexor tendon healing, *Acta Orthopaed Scand* 52:615-622, 1981.

105. Gelberman RH, Amiel D, Gonsalves M, et al: The influence of protected passive mobilization on the healing of flexor tendons: a biochemical and microangiographic study, *Hand* 13(2):120-128, 1981.

106. Johnson DP: The effect of continuous passive motion on wound-healing and joint mobility after knee arthroplasty, *Bone Joint Surg Am* 72(3):421-426, 1990.

107. van Royen BJ, O'Driscoll SW, Dhert WJ, et al: A comparison of the effects of immobilization and continuous passive motion on surgical wound healing in mature rabbits, *Plast Reconstr Surg* 78(3):360-368, 1986.

108. Forrester JC, Zederfeldt BH, Hayes TL, et al: Wolff's law in relation to the healing of skin wounds, *J Trauma* 10(9):770-780, 1970.

109. Lagrana NA et al: Effect of mechanical load in wound healing, *Ann Plast Surg* 10:200-208, 1983.

110. Arnold J, Madden JW: Effects of stress on healing wounds. I. Intermittent noncyclical tension, *J Surg Res* 29:93-102, 1976.

111. Akeson WH, Amiel D, Woo SL-Y: Physiology and therapeutic value of passive motion. In Helminen HJ, Kivaranka I, Tammi M, editors: *Joint loading: biology and health of articular structures*, pp. 375-394, Bristol, England, 1987, John Wright.

112. McCarthy MR, Yates CK, Anderson MA, et al: The effects of immediate continuous passive motion on pain during the inflammatory phase of soft tissue healing following anterior cruciate ligament reconstruction, *J Orthop Sports Phys Ther* 17(2):96-101, 1993.

113. Raab MG, Rzeszutko D, O'Connor W, et al: Early results of continuous passive motion after rotator cuff repair: a prospective, randomized, blinded, controlled study, *Am J Orthop* 25(3):214-220, 1996.

114. Simkin PA, de Lateur BJ, Alquist AD, et al: Continuous passive motion for osteoarthritis of the hip: a pilot study, *Rheumatology* 26(9):1987-1991, 1999.

115. O'Driscoll SW, Giori NJ: Continuous passive motion (CPM): theory and principles of clinical application, *J Rehabil Res Dev* 37(2):179-188, 2000.

116. Williams JM, Moran M, Thonar EJ, et al: Continuous passive motion stimulates repair of rabbit knee articular cartilage after matrix proteoglycan loss, *Clin Orthop* (304):252-262, 1994.

117. Greene WB: Use of continuous passive slow motion in the postoperative rehabilitation of difficult pediatric knee and elbow problems, *J Pediatr Orthop* 3(4):419-423, 1983.

118. Lederman E: *Harmonic technique,* Edinburgh, 2000, Churchill Livingstone.

119. Levick JR: Synovial fluid and trans-synovial flow in stationary and moving normal joints. In Helminen HJ, Kivaranki I, Tammi M, editors: *Joint loading: biology and health of articular structures*, pp. 149-186, Bristol, 1987, John Wright.

120. Skyhar MJ, Danzig LA, Hargens AR, et al: Nutrition of the anterior cruciate ligament: effects of continuous passive motion, *Am J Sports Med* 13(6):415-418, 1985.

121. O'Driscoll SW, Kumar A, Salter RB: The effect of continuous passive motion on the clearance of haemarthrosis, *Clin Orthopaed Rel Res* 176:305-311, 1983.

122. Kamm RD: Flow through collapsible tubes. In Skalak R, Chien S, eds., *Handbook of bioengineering,* New York, 1987, McGraw-Hill.

123. McGeown JG, McHale NG, Thornbury KD: Effects of varying patterns of external compression on lymph flow in the hind limb of the anaesthetized sheep, *J Physiology* 397:449-457, 1988.

124. Airaksinen O: Changes in post-traumatic ankle joint mobility, pain and oedema following intermittent pneumatic compression therapy, *Arch Phys Med Rehab* 70(4):341-344, 1989.

125. Airaksinen O, Partanen K, Kolari P J, et al: Intermittent pneumatic compression therapy in posttraumatic lower limb edema: computed tomography and clinical measurements, *Arch Phys Med Rehabil* 72(9):667-670, 1991.

126. Schmid-Schonbein GW: Microlymphatics and lymph flow, *Physiol Rev* 70(4):987-1028, 1990.

127. McHugh MP, Magnusson SP, Gleim GW, et al: Viscloelastic stress relaxation in human skeletal muscle, *Med Sci Sports Exerc* 24(12):1375-1382, 1992.

128. Magnusson SP, Simonsen EB, Aagaard P, et al: Biomechanical response to repeated stretching in human hamstring muscle in vivo, *Am J Sports Med* 24(5):622-628, 1996.

129. Magnusson SP, Simonsen EB, Aagaard P, et al: Mechanical and physiological responses to stretching with or without preisometric contraction in human skeletal muscle, *Arch Phys Med Rehabil* 77: 373-378, 1996.

130. Magnusson SP, Simonsen EB, Aagaard P, et al: Determinants of musculoskeletal flexibility: viscoelastic properties, cross-sectional area, EMG and stretch tolerance, *Scand J Med Sci Sports* 7:195-202, 1997.

131. Magnusson SP, Aagard P, Simonsen E, et al: A biomechanical evaluation of cyclic and static stretch in human skeletal muscle, *Int J Sports Med* 19(5):310-316, 1998.

132. Magnusson SP: Passive properties of human skeletal muscle during stretch maneuvers. A review, *Scand J Med Sci Sports* 8(2):65-77, 1998.

133. Taylor DC, Dalton JD, Seaber AV, et al: Viscoelastic properties of muscle-tendon units: the biomechanical effects of stretching, *Am J Sports Med* 18(3):300-309, 1990.

134. Bandy WD, Irion JM: The effect of time on static stretch on the flexibility of the hamstring muscles, *Phys Ther* 74(9):845-850, 1994.

135. McNair PJ, Dombroski EW, Hewson DJ, et al: Stretching at the ankle joint: viscoelastic responses to holds and continuous passive motion, *Med Sci Sports Exerc* 33(3):354-358, 2001.

136. Bandy WD, Irion JM, Briggler M: The effect of time and frequency of static stretching on flexibility of the hamstring muscles, *Phys Ther* 77(10):1090-1096, 1997.

137. Magnusson SP, Simonsen EB, Aagaard P, et al: Viscoelastic response to repeated static stretching in the human hamstring muscle, *Scand J Med Sci Sports* 5(6):342-347, 1995.

138. Magnusson SP, Simonsen EB, Aagaard P, et al: Contraction specific changes in passive torque in human skeletal muscle, *Acta Physiol Scand* 155(4):377-386, 1995.

139. Roberts JM, Wilson K: Effect of stretching duration on active and passive range of motion in the lower extremity, *Br J Sports Med* 33(4):259-263, 1999.

140. Warren CG, Lehman JF, Koblanski JN: Heat and stretch procedure: an evaluation using rat tail tendon, *Arch Phys Med Rehabil* 57:122-126, 1976.

141. Light KE, Nuzik S, Personius W: Low load prolonged stretch vs. high load brief stretch in treating knee contractures, *Phys Ther* 64:330-333, 1984.

142. DeFeudis FV, DeFeudis PAF: *Elements of the behavioral code,* London, 1977, Academic Press.

143. Schmidt RA: *Motor learning and performance: from principles to practice,* Champaign, Ill, 1991, Human Kinetic Books.

144. Williams HG: Neurological concepts and perceptual-motor behavior. In Brown RC, Cratty BJ, editors: *New perspective of man in action.* Englewood Cliffs, NJ, 1969, Prentice-Hall.

145. Schmidt RA: *Motor learning and control: a behavioral emphasis,* Champaign, Ill, 1982, Human Kinetics.

146. Lackner JR, DiZio P: Adaptation to Coriolis force perturbation of movement trajectory; role of proprioceptive and cutaneous somatosensory feedback, *Adv Exp Med Biol* 508:69-78, 2002.

147. Gregory JE, Brockett CL, Morgan DL, et al: Effect of eccentric muscle contractions on Golgi tendon organ responses to passive and active tension in the cat, *J Physiol* 538(Pt 1):209-218, 2002.

148. Vallbo AB, Hagbarth K-E, Torebjork HE, et al: Somatosensory, proprioceptive and sympathetic activity in human peripheral nerve, *Physiol Rev* 59(4):919-957, 1979.

149. Jami L: Golgi tendon organs in mammalian skeletal muscle: functional properties and central actions, *Physiol Rev* 73(3):623-666, 1992.

150. Matthews PBC: Muscle spindles: their messages and their fusimotor supply. In Brookhart JM, Mountcastle VB, Brooks VB, et al: *Handbook of Physiology, Section 1: The Nervous System,* vol. II: Motor Control, Bethesda, MD, American Physiological Society, 1981.

151. Valbo AB: Afferent discharge from human muscle spindle in non-contracting muscles. Steady state impulse frequency as a function of joint angle, *Acta Physiol Scand* 90:303-318, 1973.

152. Gandevia SC, McCloskey DI, Burke D: Kinaesthetic signals and muscle contraction, *Trends Neurosci* 15(2): 64-65, 1992.

153. Paillard J, Brouchon M: Active and passive movements in the calibration of position sense. In Freedman SJ editor: *The neuropsychology of spatially oriented behavior,* pp. 37-55, Homewood, Ill, 1968, Dorsey Press.

154. Lemon RN, Porter R: Short-latency peripheral afferent inputs to pyramidal and other neurones in the precentral cortex of conscious monkeys, pp. 91-103, In Gordon G, editor: *Active touch,* Oxford, England, 1978, Pergamon Press.

155. Gandevia SC, McCloskey DI: Joint sense, muscle sense and their combination as position sense, measured at the distal interphalangeal joint of the middle finger, *J Physiol* 260:387-407, 1976.

156. Ralston HJ, Libet B: The question of tonus in skeletal muscles, *Am J Phys Med* 32:85-92, 1953.

157. von-Wright JM: A note on the role of guidance in learning, *Br J Psychology* 48:133-137, 1957.

158. Matthews PBC: Proprioceptors and their contribution to somatosensory mapping: complex messages require complex processing, *Can J Physiology Pharmacol* 66:430-438, 1988.

159. Rock I, Harris CS: Vision and touch, *Sci Am* 216:96-107, 1967.
160. Isaacs KR, Anderson BJ, Alcantara AA, et al: Exercise and the brain: angiogenesis in the adult rat cerebellum after vigorous physical activity and motor skill learning, *Cereb Blood Flow Metab* 12(1):110-119, 1992.
161. Black JE, Isaacs KR, Anderson BJ, et al: Learning causes synaptogenesis, whereas motor activity causes angiogenesis, in cerebellar cortex of adult rats, *Proc Natl Acad Sci USA* 87(14):5568-5572, 1990.
162. Saxton JM, Clarkson PM, James R, et al: Neuromuscular dysfunction following eccentric exercise, *Med Sci Sports Exerc* 27(8):1185-1193, 1995.
163. Bonfim TR, Paccola CAJ, Barela JA: Proprioceptive and behavior impairments in individuals with anterior cruciate ligament reconstructed knees, *Arch Phys Med Rehab* 84(8):1217-1223, 2003.
164. Bobath B: The application of physiological principles to stroke rehabilitation, *Practitioner* 223:793-794, 1979.
165. DeFeudis FV, DeFeudis PAF: *Elements of the behavioral code,* London, 1977, Academic Press.
166. Schmidt RA: *Motor learning and performance: from principles to practice,* Champaign, Ill, 1991, Human Kinetic Books.
167. Williams HG: Neurological concepts and perceptual-motor behavior. In Brown RC, Cratty BJ, editors: *New perspective of man in action.* Englewood Cliffs, NJ, 1969, Prentice-Hall.
168. Schmidt RA: *Motor learning and control: a behavioral emphasis,* Champaign, Ill., 1982, Human Kinetics.
169. Holding DH: *Principles of training,* London, 1965, Pergamon Press.
170. Osgood CE: The similarity paradox in human learning: a resolution, *Psychol Rev* 56:132-143, 1949.
171. Fleishman EA: Human abilities and the acquisition of skills. In Bilodeau EA, editor: *Acquisition of skill,* New York, 1966, Academic Press.
172. Lederman E: Osteopathic neuromuscular rehabilitation, *Osteopathy Today* June, 8, 2002 (available at *www.cpdo.net*).
173. Skinner HB, Barrack RL, Cook SD, et al: Joint position sense in total knee arthroplasty, *J Orthop Res* 1:276-283, 1984.
174. Hurley MV, Newham DJ: The influence of arthrogenous muscle inhibition on quadriceps rehabilitation of patients with early, unilateral osteoarthritic knees, *Br J Rheumatol* 32:127-131, 1993.
175. Parkhurst TM, Burnett CN: Injury and proprioception in the lower back, *J Orthop Sports Phys Ther* 19(5):282-295, 1994.
176. Herzog W, Longino D, Clark A: The role of muscles in joint adaptation and degeneration, *Langenbecks Arch Surg* 388(5):305-315, 2003.

CHAPTER

17

Jaclyn Maurer

Nutrition for the Athlete

LEARNING OBJECTIVES

After studying this chapter, the reader will be able to do the following:

1. Estimate daily total energy needs
2. Describe the appropriate amount of carbohydrate, protein, and fat for an athlete's diet
3. Describe the appropriate protocol for carbohydrate loading
4. Identify the appropriate nutrient for consumption, before, during, and after exercise
5. Describe optimal fluid intake guidelines for exercise
6. Evaluate ergogenic aids for safety and effectiveness
7. Understand the influence of exercise on gastrointestinal function and the effect of diet
8. Describe how to evaluate the optimal body weight and composition for an athlete

Nutritional recommendations for an athlete depend on many factors including (1) type of exercise; (2) duration of exercise; (3) intensity of exercise; (4) performance goals; and, of course, (5) personal preference. Simply consuming a "sports" bar or "sports" drink does not constitute a top-notch sports nutrition diet plan. This chapter helps to alleviate the confusion about what to eat for peak performance and provides an overview of the basic and essential considerations when choosing foods to fuel an athlete.

ENERGY NEEDS

A top concern for any athlete is making sure the appropriate amount of energy (i.e., calories) is consumed to meet daily needs. This energy is used to fuel not only exercise but any other muscular activity and all the metabolic processes in the body.[1] For an athlete, determining how much energy to con-sume is the first step in designing his or her sports nutrition diet plan. The three major components of an individual's energy requirement include the following[2]:

1. Resting energy expenditure (REE): the amount of energy necessary to maintain basic body systems and body temperature at rest
2. Thermic effect of food (TEF): the amount of energy used following consumption of food/nutrients for absorption, digestion, metabolism, and storage of the food/nutrients
3. Activity energy expenditure (AEE): the amount of energy used during both activities of daily living (e.g., cooking, showering, dressing), involuntary muscular movements (e.g., shivering), and planned physical activity

The average person's total energy requirement is predominately (60% to 80%) determined by his or her REE,[2] which varies with body size and composition. A higher body weight will increase REE, while a higher muscle mass will do the same. The second component, TEF, accounts for approximately 6% to 10% of an individual's total energy requirement and varies by macronutrient composition of the diet, as well as the energy density of a meal.[2] The final component, AEE, is the most variant factor in determining an athlete's total energy requirements and typically accounts for 20% to 40% of total energy requirements, but for some elite athletes it can account for closer to half of their total energy needs.[1] This latter factor is the most essential in determining an individual athlete's energy needs and is heavily influenced by an athlete's training duration, intensity, and frequency.

CALCULATING AND MEETING ENERGY NEEDS

Most athletes want to know exactly how much energy they need to train and perform, but simply telling them they need to consume 3000 calories daily does little to support their

Table 17-1	Equations for Estimating Resting Metabolic Rate in Healthy Individuals
Equation 1	Males: REE calories = 11 × body weight in pounds
	Females: REE calories = 10 × body weight in pounds
Equation 2	Males: REE calories = 66.47 + 13.75 (weight, kg) + 5 (height, cm) − 6.76 (age, yr)
	Females: REE calories = 655.1 + 9.65 (weight, kg) + 1.84 (height, cm) − 4.68 (age, yr)
Equation 3	Males and females: 500 + (22 × lean body mass)

Data from Cunningham JJ: *Am J Clin Nutr* 33(11):2372-2374, 1980; Frankenfield DC, Muth ER, Rowe WA: *J Am Diet Assoc* 98(4):439-445, 1998.
REE, Resting energy expenditure.

Table 17-2	Activity Factors		
		Activity Factor	
Activity Level		Male	Female
Resting: Sleeping, reclining		1	1
Sedentary: Minimal movement, mainly sitting/lying down; activities include watching television and reading		1.3	1.3
Light: Office work, sitting, day consists of sleeping 8 hrs with 16 hrs of walking or standing; activities include walking, laundry, golf, ping pong, walking on level ground at 2.5-3 mph Usually includes 1 hr of moderate activity		1.6	1.5
Moderate: Light manual labor; activities include walking 3.5-4 mph, carrying a load, cycling, tennis, dancing, weeding, and hoeing		1.7	1.6
Very active: Full-time athletes, agricultural laborers, active military duty, hard laborers (mine and steel workers); activities include walking with a load uphill, team sports, climbing		2.1	1.9
Extremely active: Lumberjacks, construction workers, coal miners, some full-time athletes with daily strenuous training		2.4	2.2

Data from ESHA Research, Food Processor, version 8.3, Salem, Ore.

training and improve their performance. In addition to estimating daily energy needs, athletes need guidance in choosing foods and drinks to meet these needs. Several methods exist to measure energy needs including laboratory-based measurements; however, these methods can be complicated and time consuming with limited availability; therefore more simple prediction equations have been developed. Prediction equations have been developed to estimate an individual's REE on the basis of factors including gender, age, and body weight. Table 17-1 provides some commonly used equations. Most equations were developed using data from sedentary populations, limiting the applicability to athletes.[2,3] Once the REE is estimated, it can then be multiplied by an appropriate factor, which accounts for daily level of activity, to provide an estimate of total energy needs.[2] For an athlete, choosing the appropriate activity factor is critical and may vary with training and competition (Table 17-2).

Given that these prediction equations only provide *estimated* daily total energy needs, evaluating if these estimates are correct can occur through monitoring body weight (i.e., is weight stable or decreasing/increasing as desired? is body weight within a healthy range?), body composition (i.e. fat mass, muscle mass at appropriate levels for sport and health of athlete), and performance.

Once total energy needs are estimated, it is important for athletes to consume foods and drinks that will not only meet these energy needs but also the recommended carbohydrate, protein, and fat needs of the athlete. Tables 17-3 and 17-4 provide an overview of more specific recommendations for carbohydrate and protein intake by exercise level and duration.

SPECIFIC RECOMMENDATIONS FOR SPORT AND NUTRIENT INTAKE

Recommendations for nutrient intake vary by sport and should focus around enhancing energy stores, reducing risk of dehydration, preventing nausea and gastrointestinal discomfort, and enhancing muscle and energy recovery while replacing fluid losses.[4] Recommendations will also vary depending on weight and body composition goals of an athlete. For instance, athletes desiring muscle mass gains must first ensure that overall energy needs are met (including an increase in energy intake if necessary) and second that adequate protein is consumed at appropriate times throughout the day (more on this later).[5] For all athletes, the key to maximizing the benefit of optimal nutrient intake is timing. Macronutrients and fluid intake in relation to exercise are covered in detail next.

Table 17-3	Carbohydrate Intake Guidelines for Athletes
Exercise Intensity	Daily Carbohydrate (grams/pound body weight)
Low intensity (moderate duration)	2.3 to 3.2
Moderate to heavy intensity	3.2 to 5.5
Extreme intensity*	4.5 to 5.5+
Immediately (0-4 hr) following exercise	0.45 to 0.55

Data from Burke LM, Kiens B, Ivy JL: *J Sports Sci* 22(1):15-30, 2004.
*Elite level.

Table 17-4	Protein Intake Guidelines	
Activity Level		Protein Needs (grams/pound body weight)
Sedentary		0.36
Recreational endurance*		0.36
Recreational resistance (strength training)		0.36
Moderate-intensity endurance†		0.54
Elite female endurance athletes		0.53-0.63
Elite male endurance athletes		0.72
Resistance (strength) training athletes (consistent training, midseason, for maintenance of muscle mass)		0.53-0.63
Cross-training or intermittent, high-intensity training athletes (basketball, soccer, hockey)		0.63-0.77
Resistance (strength) trained athletes (early training or promotion of muscle mass growth, or both)		0.68-0.81

Data from Tarnopolsky M: *Nutrition* 20(7-8):662-668, 2004; Lemon PW: *J Am Coll Nutr* 19(5 Suppl):513S-521S, 2000
*4-5 times/week for 30 min at <55% VO$_2$ max.
†4-5 times/week for 40-60 minutes.

The Role of Carbohydrates and Carbohydrate Loading

Carbohydrates are the main fuel source for the brain and muscles, thereby making them an essential component of each athlete's diet. Carbohydrates are so essential to an athlete's diet that the American College of Sports Medicine, American Dietetic Association, and the Canadian Dietetic Association all confer that athletes should strive to achieve optimal carbohydrate intake for peak performance.[6] Carbohydrates can be found in most foods including grains, cereals, pasta, fruits, vegetables, dairy, nuts, and beans. Just how many carbohydrates an athlete should eat and when they should be consumed will vary by type of exercise. Prolonged or endurance exercise lasting longer than 90 minutes requires high carbohydrate consumption for optimal performance.[7] Athletes participating in such exercise should focus their dietary practices on consuming the appropriate amount of carbohydrates at key times to maintain high carbohydrate stores (glycogen) in the liver and muscles.[4,8] Depletion of these stores is an underlying factor leading to fatigue and decreased performance.[7,9] To enhance performance in endurance athletes, the strategy of carbohydrate loading to supercompensate muscle glycogen stores was introduced to endurance training in the late 1960s.[10] The original protocol called for a period of muscle glycogen depletion achieved by consuming a low-carbohydrate diet for 3 to 4 days in conjunction with intense training, followed by another 3 to 4 days, this time tapering exercise and consuming a high carbohydrate diet. This strategy has since been updated to eliminate the period of low-carbohydrate intake and instead focus on 3 to 4 days of high-carbohydrate intake in conjunction with exercise taper.[9,11,12] The main factors for athletes to focus on when trying to adopt this nutritional strategy for increasing glycogen stores before exercise are to (1) ensure a high carbohydrate intake (≈3 to 4.5 g of carbohydrates per pound of body weight daily) and (2) taper intensity and duration of training.[12]

Evidence-Based Clinical Application: Carbohydrate Loading

Recent research suggests that highly trained athletes may enhance their glycogen stores in less than 24 hours before competition while still training. When trained endurance athletes consumed a high-carbohydrate diet (≈4.5 g/lb of body weight) over the 24 hours following a 3-minute bout of high-intensity exercise, muscle glycogen supercompensation occurred.[13]

Although endurance athletes benefit from carbohydrate loading before events, athletes participating in exercise lasting less than 60 to 90 minutes should be able to load carbohydrate stores before competition by consuming 3 to 4.5 g of carbohydrates per pound of body weight and resting or reducing training load in the 24 to 36 hours preceding competition.[4]

Evidence-Based Clinical Application: Resting Values for Muscle Glycogen

In trained athletes resting values for muscle glycogen levels are between 100 and 135 mmol/kg wet weight. Following a period of carbohydrate loading, muscle glycogen stores can increase to 150 to 250 mmol/kg wet weight.[4,8]

Preexercise Carbohydrate and Glycemic Index

The preexercise meal or snack is an important part of the nutritional strategy to promote adequate glycogen stores. The preexercise meal is generally recommended to be consumed 3 to 4 hours before the onset of exercise and be high in carbohydrates, containing approximately 200 to 300 g of carbohydrate.[7] This is true not only for the endurance athlete but for athletes participating in intermittent sports like soccer matches or basketball games, which can last 1½ to 3 hours and significantly draw on glycogen stores. Even resistance-training athletes desiring muscle mass gains should consume carbohydrates in their meal or snack before exercise to provide energy from carbohydrates to fuel training while sparing protein for muscle repair and growth.[5]

Not all exercise events will permit an athlete to consume a meal containing carbohydrates 3 to 4 hours beforehand, especially if an event is early in the morning. In this circumstance, if the athlete will be engaging in exercise lasting longer than 60 minutes, consumption of carbohydrates within the hour before and also during exercise may enhance performance.[7,14] Some athletes can be weary of consuming carbohydrates in the hour preceding exercise for fear of this leading to a rapid drop in blood sugar at the onset of exercise, which could impair performance. Although this was once a prevalent theory in sports nutrition dogma,[15] subsequent research and recent reviews on the topic have concluded no effect on performance[16,17] or improved endurance performance[18] and suggest that any decline in blood sugar that may occur during the first 20 minutes of exercise is later self-corrected, causing no detriment to exercise performance.[19] On the other hand, some individual athletes may be sensitive to fluctuations in blood sugar and consuming carbohydrates in the hour leading up to exercise may negatively affect their performance. For these athletes it has been recommended that if carbohydrates are consumed within an hour of exercise, they should be in a quantity greater than 70 g and possibly with a lower glycemic index (see later).[4] Overall, athletes who are sensitive to carbohydrate intake close to the onset of exercise should experiment during their training with optimal timing for carbohydrate intake.

The glycemic index (GI) refers to the measure of how quickly a carbohydrate containing food will increase blood sugar following ingestion compared with a reference food like white bread.[20] Early research showed that foods with lower GIs consumed before exercise would allow for a more sustained release of glucose into the blood stream during exercise, thereby preventing large swings in blood sugar and improving performance. Additionally, it was thought that a lower-GI carbohydrate allowed for an increase in free fatty acids available for oxidation during exercise that would lead to sparing of glycogen for later energy use.[21] Although this was a promising theory, limitations to the use of the GI included how other macronutrients (i.e., fat and protein) affect the GI when consumed with a carbohydrate food; the influence of food preparation/processing/ripeness on GI; and the fact that the GI is based on the blood glucose response of 50 g of a carbohydrate, which is an amount that may not accurately reflect the amount of carbohydrates an athlete consumed.[22] Furthermore, research has failed to show consistently that lower-GI foods consumed before exercise improve blood glucose response during exercise, while most research evaluating performance and GI has failed to find an enhancement in performance when consuming low-GI carbohydrate versus high-GI carbohydrates before exercise.[23] Finally, the influence, if any, that the GI of a preexercise carbohydrate meal or snack may have on performance is likely overshadowed by the benefits from consuming carbohydrates during prolonged exercise.[24] As the timing of food intake preexercise nears the onset of exercise, the major concern surrounding preexercise food selection centers around tolerance.

Carbohydrate Intake during Exercise

In addition to adequate consumption of carbohydrates before exercise, consumption of carbohydrates during exercise lasting longer than 60 to 90 minutes has been shown to improve endurance performance.[8,9,14,23] This improvement in performance has been linked to the following:

- Prevention of hypoglycemia (low blood sugar)
- Provision of energy during later stages of exercise

As mentioned earlier, as glycogen stores get depleted with prolonged exercise—both endurance and moderate-intensity intermittent exercise—blood sugar levels will decrease, reducing the amount of available energy to fuel the athlete. Consumption of carbohydrates during exercise can both prevent this decrease in blood sugar and provide additional fuel when energy stores are reduced. Consumption of carbohydrates during prolonged exercise is of particular importance when adequate carbohydrates to maximize glycogen stores have not been consumed before the onset of exercise. In general it is recommended that athletes consume 30 to 60 g of carbohydrates throughout each hour of exercise[6]; however, some research suggests that smaller amounts (≈16 g/hour) are sufficient,[14] and other research suggests that more should be consumed.[23] Although research supports that the form of carbohydrate, solid or liquid, does not appear to influence the performance benefits of carbohydrate ingestion,[14] ultimately convenience and individual tolerance will dictate whether an athlete chooses to drink or eat carbohydrates. As a rule of thumb, an athlete consuming a solid form of carbohydrates (e.g., an energy bar or gel) should consume it with fluid to help improve absorption and reduce stomach distress.

Athletes participating in high-intensity stop-and-go or intermittent sports like basketball or soccer, lasting 60 minutes or longer, can also improve performance through carbohydrate supplementation during exercise. The physiology explaining this benefit is currently unknown but theorized to be associated with an influence on skeletal muscle and possibly the cardiovascular and central nervous systems.[25] The exact mechanisms supporting a benefit, as well as the optimal carbohydrate intake during intermittent sports, require future research; however, for now it appears that following the general guideline of 30 to 60 g of carbohydrates every hour will benefit performance. Athletes participating in stop-and-go sports are at an advantage over endurance athletes engaged in long-duration continuous exercise when it comes to carbohydrate consumption and availability opportunities. A soccer player can more easily pack a variety of solid and liquid forms of carbohydrates to keep on the sidelines than a runner can during a race. For both endurance and intermittent sport athletes, consuming 30 to 60 g of carbohydrates in feedings every 10 to 30 minutes will help provide a steady delivery of fuel during exercise and alleviate risk for stomach distress.[25]

Carbohydrate Intake after Exercise

In addition to consumption before and during exercise, consumption of carbohydrates following exercise is essential to replenishing exhausted glycogen stores, enhancing recovery, and preparing the body for the next event or training session. The postexercise recovery period can be one of the most opportune times for athletes to benefit from optimal sports nutrition practices, yet it can also be one of the most neglected because many athletes, especially following intense exercise, have little appetite or desire to eat and drink. The first hour postexercise is a time in which the highest rates of glycogen storage can occur.[12] Three major effects from exercise likely explain this enhanced period of storage and include the following:

1. Exercise-induced glycogen depletion activates glycogen synthase (the rate-determining enzyme for glycogen synthesis)[26]
2. Exercise-induced increase in insulin sensitivity—higher insulin will allow for higher delivery of glucose into cells[27]
3. Exercise enhancement of muscle cell membrane to delivery of glucose[12]

Evidence-Based Clinical Application: Rates of Glycogen Synthesis

The typical rate of glycogen synthesis is 4.3 mmol per wet weight/hour. Rates increase to 7.7 mmol per wet weight/hour during the first 2 hours postexercise. This increased rate highlights the importance of postexercise recovery nutrition for enhancing glycogen resynthesis and storage.[28]

Although glycogen synthesis is enhanced for a short time period following intense exercise, as mentioned earlier, it is not always practical for an athlete to consume the recommended amount of carbohydrate during this time. Fortunately, research shows that if the recovery time period between training sessions or competitions is 8 to 24 hours, athletes can delay the initiation of postexercise carbohydrate intake to a more favorable start time, keeping in mind that they must achieve the carbohydrate intake goal for recovery before the onset of their next training session or event.[12] For those athletes with short recovery periods, 4 to 8 hours, efforts should be made to initiate carbohydrate replacement immediately following exercise. This may be more achievable by athletes when the form of carbohydrate is fluid; however, all athletes should experiment with what works best for them.

In addition to timing of intake, the total amount of carbohydrate consumed after exercise affects glycogen storage.[12] To maximize glycogen stores, research recommends a daily carbohydrate consumption of approximately 3 to 4.5 g per pound of body weight (for a 150-lb athlete, this would equal 450 to 675 g daily) for athletes engaging in glycogen-depleting exercise.[29] This recommendation is only an estimate and can be lower for athletes participating in recreational exercise or exercise that does not stress glycogen stores; however, for those athletes engaged in high-intensity, long-duration training (i.e., ultra-endurance athletes), daily intake of carbohydrates greater than 4.5 g per pound of body weight is recommended.

More specifically, recommendations for immediate carbohydrate consumption include consumption of 4.5 to 5.5 g per pound of body weight immediately after and then again 2 hours following exercise (see Table 17-3).[30] Small, frequent, high-carbohydrate snacks, either solid or liquid, can help athletes meet these recommended intakes. Athletes need to remember to follow the postrecovery nutrition diet after both training and competition.

Glycemic Index and Postexercise Carbohydrate Consumption

Although research does not support choosing preexercise carbohydrates on the basis of GI, evidence supports a benefit of consuming carbohydrates with a medium- to high-GI postexercise.[12,30] The greater insulin release and faster rise of blood glucose from a medium- to high-GI carbohydrate compared with low-GI carbohydrate may explain the benefit to glycogen resynthesis, although such has not been clearly explained.[12] Worrying about the GI of a postrecovery meal or snack will not likely be a major concern for most athletes, and the majority will likely consume carbohydrates with higher GIs (e.g., sports drinks) due to the ease and comfort associated with their consumption. Overall, athletes should focus on consuming energy adequate to both replace energy expended during exercise and provide for storage.

Adding Protein to Carbohydrate Postexercise

Results evaluating whether the addition of protein to carbohydrate consumption postexercise will enhance glycogen storage are mixed.[32] Some research finds that the addition of protein enhances glycogen storage,[33] while other have not.[30,34-36] Evaluation of the different study designs suggests that timing/interval of consumption and total amount of carbohydrates consumed may explain conflicting results. Studies that provided exercisers with either a carbohydrate-alone or carbohydrate-plus-protein beverage at frequent intervals (e.g., every 15 to 30 minutes) after exercise found no difference in glycogen storage,[30,34-36] whereas studies using feeding intervals of 2 hours did.[33,37] These results suggest that more frequent consumption of carbohydrates may offset any benefit that additional protein can have on enhancing glycogen resynthesis. Additionally, with consumption of high amounts of carbohydrate (≈0.5 g of carbohydrates per pound of body weight), additional protein has not been shown to provide any further benefit to glycogen recovery.[30] Although these findings do not support a clear benefit of adding protein for enhancement of glycogen storage, they do not dismiss one potential benefit. A recent study found that when recovery time was limited for an athlete, such as occurs with back-to-back endurance events, the consumption of a carbohydrate-plus-protein beverage or snack immediately after exercise (within 10 minutes) improved glycogen recovery over that of a single-carbohydrate-alone beverage or snack consumed at the same time.[33] Until more research is done, it is not clear if consumption of protein with carbohydrate postexercise will improve glycogen resynthesis, but it likely will not limit it as long as adequate carbohydrates are consumed.

Protein Needs of Athletes

The protein needs of athletes vary by type of exercise (i.e., endurance versus resistance) and also phase of training (see Table 17-4); however, among the research community exploring the protein needs of athletes, there is no clear consensus on the value of elevated protein intake for athletes.[5] Importantly, athletes must understand the role protein plays in their diet. Protein is necessary for muscle maintenance and growth, but it is also necessary for production of enzymes (i.e., catalysts for biochemical reactions in the body); hormones like insulin and hemoglobin; and skin, hair, and part of bone.[38] Although protein can be used as an energy source, especially when carbohydrate stores or dietary intake, or both, are low, its main function is not to supply energy to the body but to supply amino acids for all the functions listed earlier. It is a huge misconception of athletes, especially athletes desiring increases in muscle mass, that dietary protein intake needs to be high in order to achieve results. In general, most athletes meet and often exceed their protein needs for muscle maintenance and growth,[5] yet many athletes may still feel they need more protein to get stronger and bigger. Interestingly, the key factor for these athletes may be the timing and composition of their protein intake. In the past few years attention has focused around consuming amino acids right before or right after resistance exercise to enhance muscle growth. Research supports a benefit for intake at both times. When healthy, recreationally active people consumed amino acids 1 hour following resistance exercise, net muscle protein growth occurred.[39-42] Furthermore, when a similar population consumed an amino acid-carbohydrate solution (consisting of 6 g essential amino acids [EAAs] and 35 g carbohydrate) immediately before or after resistance exercise, muscle growth again occurred but was higher when the solution was consumed before exercise.[43] The increased blood flow that occurs with exercise could possibly enhance the delivery of amino acids to muscle when protein is consumed before exercise and thereby translate into greater muscle mass gains.[43] Moreover, a study evaluating the effect of 25 g of protein (from a protein powder) on muscle fiber size during 14 weeks of resistance training found that when the protein drink was consumed immediately before and after exercise and in the mornings on rest days, muscle fiber size increased, leading to increases in muscle mass.[44] Clearly, timing is important in relation to muscle growth; however, whether it should be consumed before, after, or both requires future research to determine. For now, athletes training for muscle mass gains should focus on consuming protein in close relation to the onset or cessation of exercise, as well as maintaining optimal but not excessive intake during rest days.

Protein, Protein Powders, or Amino Acids?

Timing of protein intake for muscle growth is important, but which does an athlete need to consume—a whole protein, such as chicken or beans, or a protein powder or amino acid mixture? First, not all proteins and amino acids are treated equally. Dietary protein can come from animal sources and is considered complete because it contains all 20 amino acids the body needs. Protein can also come from plant sources and is often considered incomplete because, with the exception of soy, it does not contain all the amino acids. Both sources are good, but in terms of intake for muscle mass growth they may not be treated equally. Two main types of amino acids exist: essential (i.e., meaning they must be consumed from one's diet because the body cannot synthesize them) or nonessential (i.e., the body can synthesize these). Research has shown that for stimulation of muscle growth, only EAAs are necessary.[45,46] As little as 6 g of EAAs can enhance muscle protein synthesis when ingested before or after resistance exercise,[5,42,43,46] but whether this 6 g of EAAs must come from individual amino acid supplements or from a whole food source is not completely known. Either way, research has suggested that it likely does not matter if the 6 g of EAAs come from a complete protein source (e.g., chicken, soy) or as an EAA supplement.[4,46] Finances (sports supplements can be expensive), as well as the athlete's individual preference, will likely make the ultimate decision.

Should Carbohydrates Be Added to Protein?

Adding carbohydrates to the resistance training protein snack may further enhance muscle growth because carbohydrates stimulate insulin release, which has been shown to decrease muscle breakdown following exercise.[5,47] Although a promising combination, the research in this area has been complicated because some studies that add carbohydrates to a protein snack (usually as a drink) and compare it with drinks with carbohydrates or protein alone fail to control for the additional calories from the added carbohydrate.[46] This makes it difficult to determine whether the added carbohydrates or added calories are what caused the enhanced muscle growth. To help alleviate this issue, research has been done using equal-calorie drinks of EAA + protein + carbohydrates or carbohydrates alone. Results showed that the former drink stimulated muscle growth more so than the carbohydrate-alone drink.[41] The carbohydrate-induced insulin inhibition of muscle breakdown in combination with the amino acid stimulation of muscle growth may explain why adding carbohydrates to a protein can improve muscle growth.[43] Because the peak anabolic (i.e., building) effects of carbohydrates and amino acids may occur at different times, to enhance the anabolic properties of both it has been suggested that carbohydrate intake should precede amino acid intake.[41] Additionally, a complete protein (a whole food or drink protein source providing all EAAs) takes longer to digest and therefore when consumed at the same time with carbohydrate may complement the peak anabolic effect of insulin better than individual EAAs.[41,46] This is a hot topic in sports nutrition that will likely receive more attention in the future. For now, strength-training athletes will likely benefit from steering away from all- or high-protein diets and including carbohydrates at the appropriate time.

Evidence-Based Clinical Application: Protein Intake for Resistance Exercise

Practical recommendations from research suggest that 1 cup of low-fat chocolate milk or low-fat fruit yogurt will likely provide an athlete with the amount of EAA and carbohydrates necessary to enhance muscle growth. A more specific calculation for estimating quantity of protein and carbohydrate to consume is 0.045 g of EAA per pound of body weight in combination with 0.23 g of carbohydrates per pound of body weight.[48]

Protein Needs of Endurance Athletes

Endurance athletes often have different muscle mass goals than strength athletes. They mainly desire to maintain an optimal lean muscle mass that will complement but not hinder performance and therefore do not often train to promote large increases in muscle mass.[5] Because protein contributes only 1% to 6% to total energy costs during endurance exercise,[49] it is not the main dietary focus for many endurance athletes. Whether endurance exercise will increase daily protein needs depends on the intensity of training, duration of training, nutritional intake of the athlete (i.e., lower total energy or carbohydrate intake, or both, put a greater reliance on protein for energy), and state of training (i.e., with training, adaptations occur that appear to lower the body's use of protein as an energy source during endurance exercise).[49] Additionally,

research has shown that when endurance athletes consumed carbohydrates during exercise, this attenuated any increase in amino acid oxidation that would naturally occur with exercise as carbohydrate stores were used up.[50] Total energy intake is also an important factor determining how much protein an endurance athlete will oxidize during exercise. With adequate energy intake, the body's reliance on protein as a fuel source during exercise decreases.[51] These two latter points highlight the importance of an endurance athlete meeting both his or her daily total energy and carbohydrate needs for optimal performance and sparing protein for muscle mass repair and maintenance.

Overall, recreational endurance athletes—those participating in low to moderate intensity and duration exercise—likely do not have higher protein needs than the general population. Those athletes participating in moderate intensity endurance exercise (4 to 5 days weekly for longer than 60 minutes) likely have approximately 25% higher protein needs than those of the general population, while elite endurance athletes have needs approximately double those of the general population (see Table 17-4). Women's protein needs have been suggested to be close to 15% to 20% lower than those of males, although more research is necessary to confirm or refute this.[49]

FLUID NEEDS AND INTAKE GUIDELINES FOR ATHLETES

An athlete should never underestimate the importance of proper hydration. Even slight dehydration causing a loss of only 2% of body weight during exercise can negatively affect performance, especially in warm weather.[25] For a 150-lb athlete, this is only a 1½- to 3-lb weight loss. To help prevent decreased performance secondary to dehydration, it is critical that athletes develop, practice, and stick with a proper hydration plan. Such a plan includes drinking cool fluids before, during, and after exercise—not just for competition but with training as well. Additionally, athletes should make it a habit to carry fluids with them throughout the day and sip regularly, while adding fluid-rich foods (e.g., fruits, vegetables, soups) to their daily meal and snack consumption. How much fluid should an athlete consume? Although this number will vary with temperature (higher in hot, humid weather), dietary intake, and level of fitness, all athletes can benefit from the following simple guidelines for fluid replacement from the American College of Sports Medicine.[52]

Before Exercise

An athlete should consume at least 2 cups (16 to 20 oz) of cool fluid about 2 hours before exercise followed by consuming another 2 cups of cool fluid 15 to 20 minutes immediately before exercise. An athlete should remember to leave time to use the restroom before the onset of exercise, especially if he or she is participating in an event that does not allow for bathroom breaks.

During Exercise

- Consume about 5 to 10 oz of cool fluid every 15 minutes during exercise. As a rule of thumb, 1 oz of fluid equals one normal adult gulp.
- If exercise is less than 60 to 90 minutes, choose cool water as a fluid choice.
- If exercise is strenuous, performed in extreme temperatures or humidity and lasting longer than 60 to 90 minutes, choose a carbohydrate-electrolyte sports beverage. The electrolytes (mainly sodium and potassium) in a typical carbohydrate-electrolyte sports beverage aid in the absorption of fluid, while carbohydrates supply additional energy.[53]
- Overall, the athlete should always choose a beverage according to his or her individual needs, but for most, a cool temperature and appealing flavor are two important factors that help enhance consumption and ensure adequate intake.

After Exercise

- A simple way to assess fluids needs postexercise is by weighing in before and immediately after exercise. The weight lost during practice and competitions represents water weight loss.
- An athlete should consume three cups (24 oz) of cool fluid for each pound lost during exercise, with the goal of returning to preworkout or precompetition weight.
- Ensure that the postexercise fluid contains sodium. Research supports that drinks consumed after exercise may benefit from higher sodium concentrations than those found in sports drinks formulated specifically for consumption during exercise.[53] Sodium can also be consumed through solid food choices; however, fluid needs still need to be met.

 Evidence-Based Clinical Application: Fluid Replacement following Exercise

Although 2 cups of fluid are equivalent to a pound of weight loss, an athlete continues to lose fluid after exercise due to obligatory losses (i.e., continued sweating, urination) and therefore should strive to replace every pound of weight lost during exercise with 3 cups of fluid.[31,53]

Choosing the Best Sports Drink

Sports drinks come in a variety of colors with just as great a variety of ingredients. Some of the more popular types of sports drinks, typical ingredients, and optimal time of use are listed as follows:

- Carbohydrate-electrolyte replacement drink:
  - ◆ Typical ingredients: 4% to 8% carbohydrate solution, sodium chloride, and potassium.

- ◆ Optimal use: (1) during prolonged or intense exercise lasting longer than 60 to 90 minutes or exercise in hot, humid conditions where sweat losses are high; and (2) following exercise for immediate fluid and carbohydrate replacement.
- Carbohydrate-electrolyte replacement drink with protein or other added nutrients:
  - ◆ Typical ingredients: water, 4% to 8% carbohydrate solution, sodium chloride, potassium, and protein (as branch chain amino acids), as well as possibly herbs or caffeine, or both.
  - ◆ Optimal use: Research is not conclusive about the benefits of adding protein or caffeine to a sports drinks; however, if tolerated by an athlete, these ingredients could be used (1) during prolonged or intense exercise lasting longer than 60 to 90 minutes or exercise in hot, humid conditions where sweat losses are high; (2) following exercise for immediate fluid and carbohydrate replacement. To date there is no scientific support for a performance benefit or long-term safety data regarding the addition of protein or herbs to sports drinks. Caution should always be taken when consuming herbal ingredients, which can place athletes at risk for an adverse reaction or put them in violation of banned substance codes for their sport.
- Sports water:
  - ◆ Typical ingredients: water, 2.5% to 3.8% carbohydrate solution (no carbohydrate if artificially sweetened), sodium chloride, B-vitamins, vitamins E and C.
  - ◆ Optimal use: (1) general everyday fluid replacement, (2) fluid replacement during shorter duration (<60 to 90 minutes), easy to moderate intensity exercise, especially if an athlete desires a change from drinking plain water. Although sports water may encourage fluid intake in athletes, there is no scientific support that vitamins will enhance exercise performance.[54]
- Meal replacement drink:
  - ◆ Typical ingredients: mixture of water, carbohydrates, protein, and sometimes fat; tend to be concentrated source of calories.
  - ◆ Optimal use: ideal as a liquid preexercise or postexercise snack; may work well with an athlete too nervous to eat solid food before training or competition; however, caution should be taken when consumed before exercise that beverage is not consumed too close (<1 hour) to onset of exercise, which can lead to stomach distress in susceptible athletes.
- Energy drinks:
  - ◆ Typical ingredients: water, carbohydrates, caffeine, sometimes herbs, protein (amino acids), electrolytes, vitamins, and minerals.
  - ◆ Optimal use: not for use immediately before, during, or after exercise. The high carbohydrate content (sugar) in combination with carbonation prevents optimal hydration or rehydration. The high caffeine content could cause jitters and stomach distress if consumed too

close to exercise. Herbal ingredients can place athletes at risk for an adverse reaction or put them in violation of banned substance codes for their sport. Scientific support for a performance benefit and long-term safety data regarding the addition of protein to a sports drink are lacking.

Overall, the perfect sports drink does not exist. The athlete must consider several factors when choosing a sports drink including the type of exercise to be performed (e.g., if glycogen depleting, carbohydrates should be a main ingredient in the sports drink); duration of exercise; intensity of exercise; tolerability; and of course, the preference of the athlete.[53]

ERGOGENIC AIDS AND PERFORMANCE

The term *ergogenic* means having the ability to increase work. In the realm of athletics, ergogenic aids are pills, powders, drinks, bars, gels, etc., that, when consumed, can enhance an athlete's strength, endurance, recovery, body composition, or energy levels, leading to improved performance and an advantage over the athlete's competition.[55] Because athletes often supplement their dietary intake with ergogenic aids, they are also referred to as *sports supplements* and in some cases as simply *dietary supplements.* The ergogenic aids/sports supplement market is huge. In the year 2000 alone, Americans spent $16.7 billion on supplements, with athletes and active people comprising a large percentage of the buying market.[56] Furthermore, using the search engine Google on the Internet with the key words "ergogenic aids" turns up more than 68,000 hits. With so many ergogenic aids on the market today and more being added daily, it is beyond the scope of this chapter to thoroughly review even the most popular supplements. Instead, the reader is referred to recent review articles and chapters.[55-60] Following is a brief overview of the role of ergogenic aids in a sports nutrition diet plan, as well as a summary of two commonly used and potentially effective ergogenic aids: caffeine and creatine.

Ergogenic aids, while prevalently used, have a minor role, if any, in the typical athlete's sports nutrition diet plan. The key for athletes and those working with athletes is to understand that the foundation of a top-notch sports nutrition diet plan stems from choosing a variety of nutrient-dense foods (i.e., chock-full of nutrition without much added sugar and fat and without excessive calories) that help an athlete meet daily energy and nutrient needs. Complementing this with carbohydrate and fluid intake for preexercise hydration and fueling and postexercise rehydration and refueling, following the guidelines outlined earlier in the chapter, will enhance the sports nutrition diet plan. Finally, only after these previous two dietary practices have been mastered will a safe and approved supplement like caffeine be able to exert its potential ergogenic benefit.[61] No ergogenic aid or supplement will replace the benefits of sound sports nutrition dietary practices or compensate for a suboptimal diet.

In certain instances dietary supplements have a beneficial role in an athlete's diet. Those athletes with nutrient deficien-

cies (i.e., iron deficiency anemia increasing risk for fatigue or low calcium intake increasing risk for poor bone density) resulting from a combination of suboptimal energy or nutrient intake and restrictive dietary behavior, such as eliminating whole food groups like red meat, will benefit from correcting any nutrient deficiencies with diet and often dietary supplementation. However, an athlete must talk with a registered dietitian or physician before taking nutrient supplements to ensure he or she is taking the correct dosage for the appropriate amount of time because excessive intake could be detrimental to health.[56] Outside of having an overt nutrient deficiency, how can an athlete know when an ergogenic aid is safe and effective to use? Athletes can follow these guidelines, modified from the University of Arizona, College of Agricultural and Life Sciences, Department of Nutritional Sciences, Cooperative Extension,[62] to help them evaluate ergogenic aids:

Step 1: *Evaluate the source of information.* To help determine if an ergogenic aid is effective, investigate whether any research articles have been published about it in scientific peer-reviewed journals. Keep in mind that one study does not prove an ergogenic aid is effective or not. Look for a series of research studies in a large number of people from various populations over more than just a few days. Finally, beware information published by the company that sells the product or will benefit from the sale of it.

Step 2: *Look critically at who wrote the article.* Look for articles about an ergogenic aid that are written by someone who has at least a bachelor's degree and preferably an advanced degree in nutritional sciences, physiology, or both. Be cautious if the author has a personal or monetary stake in the product.

Step 3: *Critically analyze the product.* If the product sounds too good to be true, it is! Also consider the following:
- If a research study is cited, was it conducted on a healthy population or a diseased population, well-trained subjects or couch potatoes, animals or humans, men or women?
- Does the dosage seem large or unsafe? Are any safety data published?
- Does the article make conclusive statements, such as "This supplement will make you lose weight"?
- Does the product promise quick improvements in health or physical performance?
- Does the product contain some secret ingredient or formula?
- Are currently popular personalities or star athletes used in its advertisements?

Step 4: *Does any research support that the product is effective?* If there is no peer-reviewed research that the ergogenic aid is effective, especially in people similar to you (i.e., gender, sport, training level), be cautious about spending money on a product that might not even work.

Step 5: *Does any evidence indicate that the product may cause long-term health problems?* Although many athletes do so without even thinking about it, never consume a substance unless you are certain that it is safe. Ask yourself, is winning really worth your health?

Step 6: *Are there any ethical issues with taking the supplement?* Although this may be difficult to answer and this is a personal issue for each athlete, consider these few points before taking any ergogenic aid:

♦ What is the policy of your team or the governing body for your sport?

♦ Is the substance banned from use during competition by the governing body for your sport?

♦ Is taking a supplement cheating or giving you an unfair advantage?

Caffeine

Aside from giving us a kick in the morning, caffeine may have ergogenic properties for certain types of exercise. From the original work done in the 1970s to now, research has shown that small to medium amounts of caffeine (between 3 and 6 mg caffeine per kilogram of body weight) can improve endurance performance when consumed 60 to 75 minutes before exercise,[63-65] during exercise,[66] and near the end of exercise.[67] In addition, research shows that caffeine ingestion may provide benefit to exercise lasting between 1 and 6 minutes; however, it is unclear if high-intensity sprint events are beneficially influenced by caffeine ingestion.[68] The benefits of caffeine on performance have been linked to its effects on skeletal muscle, adipose tissue (increasing fat oxidation and sparing glycogen), and the central nervous system (possibly by reducing an athlete's perception of fatigue).[56] Before athletes start loading up on lattes and espressos, it is important for them to realize that not all people respond similarly to caffeine intake. Negative side effects can result from high doses of caffeine and, for some athletes, even from small to moderate amounts of caffeine. Side effects include headaches, jitters, stomach distress, and restlessness.[56] Another concern for athletes in regard to caffeine intake is the diuretic effect, or dehydrating effect, it may pose. Recent evidence suggests that ingestion of caffeine immediately before or during exercise will not encourage dehydration, but consumption after exercise of highly caffeinated beverages may slow rehydration.[69,70] For people with habitual caffeine intake, the diuretic effect of caffeine may be even lower.[71]

Creatine

Creatine is probably the most researched ergogenic aid on the market, with more than 300 studies published about it.[72] Creatine is an intriguing supplement for athletes desiring gains in muscle mass because creatine itself is used in conjunction with phosphate by the muscle to supply energy for high-intensity, short-duration (≈10 seconds or less) exercise, like sprinting or weight lifting.[56] The theory behind the ergogenic effects of creatine is that by providing the body with more creatine and thus enhancing its naturally limited stores, the body can better recover from and perform short-duration, high-intensity exercise, thereby allowing an athlete to train harder and hopefully perform better.[73] Athletes can consume creatine naturally from dietary intake (e.g., meat, fish) with typical daily consumption around 1 g, only 1 g lower than

daily needs (which are met by endogenous production predominantly by the kidney).[56,73]

Overall, reviews of the research support that creatine supplementation in strength or resistance training athletes can have positive effects on lean body mass, strength, and overall power in athletes.[74,75] Although creatine supplementation has been shown to produce quick increases in body weight, it is possible that this increased mass is due to water retention within the muscle and not actual muscle tissue growth.[56] A major factor to consider when evaluating whether creatine supplementation would benefit an athlete's sports nutrition plan is that some athletes may be creatine responders while others may not. What this means is that for reasons yet to be determined, some athletes respond better to creatine supplementation than do others.[72] A perfect example is the vegetarian resistance training athlete. Because of the naturally low dietary creatine consumption in this athlete's diet, he or she may be more likely to respond positively to creatine supplementation. Overall, creatine supplementation in resistance training athletes appears to be safe for up to 2 years and, for responders, effective in promoting performance of high-intensity, maximal exertion exercise, as well as strength resulting from resistance training.[72,74,75] The general recommended supplementation regimen consists of two phases: (1) loading phase and (2) maintenance phase. Both are accompanied by different recommended dosages. During the loading phase it is recommended that the athlete consume 20 g of creatine daily for 4 to 5 days. During the maintenance phase it is recommended that the athlete consume 1 to 2 g of creatine daily.[56] Most of the research evaluating dosages of creatine has not been of sufficient length to adequately define an appropriate maintenance phase duration, and although long-term safety data are not available, creatine supplementation within guidelines appears to be associated with minimal risk for up to 2 years.[72] Athletes should be cautious, however, of falling victim to the mantra that more is better because little, if anything, is known about the safety of high-dose, long-term creatine supplementation.[56]

GASTROINTESTINAL FUNCTION DURING EXERCISE

Gastrointestinal, or simply GI, function during exercise is an important factor to consider in relation to nutrient intake shortly before, during, and after exercise. The jostling motion in the stomach that accompanies many sports like running can limit the amount and type of food an athlete can consume within close vicinity to exercise, as well as during, to avoid GI distress (i.e., stomach distress). Exercise also affects transit time (i.e., the time it takes food to travel through the digestive tract from the mouth to the anus), by shortening it overall. Further, during exercise, blood flow to the stomach is drastically reduced because the flow is diverted toward working skeletal muscle. In combination with the decrease in blood flow, food sitting in the stomach can lead to GI distress.[76] The concentration of carbohydrates consumed during exercise can affect gastric emptying and onset of GI distress, too. Typical carbohydrate-electrolyte replacement sports drinks are approximately a 4% to 8% carbohydrate solution because this amount has been shown to optimize fluid absorption without risking slowed gastric emptying.[53] The following simple guidelines are offered to help susceptible athletes avoid GI distress and limit urgency to use the restroom during exercise[76]:

- Limit or avoid solid food within 3 hours of starting exercise. Liquid meals offer a nice alternative to fueling an athlete for exercise while reducing the risk for GI distress.
- Choose beverages with carbohydrate concentrations between 4% and 8%. This means limiting soda, fruit juices, and energy drinks within the few hours preceding exercise, during exercise, and after exercise.
- Limit high-fiber foods in the preexercise meal and during exercise.
- Limit caffeine in the preexercise meal and during exercise.
- Use the restroom before starting exercise.

These guidelines may vary with each athlete, so the key to reducing GI distress is for the athlete to practice food and fluid intake with training to identify which foods trigger distress and which foods are tolerable. Athletes should also keep in mind that competition day is not the day to try a new food or drink, no matter how appealing. If necessary, athletes should travel with appropriate food if there is concern that tolerable food may not be available at the competition destination.

DEFINING AND ACHIEVING OPTIMAL BODY WEIGHT FOR PERFORMANCE

A major goal for most athletes is achieving an optimal body weight and composition. The difference between an optimal body weight and composition and *desired* body weight and composition can sometimes be quite large. If an athlete's parents are not Mr. and Mrs. Universe, the chance that the athlete will be is limited. The ideal body weight and composition for one athlete is not the same for another, and even teammates can have different optimal body compositions due to the different demands of their positions. Although some athletes can fixate on a number they want to see flash back at them on the scale, for optimal athletic performance, athletes need to pay more attention to body composition (i.e., fat and muscle mass). A lower body fat to lean body mass ratio is an indicator of greater power output.[77]

Body composition has been related to athletic success and may be of particular importance in events that require either horizontal or vertical motion, like running and basketball, respectfully.[78] Performance in skill-based sports, such as golf, relies less on body composition; therefore it is more common to see athletes with wider ranges of body weight and composition successful at these sports than sports like basketball, where height and lean body mass describe most, but not all, of the successful players.[77] Summaries of the body composition of elite-level athletes have been published previously[78]; however, athletes should be cautious using them as "gold standards" for body composition in their sport. Although they provide guide-

BOX 17-1 Guidelines for Determining a Healthy and Achievable Body Weight

- Weight promotes overall good health.
- Weight can be maintained without severe dietary restriction or starvation.
- Weight supports healthy eating habits.
- Weight is in a range in which health risks are minimized and good health is promoted.
- Weight permits an athlete to participate in his or her sport at the intensity and level desired.
- Weight allows for *personal best* athletic performance.
- Weight considers an athlete's genetics and family history of body weight and composition.
- Weight is appropriate for the athlete's age and level of physical development.

Data from Department of Nutritional Sciences, University of Arizona, Cooperative Extension.

lines for body fat levels and muscle mass in successful athletes, the mean (the single number representing the average of several elite athletes' body fat or muscle mass) for percent body fat or muscle mass should not be viewed as a single number but rather a range, taking into consideration the variation around the mean. For example, a mean percent body fat for an elite female basketball player may be 19.2%; however, with the variation around the mean taken into consideration, the range of percent body fat in an elite female basketball player is from 14.6% to 23.8%.[78]

Although these ranges for body composition provide guidelines on optimal levels for success in a particular sport, to identify an individual athlete's optimal body composition it is best to take serial measures of his or her body composition and compare these with training load, dietary intake, and performance at the time of measurement.[77] The best performance level achieved by the athlete can provide great insight into his or her optimal body composition, as well as the dietary and training practices he or she followed to achieve this. One caveat to this formula is ensuring that the body weight and composition that corresponded with peak performance also coincided with what would be a healthy body weight for an athlete. Standards for body weight of average sedentary people may not always apply to athletes, and therefore a physician and registered dietitian can help evaluate what the optimal body weight would be for an athlete to ensure he or she is not at risk for physical problems in the future (e.g., menstrual abnormalities or bone loss) due to an unhealthy body weight or dietary intake. Refer to Box 17-1 for more guidelines on determining what a healthy and achievable body weight is for an athlete.

CONCLUSIONS

The composition and amount of nutrient (e.g., carbohydrate, protein, and fat) and fluid intake in relation to exercise (i.e., before, during, and after) can dictate how well an athlete's sports nutrition diet plan supports his or her training and enhances performance. In summary, a top sports nutrition plan includes the following:

1. Meeting daily total energy needs—these needs will vary with training load and intensity of exercise.
2. Meeting recommended nutrient intake levels— carbohydrate, protein, and fat needs differ by sport; however, all athletes need to consume adequate carbohydrates for energy and sparing of protein for structural function; sufficient protein for muscle growth, repair, and maintenance; and fat for vitamin absorption, cell structure, and additional energy.
3. Drinking adequate fluids before, during, and after all exercise training sessions and competitions.
4. Timing nutrient intake appropriately to enhance energy levels; replace used fuels during exercise; speed recovery; and support muscle repair, growth, and maintenance.
5. Defining and achieving a healthy optimal body weight and composition to support peak performance in an individual athlete's sport.

Additionally, for some athletes appropriately formulated sports drinks, bars, or gels may help deliver nutrients (e.g., carbohydrates, protein) and fluids to the athlete in preparation for exercise, for replacement of used energy stores during and after exercise, and as a supplement for high-energy needs. Ergogenic aids and sports supplements have a small, if any, role in a sports nutrition diet plan. Athletes should be informed and aware consumers and thoroughly evaluate any product before consumption and remember that no ergogenic aid or supplement will replace sound energy, nutrient, and fluid intake. Overall, the key to a successful sports nutrition diet plan is for the athlete to practice the plan like he or she would practice a sport skill or train for an event.

REFERENCES

1. Maughan RJ, Burke LM: Exercise and energy demands. In Maughan RJ, Burke LM, editors: *Handbook of sports medicine and science: sports nutrition*, Malden, Mass, 2002, Blackwell Publishing.
2. Manore M, Thompson J: Energy requirements of the athlete: assessment and evidence of energy efficiency. In Burke L, Deakin V, editors. *Clinical sports nutrition,* ed 2, Sydney, 2000, McGraw-Hill.
3. Thompson J, Manore MM: Predicted and measured resting metabolic rate of male and female endurance athletes, *J Am Diet Assoc* 96(1):30-34, 1996.
4. Burke L: Preparation for competition. In Burke L, Deakin V, editors: *Clinical sports nutrition,* ed 2, Sydney, 2000, McGraw-Hill.
5. Tipton KD, Wolfe RR: Protein and amino acids for athletes, *J Sports Sci* 22(1):65-79, 2004.
6. Position of the American Dietetic Association, Dieticians of Canada, and the American College of Sports Medicine: Nutrition and athletic performance, *J Am Diet Assoc* 100(12):1543-1556, 2000.
7. Hargreaves M, Hawley JA, Jeukendrup A: Pre-exercise carbohydrate and fat ingestion: effects on metabolism and performance, *J Sports Sci* 22(1):31-38, 2004.
8. Coleman E: Carbohydrate and exercise. In Rosenbloom CA, editor: *Sports nutrition. A guide for the professional working with active people,* ed 3, Chicago, 2000, American Dietetic Association.
9. Maughan RJ, Burke LM: Fuels used in exercise: carbohydrate and fat. *Handbook of sports medicine and science: sports nutrition,* Malden, Mass, 2002, Blackwell Publishing.
10. Bergstrom J, Hermansen L, Hultman E, et al: Diet, muscle glycogen and physical performance, *Acta Physiol Scand* 71(2):140-150, 1967.
11. Sherman WM, Costill DL, Fink WJ, et al: Effect of exercise-diet manipulation on muscle glycogen and its subsequent utilization during performance, *Int J Sports Med* 2(2):114-118, 1981.
12. Burke LM, Kiens B, Ivy JL: Carbohydrates and fat for training and recovery, *J Sports Sci* 22(1):15-30, 2004.
13. Fairchild TJ, Fletcher S, Steele P, et al: Rapid carbohydrate loading after a short bout of near maximal-intensity exercise, *Med Sci Sports Exerc* 34(6):980-986, 2002.
14. Jeukendrup AE: Carbohydrate intake during exercise and performance, *Nutrition* 20(7-8):669-677, 2004.
15. Inge K, Brukner P: *Food for sport,* Melbourne, 1986, William Heinemann.
16. Jentjens RL, Jeukendrup AE: Effects of pre-exercise ingestion of trehalose, galactose and glucose on subsequent metabolism and cycling performance, *Eur J Appl Physiol* 88(4-5):459-465, 2003.
17. Moseley L, Lancaster GI, Jeukendrup AE: Effects of timing of pre-exercise ingestion of carbohydrate on subsequent metabolism and cycling performance, *Eur J Appl Physiol* 88(4-5):453-458, 2003.
18. Kirwan JP, O'Gorman D, Evans WJ: A moderate glycemic meal before endurance exercise can enhance performance, *J Appl Physiol* 84(1):53-59, 1998.
19. Coyle EF: Timing and method of increased carbohydrate intake to cope with heavy training, competition and recovery, *J Sports Sci* 9 Spec No:29-51; discussion 51-52, 1991.
20. Jenkins DJ, Kendall CW, Augustin LS, et al: Glycemic index: overview of implications in health and disease, *Am J Clin Nutr* 76(1):266S-273S, 2002.
21. Thomas DE, Brotherhood JR, Brand JC: Carbohydrate feeding before exercise: effect of glycemic index, *Int J Sports Med* 12(2):180-186, 1991.
22. Flint A, Moller BK, Raben A, et al: The use of glycaemic index tables to predict glycaemic index of composite breakfast meals, *Br J Nutr* 91(6):979-989, 2004.
23. Maughan R: Fluid and carbohydrate intake during exercise. In Burke L, Deakin V, editors: *Clinical sports nutrition,* ed 2, Sydney, 2000, McGraw-Hill.
24. Burke LM, Claassen A, Hawley JA, et al: Carbohydrate intake during prolonged cycling minimizes effect of glycemic index of preexercise meal, *J Appl Physiol* 85(6): 2220-2226, 1998.

25. Coyle EF: Fluid and fuel intake during exercise, *J Sports Sci* 22(1):39-55, 2004.

26. Wojtaszewski JF, Nielsen P, Kiens B, et al: Regulation of glycogen synthase kinase-3 in human skeletal muscle: effects of food intake and bicycle exercise, *Diabetes* 50(2):265-269, 2001.

27. Richter EA, Mikines KJ, Galbo H, Kiens B: Effect of exercise on insulin action in human skeletal muscle, *J Appl Physiol* 66(2):876-885, 1989.

28. Ivy JL, Katz AL, Cutler CL, et al: Muscle glycogen synthesis after exercise: effect of time of carbohydrate ingestion, *J Appl Physiol* 64(4):1480-1485, 1988.

29. Burke LM, Collier GR, Beasley SK, et al: Effect of coingestion of fat and protein with carbohydrate feedings on muscle glycogen storage, *J Appl Physiol* 78(6):2187-2192, 1995.

30. Jentjens RL, van Loon LJ, Mann CH, et al: Addition of protein and amino acids to carbohydrates does not enhance postexercise muscle glycogen synthesis, *J Appl Physiol* 91(2):839-846, 2001.

31. Burke L: Nutrition recovery after competition and training. In Burke L, Deakin V, editors: *Clinical sports nutrition*, ed 2, Sydney, 2000, McGraw-Hill.

32. Maughan RJ, Burke LM: *Handbook of sports medicine and science: sports nutrition*, Malden, Mass, 2002, Blackwell Science Ltd.

33. Ivy JL, Goforth HW Jr, Damon BM, et al: Early postexercise muscle glycogen recovery is enhanced with a carbohydrate-protein supplement, *J Appl Physiol* 93(4):1337-1344, 2002.

34. Carrithers JA, Williamson DL, Gallagher PM, et al: Effects of postexercise carbohydrate-protein feedings on muscle glycogen restoration, *J Appl Physiol* 88(6):1976-1982, 2000.

35. Tarnopolsky MA, Bosman M, Macdonald JR, et al: Postexercise protein-carbohydrate and carbohydrate supplements increase muscle glycogen in men and women, *J Appl Physiol* 83(6):1877-1883, 1997.

36. van Loon LJ, Saris WH, Kruijshoop M, et al: Maximizing postexercise muscle glycogen synthesis: carbohydrate supplementation and the application of amino acid or protein hydrolysate mixtures, *Am J Clin Nutr* 72(1):106-111, 2000.

37. Zawadzki KM, Yaspelkis BB III, Ivy JL: Carbohydrate-protein complex increases the rate of muscle glycogen storage after exercise, *J Appl Physiol* 72(5):1854-1859, 1992.

38. Carroll C: Protein and exercise. In Rosenbloom CA, editor: *Sports nutrition. A guide for the professional working with active people*, ed 3, Chicago, 2000, American Dietetic Association.

39. Biolo G, Tipton KD, Klein S, et al: An abundant supply of amino acids enhances the metabolic effect of exercise on muscle protein, *Am J Physiol* 273(1 Pt 1):E122-129, 1997.

40. Tipton KD, Ferrando AA, Phillips SM, et al: Postexercise net protein synthesis in human muscle from orally administered amino acids, *Am J Physiol* 276(4 Pt 1):E628-634, 1999.

41. Borsheim E, Aarsland A, Wolfe RR: Effect of an amino acid, protein, and carbohydrate mixture on net muscle protein balance after resistance exercise, *Int J Sport Nutr Exerc Metab* 14(3):255-271, 2004.

42. Rasmussen BB, Tipton KD, Miller SL, et al: An oral essential amino acid-carbohydrate supplement enhances muscle protein anabolism after resistance exercise, *J Appl Physiol* 88(2):386-392, 2000.

43. Tipton KD, Rasmussen BB, Miller SL, et al: Timing of amino acid–carbohydrate ingestion alters anabolic response of muscle to resistance exercise, *Am J Physiol Endocrinol Metab* 281(2):E197-206, 2001.

44. Andersen LL, Tufekovic G, Zebis MK, et al: The effect of resistance training combined with timed ingestion of protein on muscle fiber size and muscle strength, *Metabolism* 54(2):151-156, 2005.

45. Tipton KD, Gurkin BE, Matin S, Wolfe RR: Nonessential amino acids are not necessary to stimulate net muscle protein synthesis in healthy volunteers, *J Nutr Biochem* 10(2):89-95, 1999.

46. Miller SL, Tipton KD, Chinkes DL, et al: Independent and combined effects of amino acids and glucose after resistance exercise, *Med Sci Sports Exerc* 35(3):449-455, 2003.

47. Biolo G, Williams BD, Fleming RY, Wolfe RR: Insulin action on muscle protein kinetics and amino acid transport during recovery after resistance exercise, *Diabetes* 48(5):949-957, 1999.

48. GSSI: Protein and amino acid supplements: do they work? *Gatorade Sports Sci Inst Sports Sci Exchange* 15(4), 2002.

49. Tarnopolsky M: Protein requirements for endurance athletes, *Nutrition* 20(7-8):662-668, 2004.

50. Riddell MC, Partington SL, Stupka N, et al: Substrate utilization during exercise performed with and without glucose ingestion in female and male endurance trained athletes, *Int J Sport Nutr Exerc Metab* 13(4):407-421, 2003.

51. Roy BD, Luttmer K, Bosman J, et al: The influence of post-exercise macronutrient intake on energy balance and protein metabolism in active females participating in endurance training, *Int J Sport Nutr Exerc Metab* 12:172-188, 2002.

52. Convertino VA, Armstrong LE, Coyle EF, et al: American College of Sports Medicine position stand: exercise and fluid replacement, *Med Sci Sports Exerc* 28(1):i-vii, 1996.

53. Shirreffs SM, Armstrong LE, Cheuvront SN: Fluid and electrolyte needs for preparation and recovery from training and competition, *J Sports Sci* 22(1):57-63, 2004.

54. Maughan RJ, Burke LM: Micronutrients: vitamins and minerals. In Maughan RJ, Burke LM, editors: *Handbook of sports medicine and science: sports nutrition*, Malden, Mass, 2002, Blackwell Publishing.

55. Ahrendt DM: Ergogenic aids: counseling the athlete, *Am Fam Physician* 63(5):913-922, 2001.

56. Maughan RJ, King DS, Lea T: Dietary supplements, *J Sports Sci* 22(1):95-113, 2004.

57. Volek JS, Rawson ES: Scientific basis and practical aspects of creatine supplementation for athletes, *Nutrition* 20(7-8):609-614, 2004.

58. Burke L, Desbrow B, Minehan M: Dietary supplements and nutritional ergogenic aids in sport. In Burke L, Deakin V, editors: *Clinical sports nutrition,* ed 2, Sydney, 2000, McGraw-Hill.

59. Antonio J, Stout JR: *Sports supplements*, Philadelphia, 2001, Lippincott Williams & Wilkins.

60. Talbott SM: *A guide to understanding dietary supplements,* Binghampton, NY, 2003, Haworth Press.

61. AIS Department of Sport Nutrition: supplements in sport—why are they so tempting? Belconnen, Australia, 2004, Australian Institute of Sport.

62. Department of Nutritional Sciences: How to Evaluate Ergogenic Aids Claims, 2004, The University of Arizona, College of Agricultural & Life Sciences, Cooperative Extension.

63. Spriet LL: Caffeine: why, when, and for what? *Gatorade Sports Sci Inst,* Chicago, 2003, Scientific Conference.

64. Graham TE, Spriet LL: Metabolic, catecholamine, and exercise performance responses to various doses of caffeine, *J Appl Physiol* 78(3):867-874, 1995.

65. Davis JM, Zhao Z, Stock HS, et al: Central nervous system effects of caffeine and adenosine on fatigue, *Am J Physiol Regul Integr Comp Physiol* 284(2):R399-404, 2003.

66. Kovacs EM, Stegen J, Brouns F: Effect of caffeinated drinks on substrate metabolism, caffeine excretion, and performance, *J Appl Physiol* 85(2):709-715, 1998.

67. Cox GR, Desbrow B, Montgomery PG, et al: Effect of different protocols of caffeine intake on metabolism and endurance performance, *J Appl Physiol* 93(3):990-999, 2002.

68. Graham TE: Caffeine, coffee and ephedrine: impact on exercise performance and metabolism, *Can J Appl Physiol* 26(Suppl):S103-S119, 2001.

69. Armstrong LE: Caffeine, body fluid-electrolyte balance, and exercise performance, *Int J Sport Nutr Exerc Metab* 12(2):189-206, 2002.

70. Van Nieuwenhoven MA, Brummer RM, Brouns F: Gastrointestinal function during exercise: comparison of water, sports drink, and sports drink with caffeine, *J Appl Physiol* 89(3):1079-1085, 2000.

71. Wemple RD, Lamb DR, McKeever KH: Caffeine vs caffeine-free sports drinks: effects on urine production at rest and during prolonged exercise, *Int J Sports Med* 18(1):40-46, 1997.

72. Clarkson P: Scientifically debatable: is creatine worth its weight? *Gatorade Sports Sci Inst,* Chicago, 2003, Scientific Conference.

73. Skinner R, Coleman E, Rosenbloom CA: Ergogenic aids. In Rosenbloom CA, editor: *Sports nutrition: a guide for the professional working with active people,* ed 3, Chicago, 2000, American Dietetic Association.

74. Nissen SL, Sharp RL: Effect of dietary supplements on lean mass and strength gains with resistance exercise: a meta-analysis, *J Appl Physiol* 94(2):651-659, 2003.

75. Branch JD: Effect of creatine supplementation on body composition and performance: a meta-analysis, *Int J Sport Nutr Exerc Metab* 13(2):198-226, 2003.

76. Fallon K: Athletes with gastrointestinal disorders. In Burke L, Deakin V, editors: *Clinical sports nutrition,* ed 2, Sydney, 2000, McGraw-Hill.

77. Maughan RJ, Burke LM: Changing body size and body composition. In Maughan RJ, Burke LM, editors: *Handbook of sports medicine and science: sports nutrition,* Malden, Mass, 2002, Blackwell Publishing.

78. Modlesky CM, Lewis RD: Assessment of body size and composition. In Rosenbloom CA, editor: *Sports nutrition. A guide for the professional working with active people,* ed 3, Chicago, 2000, American Dietetic Association.

Appendixes

The appendixes comprise a collection of cases to help the reader appreciate the clinical application of various topics discussed in the text.

Appendix A, written by Dr. Joseph Wilkes, an orthopedic surgeon, describes the process of developing a medical diagnosis. The cases presented represent a mixture of soft microtrauma and macrotrauma in an athlete population.

Appendix B, written by two physical therapists, presents cases that represent the total approach in the rehabilitation of athletes. The cases presented illustrate the athletes' progression from rehabilitation back to their sports.

Each case reviews current concepts in strength training, periodization, maintenance programs, and energy system training. Neuromuscular training concepts are illustrated with exercises on unique exercise equipment. The authors' goal is to summarize the material presented in several chapters in strength training, plyometrics, and neuromuscular training through a patient case study.

Appendixes

Approach to Differential Diagnosis in Orthopedics

OBJECTIVES

After reading this appendix, you will be able to do the following:

1. Identify the important aspects of an orthopedic medical history
2. Describe the different components of a physical examination
3. Differentiate among the various diagnostic tests used to make a diagnosis
4. Describe various treatment approaches based on the medical diagnosis
5. Understand how to develop a working diagnosis
6. Describe the correlations between the diagnosis and treatment regimens
7. Understand when to change the treatment on the basis of a reevaluation

An accurate diagnosis in orthopedics is the foundation for guiding the patient back to a maximal functional state. It consists of the medical history, physical examination, and diagnostic testing. Key to the patient history are listening, questioning, and differentiating symptoms to limit the list of orthopedic diagnostic possibilities. The physical examination involves examining the area of complaint; discriminating the findings by allowing the patient to explain what he or she is experiencing; and testing possible diagnoses using additional tests, such as magnetic resonance imaging (MRI) scans. Such tests, often ordered by the physician as a complement to the physical examination, help confirm or deny possible diagnoses. Importantly, trial treatments may be necessary, and consideration of all alternative diagnoses is warranted because a diagnosis that is not considered cannot be established. In orthopedics, as in medicine in general, the diagnosis determines the treatment.[1]

Case 1: Baseball Pitcher

An example of clinical trial treatments based on signs and symptoms was noted in a 17-year-old, male, varsity high school, right-handed pitcher who presented to the orthopedic office with shoulder pain. He was seeking treatment for his right shoulder and lateral arm pain. He had previously been treated for rotator cuff tendonitis with only mild resolution of symptoms.

History

The patient reported an insidious onset of aching pain of approximately 3 months. Initially his symptoms were only after pitching but gradually progressed to the point of pain while pitching. The pain occurred in the late cocking and acceleration phases of throwing. He also noted a gradual decrease in velocity and accuracy of his pitches. His pitching coach had observed a change in his pitching biomechanics. He reported having similar symptoms in previous seasons, although not as severe. He had been using over-the-counter ibuprofen and ice packs, which helped somewhat. He denied cervical spine and radicular symptoms. Review of his medical history was unremarkable.

Physical Examination

The patient had full range of motion (ROM) of the cervical spine and negative Spurling's test and Adson's maneuver. Active range of motion (AROM) elevation in the plane of the scapula was 170 degrees, external rotation at 90 degrees of glenohumeral abduction was 130 degrees, and internal rotation at 90 degrees of glenohumeral abduction was limited to 40 degrees. Functional internal rotation was T8. Normal glenohumeral and scapula rhythm with no scapula winging was observed during ROM testing. Palpation revealed tenderness at the subacromial space and bicipital groove, as well as the posterior rotator cuff muscles and joint capsules. Manually resisted external rotation, empty can, and subscapularis lift-off were painful with slight weakness as compared with the uninvolved shoulder. Impingement testing was positive. The apprehension and relocation tests were positive. Pulses, neurovascular, and motors were intact.

Plain radiographs consisting of axillary and outlet views of anteroposterior internal and external rotation showed the bony structures and joint spaces intact. A type II acromion was identified.

Impression

The therapist's impression of the athlete's condition was that he had right shoulder anterior glenohumeral instability with secondary rotator cuff impingement syndrome.

Plan

The athlete was advised to avoid aggravating activities (throwing) and start on nonsteroidal antiinflammatory drugs (NSAIDs) and a physical therapy program. Physical therapy consisted of modalities to decrease inflammation and pain, gentle mobilization and stretching for the posterior capsule, and a gradual initiation of glenohumeral and scapula stabilizers' strengthening. The athlete was placed on a lower body and CORE strengthening and conditioning program.

Disposition

The patient progressed through rehabilitation to performing sports-specific strengthening and an interval-throwing program. All throwing activities were monitored and supervised by the school's athletic trainer and pitching coach. The athlete was released to begin competitive pitching 6 weeks after the initial evaluation. The key component in this case was addressing the underlying system, the anterior glenohumeral instability. Preventive measures to decrease the chances of recurrence included maintenance of rotator cuff strength, posterior capsule flexibility, and correct pitching biomechanics. Emphasis was placed on lower body and CORE strengthening.

ORTHOPEDIC MEDICAL HISTORY

The purpose of a medical history is to learn the details of the patient's medical problem. A history begins with the patient's verbal account of the symptoms, the patient's assessment of the problem, and the patient's questions and concerns. Before and during the history, physicians should ensure a quiet and comfortable clinical environment with opportunities to build patient rapport. Also, as the patient recounts his or her history, the physician should consider environmental factors, such as hobbies, sporting activities, travel, and diet as possible explanations of the orthopedic problems.[1]

To engage the patient during the clinical history, the physician should introduce himself or herself, listen closely to the patient's account of the problem, and then ask open-ended questions about pertinent aspects of the medical history that will help confirm or deny diagnostic possibilities. Instead of using medical jargon, doctors should build on the patient's own words to communicate, repeating what the patient said so that clarifications in the physician's understanding of the problem can be made. Watching patient body language to ensure that questions are understood and the physician's reflection on his or her own body language to ensure an interest in the patient's medical problem is important. Establishing a satisfactory rapport ultimately assists in the physical examina-

tion and in making the appropriate diagnosis. It also helps the patient understand the explanation of the problem. Moreover, it helps the patient understand the treatment, which makes adherence to it more likely. Physicians are well trained, with one source estimating that medical professionals have approximately 100,000 words to use excluding scientific and medical vocabulary, while the average adult may have only 30,000 to 60,000 such words to use. Clear, concise communication not only helps the patient understand but helps the physician differentiate symptoms that aid in developing a list of possible diagnoses that are refined as more information becomes available.[1]

Case 2: Recreational Fisher

The following case study exemplifies the importance of gathering as much patient information as possible during the medical history. A 58-year-old male presented to an orthopedic office for evaluation and treatment of chronic swelling of his elbow. His rheumatologist referred him.

History

The patient had been previously diagnosed with rheumatoid arthritis, which had affected his knee. He presented complaining of left elbow swelling and stiffness, which had an insidious onset of approximately 3 months (Figure A-1). His rheumatologist referred him for orthopedic examination to rule out other causes for the swelling of the left elbow because it did not present as a classical case of rheumatoid arthritis. Additional history included fishing as a hobby and being punctured in the left hand with a fishing hook. The patient reported that the wound took several weeks to heal.

Physical Examination

Examination revealed circumferential swelling of the left elbow. The musculoskeletal and neurovascular systems were

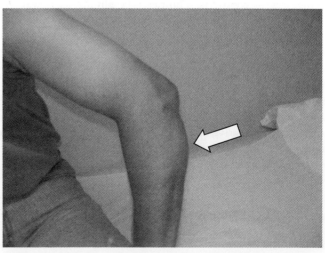

Figure A-1 Atypical swelling on the ulna aspect of the proximal forearm *(arrow)*.

intact. Active ROM was limited secondary to the swelling. He had full ROM of the shoulders, wrists, and hands. Plain radiographs showed the bony structures and joint spaces to be intact. A positive fat pad sign, anterior and posterior, was visualized on the radiographs.

Impression

The therapist believed the patient had rheumatoid joint effusion of the left elbow, although other etiologies, such as metabolic gout, nontraditional infection, and traumatic effusion, were not ruled out.

Plan

The patient was referred to an infectious disease expert for possible laboratory screening. The infectious disease physician requested that the effusion be aspirated. The aspiration returned a small amount of bloody fluid. The sample was taken to the laboratory for acid-fast bacillus culture and smear, culture and sensitivity, and fungal cultures.

Disposition

The results from the laboratory were positive for *Mycobacterium marinum*. The infectious disease physician placed him on the proper antibiotic therapy. He had a significant decrease in his symptoms after 3 weeks of drug therapy. He remained on antibiotic therapy for 10 months. At that time, all cultures were negative.

PHYSICAL EXAMINATION

The rapport and engagement between physician and patient begun during the medical history must continue in the physical examination in order to ensure an accurate diagnosis. The relaxed patient can help any physician pinpoint or eliminate various diagnoses. This is especially true for an orthopedic examination, during which muscle tightening in an anxious patient diminishes the value of the physical findings.

Physicians can help ensure the comfort of the patient by asking permission to conduct the examination and by asking the patient what he or she is experiencing during the examination. In orthopedics a focused examination is usually sufficient. This includes the area of concern, as well as adjacent and related areas as needed. The examination can be expanded as needed, or the use of special examination techniques can be employed if the findings indicate possible additional areas of involvement or if they are necessary to eliminate some possible diagnoses.

In making the diagnosis in orthopedics, an intimate knowledge of anatomy and functional aspects of an area are crucial to making the diagnosis. Being able to discriminate the origin of symptoms or signs is a function of the physician's base of knowledge, attention to the details during the examination, and use of critical thinking as the basis for understanding pathologic findings. Knowledge of pain referral patterns and

conditions that may mimic each other is also important in establishing a differential diagnosis. During the physical examination the clinician may employ most of the classical senses of sight, hearing, touch, smell, and taste, although taste has generally been supplanted by laboratory tests. As with the medical history, a physical examination can be refined in follow-up evaluations at the same visit or subsequent visits as more information becomes available.

Developing a Working Diagnosis

After completing the medical history and conducting a physical examination, the clinician should have a reasonable assessment of the medical problem and a working diagnosis or short list of possible diagnoses. Radiological evaluation is a standard part of the initial assessment of the orthopedic patient. Because of the close relationship of bone morphology to orthopedic conditions, this simple evaluation will frequently provide the information to establish the diagnosis.

Case 3: Professional Football Player

The following case emphasizes the importance of a radiological evaluation. A 25-year-old professional football player presented for evaluation and treatment of persistent right knee pain and dysfunction following autograft patella tendon anterior cruciate ligament reconstruction.

History

The patient sustained an injury to his right knee during a football game while playing defensive back. An MRI scan revealed an isolated anterior cruciate ligament tear, and subsequently the patient underwent operative reconstruction of the ligament 4 months before his visit. Despite aggressive physical therapy, he was still experiencing decreased mobility, chronic swelling, weakness, and the inability to return to football-specific activities.

Physical Examination

Pulses and neurovascular and musculoskeletal systems were intact. A low-grade joint effusion was present. Palpation of the infrapatellar tendon and fat pad was painful. AROM measured −20 degrees of extension to 110 degrees of flexion. Patella mobility was restricted both superior and inferior. Active quadriceps–vastus medialis obliquus (VMO) recruitment was fair. Gait observation revealed increased flexion of the right knee at heel strike, stance, and push-off. Plain radiographs demonstrated acceptable femoral and tibial tunnels. A low patella position was visualized on the lateral radiograph, indicating patella Baja.

Impression

The therapist believed that the patient had postoperative arthrofibrosis and patella Baja of the right knee.

Plan

The patient wanted to proceed with surgical intervention consisting of right knee arthroscopy with débridement and resection of the infrapatellar fat pad. Postoperative care consisted of continuous passive motion (CPM), home neuromuscular electrical stimulation unit (NMES) for quad-VMO recruitment, and a postoperative ROM brace locked at 0 degrees of extension for sleeping. The patient began physical therapy 1 day after his operation.

Disposition

The patient was able to achieve full, pain-free ROM of the right knee. Surgery provided resolution of the pain, swelling, and quadriceps atonia. The patient was able to return to professional football following a successful functional rehabilitation program.

DIFFERENTIATION OF THE DIAGNOSIS

If the list of potential diagnoses is limited or a firm diagnosis seems apparent, a trial treatment is begun. The response to the treatment can provide feedback for eliminating or confirming a diagnosis. Sometimes, in patients with some response to a treatment, a subtle change in the prescribed therapy may allow further differentiation of the diagnosis. Such an approach requires the clinician to use critical evaluation of treatment information along with his or her own knowledge base (clinical experience and education) to identify a more precise diagnosis.

Case 4 Tennis Player

The following case study demonstrates the importance of the continued use of diagnostic skills throughout treatment. Was what was initially diagnosed as tenosynovitis a triangular fibrocartilage complex (TFCC) tear? A 34-year-old, right-handed female presented for orthopedic examination and treatment of right wrist pain.

History

While playing tennis the patient reported falling and landing on her outstretched right arm 4 weeks before presenting for an orthopedic examination. She saw her primary care physician immediately after the injury. This physician ordered plain radiographic tests, which were read as normal. However, nonspecific wrist pain and dysfunction persisted. She denied previous injury to the wrist and reported that activities requiring her to use her wrist increased her pain. She specifically complained of weakness with gripping activities.

Physical Examination

Pulses and neurovascular and musculoskeletal systems were intact. Plain radiographs were repeated and showed the bony

structures and joint spaces intact. Palpation of the ulnar wrist was painful. Crepitus was palpable with active wrist motion. Active and passive ranges of motion were normal. Pain was elicited at the end range of active flexion over flexor carpi ulnaris and with passive flexion and radial deviation of the wrist. Resisted extension of the fourth and fifth fingers was painful. Phalen's and Tinel's tests were negative.

Impression

The symptoms indicated tenosynovitis of the right wrist and flexor carpi ulnaris and suspicion of a TFCC tear.

Plan

Conservative treatment consisting of a wrist support, NSAIDs, avoidance of aggravating activities, and a physical therapy program were initiated. The patient remained symptomatic at the 3-week follow-up appointment. An MRI scan was ordered to assess the soft tissue structures of the wrist. The MRI scan demonstrated a tear to the TFCC. An arthroscopy with débridement and repair of the TFCC was scheduled.

Disposition

Postoperative care and rehabilitation were uneventful. Eight weeks after the operation the patient was asymptomatic and able to resume activity involving the wrist at a preinjury level.

ADDITIONAL TESTS AND EVALUATIONS

Additional tests in orthopedics can assist in confirming or ruling out a particular diagnosis. Several different tests are available to assist in making a difficult diagnosis in orthopedics.

Laboratory analysis of blood, urine, and fluid can be helpful in ruling out or establishing the diagnosis of such common orthopedic problems as rheumatoid arthritis, systemic lupus erythematosus, infections, and trauma. Serum analysis; a complete blood count; rheumatologic screen, which includes a complete metabolic profile; rheumatoid factor; acetylneuraminic acid; and C-reactor protein, sedimentation rate, and then a urinalysis are tests that help pinpoint medical conditions that present as orthopedic problems. Although this is not a complete set of all tests, it gives the clinician a basis for ruling in or out many diagnoses.

Computed tomography (CT) is a scan of x-ray origin that gives an excellent assessment of bone and occult fractures. The CT scan allows evaluation in a tomographic fashion of the structure of bone in a specific area and indicates disruption of the bone's structure that is sometimes too subtle for plain radiographs.

Case 5: Pole Vaulter

The following case study illustrates the value of the CT scan in making a diagnosis. Six days after falling from a vault, a

25-year-old male presented for orthopedic evaluation and treatment of his left ankle.

History

The patient reports falling approximately 12 feet from vaulting in a track meet. He landed with the majority of his weight on the left foot and ankle on a hard surface. He was evaluated and treated in the emergency department for a lateral ankle sprain and a lateral malleolus avulsion fracture. He was placed on crutches and in an air cast ankle stirrup support and referred for an orthopedic evaluation.

Physical Examination

The patient, on crutches, was not bearing weight on the left ankle. He had an extensive swelling of the left foot. Pulses were intact. Musculoskeletal and neurovascular systems were intact. AROM of the left ankle was limited secondary to swelling. The lateral aspect of the ankle was the most tender area with palpation. A calcific chip of the lateral malleolus was visualized on plain radiographs.

Impression

The therapist suspected a left ankle sprain with a possible occult fracture of the talus and calcaneus.

Plan

The patient was placed in a fracture walker boot, and a compression sock was applied to the foot and ankle. Due to the extensive swelling in the foot, a CT scan was ordered to rule out occult fractures of the talus and calcaneus (Figure A-2).

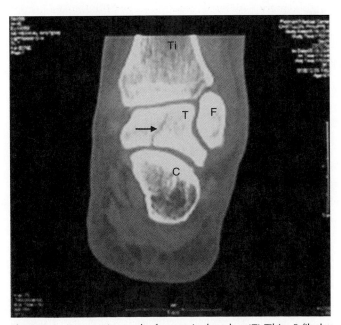

Figure A-2 *Arrow* points to the fracture in the talus. (*Ti,* Tibia; *F,* fibula; *T,* talus; *C,* calcaneus.)

Disposition

The CT scan identified a nondisplaced occult fracture of the talar dome. The patient was treated conservatively, having to use crutches without bearing weight and being in a boot for 6 weeks. Then he was started on progressive weight bearing and physical therapy and was functional after an additional 4 weeks.

The bone scan is an evaluation of the metabolic activity of bone cells of the osteocytes. Radioactive technetium is injected intravenously and then absorbed by the osteocytes, which can reveal an area of increased activity (a relative hot spot) or decreased activity (a relative cold spot). The cold spot or hot spot may need further evaluation or it may confirm a diagnosis. When the main clinical diagnostic impression is a stress factor, the bone scan gives a relative activity scale and confirms such a fracture. Otherwise, further tests are necessary to evaluate the underlying cause for increased or decreased activity in a bone area.

Case 6: Long-Distance Runner

History

The following case study clearly illustrates the use of a bone scan in diagnostic evaluation.

A 17-year-old male long-distance runner presented for orthopedic evaluation and treatment for right foot pain. The patient reported an insidious onset of right foot pain that started 4 weeks before the initial visit. The pain started around the time he had increased his mileage in preparation for an upcoming marathon. Initially the pain occurred at the end of his run, but later he was unable to compete a 1-mile run.

Physical Examination

Observation of the patient's feet in standing released pes planus bilaterally. Inspection of his running shoes showed considerable breakdown, with a collapse of the medial arch. Pulses and musculoskeletal and neurovascular systems were intact. Tenderness and puffiness were detected over the neck of the second metatarsal. The patient demonstrated full active ROM of the knee, ankle, and foot. Plain radiographs were unremarkable, demonstrating intact bony structures and joint surfaces.

Impression

The therapist thought it likely that a stress fracture of the second metatarsal had occurred.

Plan

The patient was placed on modified activity (no running) and scheduled for a three-phase bone scan. Results of the bone scan showed focal intense tracer accumulation at the base of the second metatarsal, indicating a stress fracture (Figure A-3).

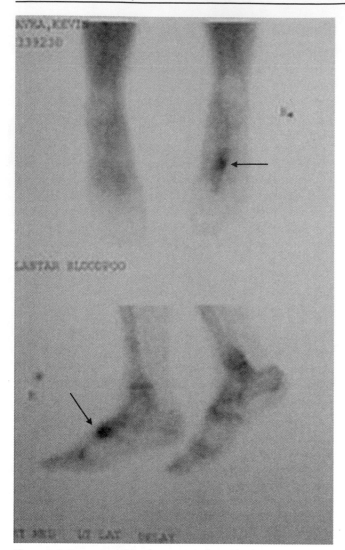

Figure A-3 Bone scan of the foot. *Arrow* shows the hot spot that indicates a stress fracture.

Disposition

The patient was treated conservatively. He was placed in a fracture walking boot full time. He was allowed to cross-train while the fracture was healing. Radiographs obtained after 8 weeks of treatment revealed that the stress fracture was healed and the athlete was asymptomatic. He was allowed to begin an interval running program and progress to competitive running. He was advised on new running shoes and given orders for custom foot orthotics to help prevent a recurrence of a stress fracture.

MRI scans provide a great deal of information about the soft tissue, bone abnormalities, blood flow, and fluid accumulation in areas. Therefore MRI can be diagnostic for avascular necrosis; some metabolic bone diseases; and disruption of structures such as meniscal tears, ligament tears, and substitution tissues (e.g., tumors).

Case 7: Basketball Player

The following case study illustrates the importance of MRI as a diagnostic tool in evaluating the knee. A 20-year-old female presented for orthopedic evaluation and treatment of a swollen and painful left knee.

History

Two months before her examination, this collegiate basketball player sustained an injury to her left knee. The patient reported that the injury occurred as she tried to change direction while running. The left foot was planted and the knee was flexed approximately 40 degrees as she attempted to cut to her left. She finished the season with conservative treatment while experiencing intermittent swelling and "catching" of the knee.

Physical Examination

A 1+ left knee joint effusion was present. The lateral joint line was tender with palpation. A palpable mass was identified on the lateral aspect of the knee. Knee AROM measured at 0 degree of extension to 115 degrees of flexion. Full flexion was inhibited by pain and swelling. Quadriceps-VMO recruitment was fair. Antonia of the quadriceps was noted. The flexion rotary test was positive (pain and palpable click present). Ligament stress tests were negative. Pulses and musculoskeletal and neurovascular systems were intact. Plain radiographs of the knee showed the bony structures and joint spaces intact.

Impression

The therapist suspected the patient had a lateral meniscal tear and a meniscal cyst.

Plan

The patient began taking NSAIDs, wearing a knee sleeve, and performing quad-VMO exercises, and had an MRI scan of the left knee.

Disposition

The MRI scan confirmed the diagnosis of lateral meniscus tear and meniscal cyst. Left knee arthroscopy with partial lateral meniscectomy and open excision of the lateral meniscal cyst was performed. Postoperative treatment and rehabilitation were unremarkable. The patient was able to resume all preinjury activities.

SUMMARY: FOLLOW-UP EVALUATIONS OF TREATMENT

Patients with orthopedic problems frequently respond slowly to treatment, creating several issues to evaluate on each subsequent visit. If the signs and symptoms remain consistent with the diagnosis, then continuation of the current treatment is appropriate; if the signs and symptoms do not remain consistent, then further investigation to fine-tune the diagnosis and the treatment is necessary.

Moreover, if the response is not as expected, the question of why must be addressed. A patient may not respond to prescribed treatment for several reasons. The physician-controlled causes of nonresponse include clinician error—either the wrong diagnosis or the wrong treatment. The patient-controlled causes include a noncompliant patient or a patient whose body is responding differently than expected.

If one of these areas can be identified, the diagnostic process and treatment can be further evaluated to correctly address the patient's problem. When to change the current treatment depends on the integration of critical analysis and the knowledge base of the physician. Each orthopedic problem may have a somewhat different presentation or response, or both, in a given patient. Taking all information of the different aspects of the evaluation including patient input and using critical analysis will lead to a more precise diagnosis. The clinician will build a knowledge base that enables more precise development of a differential diagnosis and more accurate diagnosis, resulting in more frequent prescriptions of the best treatment. This is the art of medicine.

REFERENCES

1. Coles C, Holm HA: Learning in medicine: towards a theory of medical education. In Coles C, Holm HA, editors: *Learning in medicine,* pp. 189-209, Oslo, 1993, Scandinavian University Press.
2. Kelly CK: Improving physical exams and history-taking can help you become more efficient and compassionate. In American College of Physicians, editors: *American College of Physicians observer,* Philadelphia, 2001, ACP.
3. LeBlond RF, Brower D: *DeGowin's diagnostic examination,* ed 8, p. 3, New York, 2004, McGraw-Hill.

Rehabilitation through Performance Training: Cases in Sport

LACROSSE SPORT-SPECIFIC REHABILITATION AND PERFORMANCE TRAINING

This case represents a possible cause and treatment approach for a patient with patellofemoral pain syndrome, medial collateral ligament strain, medial meniscus strain, and other diagnoses related to knee pain. Treatment is based on a finding of muscle imbalance causing poor alignment and stability of the knee, which can be affected by muscles of the hip rotators and abductors. Experts have argued widely that treatment for many of these disorders can be provided through strengthening of the vastus medialis oblique (VMO). Evidence has diminished the possibility that this muscle has an effect on patella tracking, and therefore this treatment approach should not be used as a primary treatment for patients with knee pain.[1] This appendix provides an alternate explanation and approach to treating some types of knee pain.

General Demographics

The patient is a 19-year-old Caucasian, English-speaking female who presents in the clinic with bilateral lateral knee pain that is worse on the right side than the left. The pain began 3 months ago.

Social History

M.H. is a college student who plays lacrosse and tennis. She does not smoke or drink.

Living Environment

She rents a two-story home with her two roommates.

Medical History

M.H. had right knee pain at the end of lacrosse season last year. She was seen by her pediatrician, who prescribed nonsteroidal antiinflammatory drugs (NSAIDs), which decreased the pain and allowed her to finish the season. Once lacrosse season was over, she had no more complaints of knee pain until 2 weeks into the season this year.

History of Chief Complaint

M.H. reports having pain in her right knee after the first week of lacrosse practice, which involved running 2 to 3 miles per day, and training, which included running stairs. By the end of the second week, the left knee had begun to have the same pain, but not as severe. M.H.'s parents took her back to her pediatrician, who prescribed NSAIDs again and referred her to an orthopedic surgeon. The surgeon diagnosed her with patellofemoral stress syndrome (PFSS) and instructed her to decrease running and to cease running stairs for at least 2 weeks. The surgeon also provided her with a referral to physical therapy. On evaluation in the clinic 1 week later, the patient continues to complain of knee pain with activities that require closed-chain knee extension from flexion (e.g., standing from sitting, ascending and descending stairs). She describes pain along the lateral aspect of the patella with some radiating pain inferomedially along the lateral aspect of the patella tendon.

Prior Treatment for This Condition

M.H. has treated these symptoms before with over-the-counter ibuprofen. The ibuprofen had eased her pain in the past but was not helping this time. She received Bextra from her pediatrician, which she took for the first week but felt no change in her symptoms; therefore she decided to stop taking it because she does not like taking medications. She has not been taught any exercises at this time.

Functional Status and Activity Level

M.H. is an active person. She plays lacrosse competitively and tennis recreationally. She requires no assistance with activities of daily living (ADLs).

Medications

Bextra was prescribed, but she is not taking the medication.

Hypothesis Differential: Pathology/Impairment

- Patella tendonitis—Overuse injury due to excessive running. Also pain with closed-chain extension from flexed posture.
- Patellofemoral pain syndrome—Pain with closed-chain extension from flexed posture. Lateral tracking of the patella possibly causing increased wear to the hyaline cartilage.
- Meniscal tear—Pain along the medial joint line due to overuse of the noncontractile structures to limit motion and aid in shock absorption.[2]

Tests and Measures

Gait Locomotion Balance

M.H. ambulated into the clinic without an assistive device, but excess knee flexion was noted in the midstance phase, as well as early heel off in the late stance phase of the gait cycle.

Joint Integrity and Mobility

Active motion pattern analysis reveals increased valgus motion with closed-chain knee flexion in standing.
McMurray's: Negative
Patella grind: Positive
Varus Stress: Negative
Valgus Stress: Negative

Rationale

McMurray's test, along with a negative history of any catching or locking, helps to rule out medial meniscal involvement.[2] The patella grind test is to determine patellofemoral pain and helps rule in that diagnosis.[2] Negative varus stress eliminates any possibility of lateral collateral ligament strain, and finally the negative valgus stress test rules out involvement of the medial collateral ligament.[2]

Results

This patient appears to have patellofemoral stress syndrome, but patella tendonitis has not been ruled in or out as a diagnosis. Also, the cause of the strain is, as yet, not apparent.

Manual Muscle Testing

	Right	Left
Knee		
Extension	3+/5 Pain	5/5
Flexion	4+/5	4+/5

	Right	Left
Hip		
Extension	5/5	5/5
Flexion	5/5	5/5
Internal rotation	4/5	4/5
External rotation	3/5	4/5
Abduction	3/5	4/5
Adduction	5/5	5/5

Rationale

Weakness of the knee and its proximal stabilizers should be assessed.

Results

The patient demonstrated weakness in a pattern that will allow the right knee to experience excessive valgus forces during closed-chain knee flexion.[3]

Pain Scale

M.H. rates her pain as an 8 on a visual analog scale (VAS) of 10 during and after lacrosse practice. She rates her pain as 2-3/10 at best, lying supine with the right leg elevated. The resting pain has improved since she stopped running and playing lacrosse.

Rationale

The patient's level of impairment as associated with pain should be assessed.

Result

The patient presents with pain that is consistent with an inflammatory-type injury.

Range of Motion

Knee	Right	Left
Extension	8 degrees hyperextension	8 degrees hyperextension
Flexion	140 degrees and painful	145 degrees and no pain
Thomas test	Negative	Negative
Ober test	Negative	Negative

Rationale

The patient's knee and hip range of motion (ROM) should be assessed as possible causes of or results from knee pain.

Result

Limited right knee flexion with pain at end range could be significant for patella tendonitis or PFSS, or both.

Palpation

M.H. is tender to palpation of the right knee in the superior lateral aspect of the patella. No tenderness is noted on the patella tendon or any point of the left knee.

Rationale

The therapist should attempt to correlate painful areas with anatomical causes.

Result

The tenderness correlates to patellofemoral stress syndrome and helps to rule out patella tendonitis.

Diagnosis

The patient shows numerous signs that indicate inflammation and pain of the right lateral patellofemoral joint. Signs and symptoms are consistent with patellofemoral stress syndrome.

ICD-9 CM Code: 719.46

Diagnostic Pattern

4E—Impaired Joint Mobility, Motor Function, Muscle Performance, and ROM associated with Localized Inflammation[4]

4D—Impaired Joint Mobility, Motor Function, Muscle Performance, and ROM associated with Other Connective Tissue Disorders[4]

Physical Therapy Clinical Impression: Prognosis and Plan of Care

This patient presents with tenderness and pain along an identifiable anatomical structure that has apparently been caused by increased stresses due to lacrosse. The manual muscle testing demonstrates that the patient exhibits weakness of her hip external rotators and abductors. During closed-chain knee extension from flexion and flexion from extension, these muscle groups are responsible for maintaining proper alignment of the knee over the foot. Weakness of this hip musculature, especially during weight acceptance in running and jumping, allows the knee to move medially, which increases the valgus stress and places unusual forces on the patella tendon.[5] As the knee moves into flexion the hip external rotators and abductors are being eccentrically loaded, allowing excess valgus movement of the knee. This excess movement changes the alignment of the line of pull of the quadriceps on the patella, resulting in a greater lateral force.[6] This increased force resulted in closer approximation of the patella to the lateral epicondyle of the femur and resulted in breakdown of that tissue and the resulting inflammation and pain with a flexed posture.

The first goal of intervention will be to decrease the inflammation in order to allow the healing process to progress. This process can be performed in conjunction with the next goal, which is to strengthen the right hip external rotators and abductors in order to stabilize the right knee. This strengthening process must include eccentric loading of the right hip due to the principle of specificity of training, allowing for a greater carryover effect when the patient returns to running.[7]

Expected Range of Visits

Good evidence supports that weight training 3 days per week is effective in producing strength gains; therefore this patient will be seen 3 days per week for 3 weeks for a progressive resistance training program. For the first three to four visits, iontophoresis with dexamethasone will be administered to decrease the patient's inflammation.[8] For the following visits, the patient will have a cold pack placed on the right knee after completing the exercise routine.

After 3 weeks, a decrease in pain and increase in strength should be noted due to the antiinflammatories and exercise program because it has been shown that strength gains should be apparent within the first 3 weeks of an exercise regimen.[9]

Short-term Goals (2 to 3 Weeks)

1. Decrease resting pain to 0/10 on a VAS.
2. Decrease worst pain to 5-6/10 on a VAS.
3. Increase right hip external rotation strength to 4/5 on manual muscle testing.
4. Increase right hip abduction strength to 4/5 on manual muscle testing.
5. Increase right knee flexion ROM to 145 degrees and pain free.

Long-Term Goals (6 to 8 Weeks)

1. Decrease worst pain to 0-1/10 on a VAS.
2. Increase right hip external rotation strength to 5/5 on manual muscle testing.
3. Increase right hip abduction strength to 4+/5 on manual muscle testing.
4. Increase right knee extension to 5/5 and pain free.

Functional Goals

1. Able to ascend and descend stairs without pain (4 weeks).
2. Able to transfer sit to stand and stand to sit without pain (4 weeks).
3. Able to run 2 miles without pain (6 weeks).
4. Able to run 3 miles without pain (8 weeks).
5. Able to return to lacrosse practice and games without pain (8 weeks).

Course of Treatment

Treatment consisted of a progressive resistance training program that focused on strengthening of the hip rotators and abductors. Exercises included a warm-up on the stationary bicycle followed by internal and external rotation of the right hip with resistance at the ankle supplied by pulleys, which was performed in standing with weight bearing on the left lower extremity. The patient also performed a hip stabilization exercise with weight bearing on the right lower extremity and resistance with pulleys to the left lower extremity in a series of movements that required her to maintain pelvic and trunk stability with the right hip while movement occurred through the left lower extremity.

Another exercise used the shuttle leg press system with instruction to the patient to maintain bilateral knees aligned with the feet while performing a squat across gravity. Abduction was performed on the Total Hip machine maintaining the right lower limb parallel to or slightly behind the left, and the right hip was in slight internal rotation to prevent external rotation that would allow the patient to perform the exercise predominantly with hip flexors. Finally, a series of balancing exercises were performed in order to use the hip strategy and force the patient to begin using the right hip to stabilize instead of the passive motion resistors of the knee (i.e., the capsule and ligaments). The patient was also instructed to perform sidelying hip abduction with a 10-second hold for 10 repetitions (reps) once or twice daily.

All gym exercises were performed for 10 reps for 1 set on the first day, then 3 sets of 10 on the next treatment day. The next treatment progressed to 3 sets of 12, then 3 sets of 15 on the following treatment. Finally the weight was increased one plate (10 lb), and the reps decreased to 10 for 3 sets. Then the process began again. This pattern was chosen due to evidence that strength and hypertrophic gains can be seen when training occurs between 10 and 15 reps, and 3 sets have been shown in many studies to be more effective than 1.[1] The pattern for increasing weight once per week is used in order to assure that the patient lifts 60% to 80% of his or her 1 repetition maximum (RM) within a relatively short time period. If the weight were not increased regularly, the patient would likely be working well below his or her ideal resistance and little change would be seen.

After the exercise regimen was completed, iontophoresis to the right superior lateral aspect of the patella was performed with dexamethasone as the antiinflammatory agent at 80 mA·minutes. The iontophoresis was performed for the first four visits, after which time the patient had no resting pain. From this time forward, a cold pack was placed on the patient's right knee after the exercise program for 15 minutes with elevation to prevent inflammation from becoming a problem again.

Reassessment (4 Weeks)

Staron et al[9] showed in 1994 that relative maximal dynamic strength in women can be increased with just 2 weeks of strength training of the lower extremity. Increases in strength were also shown for both sexes in the first four weeks in both the upper and lower limbs, but without significant change in muscle cross-sectional area (CSA). Therefore it was determined that neural factors, such as synaptic activity and neurotransmitter availability, are most likely responsible for these early strength gains.[9,10] An increase in strength after 4 weeks of training is therefore common, and pain arising from muscle imbalance should begin to decrease in this time period.

Manual Muscle Testing

	Right	Left
Knee		
Extension	5/5 pain free	5/5
Flexion	5/5	5/5
Hip		
Extension	5/5	5/5
Flexion	5/5	5/5
Internal rotation	4+/5	4+/5
External rotation	4/5	4+/5
Abduction	4/5	5/5
Adduction	5/5	5/5

The manual muscle tests reveal an expected pattern of strength increase considering the emphasis placed on these muscle groups in the strength training program. The left lower extremity strength gains can be attributed to the left lower limb being used to stabilize the body in stance during right leg open-chain exercise, as well as the ability for the opposite limb to experience strength gains due to increases in hormone levels, blood flow, and neural activation.[9]

Pain

Reevaluation of M.H. at 4 weeks revealed that she no longer had resting pain (0/10 on a VAS), and was able to perform community ambulation without an increase in pain. Ascending stairs no longer increased her right knee pain, either. However, she still experienced pain when descending stairs and had not attempted running at this time due to medical doctor and physical therapist recommendation. Her "worst pain" was noted when attempting to squat down and was described as 3-4/10 on a VAS.

Range of Motion

M.H. had recovered full ROM and was pain free at end range at this time.

Plan

The patient was responding well to the initial treatment plan. The inflammatory phase of healing should have been completed at this time. Therefore iontophoresis or use of a cold pack, or both, was no longer used at the end of treatment.[11] Because hypertrophic changes in the muscle are not expected until at least 6 weeks of training has occurred, the resistance training program continues to progress at this time.[9,10] If a return of pain is noted, especially after performing the gym workout or after excess physical activity at home, the phonophoresis or cold pack treatment, or both, should resume.

Goals/Prognosis Review

Long-term and functional goals remain the same at this time because the patient is progressing as expected and strength, ROM, and function are returning at a normal pace.

Reassessment (8 Weeks)

According to several journal articles, hypertrophy and fiber-type conversion, which are more permanent changes to the muscle, should occur within 8 weeks of a resistance training program.[9,10]

Manual Muscle Testing

Hip	Right	Left
Internal rotation	5/5	5/5
External rotation	5/5	5/5
Abduction	5/5	5/5

Pain

M.H. continues to have no resting pain (0/10) on a VAS and is now experiencing no pain with any activity.

Function

M.H. can transfer from sit to stand, ascend and descend stairs, and stand from a squatting position without any pain. At 6 weeks from initial evaluation, M.H. was having no pain with any activity, and hip rotation and abduction strength was equal bilaterally. At that time, she began treadmill running in our gym, progressing from a half mile run to 3 miles in the past 2 weeks. This running was performed without pain. Therefore she returned to her lacrosse practice before her last visit and completed a 2-hour practice without pain. She has also returned to playing tennis; however, she has limited herself to ground strokes from the baseline for approximately half an hour and has not experienced a return of her symptoms.

Plan

After M.H.'s last lacrosse competition, she will take a complete rest for 7 days. She will then cross-train with swimming, biking, elliptical, and resistance training. The intensity and volume will be kept low. After 6 weeks of cross-training

she will return to the clinic for a sports-specific performance evaluation to be assessed for trunk, hip, and shoulder strength, along with single-leg stance time, shuttle run time, back overhead toss, and jump height. Shoulder strength is being assessed because the upper body and extremities are involved in the sport of lacrosse, and the trunk is being assessed on the basis of the fact that trunk stabilization is especially important in a sport that involves both the upper and lower extremities. On the basis of the deficits found, M.H. will be progressed through a 3-month periodized resistance, plyometric, neuromuscular reeducation, and energy system program.

Preseason Phase (12 Weeks) 3 Macrocytes

First Macrocycle (4 Weeks)

Goals: Increase muscle strength, prepare for plyometrics, begin neuromuscular reeducation exercise, and undergo energy system training

Schedule: Mondays/Fridays—Hip and trunk strengthening, neuromuscular reeducation training, and aerobic system training

Wednesdays—Shoulder strengthening and plyometric preparation

Muscle Strength

Her trunk muscles will primarily be trained isometrically with minimal eccentric and concentric loading. Her upper and lower extremities will be trained both concentrically and eccentrically, primarily because of the stretch-shorten cycle. All strength exercises will be performed as follows: 3 sets × 8 to 12 reps. Multijoint exercises will be performed first, followed by single-joint exercises. Both the concentric and eccentric phases of the exercise will be moved through a 2 second count. One can emphasize the eccentric component by increasing the amount of time it takes to return the weight to the starting position. Initial weight will be set by her 8RM. Once she can complete 3 sets of 12 reps, her weight will be increased to allow at least 8 reps and she will work up to 12 reps again and repeat. The only exception to this is the trunk exercises, which will be progressed by increasing her holding time. There will be a 2- to 3-minute rest between sets. Following are examples of hip (Figure B-1), trunk (Figure B-2), and shoulder (Figure B-3) strengthening exercises.

Neuromuscular Retraining

The following exercises will be repeated for both legs. The athlete can move through the progression as long as she can complete the activity without a loss of balance. If she loses her balance, she must stay at that activity until she can complete it. If she can make it through the progression, increases can be made in the medicine ball weight, the speed at which she tosses the ball, and the reps, or 30 degrees of rapid head rotation can be added. The athlete should be cued to hold good hip-knee-foot alignment with a 20% contraction of the CORE.

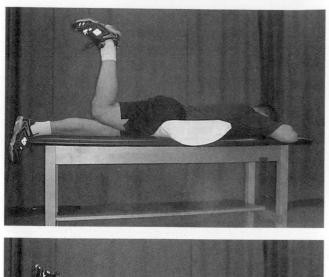

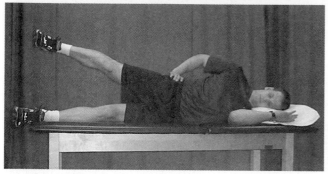

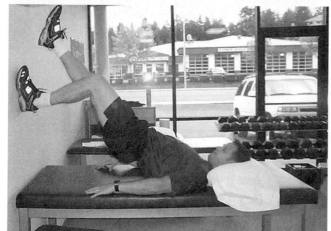

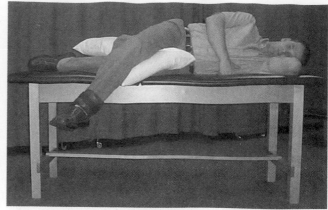

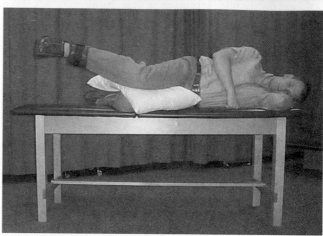

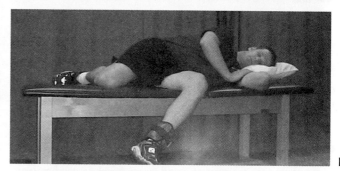

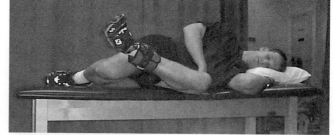

Figure B-1 Hip exercises. **A,** Hip extension. **B,** Hip abduction. **C,** 90/90 Wall hemibridges. **D,** Hip internal rotation—beginning. **E,** Hip internal rotation—end. **F,** Hip external rotation—beginning. **G,** Hip external rotation—end.

1. Athlete will start on a stable base on one leg and hold for 30 seconds.
2. Athlete will stand on leg on stable base and toss a 2-lb medicine ball straight up 6 inches × 15 reps.
3. Athlete will stand on one leg on stable base and toss medicine ball anteriorly into rebounder and catch × 15 reps (Figure B-4, *A*).
4. Athlete will remain on stable base, turn 90 degrees, stand on one leg with the near leg to the rebounder, toss the 2-lb medicine ball, and catch × 15 reps (Figure B-4, *B*).
5. Athlete will then repeat this progression while standing on a wobble board, ½ foam roller, or dynadisk (Figure B-4, *C*).

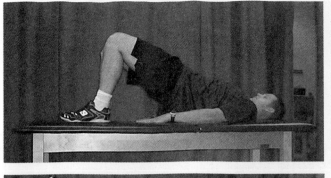

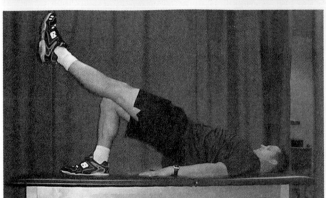

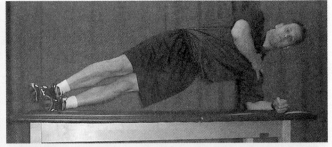

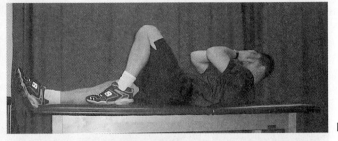

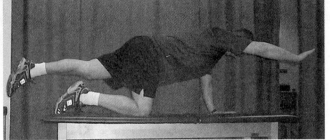

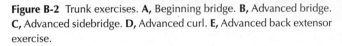

Figure B-2 Trunk exercises. **A,** Beginning bridge. **B,** Advanced bridge. **C,** Advanced sidebridge. **D,** Advanced curl. **E,** Advanced back extensor exercise.

Plyometric Preparation

The following exercises are used to prepare the body for plyometric training. The key to these exercises is to have good alignment and posture. As stated in Chapter 14, the athlete must first attain the proper alignment and then maintain it. The reader can refer to Chapter 14 for further detail.

1. Squat—Hold with proper posture and alignment × 30 seconds.
2. Squatting—Move through a squat motion going into at least 45 degrees of knee flexion while maintaining proper alignment and posture × 8 to 12 reps × 2 sets.
3. Can progress through double-leg squat to single-leg squat × 8 to 12 reps × 2 sets.
4. Forward/backward step-ups × 8 to 12 reps × 2 sets.
5. Lateral step-ups × 8 to 12 reps × 2 sets.

Ideally, by the end of the 4-week period, this athlete will be able to perform a single-leg squat and step-ups with good alignment and posture with added weight for 8 to 12 reps.

Aerobic Base Line Training

The athlete will need a foundation of endurance and overall good aerobic health. She will train three times a week, once on the bike, once on an elliptical trainer, and once on the treadmill. She will have a heart rate monitor and will train at 65% to 70% of her maximal heart rate for at least 20 minutes

working up to 40 minutes. Please see Chapter 4 for further discussion

Second Macrocycle (4 Weeks)

Goals: Increased muscle size, plyometrics support phase, advanced neuromuscular reeducation exercise, and varying energy system training

Schedule: Mondays/Wednesday/Fridays—Hip, trunk, and shoulder strengthening, aerobic and anaerobic system training, and neuromuscular retraining

Mondays/Fridays—Plyometric support exercises will precede strengthening

Muscle Hypertrophy

All hip and shoulder strength exercises will be performed for 3 to 4 sets × 6 to 12 reps. Multijoint exercises will be performed first, followed by single-joint exercises. Both concentric and eccentric phases of the exercise will be moved through a 2 count. There will be a 1- to 2-minute rest between sets. Initial weight will be set by her 6RM. Once she can complete 3 sets of 12 reps, her weight will be increased to allow at least 6 reps but no more than 12. The CORE exercises will continue with increased holding times with the addition of therapy ball exercises (Figure B-5). The shoulder exercises will continue as the same. The hip exercises will change to pulley exercises

text continued on page 315.

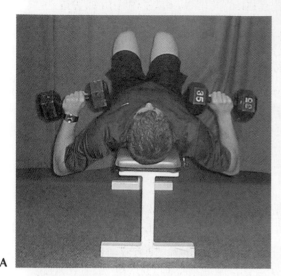

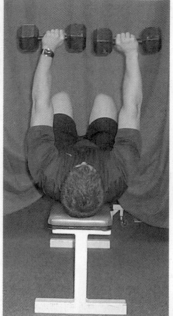

Figure B-3 Shoulder exercises. **A,** Bench and reach—beginning. **B,** Bench and reach—end. **C,** One-arm row—beginning. **D,** One-arm row—end. **E,** Mid trap lift—beginning. **F,** Mid trap lift—end.

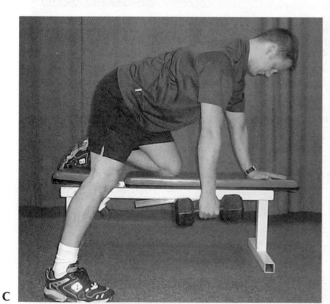

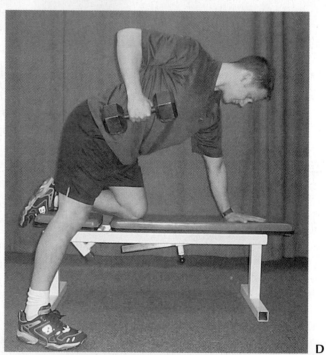

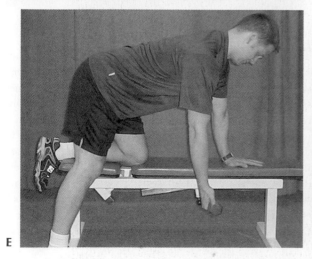

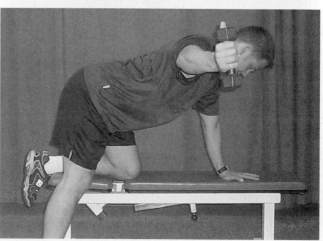

Figure B-3, cont'd G, Sidelying external rotation—beginning. **H,** Sidelying external rotation—end. **I,** Sidelying internal rotation—beginning. **J,** Sidelying internal rotation—end. **K,** Lower trap—beginning. **L,** Lower trap—end. **M,** Scapular retraction—beginning. **N,** Scapular retraction—end.

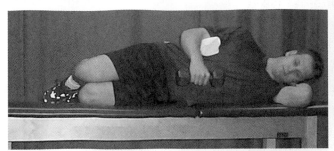

G

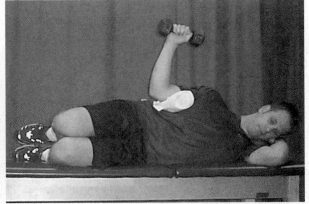

H

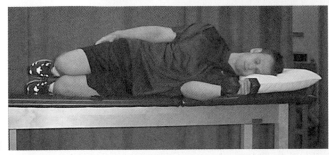

I

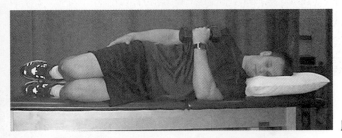

J

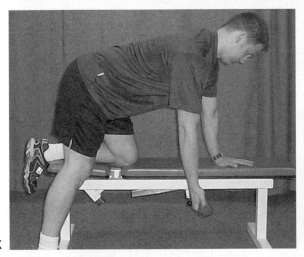

K

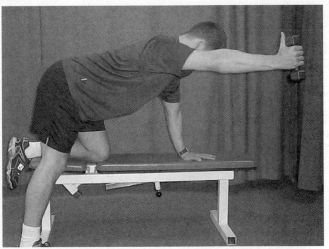

L

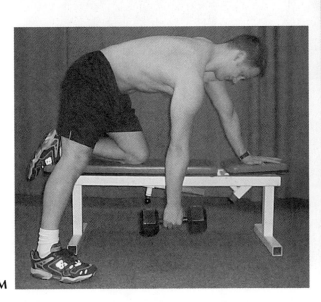

M

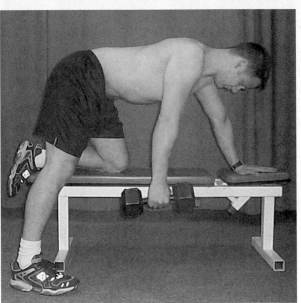

N

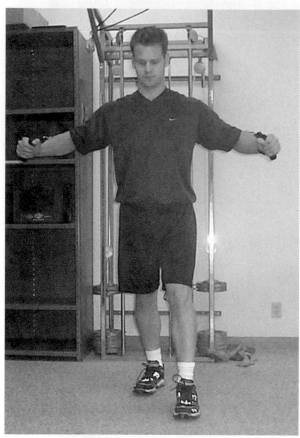

O

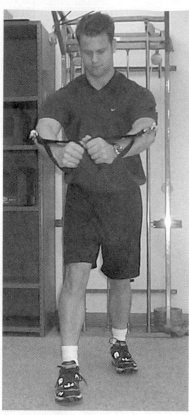

P

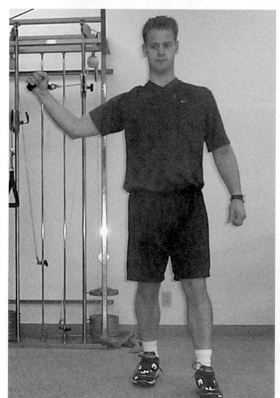

Q

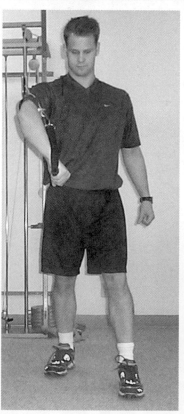

R

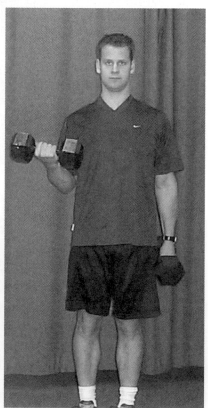

S

Figure B-3, cont'd O, Dynamic hug—beginning. **P,** Dynamic hug—end. **Q,** Diagonal shoulder exercise—beginning. **R,** Diagonal shoulder exercise—end. **S,** Bicep curl.

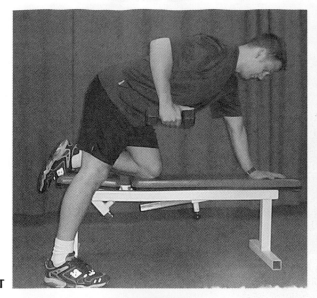

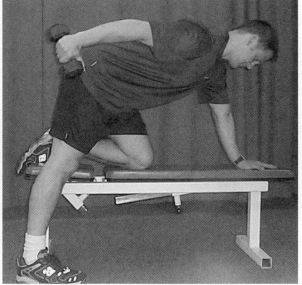

T

U

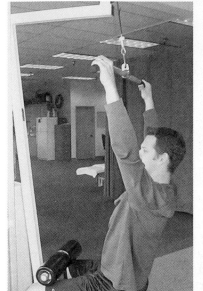

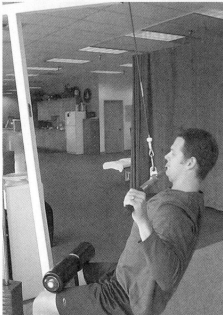

V

W

Figure B-3, cont'd T, Tricep kickback—beginning. **U,** Tricep kickback—end. **V,** Lat pulldown—beginning. **W,** Lat pulldown—end.

(Figure B-6). Following are examples of the hip pulley strengthening exercises.

Neuromuscular Retraining

The athlete will now stand on an unstable base, such as the shuttle balance. The progression from the previous macrocycle will be repeated except with the addition of the shuttle balance. On the basis of the client's ability to progress, increases can be made in the medicine ball weight, the speed at which the ball is tossed, and the reps, or 30 degrees of rapid head rotation can be added. Again, cue the athlete to hold good hip-knee-foot alignment with a 20% contraction of the CORE.

1. Patient will start on the shuttle balance on one leg and hold for 30 seconds (Figure B-7, A).
2. Patient will stand on leg on shuttle balance and toss a 2-lb medicine ball straight up 6″ × 15 reps.
3. Patient will stand on one leg on shuttle balance and toss medicine ball anteriorly into rebounder and catch × 15 reps (Figure B-7, B).
4. Patient will remain on shuttle balance, turn 90 degrees, stand on one leg with the near leg to the rebounder, toss the 2-lb medicine ball, and catch 15 reps.
5. Patient will then repeat this progression while standing on the shuttle balance and add a wobble board, ½ foam roller, or dynadisk between client and shuttle balance (Figure B-7, C).

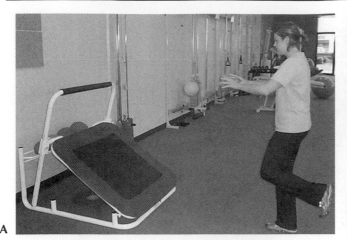

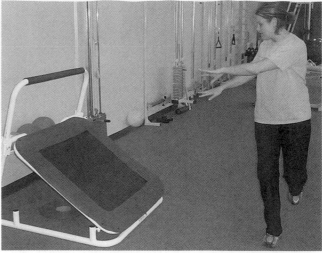

Figure B-4 Medicine ball toss anteriorly (**A**), laterally (**B**), and with unstable base (**C**).

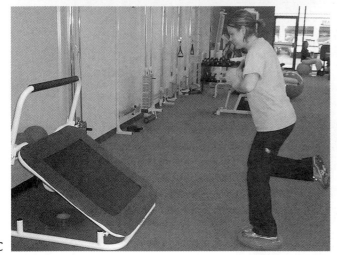

Plyometric Support

This phase is used primarily to help the athlete accommodate landing strategies. As noted in Chapter 14, the objective is to enhance proprioception and kinesthetic awareness during ground contact time. Importantly, even though lacrosse does not involve jumping as a primary component of the sport, the athlete must be able to control rapid deceleration and acceleration forces. These exercises will help her prepare for and control these forces. The athlete will start with 6 to 8 reps of each of the following exercises. She will then work up to 10 reps each. Once she can complete these reps, the therapist can call out different and random positions in which she should freeze. She can also be progressed to single-leg "freezes." She should not do more than 60 to 70 total reps in one training session.

1. Forward (FW) and "freeze"
2. Forward/Back (FW/BK) and "freeze"
3. FW/BK/FW and "freeze"
4. Lateral right (R) and "freeze"
5. Lateral left (L) and "freeze"
6. R/L/R and "freeze"
7. L/R/L and "freeze"
8. Adding a 6-inch box to these patterns represents increases in the complexity and intensity of each exercise.

After the initial 2 weeks of plyometric support training, the athlete can start to use the shuttle sled and dynamic edge. These can be considered plyometric devices that allow the athlete to use a load that is less than his or her body weight. Use these devices in conjunction with the previously described "freezes."

Shuttle Sled

For the shuttle exercise, the athlete uses the appropriate sub-maximal resistance for 3 sets of 10 reps with a 1- to 2-minute rest between sets. Once the athlete can complete the sets with good control for both single (Figure B-8, *A*) and double legs (Figure B-8, *B*), a dynadisk can be added to the foot pad (Figure B-8, *C*). A single-leg pushoff in the quadruped position (Figure B-8, *D*) or a medicine ball toss at the top of the jump can also be added (Figure B-8, *E*).

Dynamic Edge

The dynamic edge is a great way to train lateral movement with control (Figure B-9, *A*). Though M.H.'s feet never leave the ground, there is still an eccentric and concentric contraction. She will also do 3 sets of 10 reps. The resistance will again be submaximal. The athlete can also toss a medicine ball while moving back and forth on the dynamic edge (Figure B-9, *B*).

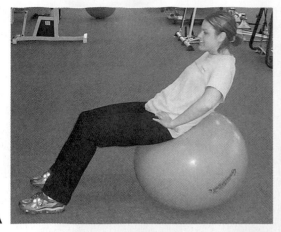
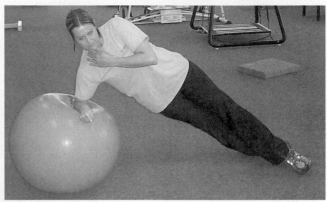
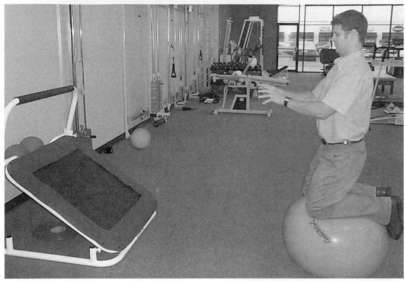

Figure B-5 Therapy ball exercises. **A,** Trunk flexion hold on ball. **B,** Sidebridge on ball. **C,** Kneel with toss on ball.

A bungee cord can be added to help the athlete learn to control valgus forces through the knee (Figure B-9, *C*). Once M.H. has control and good alignment, she will then bring in her lacrosse stick and proceed to catch the ball while moving back and forth. Head rotation will be added to enhance her vestibular ocular reflex.

Aerobic and Anaerobic System Training

Because lacrosse's energy system demands are similar to those of soccer, anaerobic system training will be added to M.H.'s sessions. She will still cross-train on the elliptical trainer, treadmill, and bike. She will begin by training for 21 minutes. She will begin at 50% of her maximum heart rate (MHR) for the first 2 minutes. On the third minute she will increase her heart rate to 80% MHR for a minute and a half. She will then come back down to the intensity where she was at 50% MHR for 2 minutes and then back up to the intensity where she was at 80% MHR. She will repeat this cycle six times. She will be progressed as tolerated through the 5 weeks. On the basis of her tolerance, her times of 50% and 80% MHR may vary within a cycle. She will continue this training three times per week.

Third Macrocycle (4 Weeks)

Goals: Increased muscle power, plyometric performance phase, advanced neuromuscular reeducation exercise, and continued variance of the aerobic and anaerobic systems
Schedule: Mondays/Wednesday/Fridays—Hip and trunk strengthening, aerobic and anaerobic system training, and neuromuscular retraining
Wednesday: Shoulder strengthening
Mondays/Fridays: Plyometric exercises will precede strengthening

Muscle Power

All hip and shoulder strength exercises will be performed for 4 sets × 4 to 6 reps. Initial weight will be set by her 4RM. Multijoint exercises will be performed first, followed by single-joint exercises. Both the concentric and eccentric phases of the exercise will be moved through a 2 count. Between sets there will be a 2-minute rest. After the initial 2 weeks of this macrocycle, the athlete's weight will be dropped by 20% to 30% of her initial 6RM. She will perform 4 sets of 4 to 6 reps at a fast speed (≤1 second each for the concentric and eccentric phases).

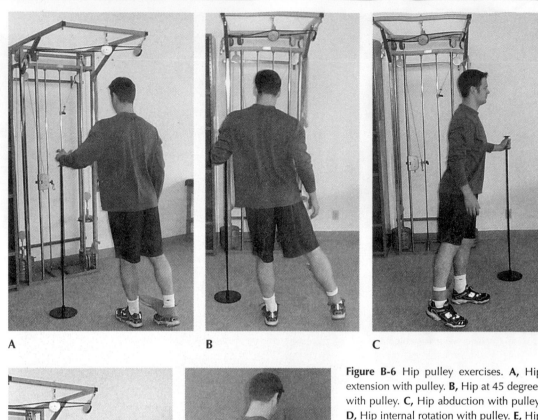

A   B   C

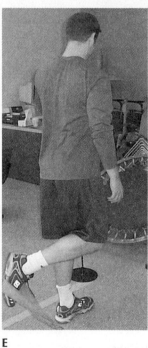

D   E

Figure B-6 Hip pulley exercises. **A,** Hip extension with pulley. **B,** Hip at 45 degrees with pulley. **C,** Hip abduction with pulley. **D,** Hip internal rotation with pulley. **E,** Hip external rotation with pulley.

The CORE exercises will continue with increased holding times and increased intensity with the ball work.

Neuromuscular Retraining

The athlete will continue to work on the shuttle balance but with the addition of jumping onto and off the platform (Figure B-10, *A*). Once M.H. can jump onto and off the platform, she can then jump onto the platform with an unstable base placed on top of it and off the platform onto an unstable base (Figure B-10, *B*). Once this is mastered, the athlete can then attempt

to catch a ball while jumping onto or off the platform with and without an unstable base. Again, an athlete can progress by increasing the medicine ball weight, the speed at which the ball is tossed, and the reps or by adding 30 degrees of rapid head rotation. Cue the athlete for good hip-knee-foot alignment with a 20% contraction of the CORE.

Plyometric Performance Phase

In this phase the athlete will be best prepared for her sport. She may progress up to 200 foot contacts with the following exer-

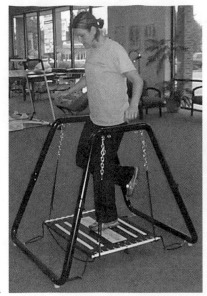
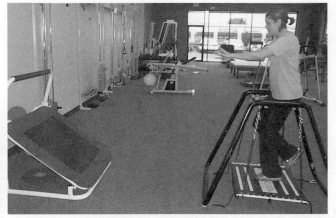
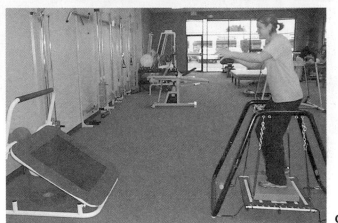

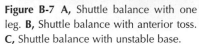

Figure B-7 A, Shuttle balance with one leg. **B,** Shuttle balance with anterior toss. **C,** Shuttle balance with unstable base.

cises. The reader is referred to Chapter 14 for a detailed description and advancement of the exercises.

1. FW/BK jumps and left/right jumps
2. Add diagonals in four-square formations
3. Staggered-ladder formation—progressive locomotive patterns
4. Two-leg-to-one-leg jumps in these patterns

The athlete will continue to use the shuttle sled and dynamic edge as in the previous cycle. The number of sets will increase to four, and the speed of the movements will increase. After the first 2 weeks of this cycle, the vertimax will be added, and this could also replace the shuttle. Figure B-11, *A* shows a picture of the vertimax with the athlete strapped in for double-limb jumping. She can also jump with one leg or jump onto an unstable surface (Figure B-11, *B*).

Aerobic and Anaerobic System Training

The athlete will continue her interval training three times a week for 30 minutes. After she completes her interval training, she will then move through various speed workouts. For example, she may move through the Edgen test (described in Chapter 14).

The athlete's foot needs to pass the lateral cones when shuffling left/right. She will complete this for 6 reps × 2 sets. She may also complete the shuffle test for 6 reps × 2 sets. She will also work on forward/backward sprints for 30 feet each way for 6 reps × 2 sets. Between all sets is a 90-second rest.

In-Season Training

Once the athlete starts her season, she will be working on technique and have sports-specific conditioning through her practices. She will still need to maintain her gains made through the off-season, though. As mentioned in Chapter 7, once the athlete begins the competition phase, the emphasis shifts to maintaining the sport-specific fitness that was developed during the preseason. Although both volume and intensity may be maintained, heavy workouts should immediately follow a competition instead of directly preceding one. During the late season, when the most important competitions are usually held, the athlete should do only a minimum of training or taper gradually by decreasing training volume but maintaining intensity so that he or she is rested without being detrained. For particularly important contests, both training volume and intensity might be decreased to peak for a maximal effort. For example, the day after her competition the athlete's workout may consist of the following:

- Skipping rope × 5 minutes as warm-up
- Plyometric exercises: 200 foot contacts total using standard exercises or shuttle and vertimax edges; double and single leg

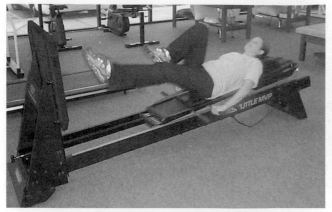

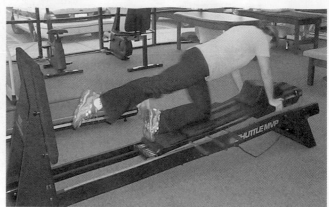

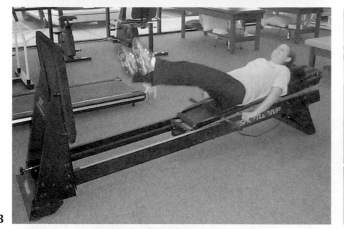

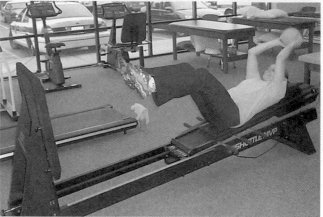

Figure B-8 A, Shuttle with single leg. **B,** Shuttle with double leg. **C,** Shuttle with dynadisk. **D,** Shuttle with quadruped single-leg push. **E,** Shuttle with medicine ball toss at top of jump.

- Hip/shoulder exercises: 8 reps of 8 RM × 3 sets moving up to 12 reps with 2-second concentric/eccentric count and 2-minute rest between sets
- Trunk exercises: advanced holding times with mat and ball work
- Advanced shuttle balance exercises 8 to 12 reps × 3 sets
- 30 minutes of interval training and 6 reps × 3 sets of lateral and forward/backward sprinting

BASEBALL SPORT-SPECIFIC PERFORMANCE TRAINING

The following is an example of a baseball specific performance program for a college center fielder. He will go through the sport-specific evaluation, start on a preseason program, and progress through his in-season workout.

Preseason Phase (12 Weeks) 3 Macrocycles

First Macrocycle (4 Weeks)

Goals: Increase muscle strength, prepare for plyometrics, begin neuromuscular reeducation exercise, and undergo energy system training

Schedule: Mondays/Fridays—Hip, trunk, and shoulder strengthening, neuromuscular reeducation training, and aerobic system training—aerobic

Wednesdays—plyometric preparation

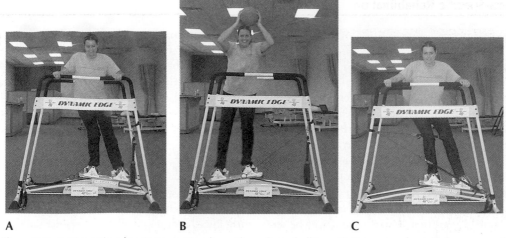

A   B   C

Figure B-9 A, Dynamic edge. **B,** Dynamic edge with medicine ball toss. **C,** Dynamic edge with bungee cord.

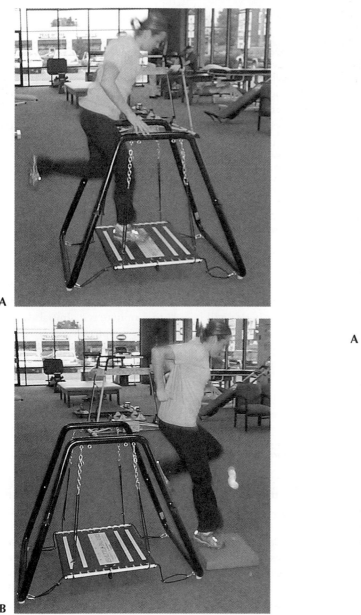

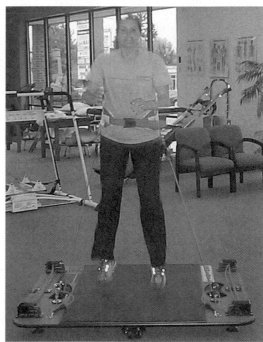

A

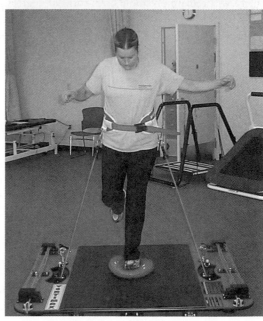

B

Figure B-10 A, Shuttle balance with jump. **B,** Shuttle balance with jump and unstable surface.

Figure B-11 A, Vertimax with double-leg jump. **B,** Vertimax with single-leg jump and unstable base.

Muscle Strength

His upper and lower extremities will be trained both concentrically and eccentrically. His trunk will be trained isometrically. All strength exercises will be performed for 3 sets × 8 to 12 reps (See Figure B-3 for the exercises for strengthening the scapular and glenohumeral rotators. See Figures B-1 and B-2 in preceding case for hip and trunk exercises). Multijoint exercises will be performed first followed by single joint exercises. Both the concentric and eccentric phase of the exercise will be moved through a 2 count. One can emphasize the eccentric component by increasing the amount of time it takes to return the weight to the starting position. Initial weight will be set by his 8RM. Once he can complete 3 sets of 12 reps, his weight will be increased to allow at least 8 reps and he will work up to 12 reps again and repeat. The only exception to this is the trunk exercises, which will be progressed by increasing his holding time. There will be a 2- to 3-minute rest between sets.

Neuromuscular Retraining

The following exercises will be repeated for both legs. The athlete can move through the progression as long as he can complete the activity without a loss of balance. If he loses his balance he must stay at that activity until he can complete it. If he can make it through the progression, increases can be made in the medicine ball weight, the speed at which he tosses the ball, and the reps, or 30 degrees of rapid head rotation can be added. Cue the athlete to hold good hip-knee-foot alignment with a 20% contraction of the CORE.

1. Athlete will start on a stable base on one leg and hold for 30 seconds.
2. Athlete will stand on leg on stable base and toss a 2-lb medicine ball straight up 6″ × 15 reps.
3. Athlete will stand on one leg on stable base and toss medicine ball anteriorly into rebounder and catch × 15 reps (see Figure B-4, A).
4. Athlete will remain on stable base, turn 90 degrees, stand on one leg with the near leg to the rebounder, toss the 2-lb medicine ball, and catch 15 reps (see Figure B-4, B).
5. Athlete will then repeat this progression while standing on a wobble board, ½ foam roller, or dynadisk (see Figure B-4, C).

Plyometric Preparation

The following exercises are used to prepare the body for plyometric training. The key to these exercises is to have good alignment and posture. As stated in Chapter 14, the athlete must first attain the proper alignment and then maintain the proper alignment. The following exercises are from Chapter 14, and the reader can refer to that chapter for further detail.

1. Squat—Hold with proper posture and alignment × 30 seconds.
2. Squatting—Move through a squat motion going into at least 45 degrees of knee flexion while maintaining proper alignment and posture × 8 to 12 reps × 2 sets.

3. Can progress through double-leg squat to single-leg squat × 8 to 12 reps × 2 sets.
4. Forward/backward step-ups × 8 to 12 reps × 2 sets.
5. Lateral step-ups × 8 to 12 reps × 2 sets.

Ideally, by the end of the 4-week period, this athlete will be able to perform a single-leg squat and step-ups with good alignment and posture with added weight for 8 to 12 reps.

Aerobic Base Line Training

The athlete will need a foundation of endurance and overall good aerobic health. He will train three times a week, once on the bike, once on an elliptical trainer, and once on the treadmill. He will have a heart rate monitor and will train at 65% to 70% of his maximal heart rate for at least 20 minutes, working up to 40 minutes. The reader can refer to Chapter 4 for further discussion

Second Macrocycle (4 Weeks)

Goals: Increased muscle size, plyometrics support phase, advanced neuromuscular reeducation exercise, and varied energy system training

Schedule: Mondays/Wednesday/Fridays—Hip, trunk, and shoulder strengthening; aerobic and anaerobic system training; and neuromuscular retraining

Mondays/Fridays—Plyometric support exercises will precede strengthening

Muscle Hypertrophy

All hip and shoulder strength exercises will be performed for 4 sets × 6 to 12 reps. Multijoint exercises will be performed first, followed by single-joint exercises. Both the concentric and eccentric phases of the exercise will be moved through a 2 count. Between sets will be a 1- to 2-minute rest. Initial weight will be set by his 6RM. Once he can complete 4 sets of 12 reps, his weight will be increased to allow at least 6 reps but no more than 12. The CORE exercises will continue with increased holding times and the addition of therapy ball exercises (see Figure B-5). The shoulder exercises will continue without change. The hip exercises will change to pulley exercises (see Figure B-6).

Neuromuscular Retraining

The athlete will now stand on an unstable base, such as the shuttle balance. The progression from the previous macrocycle will be repeated except with the addition of the shuttle balance. On the basis of his ability to progress, increases can be made in the medicine ball weight, the speed at which the ball is tossed, and the reps, or 30 degrees of rapid head rotation can be added. Again, the athlete can be cued to hold good hip-knee-foot alignment with a 20% contraction of the CORE.

1. Athlete will start on the shuttle balance on one leg and hold for 30 seconds (see Figure B-7, A).
2. Athlete will stand on leg on shuttle balance and toss a 2-lb medicine ball straight up 6 inches × 15 reps.

3. Athlete will stand on one leg on shuttle balance and toss medicine ball anteriorly into rebounder and catch × 15 reps (see Figure B-7, *B*).
4. Athlete will remain on shuttle balance, turn 90 degrees, stand on one leg with the near leg to the rebounder, toss the 2-lb medicine ball, and catch 15 reps.
5. Athlete will then repeat the above progression while standing on the shuttle balance and add a wobble board, 1/2 foam roller, or dynadisk between client and shuttle balance (see Figure B-7, *C*).

Plyometric Support

This phase is used primarily to help the athlete accommodate landing strategies. As noted in Chapter 14, the objective is to enhance proprioception and kinesthetic awareness during ground contact time. It is important to note that even though baseball does not involve jumping as a primary component of the sport, the athlete needs to be able to control rapid deceleration and acceleration forces. These exercises will help him prepare for and control these forces. The athlete will start off doing six to eight reps of each of the following exercises. He will then work up to 10 reps each. Once he can complete that the therapist can call out different and random positions to freeze in. He can also be progressed to single-leg "freezes." Keep in mind that he will not being doing more than 60 to 70 total reps in one training session.

1. Forward (FW) and "freeze"
2. Forward/Back (FW/BK) and "freeze"
3. FW/BK/FW and "freeze"
4. Lateral right (R) and "freeze"
5. Lateral left (L) and "freeze"
6. R/L/R and "freeze"
7. L/R/L and "freeze"
8. Adding a 6-inch box to these patterns represents increases in the complexity and intensity of each exercise.

After the initial 2 weeks of plyometric support training the athlete can then start to use the shuttle sled and dynamic edge. These can be considered plyometric devices that allow the athlete to use a load that is less than his body weight. The athlete may continue the "freeze" exercises in addition to the shuttle sled and dynamic edge.

Shuttle Sled

In the shuttle exercise, the athlete uses the appropriate sub-maximal resistance for 3 sets of 10 reps with a 1- to 2-minute rest between sets. Once the athlete can complete the sets with good control for both single (see Figure B-8, *A*) and double legs (see Figure B-8, *B*), a dynadisk can be added to the foot pad (see Figure B-8, *C*). A single-leg push-off can also be added in the quadruped position (see Figure B-8, *D*), or a medicine ball can be tossed at the top of the jump (see Figure B-8, *E*).

Dynamic Edge

The dynamic edge is a great way to train lateral movement with control (see Figure B-9, *A*). Although his feet never leave the ground, there are still eccentric and concentric contrac-

tions. He will also do 3 sets of 10 reps. Resistance will again be submaximal. The athlete can toss a medicine ball while moving back and forth on the dynamic edge (see Figure B-9, *B*). A bungee cord can also be added to help the athlete learn to control valgus forces through the knee (see Figure B-9, *C*). Once he has control and good alignment, the athlete will then bring in his mitt and proceed to catch the ball while moving back and forth. Head rotation will be added to enhance his vestibular ocular reflex.

Aerobic and Anaerobic System Training

Because baseball's energy demands are more anaerobic, anaerobic system training will be added to the athlete's sessions. He will still cross-train on the elliptical trainer, treadmill, and bike. He will begin by training for 21 minutes. He will begin at 60% of his maximum heart rate (MHR) for the first 2 minutes. On the third minute he will increase his heart rate to 80% MHR for a minute and a half. He will then come back down to the intensity where he was at 60% MHR for 2 minutes and then back up to the intensity where he was at 80% MHR. He will repeat this cycle six times. He will be progressed as tolerated through the 5 weeks. On the basis of his tolerance, the amount of time he spends at 60% and 80% MHR may vary within a cycle. He will continue this training three times per week.

Third Macrocycle (4 Weeks)

Goals: Increased muscle power, plyometric performance phase, advanced neuromuscular reeducation exercise, and continue variance of the aerobic and anaerobic systems
Schedule: Mondays/Wednesdays/Fridays—Hip, shoulder, and trunk strengthening; aerobic and anaerobic system training; and neuromuscular retraining
Mondays/Fridays—Plyometric exercises will precede strengthening

Muscle Power

All hip and shoulder strength exercises will be performed for 4 sets × 4 to 6 reps. Initial weight will be set by his 4RM. Multijoint exercises will be performed first, followed by single-joint exercises. Both the concentric and eccentric phases of the exercise will be moved through a 2 count. Between sets will be a 2-minute rest. After the initial 2 weeks of this macrocycle, the athlete's weight will be dropped by 20% to 30% of his initial 4RM. He will perform 4 sets of 4 to 6 reps at a fast speed (≤1 second each for the concentric and eccentric phase). He will stay between 4 and 6 reps. The CORE exercises will continue with increased holding times and increased intensity with the ball work.

Neuromuscular Retraining

The athlete will continue to work on the shuttle balance but with the addition of jumping onto and off the platform (see

Figure B-10, *A*). Once he can jump onto and off the platform, the athlete can then jump onto the platform with an unstable base placed on top of it and off the platform onto an unstable base (see Figure B-10, *B*). Once this is mastered, the athlete can then attempt to catch a ball while jumping onto or off the platform with and without an unstable base. Again, the athlete can progress by increasing the medicine ball weight, the speed at which the ball is tossed, and the reps or by adding 30 degrees of rapid head rotation. The therapist should cue the athlete for good hip-knee-foot alignment with a 20% contraction of the CORE.

Plyometric Performance Phase

In this phase the athlete will be best prepared for his sport. He may progress up to 200 foot contacts with the following exercises. The reader can refer to Chapter 14 for a detailed description and advancement of the exercises.
1. FW/BK jumps and left/right jumps
2. Add diagonals in four-square formations
3. Staggered-ladder formation—progressive locomotive patterns
4. Two-leg-to-one-leg jumps in these patterns

The athlete will continue to use the shuttle sled and dynamic edge as in the previous cycle. The number of sets will increase to four, and the speed of the movements will increase. Addition of the vertimax will occur after the first 2 weeks of this cycle, and this could also replace the shuttle sled. Figure B-11, *A* illustrates the vertimax with the athlete strapped in for double-limb jumping (see Figure B-11, *A*). He can also jump with one leg or jump onto an unstable surface (see Figure B-11, *B*).

Aerobic and Anaerobic System Training

The athlete will continue his interval training three times a week for 30 minutes. After he completes his interval training he will then move through various speed workouts. For example, he may move through the Edgen test (see preceding case) or shuttle run (see Chapter 14).

He will also work on forward sprints for 90 feet each way for 6 reps × 2 sets. A 90-second rest will occur between all sets. The athlete can also catch a baseball with his glove while performing the speed workout.

In-Season Training

Once the athlete starts his season, he will be working on technique and have sports-specific conditioning through his practices. He will still need to maintain his gains made through the off-season, though. As mentioned in Chapter 7, once the athlete begins the competition phase, the emphasis shifts to maintaining the sport-specific fitness that was developed during the preseason. Although both volume and intensity may be maintained, heavy workouts should immediately follow a competition instead of directly preceding one. During the late season, when the most important compe-

titions are usually held, the athlete should do only a minimum of training or taper gradually by decreasing training volume but maintaining intensity so that he is rested without being detrained. For particularly important games, both training volume and intensity might be decreased to peak for a maximal effort.

Because baseball games are played often throughout a week, the workout must be completed at least 48 hours before the next game if possible. For example, the day after one of his games the athlete's workout may consist of the following:
- Skipping rope × 5 minutes as warm-up
- Plyometric exercises: 200 foot contacts total using standard exercises or shuttle sled and vertimax. Double and single leg.
- Hip/shoulder exercises: 8 reps of 8 RM × 3 sets moving up to 12 reps with 2-second concentric/eccentric count and 2-minute rest between sets
- Trunk exercises: advanced holding times with mat and ball work
- Advanced shuttle balance exercises 8 to 12 reps × 3 sets

The athlete should do 30 minutes of interval training and 6 reps × 3 sets of lateral and forward/backward sprinting. This workout should be completed at least once a week.

TENNIS PLAYER WITH ACHILLES TENDON RUPTURE

This case study represents a possible treatment approach for a patient who has had Achilles tendon reconstruction following a complete transverse Achilles tendon rupture.

General Demographics:

K.K. is a 33-year-old Caucasian male who presents in the clinic after right Achilles tendon repair. K.K. currently works in sales and leads an active lifestyle. K.K. is married with two young children younger than the age of 10. He does not smoke and jogs three times per week. He was a competitive athlete while participating in collegiate football.

Medical History

K.K. has no significant medical history to report regarding his general health and right lower extremity.

History of Chief Complaint

K.K. reports attempting to play tennis for the first time in 4 years on March 23, 2004. Approximately 1 hour into the match, he attempted a drop shot, lunged forward, felt a "pop" in his right ankle, and fell forward. On April 1, 2004, K.K. underwent reconstructive surgery of his right Achilles tendon. The tendon was horizontally torn approximately $1\frac{1}{2}$ inches from the calcaneus and was reconstructed using a double-sutured technique.

On the initial evaluation date of April 27, 2004, K.K. ambulates using bilateral axillary crutches and a rocker bottom walking boot to the knee. In accordance with his physician's orders, he can household ambulate without the axillary crutches while wearing the boot. His chief complaints are of right ankle/foot swelling and calf soreness. He reports both of these symptoms are worse in the evening.

Prior Treatment for this Condition

Since surgery, K.K. has had no treatment for his right ankle.

Functional Status and Activity Level

K.K. has limited ambulation secondary to his partial weight-bearing precautions and axillary crutches. He requires assistance with ADLs and limits his community ambulation.

Medications

K.K. is not currently prescribed or taking any medications.

Hypothesis Differential—Pathology/Impairment

Achilles tendon rupture is a traumatic injury due to sport-specific body mechanics. MRI imaging and gross change in calf muscle mass anatomy confirmed Achilles tendon rupture. X-ray imaging was negative for any fractures or dislocations.

Tests and Measures

Joint Integrity and Mobility

Partial weight-bearing precautions for ambulation
Midmalleolar circumference measurements
Right: 31 cm   Left: 28 cm

Rationale

By obtaining a circumferential edema measurement, treatment to the original standard measurements can later be evaluated.

Results

The patient has considerable edema in his right ankle, which is currently limiting his ROM in all directions.

Manual Muscle Testing

Ankle	Right	Left
Dorsiflexion	3+/5	5/5
Plantarflexion	3+/5	5/5
Inversion	5/5	5/5
Eversion	5/5	5/5

Rationale

Assess weakness of the ankle and lower leg.

Results

The patient demonstrated weakness in a pattern that will affect ambulation and ADLs. This weakness is in accordance with the actions of the Achilles tendon/gastrocnemius soleus complex. K.K. does not sense any pain with dorsiflexion or plantar flexion in sitting at the time of initial evaluation.

Pain Scale

K.K. rates his pain as a 4 on a visual analog scale (VAS) of 10 in the evening when the pain is at its worst. He rates his pain at best 0-1/10, in the morning at rest while not bearing weight.

Rationale

Assess the patient's level of impairment as associated with pain.

Results

The patient presents with pain that is consistent with postoperative Achilles tendon repair and resulting edema. His chief complaint is of pain with excessive ambulation with dorsiflexion motion.

Range of Motion

Ankle	Right (Degrees)	Left (Degrees)
Dorsiflexion	−15	20
Plantarflexion	45	50
Subtalar inversion	2	5
Subtalar eversion	2	5

Rationale

The patient's ankle ROM should be assessed as a comparative measure for interventions.

Results

Limited ankle ROM dorsiflexion and plantarflexion are significant for heel-toe gait and ambulation difficulties.

Palpation

K.K. is slightly tender to palpation over the anterior talofibular (ATF) ligament and surgical incision site.

Rationale

The therapist should attempt to correlate painful-to-palpate areas with anatomical causes.

Results

Tenderness correlates to incision healing and possible ATF ligament sprain (unable to test the ATF ligament at this time secondary to edema and pain with inversion—will test when appropriate).

Diagnosis/Impression

The patient's signs and symptoms are consistent with a postoperative Achilles tendon rupture repair.

ICD-9 CM Code: Diagnostic Pattern

4E—Impaired Joint Mobility, Motor Function, Muscle Performance, and ROM associated with Localized Inflammation

4D—Impaired Joint Mobility, Motor Function, Muscle Performance, and ROM associated with Other Connective Tissue Disorders[4]

Physical Therapy Clinical Impression: Prognosis and Plan of Care

The patient presents with ROM and strength deficits of the two crucial ankle motions for proper heel-toe gait mechanics: dorsiflexion and plantarflexion. In terminal stance, normal gait requires at least 10 degrees of ankle dorsiflexion.[12] This patient is impaired significantly in muscle strength of both ankle dorsiflexion and plantarflexion, which will be a focus of the intervention once ROM has improved.

In addition to these impairments, another primary focus for intervention will be to decrease edema in the right ankle. Evidence supports that the inhibition of function due to inflammation is caused by increased pain, swelling, loss of ROM, loss of function, and weakness due to negative motor recruitment.[13] Intervention consists of neuromuscular electrical stimulation and cryotherapy. Neuromuscular electrical stimulation will proceed, and cryotherapy with elevation and compression will conclude therapeutic exercise.

Neuromuscular electrical stimulation has been shown to decrease edema through the use of muscle firing and contraction in order to initiate movement of inflammatory mediators.[14]

Cryotherapy used in conjunction with compression has been proven to decrease the intramuscular tissue temperature cooler and is faster than controls. Compression not only increases the ice contact with the skin and insulates temperature, but it also increases the density of the injured tissue and therefore reduces the amount of time necessary for fluid reabsorption.[12] Elevation allows gravity to aid in the flow of inflammatory fluid toward the direction of the heart via the lymphatic system.

These interventions at the anatomical and tissue levels will predicatively help aid in the athlete's recovery to sport sooner.

Expected Range of Visits

This patient will be treated twice per week for 4 to 6 weeks due to the type of surgical procedure and doctor's recommendations. The entirety of visits will focus on a progression of decreasing edema, increasing ROM, increasing strength and endurance, decreasing pain, and increasing function of the right ankle.

Goals

Short-Term Goal (2 to 3 Weeks)

1. Decrease worst pain to 2/10 on a VAS.
2. Decrease edema of right ankle to 30 cm (malleolar circumference).
3. Increase plantarflexion strength to 4/5 on MMT.
4. Increase dorsiflexion strength to 4/5 on MMT.
5. Increase dorsiflexion ROM to neutral (0 degrees).
6. Increase plantarflexion ROM to 50 degrees.
7. Increase inversion/eversion ROM to within normal limits (5 degrees).

Long-Term Goals (6 to 8 Weeks)

1. Decrease worst pain to 0-1/10 on a VAS.
2. Decrease edema of right ankle to approximately 28 cm (malleolar circumference).
3. Increase plantarflexion strength to 5/5 on MMT.
4. Increase dorsiflexion strength to 5/5 on MMT.
5. Increase dorsiflexion ROM to 20 degrees.
6. Increase plantarflexion ROM to 50 degrees.

Functional Goals (Time Frame to Be Noted)

1. Able to ambulate without axillary crutches, continue with walking boot (two visits).
2. Able to ambulate without walking boot (six visits).
3. Able to jog without pain (6 weeks).
4. Able to return to all sports with decreased risk of reinjury (6 weeks).

Course of Treatment

Treatment was aimed at decreasing edema, increasing ROM, increasing strength and endurance, decreasing pain, and increasing function of the right ankle. Treatment consisted of neuromuscular stimulation to the right plantarflexors, cryotherapy with compression and elevation of the right ankle, and a progressive resistive strengthening and stretching program. A home exercise program consisted of strengthening and passive dorsiflexion stretching. The home exercise program included cryotherapy, dorsiflexion towel stretch in sitting, ankle isometrics in all directions, ankle "ABCs," and aquatic therapy of toe raises on pool step.

During the first week of treatment, biphasic neuromuscular stimulation was applied to the right ankle plantarflexors with

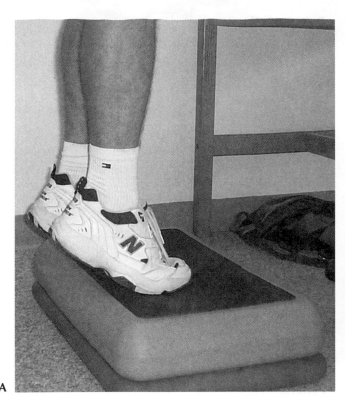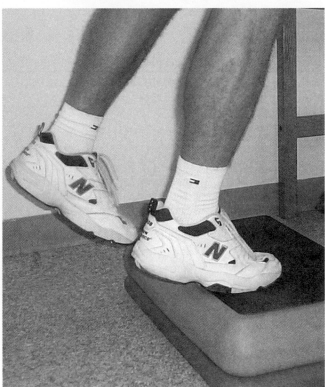

A   B

Figure B-12 A, Eccentric calf loading—beginning. **B,** Eccentric calf loading—end.

active contraction and elevation in supine. After 2 weeks, the patient complained of moderate edema following increased ambulation. Then neuromuscular stimulation was applied to the plantar aspect of the right foot (with the foot elevated in supine) to attempt to decrease the edema. Cryotherapy with compression and elevation, in supine, concluded each treatment session.

The progressive resistive strengthening and stretching program included a 10-minute warm-up on the stationary recumbent bike, followed by the use of the shuttle leg press system. Eccentric strengthening was also integrated secondary to research discussed in Chapter 13. It consisted of a double-leg calf raise and then lowering with just the right calf (Figure B-12). It was progressed as described earlier. The shuttle leg press was used to perform leg press, toe raises, and dorsiflexion stretching (see Figure B-10, *A*). Then the dynamic edge system was progressed for lower extremity strengthening and endurance (see Figure B-9, *A*). Perturbation training was added on a suspended balance board (see Figure B-7, *A*). All of the therapeutic exercises were performed without the use of any ambulatory aids.

All gym exercises were performed for 10 reps of two sets on the first day, and then three sets of 10 the next therapy day. The treatment progressed to three sets of 12 and 15 the subsequent next 2 treatment days. Once three sets of 15 were completed, during the next treatment session the weights were increased by one level of difficulty (i.e., 10 lb). This pattern is due to evidence stating that hypertrophic gains can be seen when training happens between 10 and 15 reps, with three sets being

more effective than one set.[10] In addition, the resistance of the training was increased in order to progress the patient to lifting 60% to 80% of his 1RM and increase strength gains to return to full function.

Reassessment (3 Weeks)

Joint Integrity and Mobility

Patient bears full weight without the use of any ambulatory aids.
Negative anterior talofibular ligament sprain test.
Midmalleolar circumference measurements
Right: 30.5 cm   Left: 28 cm

Manual Muscle Testing

Ankle	Right	Left
Dorsiflexion	4+/5	5/5
Plantarflexion	4/5	5/5
Inversion	5/5	5/5
Eversion	5/5	5/5

Pain Scale

K.K. reports 0/10 pain at all times. He complains of nighttime "stiffness" but no pain associated with this sensation.

Range of Motion

Ankle	Right (Degrees)	Left (Degrees)
Dorsiflexion	−10	20
Plantarflexion	50	50
Subtalar inversion	5	5
Subtalar eversion	5	5

Function

K.K. has been cleared by his physician to return to golf and tennis with caution. He should attempt these activities at approximately 50% of his effort for the sport. He currently can ambulate approximately 30 minutes before he experiences calf fatigue and increasing edema.

Plan

The patient was responding and progressing well to our treatment strategy. K.K.'s right ankle ROM and strength are increasing accordingly. Edema measurements continue to become a problem, due to patient's demand of ambulation for his ADLs. Our plan from this point on will be focused on decreasing edema and to continue strengthening and increasing the range of motion of the right ankle. Application of a compressive ACE wrap to the ankle will aim to reduce edema throughout his daily activities.

Goals/Prognosis Review

Short-term goals have been met. At this time, the long-term and functional goals will remain the same, as the patient is progressing well toward their standards.

Reassessment (7 Weeks)

Joint Integrity and Mobility

Midmalleolar circumference measurements
Right: 29.5 cm   Left: 28 cm
The patient can walk/jog 2½ miles without left ankle
    instability. He also reports playing 18 holes of golf
    yesterday with no symptoms.

Manual Muscle Testing

Ankle	Right	Left
Dorsiflexion	5/5	5/5
Plantarflexion	5/5	5/5
Inversion	5/5	5/5
Eversion	5/5	5/5

Pain Scale

K.K. reports 0/10 pain at all times. He experiences mild "calf weakness" with prolonged ambulation while ambulating longer than 1 hour.

Range of Motion

Ankle	Right (Degrees)	Left (Degrees)
Dorsiflexion	20	20
Plantarflexion	50	50
Subtalar inversion	5	5
Subtalar eversion	5	5

Function

K.K. has returned to sport (e.g., 18 holes of golf, tennis, jogging 2½ miles) with no restrictions. He can ambulate for longer than 1 hour, with only mild calf fatigue. K.K. has returned to complete function for all of his ADLs.

Plan

K.K. has stabilized his right ankle and lower extremity and has safely returned to his sporting activity. He plans to continue the progressive strengthening program at his home gym. Unilateral toe raises on a step have been added to the strengthening program previously established. At the final discharge date of 7 weeks, all long-term and functional goals have been achieved. K.K. has been discharged from physical therapy with the home exercise program. All exercises are to be performed bilaterally and 3 days per week for optimal strength gains and to prevent reinjury in the future.

REFERENCES

1. Powers CM: Patellar kinematics, part I: the influence of vastus muscle activity in subjects with and without patellofemoral pain, *Phys Ther* 80:956-964, 2000.
2. Magee DJ: *Orthopedic physical assessment*, ed 4, Philadelphia, 2002, Saunders.
3. Kendall FP, McCreary EK, Provance PG: *Muscles: testing and function*, ed 4, Philadelphia, 1993, Lippincott Williams & Wilkins.
4. American Physical Therapy Association: *Guide to physical therapist practice*, ed 2, Alexandria, Va, 2001, APTA.
5. Mascal CL, Landel RF, Powers CM: Management of patellofemoral pain targeting hip, pelvis, and trunk muscle function: 2 case reports, *J Orthop Sports Phys Ther* 33(11):642-660, 2003.
6. Powers CM: The influence of altered lower-extremity kinematic on patellofemoral joint dysfunction: a theoretical perspective, *J Orthop Sports Phys Ther* 33(11):639-646, 2003.

7. Morrissey MC, Harman EA, Johnson MJ: Resistance training modes: specificity and effectiveness, *Med Sci Sports Exer* 27(5):648-660, 1995.

8. Bertolucci LE: Introduction of anti-inflammatory drugs by iontophoresis: double blind study, *J Ortho Sports Phys Ther* 4:103-108, 1982.

9. Staron RS, Karapondo DL, Kraemer WJ, et al: Skeletal muscle adaptations during early phase of heavy-resistance training in men and women, *J Appl Physiol* 76(3):1247-1255, 1994.

10. Kraemer WJ, Duncan ND, Volek JS: Resistance training and elite athletes: adaptations and program considerations, *J Ortho Sports Phys Ther* 28(2):110-119, 1998.

11. Sussman C, Bates-Jensen BM: *Wound care: a collaborative practice manual for physical therapists and nurses*, Gaithersburg, Md, 1998, Aspen Publishers.

12. Neumann D: *Kinesiology of the musculoskeletal system foundations for physical rehabilitation*, St Louis, 2002, Mosby.

13. Merrick M, Knight KL, Ingersoll CD, et al: The effects of ice and compression wraps on intramuscular temperatures at various depths, *J Athlet Train* 28(3), 236, 238, 241-245,1993.

14. Baker LL: *Neuro muscular electrical simulation*, ed 4, Downey, Calif, 2000, Los Amigos Research & Education Institute.

Glossary

accommodative foot orthoses - Custom or off-the-shelf–type insert designed to relieve stress and shear to localize areas of the foot.

adenosine triphosphate (ATP) - A molecule composed of a ribose sugar backbone, a nitrogen and carbon chain, adenine, and three phosphate molecules; the primary energy source at rest and during low-intensity exercise.

aerobic glycolysis - The process by which glucose is broken down into pyruvate to generate ATP.

all-or-none principle - When a motor neuron is stimulated, all of the muscle fibers in that motor unit contract to their fullest extent or they do not contract at all.

alveoli - Minute, saclike clusters that make up the lungs and provide the site for gas exchange with pulmonary vessels.

anaerobic threshold - Otherwise known as lactic acid threshold; exercise intensity level (percentage of maximal oxygen consumption), which corresponds to a shift from aerobic to anaerobic pathways as the primary source of energy production; the point at which lactic acid begins to accumulate in muscle.

arteries - Blood vessels that carry blood away from the heart to the periphery.

atria - Receiving chambers of the heart, which receives blood from the periphery and transmits blood to the ventricles.

atrioventricular (AV) node - Region of the right atrium that receives electrical impulses from the sinoatrial node and transmits the impulses to the ventricles via the bundle of His.

atrioventricular (AV) valve - Valve located between the atria and ventricle that prevents the backflow of blood from the ventricles to the atria during ventricular contraction.

autonomic nervous system (ANS) - The central command center of the nervous system, which is responsible for stimulating the sinoatrial and atrioventricular nodes.

beta oxidation - Breakdown of free fatty acid chains into acetyl CoA and hydrogen.

biomechanical foot orthoses - Custom foot inserts fabricated with total contact or posting strategies to influence the foot motion.

bradycardia - A slowed heart rate typically characterized by a heart rate of fewer than 60 beats per minute.

bronchi - Second-generation airways, which terminate in the lungs.

bronchioles - Smaller, third-generation airways branching from the bronchi.

bundle of His - Cardiac muscle located in the septum that transmits electrical impulses from the atrioventricular node in the right atrium to both the right and left ventricles.

capillaries - The smallest blood vessels in the body, which connect the arterial and venous systems and provide the side for exchange of nutrients and waste products.

carbohydrate - Molecule composed of carbon, hydrogen, and oxygen. Carbohydrates are the primary substrates in aerobic glycolysis.

cardiac output (CO) - The volume of blood ejected from the left side of the heart each minute.

central fatigue - The physiological processes that occur within the central nervous system.

central pattern generator - A centrally located control mechanism that produces mainly genetically defined, repetitive actions; analogous to a motor program.

conducting zone - The region of the respiratory system that purifies, humidifies, and transports air to the lower respiratory system; no gas exchange occurs in this region.

contractility - The ability of a muscle to respond to a stimulus by shortening.

coper - Anterior cruciate ligament–deficient patient who has been able to return to high-level sporting activities for a minimum of 1 year and has not experienced knee instability.

CORE - The body's trunk inclusive of hip, pelvis, spine, and abdominal musculature.

cross-bridge cycle - The cyclic events that are necessary for the generation of force or tension within the myosin heads during muscle contraction.

cutaneous (skin) receptors - Sensory receptors located in the skin; provide afferent information to the central nervous system that is processed in conjunction with joint and muscle receptors.

diaphragm - Muscle that separates the abdominal and thoracic cavities and assists with respiration.

diastole - Period of the cardiac cycle characterized by ventricular relaxation, allowing the chambers of the heart to fill with blood.

dynamic joint stability - Ability of a joint to remain stable when subjected to rapidly changing loads it withstands during activities.

excitation-contraction coupling process - The complex signaling process from nerve depolarization to muscle contraction.

efficiency - The proportion of total available energy used to perform work.

ejection fraction - The volume of blood or fraction of end-diastolic volume (EDV) ejected from the heart with each ventricular contraction.

elasticity - The ability of a muscle to return to resting length after being stretched.

electrocardiogram (ECG) - A clinical test that records the electrical activity of the heart.

end diastolic volume (EDV) - The volume of blood in the ventricles at the end of diastole, ventricular relaxation, before ventricular contraction.

end systolic volume (ESV) - The volume of blood in the ventricles at the end of systole, ventricular contraction, before ventricular relaxation.

excitation-contraction coupling - The sequence of events by which an action potential in the sarcolemma initiates the sliding of the myofilaments, resulting in contraction.

expiratory reserve volume - The volume of air that can be expired from the lungs beyond the normal tidal volume (TV) expiration.

extensibility - The ability of a muscle to be stretched or lengthened.

Fartlek training - Endurance training program composed of continuous and interval exercise within one workout by varying training speed with the goal of enhancing aerobic capacity.

fast glycolytic (FG) fibers - Fast-twitch muscle fibers that perform primarily under glycolytic conditions.

fast oxidative glycolytic (FOG) fibers - Fast-twitch muscle fibers that have the ability to work under oxidative and glycolytic conditions.

flexibility - The range of motion in a joint or series of joints that reflects the ability of the musculotendon structures to elongate within the physical limits of the joint.

forefoot valgus - Eversion of the forefoot on the rearfoot with the subtalar joint in neutral position.

forefoot varus - Inversion of the forefoot on the rearfoot with the subtalar joint in neutral position.

Frank-Starling mechanism - The mechanical property of cardiac muscle stating that muscle contraction force is directly proportional to a muscle's length, and therefore contraction force is a function of the stretch of cardiac muscle during diastole.

free nerve endings - Joint receptor activated by high levels of noxious stimuli.

functional profile - Series of kinetic chain tests including balance, balance reach, excursion, lunge, squat, jump, and hopping in multiplanar positions.

functional progression - A series of basic movement patterns graduated according to the difficulty of the skill and an athlete's tolerance. The primary objective of functional progression in rehabilitation is an athlete's timely and safe return to competition. From a prevention standpoint, it is the optimal preparation for the specific demands of a sport.

functional residual capacity - The volume of air remaining in the lungs after a normal exhalation; equivalent to the sum of the expiratory reserve volume (ERV) and residual volume (RV).

Golgi tendon organ (GTO) - Muscle receptor that provides the central nervous system with specific force feedback.

Golgi tendon organ–like receptors - Slowly adapting joint receptor that senses extreme of a joint's normal movement range.

habituation - The negative physiologic adaptations resulting in response to a repetitive training program, creating greater difficulty adjusting to altered physiological demands.

heart rate (HR) - The number of times the heart contracts per minute.

hypertension - Abnormally high blood pressure characterized by systolic blood pressure greater than 140 mm Hg and diastolic blood pressure greater than 90 mm Hg.

hyperventilation - Increased rate and depth of breathing resulting in low levels of blood carbon dioxide.

hypotension - Abnormally low blood pressure characterized by SBP less than 70 mm Hg.

hypoventilation - Decreased rate and depth of breathing resulting in insufficient oxygen delivery to meet the metabolic requirements of the body and high levels of blood carbon dioxide.

in vitro - Study function by simulating various intracellular environments using test tubes.

in vivo - Experiments that use intact tissue and presumably do not disturb the intracellular organization of the fiber.

inspiratory capacity - The maximal volume of air that can be inspired into the lungs; equivalent to tidal volume (TV) plus inspiratory reserve volume (IRV).

inspiratory reserve volume - The volume of air that can be inspired into the lungs above the normal tidal volume (TV)

intermittent or interval training - A type of aerobic training program characterized by periods of high-intensity work interspersed with brief periods of rest.

irritability - The ability of a muscle to receive and respond to stimuli.

joint position sense - The sensation of joint position.

kinesthesia - The sensation of joint movement (both active and passive).

kinetic chain - The interplay and linkage of multiple joints when the body moves in space.

landing strategies - Landing strategies are the next progression from squats and step-ups. In essence, the landing position(s) of the body in low-intensity plyometrics is a partial-squat or what might be considered the "ready" position for an athlete.

lipolysis - The breakdown of fats into glycerol and fatty acid chains.

long, slow distance program (LSD) - Form of continuous exercise that stresses aerobic metabolic energy systems characterized by lower-intensity exercise over a long duration.

long-loop reflexes - Neuronal pathway that transmits sensory information to the brainstem and cerebellum; these reflexes are considered flexible and modifiable with training.

maximal heart rate (MHR) - The maximum number of times the heart can beat in 1 minute and can be used to determine training intensity.

maximal oxygen consumption ($\dot{V}O2max$) - The greatest amount of oxygen consumed per minute at maximum-intensity exercise.

mechanoreceptors - The sensory organs in the neuromuscular system.

metabolic equivalent (MET) - An estimate of the energy expended by the body during physical activity derived from resting energy expenditure.

minute alveolar ventilation - The amount of air capable of participating in gas exchange or the volume of air breathed each minute.

motor program - A set of motor commands that is prestructured at the executive level and that defines the essential details of a skilled action; analogous to a central pattern generator.

motor unit - A motor neuron and the muscle fibers it innervates.

muscle spindle - Low-threshold, slowly adapting muscle receptor that modulates muscle length.

muscle tonus - A state of low-level muscle contraction at rest.

muscles of expiration - Accessory muscles that assist in expelling air from the lungs during exhalation; rectus abdominis, internal oblique, external oblique, transverse abdominis, and internal intercostal muscles.

muscles of inspiration - Accessory muscles that assist in lung expansion during inspiration; external intercostal, sternocleidomastoid, serratus anterior, and scalene muscles.

myofibril - Contractile structures composed of myofilaments.

myofilaments - Contractile (thick and thin) proteins that are responsible for muscle contraction.

neuromuscular control - The subconscious integration of sensory information that is processed by the central nervous system, resulting in controlled movement through coordinated muscle activity.

noncoper - Anterior cruciate ligament–deficient patients who are unable to return to high-level sporting activities secondary to giving way of the knee.

overload principle - The principle governing exercise intensity, which implies that physiological systems must be stressed beyond their typical demand in order to achieve improved performance.

oxidative phosphorylation - The process of ATP formation from aerobic pathways.

oxygen debt - The amount of oxygen necessary to return the body to its normal, homeostatic state following a period of high-demand aerobic exercise.

pace/tempo training - A type of aerobic endurance training program at which the training intensity is just below the anaerobic/lactic acid threshold.

pacinian corpuscle - Rapidly adapting joint receptor that senses joint acceleration and deceleration.

peripheral fatigue - Involves processes associated with mechanical and cellular changes.

perturbation training - Neuromuscular training program that involves maintaining balance on unstable support surfaces; has been proven effective in improving dynamic knee stability in a potential coper population.

pes cavus - High arch foot type inclusive of plantar flexion of the forefoot on the rearfoot.

pes planus - Low arch foot type with low, inclined subtalar joint.

plyometrics - Quick, powerful movements involving prestretching or countermovement that activates the stretch shortening cycle (SSC) of muscle. Ultimately, the purpose of plyometric conditioning is to heighten the excitability of the nervous system for improved reactive ability of the neuromuscular system as a whole. Plyometrics are, in the purist sense, maximal quality efforts.

"plyometric in nature" - Younger (prepubescent and adolescent) athletes and those recovering from injury. Younger athletes may lack the strength base or physical maturity to undergo the rigors of a maximal effort plyometric workout and would benefit by performing lower-intensity exercises designed to improve movement (kinesthetic awareness and body control). Athletes recovering from injury are involved in reestablishing the neural patterns and muscular reactivity that will allow them to perform at a higher level without the risk of reinjury or additional trauma. The nature of these exercises can definitely qualify under the heading of "plyometric in nature."

postural control and dynamic stabilization - Postural control is the ability to attain alignment, whereas dynamic stabilization is the ability to maintain alignment during movement of the body including movements in place and locomotion. Training for postural control and dynamic stabilization will have a direct transfer effect that carries over to jump training, particularly during the amortization phase(s) of each repetition in a jump training set. Importantly, when an athlete can control posture at ground contact, he or she will be able to change direction "quickly and easily," with minimal wasted effort.

postural control - Regulation of the body's position in space for the dual purposes of stability and orientation.

postural orientation - The ability to maintain an appropriate relationship between the body segments and the body and the environment for a task.

postural stability - The ability to control the body's center of mass within specific boundaries.

postural stability (or balance) - The ability to maintain the projected center of mass within the limits of the base of support (referred to as the *stability limits*).

potential coper - Anterior cruciate ligament–deficient patients identified early after injury through a screening process who have the potential to develop dynamic knee stability.

pronation - Triplanar movement of the foot involving closed chain calcaneal eversion, talar adduction, and talar plantar flexion.

proprioception - The afferent information from proprioceptors (e.g., mechanoreceptors) located in the proprioceptive field that contributes to conscious sensations, total posture, and segmental posture.

pulmonary minute volume - The amount of air moved into and out of the lungs in 1 minute.

Purkinje fibers - Cardiac muscle fibers located in the ventricular walls that aid in the rapid transmission of electrical impulses from the atrioventricular node to the ventricles.

resting heart rate (RHR) - The number of times the heart beats per minute at rest; an indictor of fitness level.

rate of perceived exertion (RPE) - A subjective scale that quantifies an individual's level of exertion on the basis of the physical sensations a person experiences during physical activity.

rate pressure product (RPP) - A measure of the consumption of oxygen by myocardial muscle; a function of heart rate times systolic blood pressure.

reciprocal inhibition - The reflex relaxation of the antagonist muscle in response to the contraction of the agonist.

reflex - Rapid, involuntary response to stimuli in which a specific stimulus results in a specific motor response.

repetition maximum (RM) - The number of times an exercise can be performed until fatigue or failure; 1 RM is the amount of resistance that can be performed one time, whereas an 8 RM is the amount of weight that can be performed eight times before.

repetition training - A type of training program characterized by brief, high-intensity intervals, placing a high demand on the anaerobic system.

residual volume - The volume of air that remains in the lungs after a forced, maximal expiration.

respiration - Process of gas exchange that occurs in the alveoli of the lungs.

respiratory zone - The zone of respiratory system where gas exchange takes place.

Ruffini receptor endings - Slowly adapting joint receptors that signal static joint position, intraarticular pressure, and amplitude and velocity of joint rotations.

sarcomere - The functional unit (contractile unit) of muscle fibers.

sarcoplasmic reticulum (SR) - The specialized muscle cell organelle that stores and releases calcium.

semilunar valve - Valve that regulates the flow of blood from the ventricles, situated between the right ventricle and the pulmonary artery and the left ventricle and the aorta.

sinoatrial (SA) node - The heart's pacemaker; region in the right atrial wall that is responsible for the generation of each heartbeat.

skeletal malalignment - Skeletal malalignment inclusive of static deformities present in individual bone segments (e.g., tibial varum) and joint deformities (e.g., genu varus-valgus).

skinned fiber technique - Allows the researcher to put holes in the membrane and directly add ions to the fiber to observe force changes.

sliding filament theory of muscle contraction - The theory that explains muscle contraction as the result of the myofilaments sliding over one another.

slow oxidative (SO) fibers - Slow-twitch muscle fibers that rely primarily on oxidative metabolism to produce energy.

specific adaptation to imposed demands (SAID) principle - Adaptations resulting from a training program are specific to the energy system and muscles used or stressed during a specific activity.

spinal reflexes - Shortest of neuronal pathways; responses are typically uniform in nature and modified by the intensity of the afferent signals but are not considered modifiable by training.

steady-state - A physiologic state in which oxygen demand is equivalent to oxygen consumption.

stroke volume (SV) - The volume of blood ejected from the ventricles with each heartbeat.

supination - Triplanar motion of the foot including calcaneal inversion, talar adduction, and talar dorsiflexion.

systole - The period of the cardiac cycle characterized by ventricular contraction.

tachycardia - A rapid heart rate typically characterized by a heart rate of greater than 100 beats per minute.

task dependency - Mechanisms involved in limiting performance of an activity secondary to fatigue.

tidal volume - The amount of air inspired or expired in a normal breath at rest.

total lung capacity - The volume of air in the lungs after a maximal inspiration; equal to the sum total of tidal volume (TV), inspiratory reserve volume (IRV), expiratory reserve volume (ERV), and residual volume (RV).

total peripheral resistance - The amount of resistance to blood flow, which is a function of blood pressure and cardiac output.

trachea - The largest airway opening of the respiratory system.

transverse tubules (T tubules) - Organelles that carry the electrical signal from the sarcolemma into the interior of the cell.

triglycerides - Molecules composed of one glycerol molecule and three fatty acid chains.

triggered reactions - Longest of neuronal pathways; sensory information is processed at the cortical level of the brain and represents preprogrammed reactions; triggered reactions occur slightly quicker than voluntary reactions but may be unable to accommodate to circumstances in atypical situations.

Valsalva maneuver - A forceful exhalation against a closed airway that increases pressure in the thoracic cavity and results in decreased venous return.

valves - Muscular flaps between the chambers of the heart that function to control the volume of blood ejected from the heart and prevent the backflow of blood with each contraction.

variation - A concept of training program design that provides exposure to varied physiological demands to minimize habituation.

veins - Thinner-walled blood vessels that return blood to the heart from the periphery.

ventilation - The dynamic, time-dependent process involving the mechanical movement of air into and out of the lungs.

ventricle - The pumping chamber of the heart that receives blood from the atria and pumps blood to either the aorta or pulmonary artery.

vital capacity - The volume of air exhaled during a forced exhalation following a maximal inspiration; the sum of the inspiratory reserve volume (IRV), tidal volume (TV), and expiratory reserve volume (ERV).

voluntary reactions - Longest of neuronal pathways; sensory information is processed at the cortical level of the brain and involves the processing of multiple variables; however, responses are highly flexible.

Index

Numbers

1 RM (one repetition at maximum effort), 72, 208, 208t, 223-224, 225-226
4-square jump patterns, 240-242, 241f
4-square vs. triangle patterns, 235-236, 236t
8-to-10 repetition maximum, 208
12-minute walk/run test, 70

A

A bands, 18-19
Abdominal bracing, 206, 206f, 206t
Abdominal drawing-in stability, 204
Abilities, sensory-motor, 265t-266t
Absorbed energy at failure, 3, 3f
Acetyl-CoA, 91-92
ACLs (anterior cruciate ligaments), 1, 6-10, 98, 251-254
Acromioclavicular joints, 175-192. See also Glenohumeral, acromioclavicular, and scapulothoracic joint evaluations.
Action potential. See AP (action potential).
Action types, muscle strengthening, 226-229. See also Strength training concepts.
  concentric, 227-228
  DOMS and, 227
  eccentric, 226-227
  isometric, 228
  repeated bout effect and, 227
  SAID and, 227. See also SAID (specific adaptations to imposed demands) principle.
  stretch-shorten cycles and, 227

Active rest, 106
Active straight leg raise test. See ASLR (active straight leg raise test).
Activity energy expenditure. See AEE (activity energy expenditure).
Activity levels and factors, 280, 280t-281t
Acute changes, aerobic metabolism, 69-73, 69f-71f. See also Aerobic metabolism.
Adaptation, 73-74, 108-112, 224-266, 269-273
  environment creation, 269-273, 269f, 270t-271t, 272f
  long-term, 73-74
  vs. maladaptation, 108-112, 109f
  muscle, 224-226. See also Strength training concepts.
    aging changes and, 226
    contractile, 224-225
    exercise variables and, 225-226
    hypertrophy vs. hyperplasia, 224-225
    muscle changes and, 226
    muscle fiber type specific adaptations, 225
    neural, 224
Additions, carbohydrate vs. protein, 284-285
Adenosine diphosphate. See ADP (adenosine diphosphate).
Adenosine triphosphate. See ATP (adenosine triphosphate).
Adenosine triphosphate-creatine phosphate system. See ATP-CP (adenosine triphosphate-creatine phosphate) system.
Adenosine triphosphate-phosphocreatine system. See ATP-PC (adenosine triphosphate-phosphocreatine) system.

ADP (adenosine diphosphate), 91
AEE (activity energy expenditure), 279-280, 280t
Aerobic metabolism, 65-86
  acute changes in, 69-73, 69f-71f
    aerobic capacity and, 70-71
    central mechanisms and, 70-72, 70f-71f
    CO and, 71-72
    CV and, 69-70
    ejection fraction and, 71
    exercise intensity classification and, 71f
    maximal oxygen consumption and, 69-72, 69f
    MHR and, 70-71
    respiratory system and, 72-73
    Valsalva maneuver and, 71
    vasoconstriction vs. vasodilation, 72
  age- and sex-related considerations for, 74-76, 81-83
    children, 74-75, 81-82
    early development changes, 74-75
    males vs. females, 76
    older adults, 75-76, 82-83
  ATP and, 66-72
  BP and, 66-68
  CV anatomy and physiology, 65-66
    ANS, 66
    aortic valves, 66
    AV valves, 65-66
    heart, 65-67
    HR, 66-67
    pulmonary semilunar valves, 66
    RHR, 66-67
    SA nodes, 66
    work rate, 66-67
  EGCs and, 66
  evidenced-based clinical applications, 66-67, 70-71, 74, 78-80, 82

Note: Entries followed by *b* indicate boxes, *f* figures, *t* tables.

335

Aerobic metabolism (*continued*)
  exercise program design, 76-83
    aerobic periods and, 77
    continuous training and, 80
    conversion exercise, 77
    cool down and, 77
    dehydration and, 79
    endurance and, 76
    endurance programs and, 77-80
    exercise intensity and, 80-81
    exercise prescription principles,
      76-77
    Fartlek training and, 80
    frequency and, 80
    habituation and, 77
    heat illness and, 78
    intermittent/interval training and,
      79-80
    long slow distance programs and,
      77
    modes and, 81
    overloading and, 76-77. *See also*
      Overloading.
    pace/tempo programs and, 78-79
    program components and, 77
    repetition training and, 80
    SAID principle and, 76-77. *See also*
      SAID (specific adaptations
      to imposed demands)
      principle.
    stretch and, 77
    threshold training and, 78-79
    variables of, 80-81
    warm-ups and, 77
    work periods and, 77
  long-term adaptations of, 73-74
  processes of, 68-69, 68f-69f
  rehabilitation roles of, 65, 83
  respiratory anatomy and physiology,
    67-68
    anaerobic threshold, 68
    hypoventilation *vs.*
      hyperventilation, 67
    lung volumes, 67
    respiration, 67
    respiratory bronchioles, 67
    ventilation, 67-68
Age-related considerations, 74-76, 81-
  83, 226
Agility, 211, 212t, 253
  drills, 253
  testing, 211, 212t
Aids, ergogenic, 288. *See also* Ergogenic
  aids; Nutrition-related
  considerations.
Alactic anaerobic phosphocreatine
  production, 41-42

Alactic anaerobic systems, 40
All-or-none principle, 25
Altered neuromuscular control, 247
American College of Sports Medicine,
  79, 208, 285
American Dietetics Associations, 79
American Physical Therapy Association.
  See ATPA (American Physical
  Therapy Association).
Amino acids, essential. *See* EAAs
  (essential amino acids).
Anabolic hormones, 225
Anabolic steroids, 225
Anaerobic glycolysis. *See* LA (anaerobic
  glycolysis).
Anaerobic metabolism, 39-64
  anaerobic threshold, 68
  ATP and, 39-60
  ATP-PC system and, 39-60
  of children, 55-58, 56f
  energy continuum, 39-41, 40f-41f
  energy production and, 41-45,
    43f-44f
    alactic anaerobic phosphocreatine
      production, 41-42
    creatine and, 42-45
    ergogenic aids and, 42. *See also*
      Ergogenic aids.
    lactate clearance, 44-45, 44f
    lactic acid and lactate production,
      42-44, 44f
    turnover, 42-43
  evidenced-based clinical applications
    for, 42
  exercise response and, 45-55,
    47f-51f, 47t, 52t, 54f-55f
    anaerobic threshold, 50-52
    dynamic resistance exercise, 52
    energy power and capacity, 46-47,
      47t
    EPOC, 45-46, 45f
    incremental exercise to maximum,
      50-52, 50f-51f
    lactate changes, 47-48, 48f-49f,
      52-53, 52t
    lactate removal time frames,
      53-55, 54f-55f
    lactate threshold, 50-52
    MAOD, 46
    MLSS workload and intensity, 49
    oxygen deficit, 45-46, 45f
    pain, 53
    performance decrement, 53
    power and capacity tests, 55
    research trends for, 51
    submaximal exercise, moderate-to-
      heavy, 49

    submaximal exercise, short-and-long
      term low-intensity, 48-49
    supramaximal exercise, short-term
      high-intensity, 48
    ventilatory threshold, 50-52
    WAT, 55-57
  LA, 40-60
    of males *vs.* females, 58-59, 60f
    maximal oxygen uptake and, 40-60
    of older adults, 59-60
    rehabilitation roles of, 39
    time-continuum, 41
Anaerobiosis, 50. *See also* Anaerobic
  metabolism.
Anatomy and physiology, 65-68, 135-144
  of CORE, 134-144
  of CV system, 65-66
  of respiratory system, 67-68
Annulospiral neurons, 32
ANS (autonomic nervous system), 66
Anterior cruciate ligaments. *See* ACLs
  (anterior cruciate ligaments).
Anteversion, femoral, 155
Aortic valves, 66
AP (action potential), 16-24
Applications, 223-232, 233-234, 267-
  269, 267f-268f
  of dimensional model of MT (manual
    therapy), 267-269, 267f-268f
  for functional progressions, 233-234
  for strength training, 223-232
Architecture, 2-3, 2f, 17
  ligament, 2-3, 2f
  muscle, 17
ASLR (active straight leg raise test),
  204, 205f, 206t
Athlete's heart, 74
Athlete-specific rehabilitation topics.
  See also under individual topics.
  case collections and reviews, 293-314
    differential diagnoses (orthopedic-
      specific), 295-302
    surgical considerations, 303-314
  CORE evaluations, 175-222
    glenohumoral, acromioclavicular,
      and scapulothoracic joints,
      175-192
    trunk and hip CORE, 193-222
  muscle fatigue, muscle damage, and
    overtraining, 87-121
    detraining and overtraining
      (physiological effects),
      105-121
    muscle fatigue, 87-96. *See also*
      Fatigue, muscle.
    overuse injury and muscle damage,
      97-109

muscle physiology (exercise prescription foundations), 15-85
  aerobic metabolism, 65-86
  anaerobic metabolism, 39-64
  muscle contraction, 15-38
  nutrition-related considerations, 279-292
  orthopedic-specific differential diagnoses, 295-302
  pathophysiology (overuse injury) concepts, 123-174
    CORE anatomy and physiology, 135-144
    CORE-to-floor interrelationships, 145-174
    overhead-throwing athletes, 123-134
  physiological basis (sport-specific exercise), 223-278
  physiological foundations (sport-specific exercise), 223-278
  MT, 259-278
  neuromuscular training, 247-258
  plyometrics, 233-246
  strength training concepts, 223-232
  soft tissues (ligaments and tendons) basic science concepts, 1-14
ATP (adenosine triphosphate), 15, 20-25, 24f, 39-72, 225
ATPA (American Physical Therapy Association), 194
ATP-CP (adenosine triphosphate-creatine phosphate) system, 91
ATP-PC (adenosine triphosphate-phosphocreatine) system, 39-60
Atrioventricular valves. See AV (atrioventricular) valves.
Autonomic nervous system. See ANS (autonomic nervous system).
AV (atrioventricular) valves, 65-66

B

Back extensor endurance test, 206, 206f, 206t
Backward overhead medicine ball toss, 210-211
Balance, 126b, 211-215, 213, 214f, 214t, 266t
  testing and evaluations, 211-215, 214f, 214t
  training, 126b, 266t
  triad, 213
Balance Master (Neurocom), 214
Base of support. See BOS (base of support).

Baseball pitcher case example, 295-296
Basic positions, plyometrics, 238. See also Plyometrics.
Basic science concepts, 1-14. See also Soft tissues (ligaments and tendons) basic science concepts.
Basketball player case example, 300
BCAAs (branched chain amino acids, 111-112
Bicycle ergometers, 70f
Biochemical composition, 2-3, 2f
Biodex isokinetic dynamometers, 178t
Biomechanics, 3-4, 3f-4f, 250
Bioscaffolds, 10
Bird dog test, 205t-206t
Blood pressure. See BP (blood pressure).
Bodybuilding poses, 16f
Bone-ligament-bone complex, 3, 3f
Borg (RPE) Rate of Perceived Exertion Scale, 71f, 81
BOS (base of support), 238-239
Bottom up kinetic chain, 147-151
BP (blood pressure), 66-68
Branched chain amino acids. See BCAAs (branched chain amino acids).
Bridging test with knee extended, 205
Bronchioles, 67
By-products, metabolic, 92

C

Caffeine, 288
Calculated one repetition maximum, 208-209
Capacity tests, 55
Carbohydrate intake needs, 281-285. See also Nutrition-related considerations.
  carbohydrate loading and, 281-282
  carbohydrate roles and, 281-282
  exercise needs and, 282-283
  gylcemic index and, 282-283
  muscle glycogen and, 282-283
    resting values of, 282
    synthesis of, 283
  postexercise needs and, 283-284
  preexercise needs and, 282
  protein additions and, 283-284, 284-285. See also Protein intake needs.
Cardiac output. See CO (cardiac output).
Cardiovascular system. See CV (cardiovascular) system.
Care plans, plyometrics, 233
Case collections and reviews, 293-314. See also under individual topics.

differential diagnoses (orthopedic-specific), 295-302
surgical considerations, 303-314
Cavus foot orthosis. See CFO (cavus foot orthosis).
Cell therapy, 10
Cells/fibers, muscle, 17-18, 19f, 19t, 25-29, 26f-29f, 27t
Central balance processors, 213
Central fatigue, 92-94. See also Fatigue, muscle.
  EMG and, 93
  iEMG and, 93
  MVC and, 92
  vs. peripheral fatigue, 93. See also Peripheral fatigue.
Central mechanisms, aerobic metabolism, 70-72, 70f-71f. See also Aerobic metabolism.
Central nervous system. See CNS (central nervous system).
Centralization phenomenon, 196, 198t
CFO (cavus foot orthosis), 163
Children, 55-58, 56f, 74-75, 81-82, 100
  aerobic metabolism and, 74-75, 81-82
  anaerobic metabolism and, 55-58, 56f
  muscle damage and overuse injury in, 100
Cisterns, 18
Clearance, lactate, 44-45, 44f
Closed chain exercise, 161
CNS (central nervous system), 248-249
CO (cardiac output), 71-72
Co-contraction, 224, 253, 255t, 265t-266t
Coiled coils, 20
Collagen fiber bundles, 2-3, 2f
Collections and reviews (cases), 293-314. See also under individual topics.
  differential diagnoses (orthopedic-specific), 295-302
  surgical considerations, 303-314
Competative cycles, 107f, 108
Composite abilities, 264f, 265
Compression, 201, 201f
Computer-assisted digital video, 194
Concentric strengthening, 227-228
Conservative treatment vs. repair, 7-8
Continuous training, 80
Contractile adaptations, 15, 224-225
Contractile properties, 25-26
Contractility, 16

Contraction abilities, 264f, 265
Contraction, muscle, 15-38. *See also*
    Muscle contraction.
  evidenced-based clinical applications
      for, 36-37
  maximal oxygen uptake and, 37
  movement, muscular aspects of,
      15-29, 16f-29f, 19t, 27t
    all-or-none principle, 25
    AP, 16-24
    architectural organization, 17
    athlete-specific considerations, 29
    cisterns, 18
    contractile (twitch) properties,
      25-26
    contractility, 16
    contraction processes, 20-25,
      21f-25f
    cross-innervation, 26, 26f
    definition, 16f
    elasticity, 16
    endomysium, 17
    excitation-contraction coupling,
      21-22
    extensibility, 16
    extrafusal fibers and, 15
    fascia, 17
    fasciculi, 17, 18f
    hypertrophy, 16f
    integrated nomenclature, 26-28
    irritability, 16
    lateral sacs, 18
    macroscopic structures, 16-17,
      17f
    metabolic properties, 26
    muscle fibers/cells, 17-18,
      19f, 19t
    muscle tissue functions and
      characteristics, 15-16
    myofibrils and myofilaments,
      18-20, 19f-20f, 19t
    perimysium, 17
    sacromeres, 18-20, 24-25, 25f
    sarcolemma, 17-18
    skeletal muscle and, 15-17, 17f
    sliding filament theory, 21
    SR, 18, 19t
    straited muscles, 15
    T tubules, 18-22, 19t
    voluntary muscles, 15
  movement, neural control of
    flexibility and ROM, 35-36, 36b
    GTOs, 34-35, 34f-35f
    inverse myotatic reflex, 34-35, 35f
    nerve supply, 29-30, 30f
    neuromuscular junction, 30-31,
      30f-31f

    NMS, 31-34, 32f-34f
    plyometrics and, 34. *See also*
      Plyometrics.
    reflex control, 31-35, 32f-35f
    stretch reflex, 31
Controlled mobilization, passive, 8
Conversion exercise, 77
Cool down, 77, 106
Cooper 12-minute walk/run test, 70
Cooperative Extension guidelines,
    ergogenic aids, 287
Coordination, 266t
Copers *vs.* non-copers, 251-252, 251t
CORE concepts. *See also under individual*
    topics.
  anatomy and physiology, 135-144
  CORE-to-floor interrelationships,
    145-174
    closed chain exercise, 161
    dynamic assessments, 159-161
    evidenced-based clinical
      applications for, 146-149,
      157, 160-161, 163, 166
    foot mechanics, 159-161
    foot orthotic strategies, 161-167,
      162f-167f
    gait analyses, 159-161
    knee-foot-ankle, 145-147, 146f
    lower extremity linkage system,
      147-155, 148f-155f
    rehabilitation roles for, 145
    research trends in, 168-169
    structural malalignments, 155-159
  evaluations, 175-222
    glenohumoral, acromioclavicular,
      and scapulothoracic joints,
      175-192
    trunk and hip CORE, 193-222
Corticotrophin-releasing hormone. *See*
    CRH (corticotrophin-releasing
    hormone).
Countermovement vertical jump
    testing, 210, 210t
CP (creatinephosphate), 41
Craig's test, 207-208, 208f
Creatine, 42-45, 288
Creatinephosphate. *See* CP
    (creatinephosphate).
CRH (corticotrophin-releasing
    hormone), 112
Cross-bridging cycles, 22-24
Cross-innervation, 26, 26f
Cubes isokinetic dynamometers, 178t
Cutaneous receptors, 248
CV (cardiovascular) system, 65-70
Cycle ergometer tests, 70, 209-210
Cycles, stretch-shorten, 227

D

Damage, muscle. *See* Muscle damage
    and overuse injury.
DBP (diastolic blood pressure), 66
Decreased neuromuscular control, 247
Decrement, performance, 53
Definition, muscle, 16f
Degrees of freedom problem, 250
Dehydration, 79
Delayed-onset muscle soreness. *See*
    DOMS (delayed-onset muscle
    soreness).
Dependency, task, 93
Depth jumping, 34. *See also*
    Plyometrics.
Detraining and overtraining
    (physiological effects), 105-121.
    See also Muscle fatigue, muscle
    damage, and overtraining.
  adaptation *vs.* maladaptation,
    108-112, 109f
    mechanisms of, 109-110, 110t
    metabolism alterations, 110-111
    muscle trauma and injury, 112
    OR and, 108-109
    sympathetic *vs.* parasympathetic
      forms, 109
    UPS, 109
  detraining, 116-118, 117f
  exercise training, 105-108, 107f-108f
    cool down, 106
    individualization and, 106
    maintenance and, 106
    overload and, 105-106
    periodization and, 106-108
    principles of, 105-106
    progression and, 106
    rest/recovery/adaptation and, 106
    retrogression/plateau/reversibility
      and, 106
    SAID principle and, 105. *See also*
      SAID (specific adaptations
      to imposed demands)
      principle.
    steploading and, 106
    training plans, 107f
    warm-ups, 106
  monitoring and training logs,
    112-113
  prevention and treatment of,
    113-116
Developmental cycles, 106-107, 107f
Diagnoses (differential). *See* Differential
    diagnoses (orthopedic-specific).
Diastolic blood pressure. *See* DBP
    (diastolic blood pressure).

Dietitians of Canada, 79
Differential diagnoses (orthopedic-specific), 295-302
case examples for, 295-300
case 1 (baseball pitcher), 295-296
case 2 (recreational fisher), 296-297
case 3 (professional football player), 297-298
case 4 (tennis player), 298
case 5 (pole vaulter), 298-299
case 6 (long distance runner), 299-300
case 7 (basketball player), 300
dispositions, 296-300
follow-up evaluations, 300-301
orthopedic medical histories, 295-300
physical examinations, 295-300
plans, 296-300
Dimensional model of MT (manual therapy), 260-269, 260f, 262f, 264f, 265t-266t, 267f-268f. See also MT (manual therapy).
clinical examples for, 261, 270t-271t
early remodeling phase, 268f
fluid flow characteristic, 263
inflammatory/regeneration phase, 268f
intension and, 268-269
length adaptation characteristic, 263
manual neuromuscular re-abilitation and, 263, 265t-266t
mature remodeling phase, 268f
motor abilities complexity hierarchy and, 264, 264f
neurological dimension, 260-261, 260f, 263-266, 264f, 265t-266t, 268f
objectives of, 262, 262f
outcomes of, 260f
practical applications of, 267-269, 267f-268f
psychological dimension, 260f, 261, 267-269, 267f-268f
repair characteristic, 262-263
sensory-motor abilities, 265t-266t
signals/stimuli, 260f, 262-269, 264f, 265t-266t, 267f-268f
similarity principle and, 263
tissue dimension, 260, 260f, 262-263, 268f
Dispositions, 296-300. See also Differential diagnoses (orthopedic-specific).
Distraction test, 199, 201t
DOMS (delayed-onset muscle soreness), 97-98, 101, 227
Drop-jump screening tests, 194
Dynamic assessments, 159-161

Dynamic balance, 250
Dynamic joint stability, 247-248
Dynamic position sense, 266t
Dynamic resistance exercise, 52
Dynamic stabilization vs. static stabilization, 265t-266t
Dynamic valgus, 252-253, 263f
Dynamometers, isokinetic, 178t
Dysfunctional neuromuscular control, 247

E
EAAs (essential amino acids), 285
Early development changes, 74-75
Early phase, perturbation training, 255t
Early remodeling phase, 268f
E-C (excitation-contraction) coupling processes, 21-22, 89
Eccentric strengthening, 226-227
ECM (extracellular matrix), 2-3
EDV (end diastolic volume), 70-71
Efferent system (motor pathway)-sensory pathway interactions, 247-248
EGCs (electrocardiograms), 66
EIMD (exercise-induced muscle damage), 99
Ejection fraction, 71
Elasticity, 16
Electrocardiograms. See EGCs (electrocardiograms).
Electromyography. See EMG (electromyography).
Elongation, ultimate, 3, 3f
EMG (electromyography), 93, 250
Empty Can Testing position, 176
End diastolic volume. See EDV (end diastolic volume).
End systolic volume. See ESV (end systolic volume).
Endings, spray, 248
Endomysium, 17
Endurance-related considerations, 76, 77-80, 285
Energy, 3-4, 3f, 39-45, 40f-44f, 46-47, 47t, 68f, 279-280
absorbed, 3, 3f
continuum, 39-41, 40f-41f
density parameter, 3-4, 3f
needs, 279-280. See also Nutrition-related considerations.
activity levels and factors for, 280, 280t-281t
AEE and, 279-280, 280t
calculations for, 279-280, 280t
components of, 279

exercise intensity and, 281t
meeting of, 279-280, 280t
REE and, 279-280, 280t
TEF and, 279
power and capacity, 46-47, 47t
production, 41-45, 43f-44f
alactic anaerobic phosphocreatine production, 41-42
creatine and, 42-45
ergogenic aids and, 42
lactate clearance, 44-45, 44f
lactic acid and lactate production, 42-44, 44f
turnover, 42-43
stores, 68f
Enlarged heart, 74
Environment creation, repair and adaptation, 269-273, 269f 270t-271t, 272f
EPOC (excessive postexercise oxygen consumption), 45-46, 45f
Ergogenic aids, 43, 287-288. See also Nutrition-related considerations.
caffeine, 288
creatine, 288
energy production and, 42
evaluation guidelines for, 287-288
roles of, 287
Ergometers, bicycle, 70f
ERV (expiratory reserve volume), 67
Essential amino acids. See EAAs (essential amino acids).
ESV (end systolic volume), 70-71
Etiology, muscle damage and overuse injury, 97-99
Evaluations. See also under individual topics.
CORE, 175-222
glenohumoral, acromioclavicular, and scapulothoracic joints, 175-192
trunk and hip CORE, 193-222
of ergogenic aids, 287-288
of muscle damage and overuse injury, 99
Examinations, physical, 296-300. See also Differential diagnoses (orthopedic-specific).
Excessive postexercise oxygen consumption. See EPOC (excessive postexercise oxygen consumption).
Excessively supining foot, 165
Excitation-contraction coupling processes. See E-C (excitation-contraction) coupling processes.

Exercise intensity, 71f, 80-81, 281t. *See also* Intensity.
Exercise prescription foundations (muscle physiology), 15-121. *See also under individual topics.*
  aerobic metabolism, 65-86
  anaerobic metabolism, 39-64
  muscle contraction, 15-38
  muscle fatigue, muscle damage, and overtraining fundamentals, 87-96
  overuse injury, 97-104
  physiological effects (overtraining and detraining), 105-121
Exercise program design, 76-83
Exercise response, 45-55, 47f-51f, 47t, 52t, 54f-55f
  anaerobic power and capacity tests, 55
  anaerobic threshold, 50-52
  dynamic resistance exercise, 52
  energy power and capacity, 46-47, 47t
  incremental exercise to maximum, 50-52, 50f-51f
  lactate, 47-55
    changes, 47-48, 48f-49f, 52-53, 52t
    removal time frames, 53-55, 54f-55f
    threshold, 50-52
  MAOD, 46
  MLSS workload and intensity, 49
  oxygen deficit, 45-46, 45f
  pain, 53
  performance decrement, 53
  research trends for, 51
  submaximal exercise, 48-49
    moderate-to-heavy, 49
    short-and-long term low-intensity, 48-49
  supramaximal exercise, short-term high-intensity, 48
  ventilatory threshold, 50-52
  WAT, 55-57
Exercise training, 105-108, 107f-108f
  cool down, 106
  individualization and, 106
  maintenance and, 106
  overload and, 105-106
  periodization and, 106-108
  principles of, 105-106
  progression and, 106
  rest/recovery/adaptation and, 106
  retrogression/plateau/reversibility and, 106
  SAID principle and, 105. *See also* SAID (specific adaptations to imposed demands) principle.
  steploading and, 106
  training plans, 107f
  warm-ups, 106
Exercise variables, 225-226
Expiratory reserve volume. *See* ERV (expiratory reserve volume).
Extensibility, 16
Extracellular matrix. *See* ECM (extracellular matrix).
Extrafusal fibers, 15, 31-32
Extreme exercise intensity, 281t
Extremely active activity level, 280t

F

F actin (fibrous actin), 20
Facet scour, 199
$FADH_2$ (flavin adenine dinucleotide), 68-69
Fartlek training, 80
Fascia, 17
Fasciculi, 17, 18f
Fast oxidative glyolytic fibers. *See* FOG (fast oxidative glycolytic) fibers.
Fast twitch fibers. *See* FT (fast twitch) fibers.
Fatigue, muscle, 87-96. *See also* Muscle fatigue, muscle damage, and overtraining.
  central fatigue, 92-94
    EMG and, 93
    iEMG and, 93
    MVC and, 92
    vs. peripheral fatigue, 93
  evidenced-based clinical applications for, 88, 91-92
  mechanical manifestations of, 88
  mechanisms of, 87-88
  peripheral fatigue, 89-92
    ATP-CP system and, 91
    vs. central fatigue, 93
    components of, 90-91
    E-C coupling processes, 89
    glycolysis and, 91
    metabolic by-products and, 92
    metabolic components of, 90-91
    myofibrillar complex and, 90
    nonmetabolic components of, 90
    oxidative system and, 91-92
    sarcolemma-T-tubule system and, 89-90
    sarcoplasmic reticulum and, 89-90
    TC and, 89-90
    triad concept and, 89
  rehabilitation roles of, 87, 94
  research trends of, 93
  task dependency and, 93
  underlying causes and sites of, 88-89

Feedback, 213, 249
  specific force, 249
  vestibular, 213
  visual, 213
Females *vs.* males, 58-59, 60f, 76
  aerobic metabolism and, 76
  anaerobic metabolism and, 58-59, 60f
Femoral anteversion, 155
Femur-MCL-tibia complex. *See* FMTC (femur-MCL-tibia complex).
Fiber type specific adaptations, 225
Fibers/cells, muscle, 17-18, 19f, 19t, 25-29, 26f-29f, 27t
Fibrous actin. *See* F actin (fibrous actin).
Fine control, 266t
Fisher case example, 296-297
Flavin adenine dinucleotide. *See* $FADH_2$ (flavin adenine dinucleotide).
Flexibility and ROM (range of motion), 35-36, 36b
Floor-to-CORE interrelationships, 145-174
Flower-spray neurons, 32
Fluid flow characteristic, 263
Fluid intake needs, 285-287. *See also* Nutrition-related considerations.
  exercise needs, 286
  importance of, 285
  postexercise needs, 287
  preexercise needs, 285
  roles of, 285
  sports drink selection criteria, 286-287
FMTC (femur-MCL-tibia complex), 5-8
FOG (fast oxidative glycolytic) fibers, 26-28, 39-40, 57-58
Follow-up evaluations, 300-301. *See also* Differential diagnoses (orthopedic-specific).
Foot mechanics, 159-161
Foot orthotic strategies, 161-167, 162f-167f
Football player case example, 297-298
Footwork patterns-speed development integration, 242-244, 242t, 243f, 244b. *See also* Plyometrics.
  sample programs, aerobic *vs.* anaerobic conditioning, 244b
  sports balance training, 126b
  strength training and, 245b
  trunk conditioning and, 245b
Force, 265t-266t
Force production phase, 235
Forward/back step-ups. *See* FW/BK (forward/back) step-ups.

Four-square jump patterns, 235-236, 240-242, 241f
FRC (functional residual capacity), 67
Free nerve endings, 248
Freeze positions, 234-235, 234f, 239, 239f
Frequency, 80, 233, 236
FT (fast twitch) fibers, 25-26, 39-40
FTTR (frequency, intensity, time/duration, type/mode, and rate of progression), 233
Full Can Testing position, 176
Function assessments, 250
Functional anatomy, 136-137
Functional progressions, 233-235, 235t. See also Plyometrics.
    applications of, 233-234
    exercise-to-fatigue approaches, 233
    FTTR, 233
    guidelines for, 233
    plyosupport phase and, 233-235
    reviews of, 233-235
    routine variables and, 233
    SAID principle and, 233-234
    total foot contacts, 235t
Functional residual capacity. See FRC (functional residual capacity).
Functional stability paradigm, 248f
Functional tissue engineering, 9-10
Future directions, 10-11
FW/BK (forward/back) step-ups, 234-235, 238

G

Gaenslen's test, 200, 200f, 201t
Gait analyses, 159-161, 250
Gastrointestinal function. See GI (gastrointestinal) function.
Gene therapy, 9-10
GI (gastrointestinal) function, 288-289. See also Nutrition-related considerations.
Giving way episodes, post-initial injuries, 251t, 254
Glenohumeral, acromioclavicular, and scapulothorácic joint evaluations, 175-192
    overhead-throwing athletes, 176-185
    muscular testing, 176-181, 176f-177f, 178t-179t, 180f, 181t
    ROM testing, 176-181, 176f-177f, 178t-179t, 180f, 181t
    scapular dysfunction classification, 185-190, 186f-189f
    special tests, 181-185, 182f-185f

rehabilitation roles for, 175-176
upper quadrant glenohumeral CORE, 135-144
Global rating scores, 251t, 254
Global stabilization test norms, 205t
Global vs. local muscle systems, 137-140
Glycogen, muscle, 282-283
Glycolysis, 91
Glycolysis, anaerobic. See LA (anaerobic glycolysis).
Golgi tendon organ. See GTO (Golgi tendon organ).
Gross structures, sensorimotor system, 249f. See also Sensorimotor system.
Growth factors, 7-10
GTO (Golgi tendon organ), 34-35, 34f-35f, 248-249
Gylcemic index, 282-283

H

Habituation, 77
Half-life, lactate, 53-54
HCM (hypertrophic cardiomyopathy), 74
Healing processes, ligaments and tendons, 5f-7f, 6-10, 10f. See also Soft tissues (ligaments and tendons) basic science concepts.
Heart anatomy and physiology, 65-67
Heart rate. See HR (heart rate).
Heat generation. See Thermogenesis.
Heat illness, 78
Hip and trunk CORE evaluations, 193-222
    agility testing, 211, 212t
    anatomy and pathophysiology of, 135-144
    background perspectives of, 193
    balance testing and evaluations, 211-215, 214f, 214t
        balance triad, 213
        central balance processors, 213
        MCTSIB, 214, 214t
        perturbation reaction, 214, 216t
        vestibular feedback and, 213
        visual feedback and, 213
    evaluation sheets for, 216t-218t
    hip and trunk stabilization tests, 203-205, 205f, 205t
    hip testing, 201-203, 202f-203f, 202t-203t
    lower quadrant trunk and hip, 135-144
    mobilizer tests, 207-209, 207f, 208t-209t

power, 209-211, 210f, 210t
    stabilization tests, trunk and hip, 203-205, 205f, 205t
    trunk screening, 194-201, 195f-198f, 198t, 199f-201f
Histories. See Orthopedic medical histories.
Homeostasis, tissue, 4-5, 5f
Hop tests, 211, 211t, 212f, 250-255
HPAA (hypothalamus-pituitary-adrenal axis), 111-112
HR (heart rate), 66-67
Hyperesis, 4f, 34
Hyperplasia vs. hypertrophy, 224-225
Hypertrophic cardiomyopathy. See HCM (hypertrophic cardiomyopathy).
Hypertrophy, 16f, 74, 224-225
Hyperventilation vs. hypoventilation, 67
Hypothalamus-pituitary-adrenal axis. See HPAA (hypothalamus-pituitary-adrenal axis).

I

I bands, 18-19
IC (inspiratory capacity), 67
iEMG (integrated electromyography), 93
IGF-1 (insulin-like growth factor-1), 225
Immobilization, 5, 5f, 8
Impingement, primary vs. secondary, 183-185
Incremental exercise to maximum, 50-52, 50f-51f
Index, gylcemic, 282-283
Individualization, 106
Inflammatory/regeneration phase, 268f
Injury effects, 250-252, 251f, 251t
Injury-prevention training, 252-253, 263f
Inspiratory capacity. See IC (inspiratory capacity).
Inspiratory reserve volume. See IRV (inspiratory reserve volume).
Instability tests, 182-183
Insulin-like growth factor-1. See IGF-1 (insulin-like growth factor-1).
Intake recommendations, nutrient, 280-285, 281t. See also Nutrition-related considerations.
    carbohydrate intake needs, 281-285
    carbohydrate loading, 281
    carbohydrate roles, 281-282
    exercise needs, 282-283
    gylcemic index and, 282-283
    muscle glycogen, 282-283
    postexercise needs, 283-284
    preexercise needs, 282
    protein additions and, 283-284

Intake recommendations, nutrient
    (continued)
    fluid intake needs, 285-287
        exercise needs, 286
        importance of, 285
        postexercise needs, 287
        preexercise needs, 285
        roles of, 285
        sports drink selection criteria,
            286-287
    protein intake needs, 281, 284-286,
            284-287
        carbohydrate additions, 284-285
        EAAs, 285
        for endurance athletes, 285
        protein powders, 285
        resistance exercise and, 284-285
Integrated electromyography. See iEMG
    (integrated electromyography).
Integrated nomenclature, 26-28
Intension, 268-269
Intensity, 71f, 80-81, 235-236, 236t,
    281t
Intermittent/interval training, 79-80
Intervals, motor response, 249t
Intrafusal fibers, 31-32, 249f
Inverse myotatic reflex, 34-35, 35f
Irritability, 16
IRV (inspiratory reserve volume), 67
Isokinetic dynamometers, 178t
Isokinetic testing, 176-179, 208
Isometric manual muscle testing, 205,
    205t-206t
Isometric strengthening, 228
Isotonic repetition maximums,
    208-209, 208t

J

Joints, 175-192, 247-248
    glenohumoral, acromioclavicular, and
        scapulothoracic, 175-192
    joint position sense, 247
    joint position testing. See JPS (joint
        position) testing.
    receptors, 248
    stability, 247-248
J-point, 66
JPS (joint position) testing, 250
J-sign, 202
Jump, 240-242, 240f, 242f, 253
    drills, 253
    patterns, 240-242, 240f, 242f
        four-square, 240-242, 241f
        instructions for, 240-242, 240f-242f
        objectives of, 240
        staggered ladder, 240-242, 242f

K

Kibler scapular dysfunction
    classification, 186-187
Kinesthesia, 247-255
Kinetic chain, 147-155
    bottom up, 147-151
    top down, 151-155
Knee-foot-ankle interrelationships,
    145-147, 146f
Knock knees, 194
KOS-ADL scale, 251t, 254
Krebs cycle, 43, 47t, 68-69

L

LA (anaerobic glycolysis), 40-60
Lacrosse player case example, 304-314
Lactate, 44-55
    changes, 47-48, 48f-49f, 52-53, 52t
    clearance, 44-45, 44f
    production, 42-44, 44f
    removal time frames, 53-55, 54f-55f
    threshold, 50-52
Lactic acid, 42-44, 44f
Lactic anaerobic systems, 40
Landing strategies, 238-240, 239f-240f
Late phase, perturbation training, 255t
Lateral direction change measures,
    243-244, 243f
Lateral sacs, 18
Length, 265t-266t
Length adaptation characteristic, 263
Lewis Power Equation, 210t
Ligaments and tendons (basic science
        concepts), 1-14
    basic science, 2-5
        biology and biochemical
            composition, 2-3, 2f
        biomechanics, 3-4, 3f-4f
        bone-ligament-bone complex, 3, 3f
        collagen fiber bundles, 2-3, 2f
        ECM, 2-3
        energy absorbed at failure
            parameter, 3, 3f
        exercise effects, 5-6, 6f
        future directions of, 10-11
        hyperesis, 4f, 34
        immobilization, 5, 5f
        ligament architecture hierarchy,
            2-3, 2f
        stiffness parameter, 3, 3f
        strain energy density parameter,
            3-4, 3f
        tangent modulus parameter, 3-4,
            3f
        tissue homeostasis, 4-5, 5f

tropocollagen molecules, 2-3
ultimate elongation parameter,
    3, 3f
ultimate strain parameter, 3-4, 3f
ultimate tensile strength
        parameter, 3-4, 3f
Wolf's law, 4-5
healing processes
    ACLs, 1, 6-10, 251-254
    bioscaffolds, 10
    cell therapy, 10
    conservative treatment vs. repair,
        7-8
    FMTC and, 5-8
    functional tissue engineering, 9-10
    gene therapy, 9-10
    growth factors, 7-10
    immobilization vs. passive
            controlled mobilization, 8
    MCLs, 1-2, 2f, 6-10
    MSCs and, 10
    multiple ligament injuries, 8
    overlapping phases of, 6f
    PDGF and, 7
    reconstruction, 8-9
    SIS and, 10
    stress-exercise interrelationships, 8
    stress-strain curves and, 7f
    TGF-β and, 7-10
Light activity level, 280t
Limb symmetry index. See LSI (limb
    symmetry index).
Lipolysis, 66-68
Loading, carbohydrate, 281
Local vs. global muscle systems,
    137-140
Logs, monitoring and training,
    112-113
Long distance runner case example,
    299-300
Long loop reflexes, 249, 249t
Long slow distance programs, 77
Long-term adaptations, 73-74
Lordotic curve, 234-235
Low exercise intensity (moderate
    duration), 281t
Lower extremity linkage system,
    147-155, 148f-155f
Lower quadrant trunk and hip CORE,
    135-144
LSI (limb symmetry index), 211
Lumbar, 199, 204, 234-235
    concavity, 234-235
    multifidus segmental palpation,
        204
    quadrant rest, 199
Lung volumes, 67

M

Macroscopic structures, 16-17, 17f
Maintenance, 106
Maladaptation *vs.* adaptation, 108-112, 109f
Malalignments, structural, 155-159
Males *vs.* females, 58-59, 60f, 76
 aerobic metabolism and, 76
 anaerobic metabolism and, 58-59, 60f
Manual neuromuscular re-abilitation, 263, 265t-266t
Manual therapy. *See* MT (manual therapy).
MAOD (maximal accumulated oxygen deficit), 46
mATPase (myosin adenosine triphosphatase), 225
Mature remodeling phase, 268f
Maximal accumulated oxygen deficit. *See* MAOD (maximal accumulated oxygen deficit).
Maximal heart rate. *See* MHR (maximal heart rate).
Maximal lactate steady state workload and intensity. *See* MLSS (maximal lactate steady state) workload and intensity.
Maximal oxygen consumption, 69-72, 69f
Maximal oxygen uptake, 37, 40-60
Maximal voluntary contraction. *See* MVC (maximal voluntary contraction).
McKenzie prone prop, 199f, 199t
MCLs (medial collateral ligaments), 1-2, 2f, 6-10
MCTs (monocarboxylate transporters), 44-45, 44f
MCTSIB (modified clinical test of sensory integration and balance), 214, 214t
Mechanical manifestations, muscle fatigue, 88. *See also* Fatigue, muscle.
Mechanisms, muscle fatigue, 87-88
Mechanoreceptors, 248
Medial collateral ligaments. *See* MCLs (medial collateral ligaments).
Medical histories. *See* Orthopedic medical histories.
Medicine ball throws, 210-211
Mesenchymal stem cells. *See* MSCs (mesenchymal stem cells).
Metabolism, 39-86
 aerobic, 65-86. *See also* Aerobic metabolism.
 acute changes in, 69-73, 69f-71f
 ATP and, 66-72

BP (blood pressure) and, 66-68
 EGCs and, 66
 exercise program design, 76-83
 long-term adaptations of, 73-74
 processes of, 68-69, 68f-69f
 rehabilitation roles of, 65, 83
 respiratory anatomy and physiology, 67-68
 alterations of, 110-111
 anaerobic, 39-64. *See also* Anaerobic metabolism.
 ATP and, 39-60
 ATP-PC system and, 39-60
 of children, 55-58, 56f
 energy continuum, 39-41, 40f-41f
 energy production and, 41-45, 43f-44f
 evidenced-based clinical applications for, 42
 exercise response and, 45-55, 47f-51f, 47t, 52t, 54f-55f
 LA, 40-60
 of males *vs.* females, 58-59, 60f
 maximal oxygen uptake and, 40-60
 of older adults, 59-60
 rehabilitation roles of, 39
 time-continuum, 41
 metabolic by-products, 92
 metabolic components, 90-91
 metabolic properties, 26
MHR (maximal heart rate), 70-71
Middle phase, perturbation training, 255t
MLSS (maximal lactate steady state) workload and intensity, 49
MMT (manual muscle testing), 176
Mobilization, passive controlled, 8
Mobilizers and mobilizer tests, 135, 207-209, 207f, 208t-209t
Moderate activity level, 280t
Moderate-to-heavy exercise intensity, 281t
Modes, 81
Modified clinical test of sensory integration and balance. *See* MCTSIB (modified clinical test of sensory integration and balance).
Modified Edgren Test, 243-244, 243f
Monitoring and training logs, 112-113
Monocarboxylate transporters. *See* MCTs (monocarboxylate transporters).
Morton's extension, 165-166
Motor abilities, 264, 264f, 265t-266t
Motor pathway (efferent system)-sensory pathway interactions, 247-248

Motor relaxation, 266t
Motor response intervals, 249t
Movement, 15-38. *See also* Muscle contraction.
 muscular aspects of, 15-29, 16f-29f, 19t, 27t
 neural control of, 29-37, 29f-35f, 36b
MSCs (mesenchymal stem cells), 10
MT (manual therapy), 259-278
 dimensional model of, 260-269, 260f, 262f, 264f, 265t-266t, 267f-268f
 clinical examples for, 261, 270t-271t
 early remodeling phase, 268f
 fluid flow characteristic, 263
 inflammatory/regeneration phase, 268f
 intension and, 268-269
 length adaptation characteristic, 263
 manual neuromuscular re-abilitation and, 263, 265t-266t
 mature remodeling phase, 268f
 motor abilities complexity hierarchy and, 264, 264f
 neurological dimension, 260-261, 260f, 263-266, 264f, 265t-266t, 268f
 objectives of, 262, 262f
 outcomes of, 260f
 practical applications of, 267-269, 267f-268f
 psychological dimension, 260f, 261, 267-269, 267f-268f
 repair characteristic, 262-263
 repair timelines, 268f
 sensory-motor abilities, 265t-266t
 signals/stimuli, 260f, 262-269, 264f, 265t-266t, 267f-268f
 similarity principle and, 263
 tissue dimension, 260, 260f, 262-263, 268f
 objectives of, 259-260
 rehabilitation roles for, 259-273
 repair and adaptation environment creation and, 269-273, 269f 270t-271t, 272f
MTJ (musculotendinous junction), 97-98
Multifidus activation and atrophy, 204
Multiple ligament injuries, 8
Muscle contraction, 15-38
 evidenced-based clinical applications for, 36-37
 maximal oxygen uptake and, 37

Muscle contraction (continued)
  movement, muscular aspects of,
        15-29, 16f-29f, 19t, 27t
    all-or-none principle, 25
    AP, 16-24
    architectural organization, 17
    athlete-specific considerations, 29
    cisterns, 18
    contractile (twitch) properties,
        25-26
    contractility, 16
    contraction processes, 20-25,
        21f-25f
    cross-innervation, 26, 26f
    definition, 16f
    elasticity, 16
    endomysium, 17
    epimysium, 17
    excitation-contraction coupling,
        21-22
    extensibility, 16
    extrafusal fibers, 15
    fascia, 17
    fasciculi, 17, 18f
    hypertrophy, 16f
    integrated nomenclature, 26-28
    irritability, 16
    lateral sacs, 18
    macroscopic structures, 16-17, 17f
    metabolic properties, 26
    mitochondria, 19t
    motor unit properties, 25f
    muscle fibers/cells, 17-18, 19f,
        19t, 25-29, 26f-29f, 27t
    muscle tissue functions and
        characteristics, 15-16
    myofibrils and myofilaments,
        18-20, 19f-20f, 19t
    perimysium, 17
    sacromeres, 18-20, 24-25, 25f
    sarcolemma, 17-18
    skeletal muscle and, 15-17, 17f
    sliding filament theory, 21
    SR, 18, 19t
    striated muscles, 15
    T tubules, 18-22, 19t
    voluntary muscles, 15
  movement, neural control of, 29-37,
        29f-35f, 36b
    flexibility and ROM, 35-36, 36b
    GTO, 34-35, 34f-35f
    inverse myotatic reflex, 34-35, 35f
    myotatic reflex, 32-34, 33f
    nerve supply, 29-30, 30f
    neuromuscular junction, 30-31,
        30f-31f
    NMS, 31-34, 32f-34f

    plyometrics and, 34. See also
        Plyometrics.
    reflex control, 31-35, 32f-35f
    stretch reflex, 31
  rehabilitation roles of, 15
Muscle damage and overuse injury,
        97-104, 97-109. See also Muscle
        fatigue, muscle damage, and
        overtraining.
  ACL and, 98
  ACLs and, 98
  children and, 100
  classification of, 99-101
  clinical applications of, 99-100
  DOMS and, 97-98, 101
  EIMD and, 99
  etiology of, 97-99
  evaluations of, 99
  evidenced-based clinical applications
        for, 98, 101-102
  management of, 99
  MTJ and, 97-98
  muscle strains, 100-101
  perpetuating factors of, 98-99
  physiology of, 99
  precipitating factors of, 98
  predisposing factors of, 97-98
  rehabilitation roles for, 97
  repair of, 99-100
  research trends of, 99-100
  RICE and, 101-102
  SAID principle and, 99. See also
        SAID (specific adaptations to
        imposed demands) principle.
  therapeutic ultrasound and, 102
  tissue repair and, 101
Muscle fatigue, muscle damage, and
        overtraining, 87-121
  detraining and overtraining
        (physiological effects),
        105-121
  muscle fatigue, 87-96. See also
        Fatigue, muscle.
  overuse injury and muscle damage,
        97-104
Muscle fibers/cells, 17-29, 19f, 19t,
        26f-29f, 27t, 225
Muscle glycogen, 282-283
  resting values of, 282
  synthesis of, 283
Muscle physiological adaptations,
        224-226. See also Strength
        training concepts.
  aging changes and, 226
  contractile, 224-225
  exercise variables and, 225-226
  hypertrophy vs. hyperplasia, 224-225

    muscle changes and, 226
    muscle fiber type specific
        adaptations, 225
    neural, 224
Muscle physiology (exercise prescription
        foundations), 15-121. See also
        under individual topics.
  aerobic metabolism, 65-86
  anaerobic metabolism, 39-64
  muscle contraction, 15-38
  muscle fatigue, muscle damage, and
        overtraining fundamentals,
        87-96
  overuse injury, 97-104
  physiological effects (overtraining
        and detraining), 105-121
Muscle receptors, 248-249
Muscle spindle intrafusal fibers, 249f
Muscle strains, 100-101
Muscle strengthening action types,
        226-229. See also Strength
        training concepts.
  concentric strengthening, 227-228
  DOMS and, 227
  eccentric strengthening, 226-227
  isometric strengthening, 228
  repeated bout effect and, 227
  SAID and, 227
  stretch-shorten cycles and, 227
Muscle tissue functions and
        characteristics, 15-16
Muscle trauma and injury, 112
Muscular testing, 176-181, 176f-177f,
        178t-179t, 180f, 181t
Musculotendinous junction. See MTJ
        (musculotendinous junction).
MVC (maximal voluntary contraction),
        92
Myofibers, 224-225
Myofibrillar complex, 90
Myofibrils and myofilaments, 18-20,
        19f-20f, 19t
Myosin adenosine triphosphatase. See
        mATPase (myosin adenosine
        triphosphatase).
Myotatic reflex, inverse, 34-35, 35f

N

NADH (nicotinamide adenine
        dinucleotide), 42-60, 68-69
Nagi model of disability, 208
National Athletic Training Association,
        79
National College Athletic Association,
        Division I, 209
Nerve supply, 29-30, 30f

Neural adaptations, 224-226
Neural control, movement, 29-37, 29f-35f, 36b. *See also* Movement.
Neurocom (Balance Master), 214
Neurological dimension, 260-261, 260f, 263-266, 264f, 265t-266t, 268f. *See also* Dimensional model of MT (manual therapy).
Neuromuscular cleft, 30
Neuromuscular function assessments, 250
Neuromuscular junction, 30-31, 30f-31f
Neuromuscular re-abilitation, manual, 263, 265t-266t
Neuromuscular spindles. *See* NMS (neuromuscular spindles).
Neuromuscular training, 247-258
  altered neuromuscular control and, 247
  biomechanical gait analyses and, 250
  decreased/dysfunctional neuromuscular control and, 247
  degrees of freedom problem and, 250
  electromyography and, 250
  evidenced-based clinical applications for, 252-253
  hip strategies, 250
  hop testing and, 250-255
  injury effects and, 250-252, 251f, 251t
    ACL injuries, 251-254
    copers *vs.* non-copers, 251-252, 251t
    screening tools for, 251t
  JPS testing and, 250
  neuromuscular function assessments, 250
  observational analyses and, 250
  programs for, 252-256, 253f, 255f, 255t
    dynamic valgus and, 252-253, 263f
    injury-prevention training, 252-253, 263f
    KOS-ADL scale and, 251t, 254
    nonoperative training, 253-254
    perturbation training protocol and, 254, 255f, 255t
    postoperative training, 253-254
  proprioception, 247-248, 248f
    dynamic joint stability and, 247-248
    functional stability paradigm for, 248f
    joint position sense and, 247
    joint stability, 247-248
    kinesthesia and, 247-255

    postural control and, 247-250
    rehabilitation roles of, 247, 256
    sensorimotor system and, 248-249, 249f, 249t
      CNS and, 248-249
      cutaneous receptors, 248
      gross structures of, 249f
      GTO, 248-249
      joint receptors, 248
      long-loop reflexes, 249, 249t
      mechanoreceptors, 248
      motor response intervals, 249t
      muscle receptors, 248-249
      muscle spindle intrafusal fibers, 249f
      spinal reflexes, 249t
      spray endings, 248
      triggered reactions, 249t
      voluntary reactions, 249t
      wineglass effect and, 249
    sensory pathway-motor pathway (efferent system) interactions, 247-248
    stabilometry and, 250
    stepping strategies, 250
    strength testing and, 250
    TTDPM testing, 250
    wineglass effect and, 249
Nicotinamide adenine dinucleotide. *See* NADH (nicotinamide adenine dinucleotide).
NMS (neuromuscular spindles), 31-34, 32f-34f
Non-copers *vs.* copers, 251-252, 251t
Nonmetabolic components, 90
Nonoperative training, 253-254
Nutrient intake recommendations, 280-285, 281t. *See also* Nutrition-related considerations.
  carbohydrate intake needs, 281-285
    carbohydrate loading, 281
    carbohydrate roles, 281-282
    exercise needs, 282-283
    gylcemic index and, 282-283
    muscle glycogen, 282-283
    muscle glycogen and, 282-283
    postexercise needs, 283-284
    preexercise needs, 282
    protein additions and, 283-284
  fluid intake needs, 285-287
    exercise needs, 286
    importance of, 285
    postexercise needs, 287
    preexercise needs, 285
    roles of, 285
    sports drink selection criteria, 286-287

    protein intake needs, 281, 284-286, 284-287
    carbohydrate additions, 284-285
    EAAs, 285
    for endurance athletes, 285
    protein powders, 285
    resistance exercise and, 284-285
Nutrition plans, 290
Nutritional recommendation factors, 279, 289-290
Nutrition-related considerations, 279-292
  energy needs, 279-280
    activity levels and factors for, 280, 280t-281t
    AEE and, 279-280, 280t
    calculations for, 279-280, 280t
    components of, 279
    exercise intensity and, 281t
    meeting of, 279-280, 280t
    REE and, 279-280, 280t
    TEF and, 279
  ergogenic aids and performance, 287-288
    caffeine and, 288
    creatine and, 288
    evaluation guidelines for, 287-288
    roles of, 287
  evidenced-based clinical applications for, 281-283, 285-286
  GI function, 288-289
  nutrient intake recommendations, 280-285, 281t
    carbohydrate intake needs, 281-285. *See also* Carbohydrate intake needs.
    fluid intake needs, 285-287. *See also* Fluid intake needs.
    protein intake needs, 281, 284-287. *See also* Protein intake needs.
  nutrition plans, 290
  nutritional recommendation factors, 279, 289-290
  optimal performance body weight, 289, 289b
  rehabilitation roles for, 279, 289-290

O

Ober's test, 202, 202f
OBLA (onset of blood lactate accumulation), 52
Observational analyses, 193-194, 195f, 250
Off-season phase, 106-107, 107f, 108
OKCs (open kinetic chains), 223-224

Older adults, 59-60, 75-76, 82-83
aerobic metabolism and, 75-76, 82-83
anaerobic metabolism and, 59-60
One repetition at maximum effort. *See* 1 RM (one repetition at maximum effort).
One-leg squatting, 233-234
Onset of blood lactate accumulation. *See* OBLA (onset of blood lactate accumulation).
Open kinetic chains. *See* OKCs (open kinetic chains).
Opposite straight leg raise testing, 199
Optimal performance body weight, 289, 289b
OR (overreaching), 108-109
Orthopedic considerations, plyometrics, 237-238
Orthopedic medical histories, 295-300. *See also* Differential diagnoses (orthopedic-specific).
Orthopedic-specific differential diagnoses, 295-302
Orthotic strategies, 161-167, 162f-167f
OTS (overtraining syndrome), 109-113, 110t, 111f
Overhead-throwing athletes, 123-134
glenohumeral, acromioclavicular, and scapulothoracic joint evaluations, 175-192
rehabilitation roles for, 175-176
shoulder testing, muscular and ROM, 176-181, 176f-177f, 178t-179t, 181t
injury pathophysiology of, 123-134
180-degree rule, 130
acceleration, 124
biceps tendon superior labral complex, 128-132, 129f-131f
cocking, early *vs.* late, 124
follow-through, 124-125
internal impingement, 125-128, 125f-127f
pathophysiological cascade, 130
rehabilitation roles for, 123
scapula asymmetry, 130-132
SLAP lesions, 128-132
windup, 123-124
Overlapping healing phases, 6f
Overloading, 76-77, 105-107, 107f
Overreaching. *See* OR (overreaching).
Overtraining and detraining (physiological effects), 87-121. *See also* Muscle fatigue, muscle damage, and overtraining.

adaptation *vs.* maladaptation, 108-112, 109f
mechanisms of, 109-110, 110t
metabolism alterations, 110-111
muscle trauma and injury, 112
OR and, 108-109
OTS, 109-113, 110t, 111f
super compensation and, 110f
sympathetic *vs.* parasympathetic forms, 109
UPS, 109
detraining, 116-118, 117f
exercise training, 105-108, 107f-108f
cool down, 106
individualization and, 106
maintenance and, 106
overload and, 105-106
periodization and, 106-108
principles of, 105-106
progression and, 106
rest/recovery/adaptation and, 106
retrogression/plateau/reversibility and, 106
SAID principle and, 105. *See also* SAID (specific adaptations to imposed demands) principle.
steploading and, 106
training plans, 107f
warm-ups, 106
monitoring and training logs, 112-113
prevention and treatment of, 113-116
rehabilitation roles for, 105
Overtraining syndrome. *See* OTS (overtraining syndrome).
Overuse injury (pathophysiology) concepts. *See also under individual topics.*
CORE anatomy and physiology, 135-144
CORE-to-floor interrelationships, 145-174
overhead-throwing athletes, 123-134
overuse injury and muscle damage, 97-104. *See also* Muscle fatigue, muscle damage, and overtraining.
ACLs and, 98
children and, 100
classification of, 99-101
clinical applications of, 99-100
DOMS and, 97-98, 101
EIMD and, 99
etiology of, 97-99
evaluations of, 99
evidenced-based clinical applications for, 98, 101-102

management of, 99, 100-101
MTJ and, 97-98
muscle strains, 100-101
perpetuating factors of, 98-99
physiology of, 99
precipitating factors of, 98
predisposing factors of, 97-98
rehabilitation roles for, 97
repair of, 99-100
research trends of, 99-100
RICE and, 101-102
SAID principle and, 99. *See also* SAID (specific adaptations to imposed demands) principle.
therapeutic ultrasound and, 102
tissue repair and, 101
Oxidative phosphorylation, 68-69
Oxidative system, 91-92
Oxygen deficit, 45-46, 45f
Oxygen uptake, maximal, 37

P

P waves, 66
Pace/tempo programs, 78-79
Pain and exercise response, 53
Parasympathetic *vs.* sympathetic forms, 109
Passive controlled mobilization *vs.* immobilization, 8
Passive straight leg raising, 199, 199f
Patellofemoral pain, 147
Pathophysiology (overuse injury) concepts, 123-174, 135-144. *See also under individual topics.*
CORE anatomy and physiology, 135-144
CORE-to-floor interrelationships, 145-174
overhead-throwing athletes, 123-134
Patterns, jump, 240-242, 240f, 242f
four-square, 240-242, 241f
instructions for, 240-242, 240f-242f
objectives of, 240
staggered ladder, 240-242, 242f
PDGF (platelet-derived growth factor), 7
Performance decrement, 53
Perimysium, 17
Periodization, 106-108, 236
Periods, aerobic *vs.* work, 77
Peripheral fatigue, 89-92. *See also* Fatigue, muscle.
ATP-CP system and, 91
vs. central fatigue, 93. *See also* Central fatigue.
components of, 90-91

E-C coupling processes, 89
  glycolysis and, 91
  glycosis and, 91
  metabolic by-products and, 92
  metabolic components, 90-91
  myofibrillar complex and, 90
  nonmetabolic components of, 90
  oxidative system and, 91-92
  sarcolemma-T-tubule system and, 89-90
  sarcoplasmic reticulum and, 89-90
  TC and, 89-90
  triad concept and, 89
Peripheralization, 196, 198t
Perpetuating factors, muscle damage, 98-99
Perturbation, 214-216, 216t, 254, 255f, 255t
  reaction, 214-216, 216t
  training protocol, 254, 255f, 255t
PFK (phosphofructokinase), 53, 55-57
Phosphagen system, 40, 91
Phosphofructokinase. See PFK (phosphofructokinase).
Physical examinations, 295-300. See also Differential diagnoses (orthopedic-specific).
Physiological adaptations, muscle, 224-226. See also Strength training concepts.
  aging changes and, 226
  contractile, 224-225
  exercise variables and, 225-226
  hypertrophy vs. hyperplasia, 224-225
  muscle changes and, 226
  muscle fiber type specific adaptations, 225
  neural, 224
Physiological effects (overtraining and detraining), 105-121
Physiological foundations (sport-specific exercise), 223-278
  MT, 259-278
  neuromuscular training, 247-258
  plyometrics, 233-246
  strength training concepts, 223-232
Physiology and anatomy (CORE), 135-144
Plans, nutrition, 290. See also Nutrition-related considerations.
Plantar fasciitis, 166-167
Platelet-derived growth factor. See PDGF (platelet-derived growth factor).
Platforms/rollerboards, 255f, 255t

Plyometrics, 233-246
  basic positions of, 238
  care plans and, 233
  footwork patterns-speed development integration, 242-244, 242t, 243f, 244b
    sample programs, aerobic vs. anaerobic conditioning, 244b
    sports balance training, 126b
    strength training and, 245b
    trunk conditioning and, 245b
  frequency considerations for, 236
  functional progressions and, 233-235, 235t
    alignment and, 233-234
    applications of, 233-234
    exercise-to-fatigue approaches, 233
    FTTR, 233
    guidelines for, 233
    LOG and, 234-235
    performance phase, 234
    plyo-support phase, 233-235
    reviews of, 233-235
    routine variables and, 233
    SAID principle and, 233-234. See also SAID (specific adaptations to imposed demands) principle.
    strength phase, 234
    total foot contacts, 235t
  intensity and work volume and, 235-236, 236t
  jump patterns and, 240-242, 240f, 242f
    four-square, 240-242, 241f
    instructions for, 240-242, 240f-242f
    objectives of, 240
    staggered ladder, 240-242, 242f
  landing strategies for, 238-240, 239f-240f
  medical considerations of, 237-238
  muscle contraction and, 34. See also Muscle contraction.
  nature of, 235
  orthopedic considerations of, 237-238
  periodization and, 236
  readiness for, 237-238
  recovery and, 236
  rehabilitation roles for, 233, 244
  safety considerations of, 236-237
  squatting, 238
  SSCs and, 235-238
  step-ups, 238
  triangle vs. four-square patterns, 235-236, 236t

Plyosupport phase, 233-235
Pole vaulter case example, 298-299
Position sense, 265
Postexercise, 283-284, 287
  carbohydrate intake needs for, 283-284
  fluid intake needs and, 287
Postoperative training, 253-254
Postural control, 247-250
Powders, protein, 285
Power tests, 55, 209-211, 210f, 210t
PR intervals, 66
Precipitating and predisposing factors, muscle damage, 97-98
Preexercise, 282-285
  carbohydrate intake needs for, 282
  fluid intake needs and, 285
Prescription foundations (muscle physiology), 15-121. See also under individual topics.
  aerobic metabolism, 65-86
  anaerobic metabolism, 39-64
  muscle contraction, 15-38
  muscle fatigue, muscle damage, and overtraining fundamentals, 87-96
  physiological effects (overtraining and detraining), 105-121
Preseason phase, 106-107, 107f
Prevention considerations, 113-116
Primary sensory axions, 248
Professional football player case example, 297-298
Programs, 76-83, 244b, 252-256, 253f, 255f, 255t
  aerobic vs. anaerobic conditioning, 244b
  components of, 77
  design of, 76-83
  for neuromuscular training, 252-256, 253f, 255f, 255t
    dynamic valgus and, 252-253, 263f
    injury-prevention training, 252-253, 263f
    KOS-ADL scale and, 251t, 254
    nonoperative training, 253-254
    perturbation training protocol and, 254, 255f, 255t
    postoperative training, 253-254
Progressions, functional, 233-235, 235t. See also Plyometrics.
  applications of, 233-234
  exercise-to-fatigue approaches, 233
  FTTR, 233
  guidelines for, 233
  plyosupport phase and, 233-235

Progressions, functional (continued)
  reviews of, 233-235
  routine variables and, 233
  SAID principle and, 233-234
  total foot contacts, 235t
Progressive locomotive patterns,
    234-235
Pronation kinematics, 163
Prone instability test, 199, 200f, 201t
Proprioception, 247-248, 248f. See also
    Neuromuscular training.
  descriptions, tests, re-abilitation for,
    266t
  dynamic joint stability and, 247-248
  functional stability paradigm for, 248f
  joint position sense and, 247
  joint stability, 247-248
  kinesthesia and, 247-255
  postural control and, 247-250
Protein intake needs, 281, 284-286. See
    also Nutrition-related
    considerations.
  carbohydrate additions, 284-285
  EAAs, 285
  for endurance athletes, 285
  protein powders, 285
  resistance exercise and, 284-285
Proximal segment weaknesses, 146
Psychological dimension, 260f, 261,
    267-269, 267f-268f. See also
    Dimensional model of MT
    (manual therapy).
Pulmonary semilunar valves, 66

Q

Q waves, 66
QRS complex, 66
QT intervals, 66
Quebec Back Pain Disability Score, 204

R

R waves, 66
Range of motion. See ROM (range of
    motion) and flexibility.
Re-abilitation, 263, 265t-266t
Reactions, 249t, 266t
  reaction times, 266t
  triggered, 249t
  voluntary, 249t
Reactive-type exercises, uncontrolled,
    240
Readiness considerations, plyometrics,
    237-238
Real-time ultrasound. See RTUS (real-
    time ultrasound).

Rebound training, 34. See also
    Plyometrics.
Receptors, 248-249
  cutaneous, 248
  joint, 248
  mechanoreceptors, 248
  muscle, 248-249
Reciprocal activation, 266t
Reciprocal inhibition, 33-34
Reconstruction, 8-9
Recovery, 236
Recreational fisher case example,
    296-297
REE (resting energy expenditure),
    279-280, 280t
Reflexes, 31-35, 32f-35f, 213, 249,
    249f, 249t
  inverse myotatic, 34-35, 35f
  long-loop, 249, 249t
  reflex control, 31-35, 32f-35f
  spinal, 249t
  stretch, 31
  vestibulospinal, 213
Rehabilitation (sports-specific) topics.
    See also under individual topics.
  case collections and reviews, 293-314
    differential diagnoses (orthopedic-
      specific), 295-302
    surgical considerations, 303-314
  CORE evaluations, 175-222
    glenohumoral, acromioclavicular,
      and scapulothoracic joints,
      175-192
    trunk and hip CORE, 193-222
  muscle fatigue, muscle damage, and
    overtraining, 87-121
    detraining and overtraining
      (physiological effects),
      105-121
    muscle fatigue, 87-96. See also
      Fatigue, muscle.
    overuse injury and muscle damage,
      97-104
  muscle physiology (exercise
    prescription foundations),
    15-86
    aerobic metabolism, 65-86
    anaerobic metabolism, 39-64
    muscle contraction, 15-38
  nutrition-related considerations,
    279-292
  orthopedic-specific differential
    diagnoses, 295-302
  pathophysiology (overuse injury)
    concepts, 123-174
    CORE anatomy and physiology,
      135-144

CORE-to-floor interrelationships,
    145-174
  overhead-throwing athletes,
    123-134
  physiological basis (sport-specific
    exercise), 223-278
  physiological foundations (sport-
    specific exercise), 223-278
    MT, 259-278
    neuromuscular training, 247-258
    plyometrics, 233-246
    strength training concepts,
      223-232
  soft tissues (ligaments and tendons)
    basic science concepts, 1-14
Remodeling phase, early vs. mature,
    268f
Removal, lactate, 53-55, 54f-55f
Repair, 7-8, 99-100, 262-263, 268f-
    269f, 269-273, 270t-271t, 272f
  adaptation environment creation and,
    269-273, 269f 270t-271t,
    272f
  characteristic, 262-263
  vs. conservative treatment, 7-8
  muscle damage and overuse injury,
    99-100
  timelines, 268f
Repeated bout effect, 227
Repetition max. See RM (repetition max).
Repetition training, 80
Research trends, 51, 93, 99-100,
    168-169
Residual volume. See RV (residual
    volume).
Resistance exercise, 52, 224-225,
    284-285
Respiration, 67
Respiratory system, 67-73
Response, exercise, 45-55, 47f-51f, 47t,
    52t, 54f-55f
Response intervals, motor, 249t
Rest, ice, compression, and elevation.
    See RICE (rest, ice, compression,
    and elevation).
Resting activity level, 280t
Resting energy expenditure. See REE
    (resting energy expenditure).
Resting heart rate. See RHR (resting
    heart rate).
Resting values, muscle glycogen, 282
Rest/recovery/adaptation, 106
Reviews and collections (cases). See also
    under individual topics.
  differential diagnoses (orthopedic-
    specific), 295-302
  surgical considerations, 303-314

RHR (resting heart rate), 66-67
RICE (rest, ice, compression, and elevation), 101-102
RM (repetition max), 72
Rockerboards, 255f, 255t
Rockport One-Mile Fitness Test, 70, 71f
Rollerboards, 255f, 255t
Rolling back compression, 202
ROM (range of motion) and flexibility, 35-36, 36b, 176-181, 176f-177f, 178t-179t, 180f, 181t
Rotator cuff testing, 176
Routine variables, 233
RTUS (real-time ultrasound), 203-205
Runner case example, 299-300
RV (residual volume), 67

S

S waves, 66
SA (sinoatrial) nodes, 66
Sacral thrust, 201, 201f, 201t
Sacroiliac joint tests, 199, 200f, 201, 201t
Sacromeres, 18-20, 24-25, 25f
Safety considerations, plyometrics, 236-237
SAID (specific adaptations to imposed demands) principle, 76-77, 99, 105, 227, 233-234
Sample programs, aerobic vs. anaerobic conditioning, 244b
Sarcolemma, 17-18, 89-90
Sarcoplasmic reticulum. See SR (sarcoplasmic reticulum).
SBP (systolic blood pressure), 66
Scapula thoracic CORE, 135-144
Scapular dysfunction classification, 185-190, 186f-189f
Scapulothoracic joints. See Glenohumeral, acromioclavicular, and scapulothoracic joint evaluations.
Screening tools, 251t
Seasonal periods, total foot contacts and, 235t
Sedentary activity level, 280t-281t
Sensorimotor system, 248-249, 249f, 249t, 265t-266t. See also Neuromuscular training.
    CNS and, 248-249
    cutaneous receptors, 248
    gross structures of, 249f
    GTO, 248-249
    joint receptors, 248
    long-loop reflexes, 249, 249t

mechanoreceptors, 248
motor response intervals, 249t
muscle receptors, 248-249
muscle spindle intrafusal fibers, 249f
spinal reflexes, 249t
spray endings, 248
triggered reactions, 249t
voluntary reactions, 249t
Sensory abilities, 265, 266t
Sensory pathway-motor pathway (efferent system) interactions, 247-248
Sensory-motor abilities, 265t-266t
Sex-related considerations, 74-76, 81-83
Shock cycles, 106-107, 107f
Shuttle run, 209, 210f, 210t
Side-lying pelvic test, 205-206
Signals/stimuli component, 260f, 262-269, 264f, 265t-266t, 267f-268f. See also Dimensional model of MT (manual therapy).
Similarity principle, 263
Single-leg hop tests, 211, 211t, 212f
Single-legged squat, 194
Sinoatrial nodes. See SA (sinoatrial) nodes.
SIS (small intestinal submucosa), 10
Skeletal muscle, 15-17, 17f
Sliding filament theory, 21
Slow oxidative fibers. See SO (slow oxidative) fibers.
Slow twitch fibers. See ST (slow twitch) fibers.
Slump tests, 196-199, 199f, 201t
Small intestinal submucosa. See SIS (small intestinal submucosa).
SO (slow oxidative) fibers, 26-28, 39-40
Soft tissues (ligaments and tendons)
    basic science concepts, 1-14
    basic science, 2-5
        biology and biochemical composition, 2-3, 2f
        biomechanics, 3-4, 3f-4f
        bone-ligament-bone complex, 3, 3f
        collagen fiber bundles, 2-3, 2f
        ECM, 2-3
        energy absorbed at failure parameter, 3, 3f
        exercise effects, 5-6, 6f
        future directions of, 10-11
        hyperesis, 4f, 34
        immobilization, 5, 5f
        ligament architecture hierarchy, 2-3, 2f
        stiffness parameter, 3, 3f
        strain energy density parameter, 3-4, 3f

tangent modulus parameter, 3-4, 3f
tissue homeostasis, 4-5, 5f
tropocollagen molecules, 2-3
ultimate elongation parameter, 3, 3f
ultimate load parameters, 3, 3f
ultimate strain parameter, 3-4, 3f
ultimate tensile strength parameter, 3-4, 3f
Wolf's law, 4-5
healing processes, 5f-7f, 6-10, 10f
    ACLs, 1, 6-10, 251-254
    bioscaffolds, 10
    cell therapy, 10
    conservative treatment vs. repair, 7-8
    FMTC and, 5-8
    functional tissue engineering, 9-10
    gene therapy, 9-10
    growth factors, 7-10
    immobilization vs. passive controlled mobilization, 8
    MCLs, 1-2, 2f, 6-10
    MSCs and, 10
    multiple ligament injuries, 8
    overlapping phases of, 6f
    PDGF and, 7
    reconstruction, 8-9
    SIS and, 10
    stress-exercise interrelationships, 8
    stress-strain curves and, 7f
    TGF-β and, 7-10
rehabilitation roles for, 1, 10-11
Spatial orientation, 265, 266t
Specific adaptations to imposed demands principle. See SAID (specific adaptations to imposed demands) principle.
Specific force feedback, 249
Speed development-footwork patterns integration, 242-244, 242t, 243f, 244b. See also Plyometrics.
    sample programs, aerobic vs. anaerobic conditioning, 244b
    sports balance training, 126b
    strength training and, 245b
    trunk conditioning and, 245b
Spinal reflexes, 249t
Sports drink selection criteria, 286-287. See also Fluid intake needs.
Sports-specific rehabilitation topics. See also under individual topics.
    case collections and reviews, 293-314
    differential diagnoses (orthopedic-specific), 295-302
    surgical considerations, 303-314

Sports-specific rehabilitation topics (*continued*)
CORE evaluations, 175-222
glenohumoral, acromioclavicular, and scapulothoracic joints, 175-192
trunk and hip CORE, 193-222
muscle fatigue, muscle damage, and overtraining, 87-121
detraining and overtraining (physiological effects), 105-121
muscle fatigue, 87-96. *See also* Fatigue, muscle.
overuse injury and muscle damage, 97-104
muscle physiology (exercise prescription foundations), 15-121
aerobic metabolism, 65-86
anaerobic metabolism, 39-64
muscle contraction, 15-38
nutrition-related considerations, 279-292
orthopedic-specific differential diagnoses, 295-302
pathophysiology (overuse injury) concepts, 123-174
CORE anatomy and physiology, 135-144
CORE-to-floor interrelationships, 145-174
overhead-throwing athletes, 123-134
physiological foundations (sport-specific exercise), 223-278
MT, 259-278
neuromuscular training, 247-258
plyometrics, 233-246
strength training concepts, 223-232
soft tissues (ligaments and tendons) basic science concepts, 1-14
Spray endings, 248
Squatting, 238
SR (sarcoplasmic reticulum), 18, 19t, 89-90
SSCs (stretch shortening cycles), 227, 235-238
ST (slow twitch) fibers, 25-26, 39-40
Stability, joint, 247-248
Stabilization, 203-205, 205f, 205t, 265t-266t
dynamic *vs.* static, 265t-266t
tests, trunk and hip, 203-205, 205f, 205t
Stabilizers, 135

Stabilometry, 250
Staggered ladder jump patterns, 240-242, 242f
Staggered-leg stances, 239f
Static position sense, 266t
Static stabilization *vs.* dynamic stabilization, 265t-266t
Stationary rotational medicine ball toss, 211
Steady-level exercise, 46
Steploading, 106
Stepping strategies, 250
Step-ups, 238
Steroids, anabolic, 225
Stiffness parameter, 3, 3f
Stimuli/signals component, 260f, 262-269, 264f, 265t-266t, 267f-268f. *See also* Dimensional model of MT (manual therapy).
Strain, 3-4, 3f, 100-101
muscle, 100-101
strain energy density parameter, 3-4, 3f
ultimate, 3-4, 3f
Strength training concepts, 223-232
clinical applications, 228—229
muscle physiological adaptations, 224-226
aging changes and, 226
contractile, 224-225
exercise variables and, 225-226
hypertrophy *vs.* hyperplasia, 224-225
muscle changes and, 226
muscle fiber type specific adaptations, 225
neural, 224
muscle-strengthening action types, 226-229
concentric strengthening, 227-228
DOMS and, 227
eccentric strengthening, 226-227
isometric strengthening, 228
repeated bout effect and, 227
SAID and, 227
stretch-shorten cycles and, 227
plyometrics and, 245b. *See also* Plyometrics.
rehabilitation roles and, 223-224, 224f, 229
Stress, 7-8, 7f
stress-exercise interrelationships, 8
stress-strain curves, 7-8, 7f
Stretch, 31, 77, 227
reflex, 31
stretch shortening cycles. *See* SSCs (stretch shortening cycles).
Striated muscles, 15

Stroke volume. *See* SV (stroke volume).
Structural malalignments, 155-159
Submaximal exercise, 48-49
moderate-to-heavy, 49
short-and-long term low-intensity, 48-49
Sumo squat, wide, 239f
Super compensation, 110f
Supramaximal exercise, short-term high-intensity, 48
Surgical considerations, 303-314
SV (stroke volume), 70-71
Sympathetic *vs.* parasympathetic forms, 109
Synergistic abilities, 264-265, 264f
Synthesis, muscle glycogen, 283
Systolic blood pressure. *See* SBP (systolic blood pressure).

T

T (transverse) tubules, 18-22, 19t, 89-90
T waves, 66
Tangent modulus parameter, 3-4, 3f
Tapering, 107f, 108
Task dependency, 93
TC (terminal cisternae), 89-90
TEF (thermic effect of food), 279
Tempo/pace programs, 78-79
Tendons and ligaments (basic science concepts), 1-14
basic science, 2-5
biology and biochemical composition, 2-3, 2f
biomechanics, 3-4, 3f-4f
bone-ligament-bone complex, 3, 3f
collagen fiber bundles, 2-3, 2f
ECM, 2-3
energy absorbed at failure parameter, 3, 3f
exercise effects, 5-6, 6f
future directions of, 10-11
hyperesis, 4f, 34
immobilization, 5, 5f
ligament architecture hierarchy, 2-3, 2f
stiffness parameter, 3, 3f
strain energy density parameter, 3-4, 3f
tangent modulus parameter, 3-4, 3f
tissue homeostasis, 4-5, 5f
tropocollagen molecules, 2-3
ultimate elongation parameter, 3, 3f
ultimate strain parameter, 3-4, 3f
ultimate tensile strength parameter, 3-4, 3f
Wolf's law, 4-5

healing processes, 1-10, 251-254
ACLs, 1, 6-10, 251-254
bioscaffolds, 10
cell therapy, 10
conservative treatment *vs.* repair, 7-8
FMTC and, 5-8
functional tissue engineering, 9-10
gene therapy, 9-10
growth factors, 7-10
immobilization *vs.* passive controlled mobilization, 8
MCLs, 1-2, 2f, 6-10
MSCs and, 10
multiple ligament injuries, 8
overlapping phases of, 6f
PDGF and, 7
reconstruction, 8-9
SIS and, 10
stress-exercise interrelationships, 8
stress-strain curves and, 7f
TGF-β (transforming growth factor-beta) and, 7-10
Tennis player case example, 298
Tensile strength, ultimate, 3-4, 3f
Terminal cisternae. *See* TC (terminal cisternae).
Testosterone, 225
TGF-β (transforming growth factor-beta), 7-10
Therapeutic ultrasound, 102
Therapy, manual, 259-278. *See also* MT (manual therapy).
Thermic effect of food. *See* TEF (thermic effect of food).
Thermogenesis, 16
Thick myofilaments *vs.* thin myofilaments, 20, 20f
Thigh thrust, 200, 200f
Thomas test, 202, 202f
Threshold, 25, 50-52, 68, 78-79
anaerobic, 50-52, 68
lactate, 50-52
stimulus, 25
Threshold to detection of passive motion testing. *See* TTDPM (threshold to detection of passive motion) testing.
training, 78-79
ventilatory, 50-52
Throwing biomechanics, 187-190, 188f-189f
Tidal volume. *See* TV (tidal volume).
Time-continuum, anaerobic metabolism, 41
Timed hop testing, 251t, 254
Timelines, repair, 268f

Tissue dimension, 260, 260f, 262-263, 268f. *See also* Dimensional model of MT (manual therapy).
Tissue engineering, functional, 9-10
Tissue functions and characteristics, 15-16
Tissue homeostasis, 4-5, 5f
TLC (total lung capacity), 67
Top down kinetic chain, 151-155
Total contact orthosis, 163
Total foot contacts, 235t
Total lung capacity. *See* TLC (total lung capacity).
Total peripheral resistance. *See* TPR (total peripheral resistance).
TPR (total peripheral resistance), 71-72
Training, 76-83, 106-107, 107f, 112-113, 223-232, 247-258
components, 77
cycles, 106-107, 107f
design, 76-83
logs, 112-113
neuromuscular, 247-258
plans, 107f
strength, 223-232. *See also* Strength training concepts.
Transforming growth factor-beta. *See* TGF-β (transforming growth factor-beta).
Transition phase, 108, 1107f
Transitional ability, 266t
Transverse tubules. *See* T (transverse) tubules.
Trauma, muscle, 112
Trendelenburg gait pattern, 194
Triad concept, 89
Triangle *vs.* four-square patterns, 235-236, 236t
Triggered reactions, 249t
Tropocollagen molecules, 2-3
Tropomyosin, 20
Troponin, 20
Trunk and hip CORE evaluations, 193-222
agility testing, 211, 212t
anatomy and pathophysiology of, 135-144
background perspectives of, 193
balance testing and evaluations, 211-215, 214f, 214t
balance triad, 213
central balance processors, 213
MCTSIB, 214, 214t
perturbation reaction, 214, 216t
vestibular feedback and, 213
visual feedback and, 213
evaluation sheets for, 216t-218t

evidenced-based clinical applications for, 200, 202, 204, 207, 209, 211, 213
hip testing, 201-203, 202f-203f, 202t-203t
Craig's test, 207-208, 208f
hip motion, 201-202, 203t
Ober's test, 202, 202f
Thomas test, 202, 202f
lower quadrant trunk and hip, 135-144
mobilizer tests, 207-209, 207f, 208t-209t
1 RM, 208, 208t
8-to-10 repetition maximum, 208
calculated one repetition maximum, 208-209
isokinetic testing, 208
isometric manual muscle testing, 205, 205t-206t
isotonic repetition maximums, 208-209, 208t
observation and, 193-194, 195f
power, 209-211, 210f, 210t
countermovement vertical jump testing, 210, 210t
cycle ergometer tests, 209-210
formula for, 209
LSI, 211
medicine ball throws, 210-211
shuttle run, 209, 210f, 210t
single-leg hop tests, 211, 211t, 212f
T-test, 209
rehabilitation roles for, 193, 216
stabilization tests, trunk and hip, 203-205, 205f, 205t, 206, 206f
abdominal bracing, 206, 206f, 206t
abdominal drawing-in stability, 204
ASLR, 204, 205f, 206t
back extensor endurance test, 206, 206f, 206t
bird dog test, 205t-206t
bridging test with knee extended, 205
clinical measures, 204-205
diagnostic measures, 205
global stabilization test norms, 205t
leg loading test, 206t
local stabilization tests, 203-205
multifidus activation and atrophy, 204
Quebec Back Pain Disability Score, 204

Trunk and hip CORE evaluations,
   (continued)
   RTUS, 203-205
   screening tests, 203-204
   side-lying pelvic test, 205-206
   trunk screening, 194-201, 195f-198f,
      198t, 199f-201f, 201, 201f
   centralization phenomenon, 196,
      198t
   compression, 201, 201f
   distraction test, 199, 201t
   facet scour, 199, 201t
   Gaenslen's test, 200, 200f, 201t
   lumbar quadrant rest, 199
   McKenzie prone prop, 199f, 199t
   opposite straight leg raise testing,
      199
   passive straight leg raising, 199,
      199f
   peripheralization, 196, 198t
   prone instability test, 199, 200f,
      201t
   sacral thrust, 201, 201f, 201t
   sacroiliac joint tests, 199, 200f,
      201, 201t
   slump tests, 196-199, 199f, 201t
   special tests, 201t
   thigh thrust, 200, 200f
   trunk motion, 194-195, 198f
TTDPM (threshold to detection of
      passive motion) testing, 250
T-test, 209
Turf toe, 163
Turnover, 42-43
TV (tidal volume), 67
Twitch (contractile) properties, 25-26
Two-leg squatting, 233-234

Type IIA fibers, 224, 225
Type IIB fibers, 26-28, 224, 225
Type IIC fibers, 26-28

U

Ultimate elongation parameter, 3, 3f
Ultimate strain parameter, 3-4, 3f
Ultimate tensile strength parameter,
      3-4, 3f
Ultrasound, 102-105
   real-time. *See* RTUS (real-time
      ultrasound).
   therapeutic, 102-105
Unclassified undifferentiated fibers,
      26-28
Uncontrolled reactive-type exercises,
      240
Unexplained underperformance
      syndrome. *See* UPS (unexplained
      underperformance syndrome).
Unloading regeneration cycles, 107f,
      108
Upper quadrant glenohumeral CORE,
      135-144
UPS (unexplained underperformance
      syndrome), 109

V

Valgus, dynamic, 252-253, 263f
Valsalva maneuver, 71
Variables, 80-81, 225-226, 233
   exercise, 80-81, 225-226
   routine, 233
Vasoconstriction *vs.* vasodilation, 72
Velocity, 265t-266t

Ventilation, 67-68
Ventilatory threshold, 50-52
Vertical jump testing, 210, 210t
Very active activity level, 280t
Vestibular feedback, 213
Vestibulospinal reflex, 213
Visual feedback, 213
VO$_2$max. *See* Maximal oxygen uptake.
Voluntary muscles, 15
Voluntary reactions, 249t

W

Warm-ups, 77, 106
WAT (Wingate Anaerobic Test), 55-57
Wide sumo squat, 239f
Wineglass effect, 249
Wingate Anaerobic Test. *See* WAT
      (Wingate Anaerobic Test).
Wolf's law, 4-5
Work, 66-67, 77, 235-236, 236t
   maximal lactate steady state
      workload and intensity. *See*
      MLSS (maximal lactate steady
      state) workload and intensity.
   periods, 77
   rate, 66-67
   volume and intensity, 235-236, 236t

Y

YMCA cycle erogometer test, 70

Z

Z discs, 18-19, 18-20, 24-25